Periodontics: A Practical Approach

Periodontics: A Practical Approach

J. Bernard Kieser BDS, FDS RCS
Senior Lecturer and Honorary Consultant, Department of Periodontology, Institute of Dental Surgery,
Eastman Dental Hospital, London

WRIGHT
London   Boston   Singapore   Sydney   Toronto   Wellington

Wright
is an imprint of Butterworth Scientific

 PART OF REED INTERNATIONAL P.L.C.

First published 1990

© **J. Bernard Kieser, 1990**

British Library Cataloguing in Publication Data
Kieser, J. Bernard
  Periodontics.
  1. Dentistry. Periodontics
  I. Title
  617.6'32
  ISBN 0-7236-1823-2

Library of Congress Cataloging in Publication Data
Kieser, J. Bernard.
  Periodontics: a practical approach
  J. Bernard Kieser.
    p.   cm.
  Includes bibliographical references.
  ISBN 0-7236-1823-2
  1. Periodontics.   I. Title.
  [DLMN: 1. Periodontal Diseases – therapy.
    WU 240 K47p]
  RK361.K54   1990
  617.6'32 – dc20

Phototypeset by Scribe Design, Gillingham, Kent
Printed and bound in Great Britain by Courier International Ltd, Tiptree, Essex

Foreword

In the last twenty-five years the field of periodontology has come to be dominated by a search for a fundamental understanding of the aetiology of periodontal disease and the nature of the disease process itself. This knowledge has increasingly impinged upon the practice of clinical periodontics.

Prior to 1965 periodontal disease was considered to be of multifactorial origin, and the influences of endogenous, nutritional and occlusal factors were integral components of treatment planning. The crucial experiments of Loë and his coworkers demonstrated the cause–effect relationship between bacterial plaque and gingivitis, and thus gave a new basis for the prevention and therapy of the disease. In the following years, much research on the aetiology of periodontal disease has focused on the microbial component, and it has clearly been established that the prevention and treatment of periodontal diseases should follow concepts dictated by the nature of opportunistic bacterial infections. The overwhelming evidence implicating the role of bacteria in the aetiology and pathogenesis of periodontal disease has thus successively and profoundly influenced treatment principles. In early days, anecdotal evidence governed the art of clinical practice; today, treatment concepts have to be based upon sound scientific evidence.

In approaching the task of writing this text, Bernard Kieser sought to combine clinical experience, scientific evidence and optimal didactics in presenting a truly sound approach to periodontal treatment. He has accomplished the task he set himself by dividing this text into three components, each a separate entity, yet forming a closely interrelated whole. Hence they may be used independently as reference for those practitioners seeking to expand their knowledge and improve their skills in well-defined areas of modern periodontics. Taken together, however, these sections form an integral unit which provides a text giving the basis and understanding for the treatment of even the most complex dental cases. Such an approach in this textbook will obviously attract all who wish to base periodontal treatment upon sound scientific knowledge.

I congratulate Bernard Kieser and his coauthors on the excellence of this contribution to the periodontal literature.

Sture Nyman

List of contributors

M. Addy BDS, MSc, PhD, FDS RCS
Professor/Honorary Consultant, Department of
Periodontology, Dental School, University of Wales
College of Medicine, Cardiff

C. R. Cowell MBE, BDS, FDS RCS
Formerly Chief Dental Officer, Unilever (UKCR)
Ltd; Honorary Senior Lecturer, Department of
Community Dental Health and Dental Practice,
University College London and The London
Hospital Medical College, London

P. D. Marsh BSc, PhD
Group Head, Pathology Division, PHLS Centre for
Applied Microbiology and Research, Porton Down,
Salisbury
Also: Honorary Senior Lecturer, Department of
Clinical Pathology and Immunology, Eastman
Dental Hospital, London

R. M. Palmer BDS, PhD, FDS RCS
Senior Lecturer/Honorary Consultant, Department
of Periodontology and Preventive Dentistry, United
Medical and Dental School of Guy's and St
Thomas's Hospitals, London

A. Sheiham BDS, PhD, DHC
Professor and Head of Department, Department of
Community Dental Health and Dental Practice,
University College London and The London
Hospital Medical College, London

Preface

The traditional professional bias towards the management of the clinical features of chronic inflammatory periodontal disease has been questioned widely and the more critical aspect of microbial activity increasingly emphasized over the past two decades. The purpose of this text is to re-examine the respective roles of the patient and operator in the management of disease, to establish the problems associated with the disease as perceived by the patient and then to present a practical approach to therapy.

The rationale for periodontal therapy is primarily based upon the reparative response of periodontal tissues to plaque control. This is the basis for gingival and periodontal pocket therapy and caters for the vast majority of diseased sites. Where the pattern of past destruction precludes such plaque control, then simple pocket surgery is presented within this text as a basic surgical module applicable to all situations. Morphological hurdles created by osseous, furcation and mucogingival tissue involvement which may be encountered at operation are in turn dealt with by complex pocket surgery. The requisite additional operative measures are incorporated, as and when necessary, into the basic pocket surgical field. This proposed surgical approach thus avoids the conventional treatment planning difficulties whereby the appropriate techniques must be selected from the bewildering array currently available to cater for the varying degrees of breakdown present in any one case. The need for very careful attention to technical detail, reinforced by the supplementary 'practical hints and precautions' in surgical technique, creates a disproportionate and misleading emphasis upon surgery in this text which should be kept in perspective. The occlusal, restorative, endodontic and prosthetic aspects of periodontics are approached with individual patient needs very much in mind.

The practical emphasis of this text is exemplified by the format of the introductory chapters comprising Part I, and the separation of treatment philosophy, principles and methods, which form Part II, from the corroborative research findings in Part III. This approach is designed to facilitate an unimpeded examination and understanding of the subject, whilst maintaining a close link with the readily accessible documentary support provided in the comprehensive review chapters. Each of the parts can similarly also be studied quite independently as individual entities.

This text stems from my 25 years in clinical periodontology which has spanned three successive phases. Clinical appointments were held at The London Hospital, then The Royal Dental Hospital, London and finally, at the Institute of Dental Surgery, London. During much of this time private practice restricted to periodontics, has also been conducted in London.

The approach to therapy expounded here has evolved by a combination of clinical observation and assessment over the years, supported by a continuing critical appraisal of the literature. The contribution to this evolution by colleagues with whom I have been privileged to work has been considerable. The formative years owe much to Jack Lozdan and Aubrey Sheiham whilst that of re-evaluation was helped by Ian Davies, Greg Seymour and Esmonde Corbet. Finally, the reinforcement and consolidation was developed by postgraduate student seminars and most significantly, the supervised student research findings over the past decade.

I am deeply indebted to Richard Palmer who, in addition to contributing several chapters, gave invaluable advice and guidance during the preparation of the manuscript. Richard Ibbetson's help in the chapters devoted to occlusion and restorative dentistry is also acknowledged. The expert contributions of Philip Marsh, Aubrey Sheiham and Martin Addy, so essential to the completeness of this work, are also greatly appreciated. Special thanks must go to Colin Cowell for his encouragement, patience and skill and not least, stamina, in editing the finished product. The most taxing and seemingly endless transcription of innumerable drafts of the manuscript by initially Jenny Hauptmann, and then

Anne Hallowes, together with the skillful artwork of Angela Christie is also acknowledged with gratitude. Finally, the individual undertaking of such a text by one so committed to clinical practice, would not have been possible without enormous family sacrifices. The tolerance, forebearance and support of Jenny, Nigel and Samantha during the creation of this book must be recorded and it is to them that this text is rightly dedicated.

J. Bernard Kieser

Contents

Part I The nature of disease

1

A clinical perspective of periodontal disease

C. R. Cowell and J. B. Kieser

Research and knowledge of the periodontal lesion
Chronic inflammatory periodontal disease (CIPD)
Alternative strategies
Clinical evaluation of periodontal disease

The microbial insult
Data-handling and periodontal research
The clinical implications
Further reading

Research and knowledge of the periodontal lesion

The control of any disease must be founded ultimately upon a clear understanding of that disease yet, in spite of the resources expended internationally on periodontal research, the true nature of the advancing periodontal lesion remains a tantalizing enigma. The principal concern of this book about the management of chronic inflammatory periodontal disease (CIPD) is the control of the advancing destructive lesion, with its accompanying loss of attachment and supporting bone for the teeth.

An imperfect state of knowledge is inevitable and has always been so where the treatment of disease is concerned. The clinician must always be aware of 'state of the art' research but cannot afford the luxury of waiting until the scientist's appetite for data has been sated before treating patients affected by the disease. At the same time, clinicians must beware of becoming so attached to traditional therapeutic techniques that they cling to them when knowledge gained from research has rendered them redundant. This risk is especially high in periodontics where a strong mechanistic emphasis has predominated for so long.

The other extreme, of embracing wholeheartedly every new idea on the basis of one or two research papers, can work to the detriment of patients. Research papers that represent a 'watershed' in knowledge do occur but they are very rare.

Thus, the conscientious clinician has a difficult path to follow and must be aware of current research

fashions with their inevitable pitfalls. This is an ongoing process and the review of researched knowledge, forming Part III of this book, is intended to provide a rational basis for the therapeutic regime advocated.

Chronic inflammatory periodontal disease (CIPD)

The term 'periodontal disease' is used frequently in the dental literature to embrace all the diseases that affect the periodontium. This book deals with those forms of disease induced by bacterial plaque and where the unqualified term periodontal disease is used within the text it can be taken to refer to CIPD, to avoid prolixity or the proliferation of acronyms.

Periodontal care

Although this book is about periodontal therapy, readers should realize that this constitutes only part of periodontal care, which involves prevention as well as cure. Periodontal therapy, as described in much of this text, is necessary for only a small part of the total population and it is hoped that this text will create a greater awareness of the part therapy plays within the wider spectrum of periodontal care. It should also be appreciated that similarities exist between the techniques used for preventing disease in the individual and those used in the management of much of the disease encountered in clinical practice. However, prevention must also be concerned with populations, for which alternative

1

strategies exist. Some of the concepts arising from these strategies depart from the classic medical model with its emphasis upon the individual and on the one-to-one relationship between clinician and patient.

Alternative strategies

Rose, working within community medicine, has analysed the problems involved in dealing with the non-infectious diseases. He describes two basic strategies used for the prevention of disease and calls these 'the high risk strategy' and 'the population strategy'. It does seem that the clarity of this approach could well be applied to periodontal disease.

The high risk strategy

The high risk strategy is the conventional medical approach to disease control and is based firmly upon studies involving the individual (case-control) or groups of individuals (cohorts). It attempts to diminish the risk distribution by trying to identify those individuals who will develop the disease, ideally before the clinical manifestations of disease appear. The strategy presupposes the existence of a screening method capable of discriminating between susceptible individuals and the rest of the population.

The objective of this strategy is to design intervention appropriate to the selected individuals and, by so doing, avoid any diffusion of valuable resources throughout the population. The strategy should, therefore, prove to be cost-effective as it concentrates the care where the need, and consequently the benefit, is bound to be greater. However, although the screening process has a low cost per individual, its overall cost may be appreciable. Furthermore, assuming that an efficient screening method has been developed, its success does depend upon a high proportion of the population taking advantage of it. In practice, the uptake of any screening procedure is often greatest among those who have the least need of care. In general, it appears that screening has frequently to rely on the early signs of disease for discrimination. Although this often makes it possible to affect outcome it cannot, by definition, be regarded as being effective for prevention.

Screening for a high risk group, susceptible to periodontal destruction, has certainly failed to achieve any sustained success. If plaque is the ultimate cause of periodontal disease and gingival inflammation is its earliest manifestation, then both plaque and gingival inflammation are much too widely distributed to discriminate sufficiently between those who will experience periodontal destruction of any magnitude and those who will not. Even the detection of the early signs of periodontal attachment destruction appears to have poor predictive value for future disease experience in individuals.

Rose has also pointed out that a large number of people at low risk in the population may give rise to more cases in total than the small number at high risk. This relatively common situation thus limits the utility of the high risk approach to prevention, although the principal drawback of the high risk strategy is that it does nothing to tackle the underlying cause of the disease it proposes to control.

The population strategy

The population strategy is the public health approach to the prevention of disease which attempts to improve the whole distribution of a disease by controlling the factors that determine incidence. Such a major population change cannot be achieved for many chronic or non-infectious diseases without changing behaviour or altering commonly accepted views held by a population (societal norms). This strategy will, therefore, not achieve immediate results and may be difficult to accept by both clinician and layman used to the idea of treatment followed by cure at the individual level. It must be appreciated that it cannot hope to achieve immediate results and, further, that its achievements cannot be replicated at the individual level.

Rose points out that the population strategy is radical in its attempt to remove the underlying causes of disease and thus eventually lower its prevalence in a population. It, therefore, has a large potential for the population as a whole. This potential is often greater than the clinician would expect from data derived from individuals. He gives an example of this effect, taken from the Framingham study on coronary heart disease. This showed that a lowering of the blood pressure distribution by only 10 mmHg in the whole population, would correspond to a 30% reduction in the total attributable mortality.

Prevention strategies and dental care

An example of the two strategic approaches to dental care can be seen in the reduction in the incidence and prevalence of dental caries in children and young adults due to fluoride. It appears that the widespread use of fluoride toothpaste may have achieved an even greater population effect than the fluoridation of drinking water in reducing the incidence of dental caries. A forecast of the effect of fluoride toothpastes, taken from the controlled clinical trials of those pastes, would have suggested a 20–30% reduction in caries. The actual reductions throughout the world have exceeded this level which is in line with Rose's observations. In contrast to this 'population strategy', the strategy adopted by dental practice could be compared to a 'high risk strategy' in that it uses frequent screening of patients plus intervention. This policy has been shown by national population surveys of dental health in the UK to have lowered the existence of untreated decay, but has made little impact upon the prevalence of dental caries.

Although it was stated earlier that plaque could not be used to discriminate between the high risk and low risk individuals, the reduction of plaque can have an effect at the population level. As a population strategy for the control of periodontal disease it does make relatively small changes in plaque levels worthwhile because of the overall benefit to be gained in periodontal health. This effect of minor improvements in oral hygiene in terms of reduced edentulousness was forecast some years ago, from a statistical model constructed from epidemiological data by Sheiham and Smales. For the ten years from 1968 to 1978 there has been a reduction in edentulousness in the UK as shown by a national survey. It has also been shown by Sheiham and co-workers that, over the 14 years from 1966 to 1980 there has also been an accompanying improvement in periodontal health, as demonstrated on one group of UK workers. Thus, there is circumstantial evidence to support the forecast made by Sheiham and Smales of the population effect of small reductions in plaque.

When positive results are achieved with population studies it is only to be expected that clinicians will wish to apply this information to individual patients. Unfortunately, it is impossible to guarantee the same level of success on a one-to-one basis because 'a preventive measure which brings much benefit to the population offers little to each participating individual'. This is known as the 'prevention paradox' and may be difficult for the clinician to accept as a viable concept, although the evidence has been around for a long time in public health. This may lead to poor motivation of both clinician and patient who expect to see a short-term result that can be measured at the level of the individual.

There will be a need for both strategies whilst the disease exists because the patients affected will need both therapy and prevention of further destruction. There are few who would argue against early intervention when the disease can be identified for, at the very least, patients must be given the choice of raising the standards of periodontal health in their mouths. However, as Rose has stated 'the priority of concern should always be the discovery and control of the causes of incidence'.

Clinical evaluation of periodontal disease

Pattern of attachment loss

Although the need for clean teeth has long been appreciated, the importance of poor oral hygiene as a cause of periodontal disease was first highlighted by the international epidemiological investigations undertaken by Russell. The incrimination of bacterial plaque in the initiation and reversal of gingival inflammation was then demonstrated by Löe and his co-workers in a series of experimental gingivitis studies. These studies showed that changes occurred in the microflora as the inflammation progressed. The way then seemed clear for the concept of the classic model of periodontal disease in which gingivitis would be followed by periodontitis, causing a slow destruction of attachment and an associated resorption of bone, with the eventual loss of teeth after many years. However, it has become increasingly difficult to reconcile this model with observations on the natural history of periodontal disease.

There is a lack of longitudinal data on normal populations, but it does appear that the estimated mean rates of attachment loss pose no great threat to the dentition for most people. However, mean data can obscure wide individual variations, for it is clear that some individuals do experience rates of attachment loss which can lead to tooth loss. The areas of destruction seldom affect every tooth, or even all parts of an affected tooth, to the same extent. Thus it is possible to have severe loss of attachment on one aspect of a tooth with minimal destruction elsewhere. What is more, the periodontal destruction in this group of people may not progress in a linear fashion, as believed traditionally, but in relatively short bursts of unknown periodicity and, as yet, indeterminate cause.

The pattern of tissue breakdown would seem to indicate a powerful local factor and whilst a specific bacterial species, or sub-species, may be responsible, an equally plausible explanation would be the combination of certain bacteria with some systemic exciting factor. Support for the latter hypothesis is provided by the tendency for lesions to be grouped in certain individuals. However, this could be due to the greater opportunity for new site infection arising from bacteria already present in existing pockets within the same mouth. The problem of site specificity cannot be resolved at present.

Destructive activity

The periodicity of the acute bursts of destructive activity within the natural history of the disease, which has a span of decades, presents formidable problems for experimental design and also for therapy. However, the possibility does exist that patients might be aware of the onset of these acute episodes, and if this is so this facility could then be used to not only monitor the progress of the disease but also time therapeutic intervention.

It is unlikely that destructive lesions arise *de novo* and it is probable that a background state of chronic inflammation is a necessary precursor. The evidence offered to support the contrary thesis of periodontal destruction in the absence of gingival inflammation is unconvincing. The predisposing gingival inflammation may have very strict, but as yet undefined, determinants which render a specific site susceptible to the effect of an exciting cause of systemic origin resulting in a very localized destructive lesion. For example, although unsubstantiated as yet by controlled investigation, it is not an uncommon clinical experience to observe a patient with an apparently stabilized periodontal condition that deteriorates rapidly following a stressful life event. On the other hand, the clinician can only wonder why, in the presence of so much microbial insult, so few people experience appreciable loss of attachment and such losses that do occur affect a comparatively small number of sites. Furthermore, even when this apparently 'at risk' group has been identified, it is still not possible to predict in which of these individuals, and in turn at which sites, the inflammatory reaction will have an adverse outcome.

Attachment levels

Research into the natural history of periodontitis and the cause of periodontal destruction has encountered many practical and conceptual barriers, not least being the measurement of disease progress. Whilst no great problem arises in detecting past attachment loss of clinical importance by probing or radiographs, these measures have been found to be unreliable for actually measuring incremental losses and in identifying the periodicity of such loss. Moreover, it is important to know to what extent the changes attributed to disease are, in reality, due to measurement error. Attempts to overcome false positive results by increasing the size of minimal incremental measurement (i.e. ignoring any incremental change under, say, 2 mm) will only serve to increase the number of false negative results. Until a reliable and reproducible method of attachment, or bone height measurement is developed, the confidence attached to incremental measurement will be limited, especially when measured over relatively short periods of time.

Other clinical parameters

The other clinical parameters used in periodontal disease of gingival redness, swelling and bleeding on probing are also not indicative of periodontal destruction. As stated previously, they merely reflect the inflammatory reaction to microbial insult without giving any indication of the likely outcome. Indeed, even when combined with past evidence of attachment loss, as measured by pocketing, they have poor predictive value. It is misleading to combine the signs of inflammation from the gingival margin with those at the dento-epithelial junction located at the base of pockets. Only when the inflammation at the gingival margin has been eliminated can any attempt be made to establish the state of affairs at the deeper levels of the dento-epithelial junction. Finally, it must be reiterated that as the use of mean data will dilute true changes at a few isolated sites when the majority of sites show no change, individual site assessment must be retained for the evaluation of periodontal therapy.

The microbial insult

Early research

A great deal of interest has been focused upon the harmful nature of bacterial plaque in the hope that one organism, or group of organisms, could be incriminated in periodontal destruction and thereby support the concept of a specific plaque hypothesis. Much of the early work in periodontal microbiology suffered from the use of pooled samples and the failure to distinguish between the micro-ecology adjacent to the dento-epithelial junction and that coronal to this crucial area. Furthermore, in common with clinical parameters, use was made of mean data that could swamp any site-dependent low level effect. In addition to this, much of the data was derived from cross-sectional sampling without verifying that these samples were a true reflection of the micro-ecology of the periodontal pocket.

Current research

Current knowledge of periodontal microbiology is reviewed in Chapter 5 and appears to offer insufficient support for a specific plaque hypothesis at the present time. Evidence appears to favour a non-specific plaque hypothesis in which complex mixed groups of bacteria co-exist. Many of the technical problems inhibiting microbiological research have been overcome and increasing amounts of correlative data are appearing in the literature. However, to date, these relate more to low prevalence juvenile periodontitis than to chronic inflammatory periodontal disease. The problem of establishing reliable evidence of causation, in addition to correlation, is still to be overcome.

Data-handling and periodontal research

Site or subject

Periodontal research workers have, for some time, been unhappy with the diluting effect of using mean data which can swamp important site-dependent phenomena. This is especially so because there may be few affected sites present in any one mouth and only a proportion of these may be active at any one time. However, the proposal that the sites should be treated as independent variables has provided a topic for active and controversial debate. It is true to say that any error in this regard could risk the validity of a study. Critiques of the situation by Imrey and Osborn have suggested that the subject rather than the tooth should be treated as a unit for data analysis. However, it should be possible to form sub-groups of these subjects for analysis, if required, by the number of periodontally affected sites in their mouths.

The problems of experimental design are simplified when two matched groups are compared, as in a controlled trial. Balancing of the two groups enables any confounding factors to affect both groups equally and allows test and control to be compared with greater clarity. Finally, because periodontal disease has such a prolonged natural history and involves mainly adults it is difficult to design a study of any realistic length without encountering problems due to the loss of subjects from a variety of causes. When this becomes too great it will affect the results adversely and may make the study worthless.

The clinical implications

Working hypotheses

In the light of the conflicting currents of periodontal research and the difficulties confronting the research workers the clinician is forced to take a subjective view of how much credence to place on current research knowledge. There is as yet no definitive view to fall back on but rather collective clinical research findings which undergo gradual changes over the years. The clinician is, however, faced with patients who already have evidence of past disease. Fortunately, those people who face the loss of their teeth from periodontal disease appear to represent a relatively small proportion of the total population.

It should be accepted at the outset that whilst clinical signs of inflammation are not necessarily indicative of attachment destruction they are certainly not representative of periodontal health. Accordingly, the therapeutic rationale expounded in this text is based upon the working hypothesis that a dento-epithelial junction without signs of inflammation will remain stable and be highly unlikely to sustain further loss of attachment (*cf.* Chapter 26). The risk of inexplicable tissue breakdown occurring under these conditions is extremely small and will involve very few individuals. This hypothesis can then be accepted as a reasonable clinical objective and should be adopted until refuted.

If it is further accepted that the cause of the inflammation is a mixed microbial mass accumulation then the management of both marginal gingival and subgingival inflammation must revolve about the control of this mass. The former must remain the responsibility of the patient but subgingival plaque control requires professional help by means of subgingival root surface debridement. Although there is no conceptual reason why the supragingival plaque and its products could not be controlled by chemical means there are many practical hurdles to overcome. The use of chemicals for plaque control is discussed in Chapter 35.

Clinical objectives

It is not possible to view directly the root surface at the dento-epithelial junction so that the success of subgingival debridement can only be judged by the subsequent absence of the clinical signs of inflammation, i.e. bleeding. This judgement can only be made with any certainty when there are no confounding signs of inflammation at the gingival margin. It follows then that the essential initial objective of therapy is the resolution of marginal gingival inflammation. This requires no professional intervention other than evoking the necessary behavioural response from the patient, although in some instances attention to plaque retentive factors at the gingival margins may be necessary.

Once marginal tissue health has been achieved the remaining therapeutic problems are concerned with the removal of subgingival plaque and any associated plaque retentive calcified products upon the subgingival root surface. The greater the attachment loss the more difficult is subgingival debridement due to both the resulting pocketing and, more especially, involvement of the furcation areas of posterior teeth. Furthermore, it is not only the debridement of the root that presents a problem but also the need to control bacterial recolonization. These factors then become central to the success of therapy. On the other hand, it should be emphasized that the presence of some subgingival plaque and its accompanying inflammation may be acceptable. This is when it is associated with either a stable situation, with no further loss of attachment, or a net rate of destruction that is compatible with tooth retention for the patient's lifetime. However, until these tolerable levels of disease can be clearly established and this group of patients identified then the objective of 'no plaque-induced inflammation' in the individual patient must remain. This constitutes the basis of the practical approach to periodontics presented here.

Further reading

Chilton, N. W. (Editor) (1986) Conference on clinical trials in periodontal diseases. *J. Clin. Periodontol.* **13**, 336–549

Ekanayaka, A. (1984) Tooth mortality in plantation workers and residents in Sri-Lanka. *Comm. Dent. Oral Epidemiol.* **12**, 128–135

Imrey, P. B. (1986) Considerations in the statistical analysis of clinical trials in periodontitis. *J. Clin. Periodontal.* **13**, 517–528

Löe, H., Theilade, E. and Jensen, S. B. (1965) Experimental gingivitis in man. *J. Periodontol.* **36**, 177–187

Osborn, J. (1987) Choice of computational unit in the statistical analysis of unbalanced clinical trials. *J. Clin. Periodontol.* **14**, 519–523

Rose, G. (1985) Sick individuals and sick populations. *Int. J. Epidemiol.* **14**, 32–38

Russell, A. L. (1963) International nutrition surveys: a summary of preliminary dental findings. *J. Dent. Res.* **42**, 233–244

Sheiham, A. and Smales, F. C. (1977) Some results from a computer model for predicting the long-term effects of periodontal therapy upon tooth loss in large populations. *J. Periodont. Res.* **14**, 248–249

Sheiham, A., Smales, F. C., Cushing, A. M. and Cowell, C. R. (1986) Changes in periodontal health in a cohort of British workers over a 14-year period. *Br. Dent. J.* **160**, 125–127

Todd, J. E. and Walker, A. M. (1980) *Adult Dental Health, Vol. 1. England and Wales 1968–1978.* HMSO, London

2

The periodontium

R. M. Palmer

The dentogingival junction
Periodontal ligament, cementum and bone

Further reading

The periodontium comprises the gingiva, periodontal ligament, cementum and alveolar bone (Figure 2.1). Many diseases may affect these tissues but this text is primarily concerned with chronic inflammatory periodontal diseases (hereafter simply referred to as periodontal disease) caused by bacterial plaque.

An understanding of the structure and biology of the periodontal tissues is fundamental to an appreciation of the changes in inflammatory disease

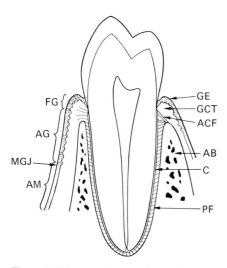

Figure 2.1 The periodontium. Key: AB, alveolar bone; ACF, alveolar crest fibres; AG, attached gingiva; AM, alveolar mucosa; FG, free gingiva; C, cementum; GE, gingival epithelium; GCT, gingival connective tissue; MGJ, mucogingival junction; PF, principal fibres of periodontal ligament

and the response of those tissues to therapy. The intention of this review is to highlight those features of the periodontium which are of direct relevance to periodontal disease rather than to provide a comprehensive description of the periodontium which can be found in many dental anatomy textbooks.

The dentogingival junction

The eruption of the teeth into the oral cavity produces a break in the continuity of the surface epithelium and provides a surface on which bacteria are not removed by the process of desquamation. The unique nature of the dentogingival junction makes this site particularly vulnerable to bacterial assault. However, it also has certain anatomical and physiological properties which are protective.

The structure of the dentogingival junction is illustrated in Figure 2.2 A. The gingival epithelium consists of the junctional epithelium, the oral sulcular epithelium and the external oral epithelium. The junctional epithelium is non-keratinized and forms the attachment to the tooth surface. In health it is situated on the enamel with its apical termination at the cement–enamel junction. The sulcular epithelium lines the gingival sulcus, which is about 0.5 mm deep in histological sections of healthy gingiva. Morphologically, it resembles the external oral epithelium in its coronal part and the junctional epithelium in its apical part.

The external oral epithelium covers the external surface of the gingiva from the gingival margin to the mucogingival junction. It is keratinized and there are well-developed rete ridges which interdigitate with the underlying gingival connective tissue,

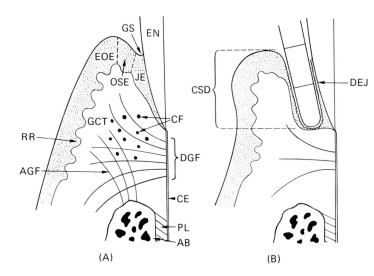

Figure 2.2 (A) The dentogingival junction, and (B) the effect of probing. Key: AB, alveolar bone; AGF, alveologingival fibres; CF, circular fibres; DGF, dentogingival fibres; CE, cementum; EN, enamel; EOE, external oral epithelium; OSE, oral sulcular epithelium; JE, junctional epithelium; GCT, gingival connective tissue; GS, gingival sulcus; PL, periodontal ligament; RR, rete ridges; CSD, clinical sulcus depth. Note: split within junctional epithelium produced by probe whilst epithelial attachment to enamel (DEJ, dento-epithelial junction) remains intact

in contrast to the very flat epithelio-mesenchymal tissue junction of the junctional epithelium. The intersections of the rete ridges produce the stippling of the gingival surface, a feature which should not be regarded as indicative of healthy tissue. The shallow gingival groove which is often apparent about 1 mm from the gingival margin demarcates the free gingiva and corresponds with the epithelial attachment to the tooth surface. The attached gingiva is theoretically measured from this groove to the mucogingival junction but, in practice, is normally estimated by subtracting the clinical sulcus depth from the measured width of keratinized tissue.

Junctional epithelium

The junctional epithelium is of particular interest as it is through this structure that the inflammatory process of periodontal disease is mediated. This is because its properties are fundamentally different from those of the external oral epithelium. The cells of the junctional epithelium are joined together by desmosomes like any other epithelial tissue, but these attachments are few when compared with the external oral epithelium. The intercellular spaces are wider in the junctional epithelium which further contributes to its relative fragility. Its attachment to the tooth surface is via specialized cell junctions, hemidesmosomes, and a basal lamina which forms a relatively strong attachment mechanism. Thus, a periodontal probe can pass readily beyond the base of the sulcus into the junctional epithelium creating a split within this structure but leaving the attachment to the tooth intact (Figure 2.2 B).

These features probably contribute to the greater permeability of the junctional epithelium compared with the relatively impermeable external oral epithelium. This permeability may be further increased because of the reported absence of membrane coating granules. These granules are visible ultrastructurally in other epithelial cells and may be responsible for membrane thickening and impermeability in both keratinized and non-keratinized epithelium. In addition, permeability is increased by the migration of phagocytes through the junctional epithelium into the gingival sulcus. This can be demonstrated in clinically healthy gingiva, and could be considered as physiological, as it is also seen in germ-free animals. However, it is considerably increased in inflammation and will be considered in more detail in the following chapter. The passage of substances through the junctional epithelium has been shown to be bi-directional. Substances such as enzymes, bacterial endotoxin and specifically labelled proteins have been shown to pass from the gingival sulcus into the gingival connective tissue. In contrast, gingival fluid passes from the connective tissue into the sulcus, increasing in volume with inflammation. This phenomenon was originally demonstrated using a fluorescein dye injected intravenously and observing its appearance in the gingival sulcus.

The cells of the junctional epithelium also have a much greater turnover rate than cells of the gingival epithelium and they are reported to be completely renewed within about 5 days. This rapid renewal is achieved by a higher rate of cell division and with a greater ratio of basal cell area to desquamation area than exists in external oral epithelium. This means that the junctional epithelium has a very high repair potential.

The properties of the junctional epithelium were

thought to be unique because it is derived initially from the reduced enamel epithelium which covers the crown of the tooth before eruption. However, this epithelium is replaced rapidly by the cells of the gingival epithelium following eruption. There is also rapid regeneration of the junctional epithelium after surgical excision from the basal cells of the external oral epithelium and it will form readily on enamel, dentine or cementum.

The type of epithelium which develops in a particular situation is dependent upon the inductive influence of the underlying connective tissue rather than any inherent property of the epithelial cells. At the dentogingival junction the junctional epithelium and the gingival epithelium share a common connective tissue and therefore the failure of junctional epithelium to keratinize may relate to the presence of the tooth.

Experiments have shown that the junctional epithelium has the potential to keratinize and it has therefore been suggested that the features of this epithelium are due to the presence of mild inflammatory changes in the subjacent connective tissue which are usually present in clinically healthy tissue.

Gingival connective tissue

The gingival connective tissue consists principally of collagen fibres, fibroblasts and ground substance. It contains a rich anastomosis of blood vessels originating from the periodontal ligament, bone and gingiva. A complicated plexus of vessels is found in association with the junctional epithelium. The normal gingival connective tissue usually contains a small population of inflammatory cells.

The collagen is mainly type 1 with some type 3. The turnover of collagen in the gingiva and periodontal ligament is much higher than other connective tissues which probably reflects the need for continuous adaptation. The collagen is secreted and resorbed by fibroblasts and these processes may occur simultaneously in the same cell. Resorption is carried out by phagocytosis of collagen fibrils and subsequent intracellular breakdown by lysosomal enzymes. Any imbalance between these functions can rapidly lead to collagen loss, which also applies to the collagen of the periodontal ligament.

The collagen in the gingiva consists mainly of fibrils about 5 μm in diameter forming the following important anatomical groups (Figure 2.2) which support the dentogingival junction:

(1) Dentogingival fibres radiate from the root surface into the lamina propria of the gingiva curving upwards beneath the gingival sulcus, horizontally outwards and apically between the gingiva and alveolar bone.
(2) Alveologingival fibres pass from the alveolar bone crest vertically into the gingival lamina propria.
(3) Circular fibres encircle the tooth above the alveolar crest.
(4) Transeptal fibres pass horizontally from one tooth root to another in a mesiodistal plane above the crest of alveolar bone (Figure 2.3).

Periodontal ligament, cementum and bone

Periodontal ligament

The periodontal ligament, which consists of collagen fibres, ground substance and blood vessels, forms a visco-elastic supporting mechanism for the tooth. When a force is applied to the tooth there is an

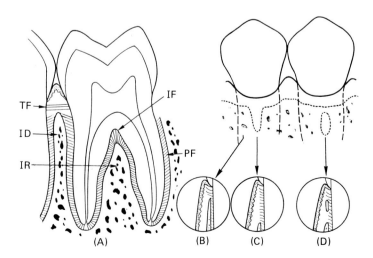

Figure 2.3 (A) Diagrammatic section through molar teeth to show periodontal ligament fibres. Key: principal fibres (PF), inter-radicular fibres (IF) and transeptal fibres (TF) and the related interdental (ID) and inter-radicular (IR) alveolar septum. (B–D) Anatomical variants at the dentogingival junction. (B) Normal situation, (C) bony dehiscence, and (D) fenestration

initial rapid displacement followed by a slow creep phase. It is highly adaptable to changing forces, contains sensory nerve endings which are important in controlling masticatory forces and is involved in the eruption of the tooth. The principal collagen fibres are inserted into the alveolar bone and root cementum. They are obliquely orientated in the main body of the ligament, but at the apex and within furcations they are radially arranged and at the alveolar crest there are horizontal and alveolar crest groups (Figures 2.1 and 2.3). The ligament is 0.2 mm in width on average and this, together with the height and quality of the ligament, allows for normal tooth mobility. However, the ligament is readily adaptable to increased forces and responds by an increase in width gained by alveolar bone resorption. This results in a tooth with increased mobility which is better adapted to withstand the increased forces.

The fibroblasts of the ligament appear to differ from those of the gingival connective tissue. Their developmental origin is supposedly from the investing layer of follicle which surrounds the tooth germ and is continuous and probably derived from the dental papilla. The formation of the periodontal ligament is intimately related to root formation, which is mapped out by the epithelial sheath of Hertwig. Following induction of odontoblasts from the dental papilla and the deposition of predentine, the root sheath undergoes fragmentation. This allows mesenchymal cells of the investing layer of follicle to migrate to the root surface and differentiate into cementoblasts. These cells form cementum incorporating the principal fibres of the ligament.

The ligament near the root surface contains the fragmented epithelium from the root sheath which form the epithelial cell rests of Malassez. The function of these cell rests is unknown but they have been implicated in several interesting hypotheses. For example, it has been suggested that they may be involved in the maintenance of the periodontal ligament width by inhibiting ingrowth of alveolar bone. In addition, they proliferate in areas of inflammation such as in the formation of the epithelial lining of dental cysts. They may therefore contribute to the epithelial ingrowth into the inflamed connective tissue in periodontal disease. Some recently published work has also suggested that the epithelial cells from Hertwig's root sheath, at the time of fragmentation, undergo a mesenchymal transformation and give rise to cementoblasts.

The turnover of collagen in the periodontal ligament is higher than in other connective tissues which may be a reflection of the greater functional demands placed upon it. For example, in mouse molars the half-life of collagen in the periodontal ligament is reported to be 1 day. The turnover is evenly distributed throughout the ligament and is not higher in the central zone which was once thought to contain an intermediate plexus. The ligament nearest the bone contains most of the blood vessels and has a population of perivascularly located fibroblasts which proliferate early in experimental wound healing. This part of the ligament also contains osteoblast precursors. The ligament nearest the tooth surface contains cementoblast precursors which may not proliferate so rapidly following wounding. The distinct populations of fibroblasts which exist in the periodontal ligament and gingival connective tissue may have a great bearing on the healing following peridontal treatment and partly explain the limited potential for regeneration of lost support.

Cementum

Cementum provides the mineralized connective tissue attachment of periodontal ligament fibres to the root surface. It is similar in composition to bone and is certainly less hard than dentine or enamel. It, too, is capable of adapting to changing functional demands by apposition, resorption and repair. These functions depend on the viability of its surface cells. At the cervical margin the cementum may overlap the enamel for a short distance, just meet the enamel or, less commonly, there is a gap with exposure of dentine. Cementum is classified according to whether or not it incorporates cementocytes, and whether it contains intrinsic fibres formed by cementocytes and/or extrinsic fibres of the periodontal ligament. Cementum which overlaps enamel is called afibrillar cementum as it does not have any periodontal ligament fibres inserted into it or intrinsic collagen fibres. The cementum in the coronal part of the root is deposited slowly with the cementoblasts remaining on the surface. This acellular cementum is 20–50 μm thick and shows resting incremental lines. Where the periodontal ligament is inserted into it as Sharpey's fibres it is termed extrinsic fibre cementum. Differences in fibre alignment can be discerned in the incremental layers. This cementum may also contain smaller intrinsic fibres and is then called mixed fibre cementum. In the apical and furcational parts of the root the deposition of cementum is usually more rapid which results in the incorporation of cells, forming cellular cementum. The incorporated cementocytes are housed in lacunae and have cell processes in canaliculi directed mainly towards their nutrient supply in the ligament. As the cementum increases in thickness these cells gradually lose their viability. Cellular cementum contains more intrinsic fibres and the increments are uneven, producing an irregular surface. The thickness of cementum increases throughout life and may reach several hundred μm in thickness in the furcations of multirooted teeth and in the apical regions. Localized over-production of cementum produces cemental spurs. In addition, areas of cementum undergo intermittent resorption and repair which may produce irregularities of the root surface.

Alveolar bone

The alveolar bone exists to support the teeth and it resorbs following loss of the teeth. The crest of the alveolus is situated 2 mm on average apical to the cement–enamel junction in health but there is considerable variation. For example, the alveolar bone may be absent over certain root surfaces in the commonly encountered normal anatomical variations which are called dehiscences and fenestrations. Dehiscences are localized marginal deficiencies and fenestrations are 'windows' in the alveolus overlying root surfaces (Figure 2.3 C and D). These features are usually associated with teeth which are outside the line of the arch and commonly also have a thin covering of gingival tissue.

The periodontal ligament is inserted into the cribriform plate or lamina dura of the socket wall. This often appears radiographically as a thin white line in contrast to the black space of the periodontal ligament. Loss of this radiographic appearance is often taken as evidence of bone resorption, but it must be remembered that it may also be altered simply by changing the angulation of the radiograph.

Bone is highly labile and undergoes continuous remodelling so that it is able to adapt to different functional demands and to adapt during movement of teeth. Consequently, any disturbance of deposition or resorption of bone rapidly produces changes in its volume and density. In particular, the alveolar bone is resorbed rapidly in areas adjacent to inflammation. Resorption is mediated by multinucleate osteoclasts which are located within resorption bays or Howship's lacunae. The secretion of lysosomal enzymes is important in this process.

Further reading

Berkowitz, B. K. B., Moxham, B. J. and Newman, H. N. (1982) *The Periodontal Ligament in Health and Disease.* Pergamon Press, Oxford

Listgarten, M. A. (1972) Normal development, structure, physiology, and repair of gingival epithelium. *Oral Sciences Reviews,* Vol. 1, pp. 3–68. Munksgaard, Copenhagen

Melcher, A. H. and Bowen, W. H. (1969) *Biology of the Periodontium.* Academic Press, London

Osborn, J. W. (1981) *Dental Anatomy and Embryology. A Companion to Dental Studies,* Vol. 1, Book 2. Blackwell, Oxford

Osborn, J. W. and Ten Cate, A. R. (1983) *Advanced Dental Histology. Dental Practitioner Handbook.* Wright, Bristol

Ten Cate, A. R. (1985) *Oral Histology: Development, Structure and Function.* C. V. Mosby, St Louis

3

Pathogenesis of chronic inflammatory periodontal disease (1)

R. M. Palmer

Introduction

The inflammatory response to bacterial plaque at the dentogingival junction is a fundamental defence mechanism against bacterial infection and as such differs little from many other inflammatory responses. This defence is extremely effective as periodontal disease is generally slowly progressive taking many decades to produce loss of a tooth. There is usually minimum discomfort to the patient and only rarely is any systemic ill effect produced. However, both the inflammatory and immune responses involved have protective and destructive effects. The balance between these effects can differ between patients and accounts, in part, for individual variation in susceptibility to disease.

The inflammatory response is initially acute but, as the adherent bacterial mass is not readily removed by host defence, it develops into a classic chronic inflammation. The hallmark of chronic inflammation is coincident destruction and repair, in which a delicate balance exists, resulting in different rates of tissue destruction. In addition, acute inflammatory episodes may be superimposed upon this chronic state and may cause more rapid loss of tissue at times. These features of the disease may be seen clinically where periodontal lesions may be stable, progress in a slow, uniform fashion or undergo periods of more rapid activity. Resolution of these acute inflammatory bursts may, therefore, produce an apparent improvement in clinical measurements of pocket depth and attachment levels.

The distribution and rapidity of progression of periodontal disease may be associated with certain pathogenic bacteria, which are considered in Chapter 5, and to the host response to plaque bacteria which is dealt with in this chapter.

Development of plaque induced inflammation

Healthy normal gingiva usually contains a small population of inflammatory cells including phagocytes, lymphocytes and plasma cells which increase dramatically in number with the development of inflammation. Previous research has highlighted the potentially damaging effects of these cells and each in turn has assumed a prominent position in the various hypotheses proposed for the immunopathogenesis of periodontitis. Inflammatory cells are involved primarily in the defence of the periodontium and may be individually more numerous at different stages of the disease process. The development of the inflammatory lesion of periodontal disease from previously healthy gingiva has been divided into several stages. This provides a convenient model to describe the cell types and their beneficial and potentially harmful effects. It should be stressed that many of the proposed harmful effects have not been shown to occur in the disease and certainly may not be operative at the stage of the disease in which they are described. The proposed stages are:

(1) initial lesion
(2) early lesion
(3) established lesion
(4) advanced lesion

The first three lesions are characterized by histological features and the fourth by additional clinical features.

Initial lesion

This lesion occurs theoretically within 2–4 days of plaque accumulation in previously healthy gingiva and is characterized by an acute inflammation in the connective tissue subjacent to the junctional epithelium (Figure 3.1 A). It occupies no more than 5–10% of the gingival connective tissue volume and therefore the gingiva appear clinically healthy. In fact, the histology of the initial or early lesion can often be demonstrated in biopsies of clinically healthy gingiva. The acute inflammation results in increased exudation of serum, which can be detected as an increase in gingival fluid, and an increased emigration of phagocytes from blood vessels and through the junctional epithelium to the site of bacterial challenge. The phagocytes are

therefore the first line of defence in the prevention of bacterial penetration of the tissue. They are found in the gingival sulcus forming a defensive zone between the plaque and the tissue. The permeable junctional epithelium allows the ingress of bacterial substances which establishes a chemotactic gradient for the phagocytes. In addition the permeability of the junctional epithelium may be increased by enzymes derived from bacteria or the host. Even at this early stage of inflammation collagen loss may be detected around the blood vessels. This highlights the rapidity with which collagen may be lost and may be due to host or bacterial collagenases or to an imbalance of collagen turnover. It has been generally thought that the inflammation is mediated by bacterial products rather than by invasion of viable bacteria, although some studies have shown bacteria within the tissue in more advanced disease (see Chapters 5 and 29 – Curettage).

The early lesion

This is seen to occur within 7–10 days of plaque accumulation and has all the features of the initial lesion with the additional appearance of lymphocytes which are mainly T cells (Figure 3.1 B). The

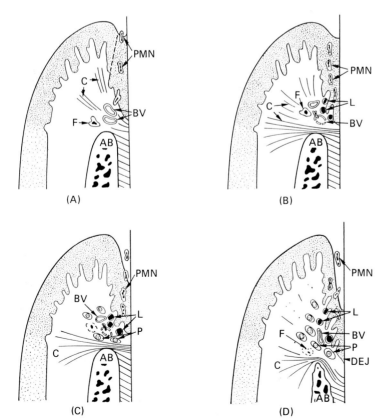

(A)

(B)

(C)

(D)

Figure 3.1 Stages of the inflammatory lesion as described by Page and Schroeder. (A) The healthy dentogingival junction. (B) The initial lesion. (C) The established lesion, and (D) the advanced lesion. Key: AB, alveolar bone; BV, blood vessel; C, collagen fibres; F, fibroblast; L, lymphocyte; P, plasma cell; PMN, polymorphonuclear leucocyte; DEJ, dento-epithelial junction

lesion has increased in size and occupies 5–15% of the gingival connective tissue. Within the inflammatory focus the collagen loss may be as great as 60–70% and the fibroblasts show cellular alterations which suggest an impaired function. There is also early proliferation of the basal cells of the junctional epithelium.

The established lesion

The additional feature of this lesion (Figure 3.1 C) is the appearance of plasma cells and B lymphocytes. The B lymphocytes are capable of reacting to specific antigens by producing plasma cells which secrete antibody. The lesion is larger and there is collagen loss over a greater area but there is still no loss of collagen attachment to the root surface. Epithelial proliferation of the junctional epithelium extends laterally into the inflammatory focus and may begin to resemble pocket epithelium. It was originally suggested that this lesion will develop within 2–4 weeks of plaque accumulation and would therefore coincide with the clinical appearance of gingivitis. At this stage the gingiva appears red and oedematous and bleeds on probing. The sulcus depth is increased due to swelling of the gingiva and some loss of epithelial attachment. Clinically the tissue would have a decreased resistance to periodontal probing. The mechanism by which the coronal part of the junctional epithelium detaches is not known but may be due to bacterial colonization and proliferation along the tooth surface in conjunction with enzymatic degradation. This would result in the plaque extending subgingivally and the formation of a gingival pocket without loss of connective tissue attachment to the root surface. These changes may, however, provide conditions which favour colonization and growth of periodontopathic bacteria. The established lesion may remain indefinitely as a stable lesion of gingivitis or progress to periodontitis.

The advanced lesion

The advanced lesion is characterized by the same histological cell types as the established lesion but with the clinical criteria of periodontal pocketing as a result of loss of connective tissue attachment to the root surface (Figure 3.1 D). The bacterial plaque has extended apically separating the soft tissues from the root surface and the junctional epithelium has migrated apically (the junctional epithelium at the base of the pocket will be referred to as the dento-epithelial junction in the rest of this book). The detached epithelium forms the epithelial lining of the periodontal pocket which proliferates extensively within the inflamed connective tissue. At the inner surface lining the pocket, the epithelium may be very thin, attenuated and in some areas

ulcerated. The inflammatory focus also contains many thin-walled blood vessels which are readily ruptured by periodontal probing. The inflammatory cell infiltrate forms a defensive zone which extends into the connective tissue in a radius from the plaque for about 1.5–2.5 mm. This is surrounded by a zone of inflammation-free fibrous tissue which effectively walls off the lesion and is a hallmark of chronic inflammation. The underlying bone resorbs to accommodate the lesion. Generally there are no signs of active bone resorption and very few osteoclasts. The bone and periodontal ligament are essentially free of inflammation. These features may be more consistent with the stable lesion of periodontitis or certainly one that is very slowly progressive and will be discussed further in the section on disease progression.

Many hypotheses have been put forward in an attempt to explain the pathogenesis of periodontitis based upon the properties of the inflammatory cells within the lesion and their interactions. It is therefore worthwhile reviewing the basic protective mechanisms and the potentially harmful effects produced by these cells.

Phagocytes and acute inflammatory response

The phagocytes are cells of the innate or non-specific immune system whose basic function is to engulf and destroy bacteria and bacterial products. There are two types of phagocytes, neutrophil polymorphonuclear leucocytes and macrophages, both of which are highly motile cells and capable of:

(1) *Chemotaxis* – directional migration, as opposed to random movement, along a chemical gradient. The gradient may be provided by bacterial products, in particular formyl–methionyl peptides or by activated serum components within the gingival sulcus.
(2) *Phagocytosis* – the engulfing of the bacteria by the cell plasma membrane to form a phagosome. Before this, the phagocyte must recognize the bacteria as foreign material and have a method of adherence. This is also enhanced by serum factors.
(3) *Bacterial killing* – this is accomplished by a battery of powerful enzymes and products, such as hydrogen peroxide, together with halide ions and myeloperoxidase which provide a very effective microbicidal combination. Killing is usually intracellular by fusion of lysosomal granules to the phagosome to produce a phagolysosome. Alternatively, enzymes may be secreted into the extracellular environment. These enzymes include lysozyme, collagenase, proteases and elastase which are potentially

damaging to the host tissue whether secreted or released during phagocytosis or following cell death. Much of the tissue damage in abscesses is due to extracellular release of lysosomal enzymes.

The function of phagocytes is considerably enhanced by serum factors such as complement, and antibodies which are produced by plasma cells. Complement is a series of factors which are activated in an amplification cascade to cause, ultimately, bacterial cell lysis by disruption of the cell membrane. Complement activation may occur by complexes of antigen and antibody, in the so-called classic pathway or by bacterial cell components such as endotoxin, a component of Gram-negative bacterial cell walls, via the alternative pathway. Several activated complement factors are generated within the cascade; these increase vascular permeability by stimulating the release of substances such as histamine from mast cells, increase phagocyte chemotaxis and provide an adherence mechanism between bacterial cells and phagocytes. Activated complement components have been demonstrated in gingival fluid. Therefore, complement activation may enhance the function of the phagocytes but at the same time increase the inflammation.

The majority of phagocytes are neutrophil polymorphonuclear leucocytes which have a short lifespan with a circulatory half-life of 6–7 h. Their function within the gingival sulcus is enhanced considerably by the fact that they can operate aerobically and anaerobically. However, their function may be inhibited by bacterial leucotoxins, and phagocytosis of bacteria within an adhesive mass covered by extracellular polysaccharide may be difficult. Nevertheless, the neutrophils often form a barrier covering the apical border of the plaque and many of them contain phagocytosed microorganisms. In animals which have been depleted of neutrophils, plaque microorganisms extend subgingivally very rapidly producing gross tissue destruction.

The other type of phagocyte is the longer-lived macrophage. This is, additionally, a very important cell in the specific immune response as it presents antigens to lymphocytes in a form which they are able to recognize. It is an important producer of prostaglandins which promote bone resorption and of interleukin 1 which is a molecule which communicates with lymphocytes and has many important biological activities. These include the stimulation of bone resorption and the production of collagenase by fibroblasts. Macrophage activity may be enhanced by a lymphokine called macrophage activating factor (MAF) produced by lymphocytes. This increases the phagocytic and killing ability of the cell but it also increases the secretion of prostaglandins

and collagenase. Although such activities may be associated with increased tissue destruction, there is also considerably more periodontal disease in individuals who have defects in their macrophage or neutrophil function. Therefore, a delicate balance must exist where either increased or decreased function may result in more severe disease.

Lymphocytes and plasma cells

Lymphocytes are involved in specific immunity. They can be divided into T and B lymphocytes. The T lymphocytes appear earlier in the lesion and are involved in cell-mediated immunity. Subpopulations of T cells include: (1) T helper cells which enhance the B lymphocyte response and the function of macrophages; (2) T suppressor cells which damp down the response of T helper cells, B cells and antigen presenting cells; (3) cytotoxic T cells which can kill other cells. They produce their effects through a number of factors called lymphokines which have a wide range of biological activities. These include macrophage activating factor (MAF) which increases the killing ability of this cell, migration inhibition factor (MIF) which keeps the phagocytes at the inflammatory focus, osteoclast activating factor (OAF, which has recently been characterized and is homologous to interleukin-1 beta) which stimulates osteoclasts to resorb bone, and lymphotoxin which is cytotoxic to many cells. It has been suggested that fibroblasts may be killed by lymphotoxin. Some fibroblasts in periodontitis showing signs of severe damage have been described in close association with lymphoid cells, which may be cytotoxic T cells or belong to a group of cells described as natural killer cells. In direct contrast, another lymphokine, fibroblast activating factor (FAF) stimulates proliferation of fibroblasts and the production of collagen. This may therefore be important in the healing and fibrosis which accompanies periodontitis.

It has been shown that the majority of lymphocytes in childhood gingivitis are T cells. The ability of T cells from patients with periodontitis to respond to plaque antigens has been reported and was previously used as evidence of the importance of cell-mediated immunity in periodontitis. A major role for cell-mediated immunity in periodontitis currently seems unlikely but further appreciation of the complex interactions between this limb of the immune system and the humoral and non-specific systems does not rule out this possibility.

Responsibility for humoral immunity is the function of B lymphocytes which mediate their effects through antibodies produced by plasma cells. The B cells react more rapidly on a second challenge by an antigen as they produce memory cells on their first encounter. Antibodies react specifically with the corresponding antigen to produce an immune complex. This may enhance phagocytosis by neutralizing noxious antigens, provide a method of adherence to the phagocyte and activate complement. The enhancement of phagocyte function is beneficial but may be associated with tissue damage as discussed in the previous section. Antibodies to suspected periodontopathic bacteria have been detected in serum indicating a systemic response and in high levels in gingival fluid indicating an additional local production within the lesion. It has been suggested that many of the antibodies produced in the lesion of periodontitis are non-specific. This is possible because certain components in plaque such as endotoxin, levan and dextran are non-specific stimulators of B cells. They are called mitogens and produce polyclonal B cell stimulation. If most of the antibodies are non-specific then they cannot produce immune complexes with possible beneficial effects. A major drawback resulting from this type of stimulation is the production of many B cell lymphokines which have the same potent biological effects as T cell lymphokines in producing tissue destruction.

More recently, the application of laboratory tests with increased sensitivity have shown that many of the antibodies found in gingival fluid are directed against suspected pathogens.

Clinical features of chronic inflammatory periodontal disease

The inflammatory response in chronic gingivitis produces changes in the colour, contour and consistency of the gingival tissues. They change from a pale pink colour to red, and the thin scalloped margin becomes swollen and oedematous. On examination with a periodontal probe the tissues bleed readily and an increase in probing depth from the normal 1–2 mm may be recorded. The depth to which the probe passes into the sulcus or pocket measured from the gingival margin is called the probing depth and is not an accurate representation of the actual histological pocket depth. In the previous chapter it was explained how the probe causes a split within the junctional epithelium in healthy tissue. The decreased resistance of the tissues caused by inflammation allows the probe to pass beyond the junctional epithelium into the underlying inflammatory focus. The depth to which a probe passes into the gingival sulcus/pocket is therefore dependent upon the inflammatory status of the tissue, the probing force, the diameter and profile of the probe tip and the angulation of the probe. Swelling of the gingival margin and any accompanying fibrosis in chronic gingivitis will also increase the probing depth. Pocketing which results

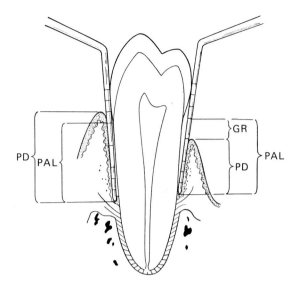

Figure 3.2 Relationship between the clinical measurements of probing depth (PD), probing attachment level (PAL) and gingival recession (GR)

from hyperplasia or swelling of the gingiva without loss of connective tissue attachment is called false pocketing.

Chronic periodontitis is diagnosed when loss of connective tissue attachment accompanies the inflammatory changes. Attachment loss is measured clinically as the distance the probe passes into the pocket from the cement enamel junction (Figure 3.2). This is referred to as the clinical attachment level or the probing attachment level (PAL). In clinical trials, changes in the PAL are often measured from a more convenient fixed landmark such as an occlusal overlay. Because of the aforementioned inaccuracies of clinical probing it is difficult to be certain when early connective tissue attachment loss has actually occurred. This is also a problem when trying to measure incremental loss of attachment to determine the progression of periodontitis. On the other hand, gingival recession is an unequivocal manifestation of attachment loss and may occur in conjunction with a healthy or inflamed gingival margin and with normal or increased probing depth values (*cf.* Chapter 13).

Clinical recording of probing depths and gingival recession is usually carried out at six points around each tooth at the mesio-, mid- and distobuccal and mesio-, mid- and distolingual aspects. In addition, any bleeding or exudation of pus is noted. Where the disease has progressed to involve the furcation areas of multirooted teeth, the horizontal probing depth into the furcation is also recorded. The degree of furcation involvement may be classified by degrees or graded as grade 1 where this measure-

NAME ___Mr. O.A.___   Date ___Nov. 84 INITIAL CHARTING___

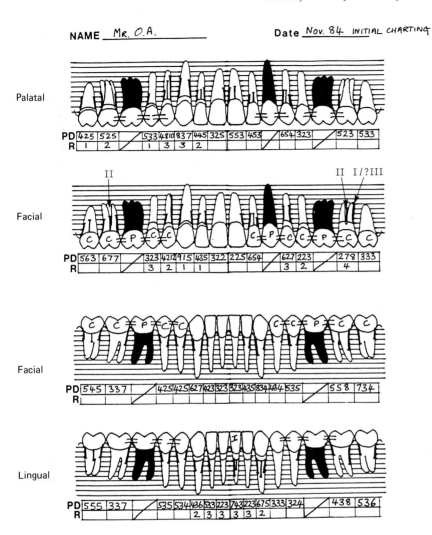

Palatal

PD | 425 | 525 | / | 533 | 410 | 837 | 445 | 325 | 553 | 453 | / | 654 | 323 | / | 523 | 533
R | 1 | 2 | / | 1 | 3 | 3 | 2 |

II   II   I/?III

Facial

PD | 563 | 677 | / | 323 | 421 | 915 | 435 | 322 | 225 | 654 | / | 627 | 223 | / | 278 | 333
R | | | / | 3 | 2 | 1 | 1 | | | | / | 3 | 2 | / | 4 |

Facial

PD | 545 | 337 | / | 425 | 425 | 627 | 423 | 323 | 323 | 435 | 834 | 484 | 535 | / | 558 | 734
R |

Lingual

PD | 555 | 337 | / | 535 | 534 | 436 | 533 | 223 | 743 | 223 | 675 | 333 | 324 | / | 438 | 536
R | | | / | | | 2 | 3 | 3 | 3 | 3 | 2 |

Notes

Figure 3.3 Periodontal charting. Anatomical type periodontal chart of patient radiographed as shown in Figure 3.4. Key: PD, probing depths; R, recession; C, crown; P, pontic; =, teeth joined; I, mobility grade I; Blacked out areas indicate missing teeth. Notes: 14, 27 Root filled. 23 Retained root. Furcation involvement: 17 Grade II buccal; 27 Grade II buccal, Grade I distal, (but ? Grade III buccal to distal)

ment is less than 3 mm, grade 2 if greater than 3 mm but not completely through, or grade 3 if it is completely through (*cf.* Chapter 18). As the disease becomes more advanced there is an increase in the tooth mobility (*cf.* Chapter 23). This may be recorded on a scale of 0–3 where 0 = normal physiological mobility, 1 = less than 1 mm, 2 = greater than 1 mm, and 3 = mobility in an apical direction. The recordings may be made on a periodontal chart as shown in Figure 3.3 or more simply, as in Figure 12.1.

Alveolar bone loss is usually assessed by radiographic examination. In the early stages of disease routine bitewings may be adequate and by using exactly the same technique, but with the film positioned vertically (vertical bitewings), the bone loss in moderate disease may be examined. Periapical radiographs are necessary for evaluating bone loss in more advanced disease. The paralleling technique is preferable to the more commonly used bisecting angle technique as it minimizes distortion (Figure 3.4 A). It also increases the reproducibility of

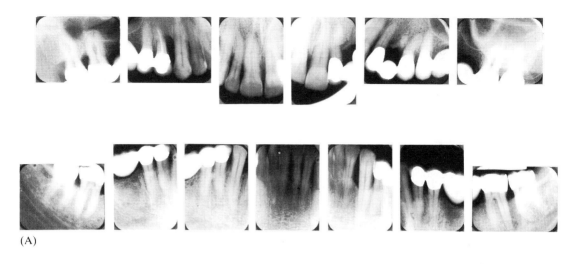

(A)

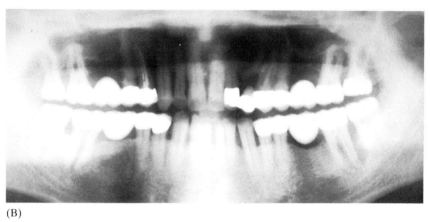

(B)

Figure 3.4 Radiographic presentation of patient with charting demonstrated in Figure 3.3 using (A) paralleling, and (B) orthopantomographic techniques and of another case (C and D, by courtesy of Oral Hygiene Centre, London, W1). Note slight distortion and reduced clarity with the latter technique but it is nevertheless suitable for periodontal diagnostic purposes.

sequential radiographs when evaluating the effects of treatment and modifications of the technique have been used by some researchers in an attempt to determine disease progression. Rotational tomograms such as the orthopantomogram are liable to the most distortion (Figure 3.4 B), but do provide a convenient overall radiographic assessment of the periodontal status and are popular with many clinicians.

It should be appreciated that radiographs are useful in confirming clinical findings but, in most instances, prove to reveal limited additional information in terms of disease severity. Accurate radiographs are considered critical in assessing root morphology and endodontic status, and when complex furcation therapy involving root resections are contemplated. However, in many of these circumstances the definitive decision on treatment may have to be deferred until additional clinical information is obtained at the time of surgical exposure. Similarly, the radiographic finding of post-treatment bone regeneration in intrabony defects is dependent upon sequential reproducible radiographs and even then, only as a gratifying confirmation of the improvement recorded by the clinical measurements.

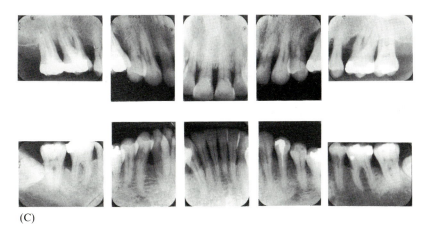

(C)

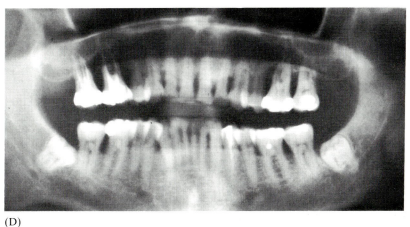

(D)

Figure 3.4 (*cont.*)

Further reading

Fowler, C., Garrett, S., Crigger, M. and Egelberg, J (1982) Histologic probe position in treated and untreated human periodontal tissues. *J. Clin. Periodontol.* **9**, 373–385

Genco, R. J. and Slots, J. (1984) Host responses in periodontal diseases. *J. Dent. Res.* **63**, 441–451

Listgarten, M. A. (1980) Periodontal probing: What does it mean? *J. Clin. Periodontol.* **7**, 165–176

Listgarten, M. A. (1986) Pathogenesis of periodontitis. *J. Clin. Periodontol.* **13**, 418–425

Löe, H., Anerud, A., Boysen, H. and Smith, M. (1978) The natural history of periodontal disease in man. *J. Periodontal.* **49**, 607–620

Page, R. C. (1986) Pathogenesis of gingivitis. *J. Clin. Periodontol.* **13**, 345–355

Page, R. C. and Shroeder, H. E. (1976) Pathogenesis of inflammatory periodontal disease. A summary of current work. *Lab. Invest.* **33**, 235–249

Page, R. C. and Schroeder, H. E. (1981) Current status of the host response in chronic marginal periodontitis. *J. Periodontol.* **52**, 477–491

Page, R. C. and Schroeder, H. E. (1982) *Periodontitis in Man and Other Animals. A Comparative Review.* Karger, Basel

Seymour, G. J., Powell, R. N. and Davies, W. I. R. (1979) The immunopathogenesis of progressive chronic inflammatory periodontal disease. *J. Oral Pathol.* **8**, 249–265

4

Pathogenesis of chronic inflammatory periodontal disease (2)

R. M. Palmer

Disease progression

The classic picture

Chronic inflammatory periodontol disease has classically been divided into gingivitis, in which inflammation is confined to the marginal gingival tissue, and periodontitis, where the disease has progressed to involve loss of connective tissue attachment between the root surface and alveolar bone. Gingivitis does not inevitably progress to periodontitis and although periodontitis is usually preceded by gingivitis this is not invariable. Examination of the dentition of many individuals shows areas of gingivitis, periodontitis and healthy gingiva within the same mouth, often with some degree of symmetry. In addition, certain teeth and tooth surfaces show a greater susceptibility to disease than others. For example epidemiological data indicate that, in general, the canines and premolars are more resistant to periodontal disease than the rest of the dentition. Much of the variation may be explained in terms of plaque distribution and tooth morphology, and the part played by the local and systemic immune responses and the presence of specific microorganisms. Factors which impede plaque removal or enhance plaque retention may predispose certain tooth surfaces to more disease. These predisposing factors include calculus, deficient or overhanging restoration margins, removable or fixed prostheses and crowded or malpositioned teeth or position in the dental arch. These factors make it difficult or sometimes impossible for the patient to remove plaque from the tooth surface and may allow an ecological niche to be provided for pathogenic bacteria. Similarly, once pocketing has occurred this predisposes the site to further disease.

Patterns of attachment loss

Certain factors have been used to explain the variable pattern/morphology of the pockets and associated loss of bone in periodontitis. Pockets with their base coronal to the bone margin are called suprabony pockets and are usually associated with even or horizontal loss of bone (Figure 4.1). Pockets which extend apical to the bone crest are called intrabony pockets, and these involve angular or

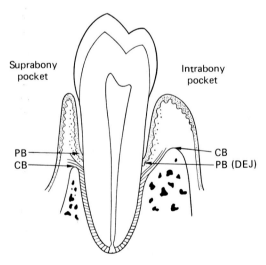

Figure 4.1 Relationship of the base of the pocket (PB) to the crest of the alveolar bone (CB) in suprabony and intrabony pockets. Note the pocket base is formed by dento-epithelial junction (DEJ)

vertical bone loss. The simplest explanation of why a particular pattern of bone destruction predominates relates to the surrounding osseous anatomy and the dimensions of the inflammatory lesion. Thus, in situations where the alveolar bone morphology is thin, its complete loss is inevitable and a suprabony pocket results. In areas where the alveolar bone is thick the inflammatory lesion, which has a radius of about 1.5–2.5 mm extending from the plaque on the tooth surface, can be accommodated by partial loss of bone and the production of an angular defect. This can be verified clinically where intrabony defects are only seen where room is provided for them by the thickness of the bone and are thus more frequent in the molar interdental areas. In much the same way, the anatomy of the gingival tissue may dictate the degree of recession or pocketing. Thus, thin gingiva is more susceptible to recession and the mechanisms responsible are considered in Chapter 13.

Active disease

However, the foregoing discussion does not address the problem of why there may be progression to periodontitis initially and how progression occurs once disease is established. The term periodontitis suggests inflammation involving the periodontal ligament and bone. For the most part this would appear to be inaccurate because, as stated in the description of the histological features of the advanced lesion in the previous chapter, the inflammatory lesion of periodontitis is walled off from the underlying periodontal ligament and bone by fibrous tissue. These tissues are free of inflammation and there is little evidence of active bone resorption. This lesion may be stable or extremely slowly progressive and its cellular composition may differ little from a well-established gingivitis.

However, it has been suggested that the lesion of periodontitis is dominated by B lymphocytes and plasma cells in contrast to gingivitis which is T cell dominated. A hypothesis has therefore been proposed which suggests that the change from gingivitis to progressive periodontitis involves a conversion from a T cell dominant lesion to a B cell dominant lesion. Certainly there is evidence that childhood gingivitis contains mainly T lymphocytes, but the situation in long-standing adult gingivitis may be quite different. There are many plasma cells and B lymphocytes in the advanced lesion but it is questionable whether this lesion is consistent with more recent concepts of disease progression.

These concepts have evolved from information gained by repeated clinical measurements of pockets in untreated periodontitis over periods of 1–6 years. They have shown that the majority of periodontitis lesions are stable and that only a small percentage

(probably less than 5%) undergo progression. Sites that show progression during this time may subsequently remain stable for many years. It has been proposed that progression of disease therefore occurs in bursts which may last only a few days or weeks. The clinical measurements can at best only detect when there has been an active phase at some time between two sets of measurements and, as yet, there is no parameter which can accurately detect current disease progression or predict this event. There is even some controversy as to whether even some large changes in probing depths are due to errors in measurement. It is not surprising, therefore, that practically all specimens of human periodontitis which have been examined histologically may be examples of the stable or slowly progressive lesion of periodontitis.

It has been suggested that the diagnosis of periodontitis should refer to an inflammatory disease of the periodontium characterized by the presence of periodontal pockets and active bone resorption with acute inflammation. This type of lesion is readily demonstrated in experimental periodontitis in various animal species and is usually induced by placing plaque retaining ligatures subgingivally. The experimental periodontitis models in animals are different from periodontitis in humans and are the equivalent of a persistent acute inflammatory lesion. It has been proposed that progression of human periodontitis occurs within similar but short periods of acute inflammation characterized by a rapid increase in the number of phagocytes and the release of many damaging enzymes. The phagocytes may be retained in the periodontal tissue due to a disruption of the chemotactic gradient caused by ulceration of the pocket wall or perhaps by tissue invasion and proliferation of pathogenic bacteria. The rarity of histological evidence of this proposed event would also be explained by the low statistical probability of obtaining a specimen in the active phase. The inflammation may extend and destroy the fibrous zone of the chronic lesion and cause active bone resorption. Acute periodontal abscesses result in rapid and extensive tissue destruction and may represent the extreme end of a spectrum of progressive lesions.

Bone resorption may be detected after the event on radiographic examination. More sophisticated radiographic techniques such as subtraction radiography and computer-assisted image analysis have been used to measure very small changes in bone mass but rely heavily on highly reproducible radiographic images. These techniques are not able to detect current disease progression although application of bone-seeking radiopharmaceuticals such as technetium-99m–methylene disphosphonate may overcome some of the difficulties.

Progression of periodontitis may, therefore,

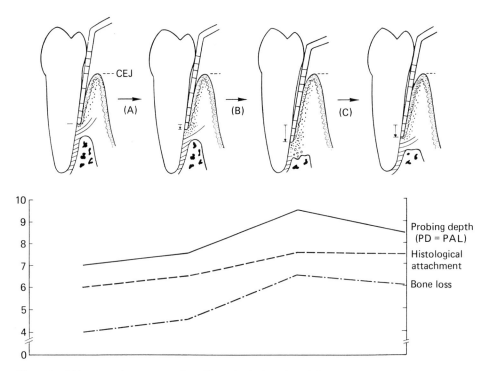

Figure 4.2 Diagrammatic representation of hypothetical models of disease progression. (A) Slow progression –
undetectable clinically and radiographically in the short term. (B) Progression to active lesion – extension of inflammation
with destruction of fibrous wall of chronic lesion. (C) Resolution of acute inflammation – reversion to stable or slowly
progressive lesion. For simplicity the gingival margin has been retained at the cemento-enamel junction (CEJ) so that
probing depth (PD) and probing attachment levels (PAL) are the same

involve slow continuous activity which would be
very difficult to measure clinically in the short term,
or may result from rapid bursts of activity interspersed with periods of stability (Figure 4.2). The
bursts of activity may be associated with an
imbalance in the pocket bacteria or the host
response. Another factor which has also been held
responsible for increased disease progression is
trauma from occlusion. It is worthwhile briefly to
consider the available evidence for this.

Occlusion as a factor

It has been established that forces from occlusion do
not cause gingivitis, periodontitis or the progression
of gingivitis to periodontitis, but they may possibly
cause accelerated progression of established
periodontitis. Increased forces, when applied to a
healthy periodontium, cause bone loss and widening
of the ligament which results clinically in increased
mobility. The radiographic appearance is similar to
a very narrow intrabony lesion as there is funnel-
shaped widening of the coronal part of the ligament

space. It is not surprising therefore, that it has been
suggested that occlusal trauma and periodontitis are
co-destructive, as they have several features in
common. Unfortunately, experiments in different
animal species having teeth subjected to both
periodontitis and excessive occlusal forces were
inconclusive, often with quite opposing results. The
design of such experiments is extremely difficult and
no model has been found to date which will mimic
satisfactorily the human situation. In the various
animal models an experimental periodontitis is
induced around the teeth using plaque retaining
devices and this produces either rapidly and
continuously progressive disease or a progressive
phase which lasts for only the first few weeks of the
experiment and is stable by the time the occlusal
forces are applied. It would appear that neither case
would pertain to the human situation. In addition,
the applied forces have been excessive in magnitude
and/or duration. It may be concluded from the
available evidence that co-destruction may occur
only under very special circumstances, probably
involving the superimposition of a developing lesion
of occlusal trauma on a tooth undergoing a burst of

disease activity. Fortunately, from the clinical point of view, most would agree that if plaque-induced periodontitis is treated then the forces from occlusion cannot be co-destructive.

Other types of periodontitis

The preceding account of chronic inflammatory periodontal disease has been mainly concerned with the most common periodontitis, sometimes referred to as adult periodontitis. The recognition that certain individuals have more aggressive forms of the disease which often affect them at a much earlier age suggests that the blanket diagnosis of periodontitis is too broad. Thus, juvenile periodontitis or periodontosis has been recognized as a specific disease entity for many years and, more recently, further types such as rapidly progressive and prepubertal periodontitis have been described. In addition, certain systemic diseases modify the inflammatory response to bacterial plaque and may cause increased severity of disease.

Juvenile periodontitis

Juvenile periodontitis is a condition affecting young individuals with a suggested onset around puberty. Patients over the age of 25 years who present with similar features of the disease are often classified as post-juvenile periodontitis. The condition is relatively uncommon with an incidence in teenagers of about 1:1000. Earlier reports suggested that females were more likely to be affected than males, but currently it is thought that the sex incidence is about equal. The permanent incisors and first molars are the teeth most commonly affected, and therefore it is often referred to as localized juvenile periodontitis (LJP). A more generalized form of the disease affecting almost the entire dentition has been recognized, but this may be confused with rapidly progressive periodontitis. The gingival tissues around the affected teeth often appear healthy and the disease is only detected on probing or radiographic examination. Occasionally, the patient presents with drifting and spacing of incisor teeth and may complain of increased mobility. The pattern of disease is often remarkably symmetrical and the radiographic appearance of deep angular bone defects around affected teeth has been described as a mirror image pattern. In the early stages of the disease subgingival plaque may be very sparse and loosely adherent with no evidence of calcification. Although the lesions are rapidly progressive in the early stages they may slow or 'burn out' and assume characteristics more consistent with adult periodontitis.

The disease has a familial distribution and is usually associated with a specific bacterium and host defence defect. The bacterium most closely associated with this disease is *Actinobacillus actinomycetemcomitans* (see Chapter 5). This organism produces a powerful leucotoxin which affects the phagocytes and may enhance the bacteria's ability to invade tissue. Patients with juvenile periodontitis often have circulating antibodies to the bacteria and its leucotoxin. The majority of individuals also have a functional defect in either neutrophils or macrophages, which is insufficient to cause systemic disease but may enhance local tissue destruction. It is difficult to explain the site distribution but this may relate to the stage of eruption of the permanent teeth at the age of onset or possibly to some defect in the attachment of collagen fibres to cementum. The unique features of the disease would suggest that the treatment required may be different from that administered for adult periodontitis and often involves the use of antibiotics. This will be discussed in more detail in Chapters 5 and 35.

Rapidly progressive periodontitis

This condition appears to be less common than juvenile periodontitis but some patients may have previously suffered from juvenile periodontitis. The age of onset is usually between puberty and 30 years. Lesions are severe and generalized with evidence of rapid bone destruction. Gingival tissue may appear acutely inflamed or relatively normal, possibly corresponding to whether the disease is in an active or stable phase, although there is no evidence to support this hypothesis. Many of the patients have functionally defective phagocytes. It is suggested that some of the affected individuals have constitutional symptoms such as malaise and weight loss. The currently available knowledge of this condition makes diagnosis considerably more difficult than localized juvenile periodontitis. It is possible that this disease is a generalized form of juvenile periodontitis or represents the extreme in susceptibility of the adult periodontitis group.

Prepubertal periodontitis

This is an extremely rare condition which affects the primary dentition and may have a genetic basis. It has been described in a generalized form in which acute inflammation and rapid destruction of the periodontal tissues are associated with profound functional defects in the phagocytes. The defects in the phagocytes are confined to the neutrophils or macrophages but not both. Individuals are prone to repeated systemic infections and the periodontitis may be refractory to treatment. The permanent dentition may be subsequently affected. The localized form is less severe and more amenable to treatment.

Influence of systemic conditions

Most patients presenting with periodontal disease have no recognizable systemic condition to account for any increased susceptibility. However, some systemic disorders are positively associated with severe periodontal disease. These disorders may affect the phagocytes, the lymphocytes, the vascular response or the healing ability of the periodontium.

The phagocytes most commonly affected are the neutrophils. In conditions such as agranulocytosis or cyclic neutropenia, where there is a significant reduction in neutrophils, individuals suffer from severe periodontitis in association with other serious and perhaps life-threatening infections. In less profound functional defects of neutrophils, such as the reduced chemotaxis and phagocytosis reported in some diabetics and reduced phagocytosis in Down's syndrome, there is often severe periodontitis. Uncontrolled diabetics, for instance, are reported to suffer from recurrent multiple periodontal abscesses. The balance in the number and function of the phagocytes in maintaining periodontal health appears to be critical.

Individuals whose lymphocyte function has been depressed for the prevention of organ transplant rejection seem to have little difference in periodontal disease experience compared with control patients. However, the leukaemias are often associated with gross gingival enlargement due to the accumulation of neoplastic leucocytes within the gingival tissue and an increased tendency to infections such as acute necrotizing gingivitis (*cf.* Chapters 5 and 25). Acute monocytic leukaemia is reported to be most frequently associated with an increased manifestation of periodontitis. Persons suffering from HIV may also present with severe periodontitis or acute necrotizing gingivitis causing extensive destruction of the periodontal tissues. Some authorities have suggested that HIV periodontitis should be considered as a specific periodontal disease entity.

The severity of gingival inflammation may be enhanced by factors affecting the vasculature. The most common conditions are those associated with hormonal changes such as puberty and pregnancy. In pregnancy the increase in progesterone is responsible for the heightened gingival response to plaque. This results in a pregnancy gingivitis and occasionally in localized areas there is proliferation of the vasculature and inflammatory cells producing a pregnancy epulis. Similar responses have previously been observed with some patients taking contraceptive pills.

The classic impairment of the healing response occurs in vitamin C deficiency. This is extremely rare in the UK but is seen typically in individuals with bizarre dietary habits, such as chronic alcoholics. Vitamin C is essential for the formation of collagen and deficiency results in scurvy. Gross inflammatory changes and destruction of the periodontal tissues leads to fairly rapid exfoliation of the teeth. Fibrous and inflammatory gingival enlargement or hyperplasia, particularly affecting the interdental papillae, is a fairly common side effect in patients taking phenytoin (anti-epileptic), cyclosporin (immunosuppressant) and nifedipine (antihypertensive).

It should be emphasized that the preceding diseases are rare but occasionally it is periodontal examination that leads to the diagnosis of an underlying systemic disorder. The conditions do, however, emphasize how the delicate balance between bacterial insult and host defence can be altered in favour of increased disease progression.

Further reading

Genco, R. J., Christersson, L. A. and Zambon, J. J. (1986) Juvenile periodontitis. *Int. Dent. J.* **36**, 168–176

Goodson, J. M., Haffajee, A. D. and Socransky, S. S. (1984) The relationship between attachment level loss and alveolar bone loss. *J. Clin. Periodontol.* **11**, 348–359

Goodson, J. M., Tanner, A. C. R., Haffajee, A. D., Somberger, G. C. and Socransky, S. S. (1982) Patterns of progression and regression of advanced destructive periodontal disease. *J. Clin. Periodontol.* **9**, 472–481

Hausmann, E. and Jeffcoat, M. (1988) A perspective on periodontal disease activity. *J. Clin. Periodontol.* **15**, 134–136

Janssen, P. T. M., Faber, J. A. J. and van Palenstein Helderman, W. H. (1987) Non-Gaussian distribution of differences between duplicate probing depth measurements. *J. Clin. Periodontol.* **14**, 345–349

Page, R. C., Altman, L. C., Ebersole, J. L., Vandesteen, G. E., Dahlberg, W. H., Williams, B. L. and Osterberg, S. K. (1983) Rapidly progressive periodontitis. A distinct clinical condition. *J. Periodontol.* **54**, 197–209

Page, R. C., Bowen, T., Altman, L., Vandesteen, E., Ochs, H., Mackenzie, P., Osterberg, S., Engel, L. D. and Williams, B. L. (1983) Prepubertal periodontitis I. Definition of a clinical disease entity. *J. Periodontol.* **54**, 257–271

Polson, A. M. (1986) The relative importance of plaque and occlusion in periodontal disease. *J. Clin. Periodontol.* **13**, 923–927

Polson, A. M. (1980) Interrelationship of inflammation and tooth mobility (trauma) in pathogenesis of periodontal disease. *J. Clin. Periodontol.* **7**, 351–360

Saxen, L. (1980) Juvenile periodontitis. *J. Clin. Periodontol.* **7**, 1–19

Schenker, B. J. (1987) Immunologic dysfunction in the pathogenesis of periodontal diseases. *J. Clin. Periodontol.* **14**, 489–498

Seymour, G. J. (1987) Possible mechanisms involved in the immunoregulation of chronic inflammatory periodontal disease. *J. Dent. Res.* **66**, 2–9

Seymour, G. J., Crouch, M. and Powell, R. N. (1981) The phenotypic characterization of lymphoid cell subpopulations in gingivitis in children. *J. Periodont. Res.* **16**, 582–592

Seymour, G. J., Powell, R. N. and Davies, W. I. R. (1979) Conversion of a stable T-cell lesion to a progressive B-cell lesion in pathogenesis of chronic inflammatory periodontal disease: an hypothesis. *J. Clin. Periodontol.* **6**, 267–277

Socransky, S. S., Haffajee, A. D., Goodson, J. M. and Lindhe, J. (1984) New concepts of destructive periodontal disease. *J. Clin. Periodontol.* **11**, 21–32

5

The microbiology of periodontal disease

P. D. Marsh

Introduction

Although it is more than 300 years since Leeuwenhoek implicated microorganisms with oral malodours and inflammation of the gums, it is only in the last two decades that any real progress has been made in identifying and characterizing the bacteria associated with the gingival crevice in health and disease. Recent studies suggest that each form of periodontal disease is associated with distinct mixtures of a relatively limited number of bacterial species. The predominant organisms in disease are frequently found to be obligately anaerobic or carbon dioxide-requiring Gram-negative rod, spiral or filament-shaped bacteria, some of which appear to be specifically associated with the periodontal pocket. However, many of these bacteria are also found on occasions at healthy sites (albeit in low numbers). Thus, periodontal diseases, unlike many classic infections, result from an imbalance in the proportions of the resident (commensal) flora of the gingival crevice.

The challenge posed by microbiological studies of periodontal diseases, therefore, centres around determining:

(1) the causative organism(s) of disease at sites where there is a pre-existing 'background' of commensal bacteria, which is both complex and variable in composition,
(2) the role of the individual bacterial species in disease,
(3) the factors responsible for the transition of the

normal flora from having a commensal to a pathogenic relationship with the host.

In addition, it is equally important to determine the relationship between the pocket bacteria and the host defences. However, for the most part, this aspect will fall beyond the scope of this chapter.

It is implicit from the above that, in order to interpret the results of a microbiological study of a periodontal disease, it is necessary first to characterize the resident flora of the (healthy) gingival crevice and to define the major ecological determinants of this site. To do so necessitates the sampling of bacterial plaque; a brief reference to the techniques and difficulties involved would, therefore, be instructive.

Methods of sampling and quantifying subgingival plaque

The problems of sampling

Plaque from the gingival crevice and periodontal pocket has proved to be the most difficult to sample because of the anatomy and anaerobic nature of the site. The flora will be shown later to be comprised of high numbers of obligately anaerobic bacteria, including spirochaetes, most of which will rapidly lose their viability if exposed to air. In disease, the anatomy of the site means that those organisms at the base of the pocket, near the advancing front of

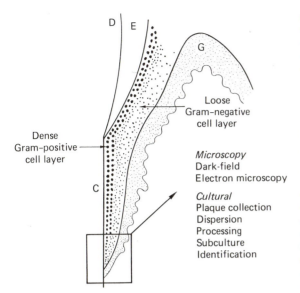

Figure 5.1 Anatomy of the periodontal pocket. A diagrammatic representation of a periodontal pocket to illustrate (a) the difficulty in sampling the advancing front of the lesion without removing bacteria from other sites in the pocket and (b) the stages in plaque processing. Key: G, gingiva; E, enamel; D, dentine; C, cementum

the lesion, are likely to be of most interest (Figure 5.1). It is important, therefore, not to include in a sample, organisms from other sites within the pocket as this might obscure significant relationships between specific bacteria and disease. To overcome these problems a number of methods have been developed, all of which have their particular advantages and drawbacks. For example, a simple approach has been to insert paper points into pockets but the number of organisms removed from the root of the tooth or from epithelial surfaces by this method will be small. Samples have also been taken by irrigation of the site and retrieval of the material through syringe needles; this has the disadvantage of removing plaque from the whole depth of the pocket.

Particularly sophisticated methods employ a broach tipped with calcium alginate fibres, which can be kept withdrawn in a protective cannula sheath until in position near the base of the pocket and, if necessary, the broach can be flushed continuously with oxygen-free gas. Perhaps the most frequent approach has been to use a curette or scaler after the supragingival area has been cleared. The scaler tips can be detached and placed immediately in gas-flushed tubes containing reduced (anaerobic) transport fluid for delivery to the laboratory. Alternatively, when periodontal surgery is needed,

plaque can be removed from surfaces exposed by flap reflection. It is important to realize, particularly when comparing microbiological studies in which different sampling procedures have been used, that the results will, to a certain extent, be biased by the methods adopted.

Storage and transportation

Samples must be brought to the laboratory for processing as quickly as possible in transport fluids specially-designed to reduce the loss of viability of obligately anaerobic bacteria during transit. Plaque by definition is a complex mixture of a range of microorgansisms which are bound tenaciously to one another. These clumps and aggregates of bacteria must therefore be dispersed efficiently (ideally to single cells) if the specimen is to be diluted and counted accurately. One of the most efficient dispersion methods for subgingival plaque is to vortex samples with small glass beads in a tube filled with carbon dioxide.

Bacterial identification

Once dispersed, samples are usually serially diluted and aliquots spread on to agar plates. These plates are chosen to grow either the maximum number of bacteria or, using selective media, only a limited number of species that are present perhaps in low numbers. The identity of the bacteria on these plates cannot be confirmed by their colonial appearance or mere presence on a particular medium, and further tests are required. The first stage of identification usually involves colony counting whereby colonies with a similar appearance are counted and subcultured for further tests. The first level of discrimination involves the Gram-staining of subcultured colonies. Bacteria are then grouped according to whether their cells are Gram positive or Gram negative, and are rod, filamentous or coccal-shaped. This dictates which further tests will be necessary to achieve speciation.

Some bacteria can be identified using simple criteria, for example sugar fermentation tests, while others, particularly the obligately anaerobic species, require a more sophisticated approach such as the use of gas-liquid chromatography to determine their pattern of fermentation products. The identification of an organism is only successful when it is based on a sound classification scheme. A great deal of emphasis is currently being placed on improving the classification (taxonomy) of plaque bacteria because, without valid subdivisions, the association of species with particular diseases will never be made. The commonly isolated genera from dental plaque

Table 5.1 Some of the commonly isolated bacterial genera[a] from dental plaque

Gram-positive cocci	Gram-negative cocci
Streptococcus	*Branhamella*
Peptostreptococcus	*Neisseria*
	Veillonella
Gram-positive rods	**Gram-negative rods**
Actinomyces	*Actinobacillus*
Arachnia	*Bacteroides[b]*
Bifidobacterium	*Campylobacter*
Corynebacterium (formerly	*Capnocytophaga*
Bacterionema)	*Centipeda*
Eubacterium	*Eikenella*
Lactobacillus	*Fusobacterium*
Propionibacterium	*Haemophilus*
Rothia	*Leptotrichia*
	Selenomonas
	Treponema
	Wolinella

[a] Most genera contain more than one species.
[b] It has been proposed that *B. gingivalis* be transferred to the new genus *Porphyromonas*

are listed in Table 5.1. Most of these genera consist of more than one species, not all of which are found in the gingival crevice (see a later section and Table 5.3).

Alternatives to culturing

As an alternative to cultural studies, the principal morphological groups of bacteria found in plaque can be recognized using light microscopy. Phase-contrast and dark-field illumination techniques have been used to quantify the numbers of motile bacteria in 'dispersed' subgingival plaque without the need for serial dilution. These bacteria include spirochaetes, which are extremely difficult to cultivate by conventional means. As the numbers of spirochaetes and motile organisms have been related to the severity of some periodontal diseases, and because microscopy is a relatively cheap and rapid method, it had been hoped that these techniques could be used in the clinic to monitor the progress of patients undergoing treatment. However, a major disadvantage of microscopy is that most of the putative pathogens cannot be recognized by morphology alone. To overcome this problem, antisera (monoclonal or specific polyclonal) are being raised against a limited number of bacteria believed to be implicated in disease so that their numbers in plaque can be quantified rapidly by standard fluorescence microscopy or ELISA techniques. This approach would obviate the need for many of the lengthy and labour-intensive steps

described above but to date only a limited number of specific antisera have been produced. Likewise, gene (DNA) probes have also been made against some putative periodontal pathogens, and they can be used to screen plaque for the presence of the species. Electron microscopy has proved useful for studying plaque formation and it has also been used to show that bacteria may invade gingival tissues in aggressive forms of periodontal disease. Immunocytological techniques have made it possible to identify some of the invading bacteria.

Microbial ecology of the gingival crevice

In order for microorganisms to persist in the mouth, cells have to adhere to and be retained at surfaces. Thus, although saliva contains approximately 10^8 bacteria/ml, these organisms are derived from mucosal and enamel surfaces and are lost by swallowing before they are able to maintain their presence by cell division. A unique feature of the mouth is the presence of non-shedding tooth surfaces for microbial colonization. Elsewhere, in the body, desquamation ensures that the bacterial load on mucosal surfaces is light and indeed only a few species of bacteria are usually able to adhere. In contrast, relatively thick films of microorganisms (dental plaque) are able to accumulate on teeth, particularly at sites like fissures, approximal regions and the gingival crevice. All these areas offer protection to bacteria from, for example, saliva, mastication or crevicular fluid flow. The bacterial composition of dental plaque varies from site to site on the tooth surface. Nevertheless, the major factors influencing the microbiology of the gingival crevice can be defined and are discussed below.

The affinity of the organisms for the habitat

Gram-positive bacteria preferentially colonize the enamel surface by means of a range of specific molecular interactions between 'adhesins' on their cell surface (e.g. lipoteichoic acid, glucosyltransferase, dextran-binding proteins, etc.) and components in the acquired pellicle on the enamel (e.g. blood group reactive proteins, lysozyme, antibodies). Factors in crevicular fluid and, to a lesser extent, saliva will adsorb on to enamel (or cementum) and influence the adhesion of plaque bacteria in the gingival crevice. This film of Gram-positive cells is relatively thin (<60 μm) and cultural studies have shown the bacteria to belong to only a limited number of species, namely *Streptococcus sanguis*, *Actinomyces viscosus*, *A. naeslundii* and

A. israelii. The subsequent accumulation of Gram-negative bacteria is dependent on the presence of this layer of Gram-positive cells. A number of *Bacteroides*, *Capnocytophaga*, *Fusobacterium*, *Eikenella* and *Veillonella* species can attach specifically to streptococci and actinomyces by the process of co-aggregation. Co-aggregation involves lectins which are carbohydrate-binding proteins that interact with the complementary carbohydrate-containing receptor on another cell. Electron microscopy studies have shown that the Gram-negative bacteria form a loose layer over the surface of the Gram-positive bacteria. This loose layer is in contact with the gingival epithelium and contains a number of bacterial associations. The most common of these associations involves the attachment of coccal-shaped bacteria to one end of a filamentous cell, and have been termed 'corn-cobs'. The bacterial components have been identified as *Corynebacterium* (formerly *Bacterionema*) *matruchotii* with *Strep. sanguis* and *Eubacterium sabbureum* with *Veillonella alkalescens*.

Crevicular fluid

Serum components can reach the mouth by the flow of fluid through the junctional epithelium of the gingiva, the rate of which is markedly increased during periodontal disease. This fluid can influence the ecology of the site in a number of ways. Its flow will remove non-adherent bacteria but will also act as the primary source of nutrients for the indigenous microorganisms, providing a range of proteins, glycoproteins and lipoproteins, including albumin, transferrin, haemopexin and haptoglobins. Many bacteria from subgingival plaque are proteolytic and synergistically interact to break down some of these proteins to provide essential peptides and amino

acids, as well as haemin for the growth of black-pigmented *Bacteroides* spp. Carbohydrates are obtained primarily from the metabolism of the oligosaccharide side chains of glycoproteins. Other growth factors that can be present include urea, α_2-globulin for *Treponema denticola* and hormones (progesterone, oestradiol) for *Bacteroides intermedius* (Table 5.2). Part of the diversity of the flora of the gingival crevice can be attributed to the development of food chains whereby the products of metabolism of one cell become the primary nutrients of another; some examples are listed in Table 5.2.

Crevicular fluid can also influence the pH of the site which, in turn, will markedly affect the proportions and types of bacteria able to grow. Measurements of the crevice during health have shown the pH to be around neutrality (pH 6.90 ± 0.23 in nine sites) but at sites where the gingival index (GI) increases the pH of crevicular fluid becomes more alkaline (pH 8.66 ± 0.44 in ten sites with a GI = 2). The most likely explanation for this is the bacterial production of ammonia from deamination and the elevated supply of urea during inflammation. The growth and enzyme activity of *Bacteroides gingivalis*, one of the Gram-negative species associated with severe forms of periodontal disease, is favoured by alkaline conditions.

The host is also able to interact with the bacteria in the gingival crevice via crevicular fluid in another way. Crevicular fluid contains most of the humoral and cellular components found in the blood (see Chapter 2). Several putative periodontal pathogens have been shown in the laboratory to have the ability to modulate the host defences by (1) reducing the effectiveness of polymorphs, (2) producing proteases that cleave immunoglobulins and complement, and (3) inducing suppressor T cells (see Table 5.8). There exists, therefore, a delicate interplay

Table 5.2 Some examples of nutritional interactions within the gingival crevice

Factor	Source	Beneficiary
Carbohydrates	Glycoproteins	Saccharolytic bacteria
Haemin	Crevicular fluid	Black-pigmented *Bacteroides*
Peptides	Crevicular fluid	Asaccharolytic bacteria
Hormones	Crevicular fluid	*Bacteroides intermedius*
Isobutyrate	*Fusobacterium*	Spirochaetes
Putrescine/spermine	*Fusobacterium*	Spirochaetes
Succinate	Gram-positive rods	Spirochaetes
H_2, formate	*Fusobacterium*/*Bacteroides*	*Wolinella*
Vitamin K	Crevice bacteria	Black-pigmented *Bacteroides*
Lactate	Crevice bacteria	*Veillonella*/spirochaetes
Protohaeme	*Wolinella*	*B. gingivalis*

The nutritional requirements of the bacterial flora of the gingival crevice are satisfied directly by crevicular fluid and by the establishment of food chains between various organisms

between the encouragement of bacterial growth by crevicular fluid and the attempted control of this flora by the host defences. Some evidence of this interplay can be inferred from the detection of a number of lysosomal and bacterial enzymes found free in crevicular fluid.

The redox potential of the site

The normal gingival crevice and the periodontal pocket are the most anaerobic sites in the mouth. This, coupled with the provision of essential nutrients by crevicular fluid, enables this site to be colonized by many obligately anaerobic bacteria. The redox potential (*Eh*) is a measure of the degree of anaerobiosis at a site, and the *Eh* of a healthy gingival crevice is higher (i.e. less anaerobic; mean value = +73 mV) compared with periodontal pockets (mean value = −48 mV) in the same individuals. Other studies have reported lower values for both sites which is to be expected as spirochaetes are recovered almost exclusively from this area in the mouth.

The microbiology of the gingival crevice

The bacteriology of the normal gingival crevice differs from that of other sites on the tooth surface. The flora in health is sparse and in one study of seven subjects, only 10^3–10^6 colony forming units (cfu) were obtained per crevice. The proportions of the major bacterial groups found within the healthy crevice are listed in Table 5.3. Unlike the flora of fissures and approximal surfaces, more obligately

Table 5.3 The predominant cultivable flora of the healthy gingival crevice

Bacterium	Mean percentage of total flora	Range	Percentage isolation frequency
Streptococcus	40	2–73	100
Peptostreptococcus	1	0– 6	14
Actinomyces	35	10–63	100
Gram-positive anaerobic rod	10	0–37	86
Neisseria	0.3	0– 2	14
Veillonella	2	0– 5	57
Haemophilus[a]	0	0	0
Gram-negative anaerobic rod	13	8–20	100

Spirochaetes have also been detected by dark-field microscopy
[a] Other studies have recovered haemophili from the gingival crevice quite commonly but in low numbers

anaerobic bacteria are recovered (particularly Gram-negative rods/filaments and spirochaetes) from the gingival crevice although their proportions are markedly increased in disease. Other studies have shown the presence of few motile organisms and black-pigmented *Bacteroides* in health although the isolation frequently of the latter is higher in adults than children. The most commonly found black-pigmented *Bacteroides* spp. in the normal gingival crevice is *B. melaninogenicus* while *B. intermedius* has also been recovered on occasions; *B. gingivalis* is rarely isolated from healthy sites. Other commonly isolated obligately anaerobic species of bacteria are *Fusobacterium* spp., non-pigmented *Bacteroides* spp., *Leptotrichia buccalis*, *Propionibacterium* spp., *Arachnia propionica*, *Eubacterium* spp. and *Bifidobacterium* spp. The predominant spirochaetes are of both small and medium size and it has been reported recently that they can be present at healthy sites even in prepubertal children. The microflora of subgingival plaque taken from sites with various forms of periodontal disease will now be described in detail.

The microbiology of periodontal diseases

Evidence for the aetiological role of microorganisms

Unequivocal evidence that bacteria are specifically implicated in periodontal diseases has come from gnotobiotic animal studies. Germ-free animals rarely suffer from periodontal disease although, on occasions, food can be impacted in the gingival crevice producing inflammation. However, inflammation is much more common and severe when specific bacteria, particularly some of those isolated from human periodontal pockets, are used in pure culture to infect the animals. These bacteria include streptococci and *Actinomyces* spp. but are more commonly Gram-negative, for example, *Actinobacillus*, *Bacteroides*, *Capnocytophaga*, *Eikenella*, *Fusobacterium*, and *Selenomonas* spp. Furthermore, periodontal disease is arrested when an antibiotic active against the particular organism is administered to the infected animal. In humans, evidence for the role of microorganisms has also come from plaque control and antibiotic-treatment studies. However, these latter types of studies give no information as to whether disease results from the activity of (i) a single, or only a limited selection, of species (the specific plaque hypothesis), or (ii) any combination of a wide range of plaque bacteria (the non-specific plaque hypothesis). In order to test these 'hypotheses' a large number of cross-sectional epidemiological studies have been performed on patients with particular forms of periodontal disease. A disadvantage of this type of study is that true 'cause-and-effect' relationships can never be determined. Organisms that appear to predominate at diseased sites might be present as a result of the disease rather than having actually initiated it. With the exception of gingivitis, longitudinal studies (which do not suffer from this drawback) are not usually possible because of the lengthy natural history of some forms of periodontal disease and the difficulties in predicting subjects and sites likely to become affected. Despite these problems of study design, coupled with the technical difficulties mentioned earlier, genuine progress has been made in our understanding of the microbiology of periodontal diseases. This will be outlined briefly in the following sections although it will be possible here to describe only the major trends. Much of the confusing and at times contradictory literature has been simplified for clarity.

Gingivitis

Chronic marginal gingivitis

Chronic marginal gingivitis is a reversible, inflammatory response to dental plaque. Initially, many regarded gingivitis as resulting from a non-specific proliferation of the normal gingival crevice flora due to poor oral hygiene. Certainly, the number of bacterial cells in plaque associated with gingivitis is increased substantially by 10–20-fold compared with healthy control sites. However, this increase in plaque mass is associated with increases in the proportions of only a limited number of bacterial types which are mainly *Actinomyces* spp., plus certain facultatively and obligately anaerobic Gram-negative rods. This has prompted a number of 'experimental' gingivitis studies in humans.

Experimental gingivitis

The finding that gingivitis develops in a predictable and reproducible manner in volunteers who refrain from any oral hygiene measures has allowed the design of longitudinal studies to determine the bacteriological events that lead to disease. As the plaque mass begins to increase, there is a shift from a streptococci-dominated plaque to one in which *Actinomyces* spp. predominate. Results from one study of 25 subjects suggested that specific relationships might exist between certain bacteria and particular stages in the development of gingivitis. When the gingivitis score was plotted as a function of the plaque score (Figure 5.2), the gingivitis score increased in two large increments. For example, proportions of *A. israelii* increased significantly from 13 to 26% of the total cultivable flora with the onset of a non-bleeding gingivitis (GI = 1.0; plaque

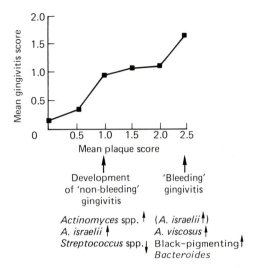

Figure 5.2 Bacteriology of human experimental gingivitis. The relationship between plaque and gingivitis scores in young adults during a 21-day period without oral hygiene. Statistically significant changes in the flora are indicated. (From Loesche and Syed (1978) *Infect. Immun.*, **21**, 830–839)

index (PI) = 1.0). This was also associated with an increase in the percentage viable counts of *A. viscosus* from 7 to 14% of the flora. When the gingivitis progressed to a bleeding stage (GI = 2.0; PI = 2.5) a black-pigmenting *Bacteroides* sp., possibly *B. gingivalis,* increased from 0.01 to 0.2% of the flora.

The effect that bleeding might have on the composition of the flora is of interest as black-pigmented *Bacteroides* spp. require haemin for growth and this can be obtained from the enzymic hydrolysis of blood proteins. Perhaps significantly, in laboratory studies, strains of *B. gingivalis* were found to have the greatest hydrolytic activities of the black-pigmented *Bacteroides* species.

In a more recent study of experimental gingivitis, in which the most comprehensive bacteriological analysis of plaque to date has been performed (although this did restrict the study to only four adult subjects), 166 different bacterial groups (taxa) were recovered. Of these, 73 taxa showed a positive correlation with gingivitis, 29 were negatively correlated while the remainder either showed no correlation or were regarded as being present as a result of gingivitis. This last conclusion emphasizes the value of longitudinal studies. The flora of the four individuals were extremely variable although certain trends did emerge which were reproducible in replicate experiments. The flora became more diverse with time as gingivitis developed and progressed, and the most likely aetiological agents

Table 5.4 Bacteriology of experimental gingivitis in young adult humans

Primary agents in gingivitis	% viable count
Actinomyces israelii	1.4
Actinomyces naeslundii[a]	2.7–6.9
Actinomyces naeslundii/viscosus	4.0
Actinomyces odontolyticus[a]	1.7–3.7
Propionibacterium acnes	1.4
Lactobacillus sp.	2.1
Streptococcus anginosus	5.5
Streptococcus mitis	1.0
Peptostreptococcus micros	1.4
Anaerobic coccus	0.6
Bacteroides oris	1.2
Veillonella parvula	11.7
Treponema sp.	+[b]
Fusobacterium nucleatum	4.4

[a] More than one biotype was recognized
[b] Present, but not enumerated

were considered to be a number of *Actinomyces* spp., a *Lactobacillus* sp., *Strep. anginosus* (similar to *Strep. milleri*), *F. nucleatum*, *V. parvula*, and a non-typable spirochaete (a *Treponema* sp.). A fuller list of the likely causative bacteria is given in Table 5.4. In addition, *B. intermedius*, curved rods (*Campylobacter* and *Wolinella* spp.), *S. sanguis*, *Peptostreptococcus anaerobius*, certain *Eubacterium* spp., and other spirochaetes were isolated in increased numbers in naturally-occurring gingivitis in adults and children. No species are uniquely associated with gingivitis.

Modifying factors

There are also exaggerated forms of gingivitis that are associated with HIV infection, pregnancy, puberty, menstruation, stress or the use of oral contraceptives. The factors responsible for an exaggerated gingivitis in pregnancy have been investigated and linked to an increase in the proportions of the black-pigmented *Bacteroides* sp., *B. intermedius,* during the second trimester. Steroid hormones can be detected in crevicular fluid and, following laboratory studies, the rise in numbers of *B. intermedius* was attributed to the preferential ability of this species to metabolize progesterone and oestradiol. Both of these hormones were able to replace the normal growth requirement for vitamin K by this species.

Acute necrotizing gingivitis (ANG)

Vincent's infection, or ANG, is a painful acute condition of the gingivae. Patients suffering from it may be under acute emotional stress or may be debilitated by another illness. Unlike chronic marginal gingivitis, microorganisms can be seen invading the host tissues of patients with ANG. In smears of the affected tissues the invading organisms resemble spirochaetes and fusiform bacteria. Early electron microscopic investigations showed that the invading organisms consisted primarily of large and intermediate-sized spirochaetes which were present in the lesions in high numbers and in advance of other organisms. Surprisingly, there have been few bacteriological studies of ANG using modern anaerobic techniques. Recently, in a study of 22 ulcerated sites in eight patients, a heterogeneous collection of microorganisms were isolated. Various spirochaetes (*Treponema* spp.) were found in high numbers (approximately 40% of the total cell count) confirming the previous electron microscope studies. However, the most surprising finding, in view of the fuso-spirochaetal pattern characteristically observed, was the relatively low levels of *Fusobacterium* spp. and the prevalence of *B. intermedius* which averaged 3 and 24% of the total cultivable flora, respectively (Table 5.5). Metronidazole was effective in eliminating the fuso-spirochaetal complex from infected sites and this was associated with an obvious and rapid clinical improvement. This study also concluded that disease was a result of an overgrowth of the normal flora by obligately anaerobic species as a result of selection through the availability of host-derived nutrients in individuals who had undergone stress.

Table 5.5 Bacteriology of acute necrotizing ulcerative gingivitis[a]

Implicated bacterial species	Mean % viable count
B. intermedius	24.0
Veillonella spp.	3.5
Fusobacterium spp.	2.6
A. odontolyticus	2.3
S. sanguis	2.4
A. viscosus	1.5
B. gingivalis	<1.0
Capnocytophaga	<1.0
	Mean % microscopic count
Treponema spp.	30.2
Large treponeme	9.9
Selenomonads	6.9
Motile rods	2.2

[a] 22 ulcerated sites in eight patients

Viral gingivitis

The majority of cases of gingivitis are bacterial in origin but, occasionally, viral gingivitis is seen, usually in young people. The commonest form of viral gingivitis is acute herpetic gingivitis (AHG) due to infection with *Herpes hominis* Type 1 (HSV 1).

Chronic periodontitis

Gingivitis is probably a precursor of chronic periodontitis but comparatively few sites with gingivitis progress to more severe forms of periodontal disease. The nature of the stimuli that lead to chronic periodontitis are at present unknown but an interaction between the bacteria, their products, and the host defences will be involved (see Chapters 3 and 4). Despite a large number of studies designed to compare the flora of the healthy gingival crevice with that of pockets in the same mouth, no clear picture has emerged of any specific bacteria that could be implicated uniquely with disease. It would seem logical to regard bacteria located at the advancing front of the lesion to be the most important. However, one of the major technical problems leading to unwanted variation is to sample this area without removing bacteria from other parts of the pocket (see Figure 5.1).

Implicated microorgansisms

All studies agree that the flora from the pockets of patients with chronic periodontitis is diverse and is composed of a wide range of obligately-anaerobic Gram-negative rod and filament-shaped bacteria, many of which are asaccharolytic but proteolytic. These bacteria are often difficult to grow and identify in the laboratory and there is little agreement or convincing evidence as to which bacteria are the primary pathogens. Patients diagnosed as having the same clinical conditions can yield microfloras that are markedly different. For example, in a study of 'early periodontitis', peptostreptococci predominated in one pocket while black-pigmented *Bacteroides* spp. and *A. israelii* were recovered in high numbers from another. Dark-field microscopy has shown that many of the bacteria in plaque from patients with periodontitis are motile and that spirochaetes can be present in elevated numbers. Indeed, for a long time, it was believed that the numbers of these bacteria correlated with the severity of the disease process, but this association is now less clear. Some of these motile organisms have now been identified in cultural studies and shown to be *Wolinella recta* and *Selenomonas sputigena*.

A major problem in studies of chronic periodontitis has been in the manipulation of the large amounts of microbiological data. A significant advance was made when cluster analysis techniques implicated certain *combinations* of bacteria with disease. However, a further complication in determining the aetiology of periodontitis arose when it was found that on occasions very different mixtures (consortia) of bacteria could produce an apparently similar pathological response. Examples of these groupings are shown in Table 5.6; in cases of advanced periodontitis the clusters were apparently dominated by either *B. gingivalis* or *F. nucleatum*. Thus, unlike localized juvenile periodontitis, complex *mixtures* of interacting bacteria are associated with disease.

Other studies have recovered different and sometimes even more complex mixtures of bacteria. For example, in one comprehensive study of plaque from 38 sites in 22 subjects diagnosed as having 'moderate periodontitis', 22 bacterial taxa (recognized by cultural characteristics) and five types of spirochaete (distinguished on the basis of their morphology using microscopy) were considered as possible causative agents. However, some species have been found consistently in high numbers in the majority of diseased sites in a variety of studies. These include *F. nucleatum*, black-pigmented *Bacteroides* spp., but particularly *B. gingivalis* (from deep pockets) and *B. intermedius* (from less deep pockets; see Table 5.6), *Wolinella recta* and spirochaetes. The latter remain as yet poorly characterized because of difficulties associated with their isolation and cultivation in the laboratory and much remains to be learned about their disease potential. Mycoplasmas have also been isolated more frequently in patients with severe chronic periodontitis but again little is known of their aetiological significance.

Table 5.6 Bacterial species which discriminated between clusters of sites with different forms of chronic periodontitis

Bacterium	Cluster				
	'Minimally inflamed' periodontitis	'Advanced' periodontitis			
	1	*2*	*3*	*4*	*5*
Actinomyces sp.	2[a]	0	0	0	0
B. intermedius	12	0	0	0	0
E. corrodens	6	0	0	0	0
F. nucleatum	8	31	23	3	16
W. recta	0	0	12	3	4
'*B. forsythus*'	3	1	7	4	15
Peptostreptococcus sp.	0	7	0	1	0
B. gingivalis	0	3	0	39	21

[a] Median percentage viable count within a cluster

Summary

In summary, chronic periodontitis is associated with complex, mixed cultures of predominantly obligately anaerobic Gram-negative rod and filament-shaped bacteria. The composition of these mixtures can vary with the depth of the pocket and with the severity of the disease. It also appears that floras with a radically-dissimilar composition can produce an apparently similar pathological condition. However, this variation may merely reflect the lack of precision in clinical diagnosis or sample taking, or both. It may also reflect differences in the level of disease activity in the pocket at the time of sampling and this will be discussed in a later section.

Juvenile periodontitis

Localized form

Juvenile periodontitis is a rare condition which usually occurs in adolescents. It is a familial disease in which there is a distinct pattern of alveolar bone loss which is characteristically localized, for as yet unknown reasons, to the first permanent molars and the incisor teeth and hence is referred to as localized juvenile periodontitis (LJP). In contrast to most other forms of periodontal disease, perhaps remarkably so in view of the aggressive nature of the tissue destruction, the plaque associated with juvenile periodontitis is sparse. Few cells are present (approximately 10^6 colony forming units per pocket) belonging to only a limited number of species. In particular, large numbers of Gram-negative rods were isolated in early studies that were not obligately anaerobic but required carbon dioxide for growth (capnophilic). Subsequent studies identified these bacteria as *A. actinomycetemcomitans* (there has been a proposal that this organism should be reclassified as *Haemophilus actinomycetemcomitans*) and *Capnocytophaga* spp. This finding had important implications in treatment design because tetracycline has been shown in clinical studies to be effective in both eliminating *A. actinomycetemcomitans* from infected pockets and resolving the clinical condition. This is in contrast to other forms of chronic inflammatory periodontal disease when metronidazole would be chosen because of its specific action against obligately anaerobic bacteria.

More recent work has generally confirmed the importance of *A. actinomycetemcomitans* but failed to support the role of *Capnocytophaga* in disease. In one study of 403 subjects, 17% of healthy adults harboured low levels of *A. actinomycetemcomitans* while 97% of localized juvenile periodontitis patients had elevated numbers of this species. Three serotypes have been described; serotype *b* strains are found more commonly in LJP patients compared

with either serotype *a* or *c* strains. Other evidence supporting the key role of this organism in LJP has come from treatment studies. A positive correlation was found between elimination of *A. actinomycetemcomitans* from pockets and resolution of LJP while recurrence of the disease was related directly to the reappearance of this organism. Histological studies have shown *A. actinomycetemcomitans* invading gingival connective tissues while immunological findings have also provided additional evidence for the key role of this organism. LJP patients have high levels of antibodies in serum, saliva and crevicular fluid directed specifically against *A. actinomycetemcomitans*.

Unlike those found at healthy sites, the majority of *A. actinomycetemcomitans* strains recovered from LJP patients produce a leucotoxin and this appears to be a major virulence factor. This leucotoxin could impair local host defences by destroying the polymorphonuclear leucocytes. Thus, in contrast to most other forms of periodontal disease, LJP appears to result from the activity of a relatively specific microflora dominated by a single species. However, it should also be pointed out that there are sites in which *A. actinomycetemcomitans* is not necessarily the predominant organism, while the organism cannot be isolated from the pockets of a small number of LJP patients.

In children there is also a condition termed localized pre-pubertal periodontitis. Organisms such as *A. actinomycetemcomitans*, *B. intermedius* and *Capnocytophaga* have been isolated.

Generalized form

As stated earlier, although the disease is usually localized to certain sites, a severe 'generalized' form of juvenile periodontitis has been described (see Chapter 3). In one of the few microbiological studies, two unclassified *Treponema* species were closely associated with disease as were other bacteria, including *F. nucleatum*, several species of *Eubacterium*, lactobacilli, *Peptostreptococcus* spp., *B. intermedius* and *Selenomonas* spp. The significance of these species in disease has yet to be determined.

HIV periodontitis

HIV patients can suffer from an unusually severe and rapid form of periodontitis. The disease is generalized, and is associated with pain and spontaneous bleeding. Preliminary studies suggest that the isolation frequency of *B. gingivalis*, *B. intermedius*, *F. nucleatum*, *A. actinomycetemcomitans*, *E. corrodens*, *Wolinella* spp. and *Candida albicans* is higher than at control sites. More studies will be necessary to fully characterize the flora of these lesions.

The habitat and source of periodontopathic bacteria

One of the most intriguing questions in periodontology concerns the reservoir or natural habitat of the bacteria implicated in disease. Usually these bacteria are found only occasionally and in low numbers in the healthy gingival crevice. It is possible that they might be more widespread but in numbers below those capable of detection by conventional techniques. However, if there is a change in the local environment, for example as a result of trauma, an alteration in the immune status of the host, or an increase in crevicular fluid flow following plaque accumulation due to poor oral hygiene, then the growth of periodontopathic bacteria might be favoured at the expense of other species. This could lead to a shift in the proportions of the resident subgingival microflora in an analogous way to the increases in *S. mutans* and *Lactobacillus* spp. seen prior to caries development following the repeated ingestion of dietary carbohydrates. Evidence for this has come from a laboratory study in which subgingival plaque was passaged repeatedly through human serum (as a substitute for crevicular fluid). Eventually the microflora became dominated by species associated with periodontal destruction, such as black-pigmented *Bacteroides*, peptostreptococci, *Fusobacterium* spp. and spirochaetes, many of which were not detected in high numbers in the original plaque samples. In this way, periodontal diseases can be regarded as endogenous infections caused by an imbalance in the composition of the resident microflora at a site due to an alteration in the ecology of the crevice.

Some periodontopathic bacteria can also attach to mucosal surfaces and recent studies of human volunteers have isolated *B. melaninogenicus* and *B. intermedius* from the dorsum of the tongue and from tonsils. Spirochaetes and various motile organisms were also recovered from tonsils while *Fusobacterium* spp. were found on the tongue, tonsils and buccal mucosa. In contrast, *Capnocytophaga* spp. and *A. actinomycetemcomitans* were never isolated from any mucosal surface. Following an experimental gingivitis study with these volunteers, in which the plaque flora from diseased sites were compared with the mucosal carriage of the above bacteria, it was proposed that the dorsum of the tongue may act as a nidus for certain periodontopathic bacteria.

It has also been suggested that some forms of periodontal disease should be regarded as exogenous infections because the causative bacteria (e.g. *B. gingivalis*) are not widely distributed in the normal mouth and should not, therefore, be regarded as members of the indigenous microflora. Intriguingly, there has been a single recent report of a child with Papillon–Lefèvre syndrome who was consistently re-infected with *A. actinomycetemcomi-*

tans. When *Actinobacillus* strains from possible sources of infection were compared using restriction endonuclease mapping of the bacterial DNA it appeared that the child had acquired its biotype of *A. actinomycetemcomitans* from the family pet dog. Further studies will be necessary to determine whether other episodes of *Actinobacillus*-associated periodontal destruction in children also represent a zoonosis.

Bacteria and disease activity

After the careful clinical monitoring of a number of pockets it was proposed recently that destructive periodontal disease may not develop at a slow, continuous rate but in fact progresses in bursts by recurrent acute episodes. Such 'active' phases, which may last for days or weeks, are then followed by periods of quiescence and even healing. Studies, in which sudden changes in probing depth were presumed to indicate disease activity, have suggested that the flora may change with each of these 'phases'. In one study of 19 subjects, 50 sites considered to exhibit *active* destructive periodontal disease were more likely to have elevated levels of *W. recta*, *B. intermedius* and '*B. forsythus*' (a newly-proposed *Bacteroides* species with an unusual filamentous cell morphology). Others have found the presence of *B. gingivalis*, *B. intermedius* and spirochaetes to be good markers (but not, so far, predictors) of 'active' sites. In a longitudinal study of localized juvenile periodontitis, periods of disease activity were reflected in a less diverse flora in which the numbers of *A. actinomycetemcomitans* and *E. corrodens* only, were statistically significantly higher than during inactive periods (Table 5.7). If these

Table 5.7 Longitudinal study of active and inactive lesions of subjects with localized juvenile periodontitis

Bacterial species	Mean $\log_{10}$ viable count	
	Inactive	Active
B. intermedius	1.9	1.5
C. ochracea	2.1	1.6
C. gingivalis	1.5	1.0
E. corrodens	0.2	1.9
F. nucleatum	3.3	3.4
S. mutans	0.2	
S. sanguis	0.9	
A. viscosus	0.9	
A. naeslundii	0.7	
A. actinomycetemcomitans	1.5	3.5
Total counts	5.1	5.2

findings are confirmed in subsequent studies, it will be essential for plaque sampling to occur only during periods of disease activity. More refined and reliable criteria (e.g. the presence of enzymes or tissue breakdown products in crevicular fluid) for establishing the state of pocket at the time of sampling will greatly improve the likelihood of determining the association of specific bacteria with disease.

Direct proof that specific bacteria can be responsible for initiating periods of disease activity was obtained when *B. gingivalis* was implanted into the pockets of a monkey periodontitis model. Although there was an existing complex subgingival microflora present, significant bursts of bone loss occurred almost exclusively at those sites implanted with *B. gingivalis*.

Bacterial damage to the gingival tissues

Bacterial invasion

Despite the frequent massive presence of bacteria in the periodontal pocket, microbial invasion of the host tissues appears to be rare (*cf.* Chapter 29). An exception to this is in acute necrotizing gingivitis where there is a consistent (but superficial) invasion of the gingival connective tissues by spirochaetes. It has also been reported recently that bacteria can invade tissues in other acute forms of periodontal disease, e.g. localized juvenile periodontitis, and in the late stages of severe chronic periodontitis. The bacteria have been detected using scanning and transmission electron microscopy of sectioned tissue while immunocytological techniques have been used to identify the invading organisms. In juvenile periodontitis, invasion of both gingival epithelium and adjacent connective tissues has been described, the organisms including numerous coccobacillary-shaped bacteria and *Mycoplasma*-like organisms. Other studies claim to have specifically identified cells of *A. actinomycetemcomitans* in the host tissues.

In advanced cases of periodontitis, tissue invasion by a number of bacterial morphotypes has been seen in some but not all of the sites examined. Most bacteria appear to be Gram negative and include cocci, rods, filaments and spiral-shaped cells although some Gram-positive bacteria have also been observed. The microorganisms are usually located in enlarged epithelial intercellular spaces but when found in the underlying connective tissue there is evidence of severe (host) cell damage and collagen breakdown. It should be stressed however that, although bacterial *invasion* has been observed, it is not a common occurrence and may sometimes only represent bacterial *translocation* (passive entry) into the gingival tissues instead. Moreover, it can be extremely difficult to locate bacteria in the tissues and considerable care has to be taken not to 'contaminate' any tissue specimen with pocket bacteria during its sampling and processing.

Possible mechanisms of tissue damage

As bacteria appear not to invade the gingival tissues to any significant degree, tissue damage must be mediated by surface components and extracellular products of bacteria (Table 5.8). There are two schools of thought as to how these bacterial products might cause destruction of gingival tissue. In one, damage is believed to result from the *direct* action of bacterial enzymes and cytotoxic products of metabolism on the tissues. In the other, bacterial components are only *indirectly* responsible, causing tissue destruction as the inevitable side effect of the protective host inflammatory response to the plaque antigens (Chapters 3 and 4).

A range of species, but particularly *B. gingivalis*, *B. intermedius*, *Capnocytophaga* spp., *A. actinomycetemcomitans* and *Peptostreptococcus* spp. synthesize between them a number of cell surface or extracellular enzymes that could potentially weaken the integrity of the periodontal tissues. The enzymes include collagenase, hyaluronidase, a trypsin-like protease, and chondroitin sulphatase. In Gram-negative species, these enzymes are also located on vesicles that are shed from the bacterial cell surface during growth, enhancing the likelihood of tissue penetration by these enzymes. Once the integrity of the tissues is impaired, further damage might arise from the increased penetration of cytotoxic bacterial metabolites such as indole, amines, ammonia, volatile sulphur compounds (e.g. H_2S), and butyric and propionic acids. *Bacteroides gingivalis* has been shown to have the greatest proteolytic activity of the Gram-negative bacteria isolated in high numbers from sites affected by periodontal diseases. It is perhaps not surprising, therefore, that *B. gingivalis* was also the most virulent species when inoculated into animals in a simple pathogenicity test. Other components able to cause direct tissue damage include surface antigens, such as the lipoteichoic acid of some Gram-positive bacteria and endotoxin (lipopolysaccharide, LPS), of Gram-negative cells. LPS has been shown in laboratory studies to stimulate bone resorption. Molecules of even greater biological activity are being identified in some Gram-negative bacteria. One example of this is the capsule of *A. actinomycetemcomitans* which is 1000-fold more potent at causing bone resorption *in vitro* than the purified lipopolysaccharide of this organism.

The most likely situation is that both the direct and indirect mechanisms of tissue damage operate *in vivo* with only a limited number of bacteria (e.g. *B. gingivalis*, *A. actinomycetemcomitans*) having the capacity to act as primary pathogens.

Pathogenic synergism and periodontal disease

One of the most consistent and controversial features of the microbiology of periodontal diseases is the isolation of complex mixtures of bacteria from diseased sites. Particularly in chronic periodontitis, the composition of these mixtures can differ considerably both between and within studies of patients presenting with apparently similar clinical features. These variations might be explained by (a) differences in sampling and plaque-processing methods, (b) difficulties in accurately diagnosing the clinical condition, or (c) plaque being sampled during both 'active' and 'inactive' phases of the disease. However, for the establishment of disease, an organism must gain access to and adhere at a susceptible site, multiply, overcome or evade the host defences, and then produce or induce tissue damage. A large number of virulence traits are needed, therefore, for each stage in the disease process (Table 5.8), and it is unlikely that any single organism will produce all of these factors optimally or in every situation.

An alternative explanation for some of the observed variations in floras associated with periodontal disease could be that tissue destruction is a result of consortia of interacting bacteria and that periodontal disease is a particularly striking example of a synergistic infection whereby organisms which are individually unable to satisfy all of the requirements necessary to cause disease, combine forces to do so. Thus, although only a few species (e.g. *B. gingivalis, B. intermedius, A. actinomycetemcomitans*) produce enzymes that cause tissue damage directly, the persistence of these 'primary pathogens' in the pocket may be dependent on a number of organisms to provide means of attachment (e.g. receptors on streptococci and *Actinomyces* spp.) or essential nutrients such as vitamen K (Table 5.2). Similarly, the bacteria that support the growth of the 'primary pathogens' may well require other organisms to suppress or inactivate the host defences or to inhibit competing organisms (e.g. by bacteriocin production) to ensure their survival. Bacteria could also have more than one function in the aetiology of periodontal disease and a schematic diagram illustrating this pathogenic synergism is shown in Figure 5.3. Some evidence to support this proposal is provided by infection studies in animals and recent laboratory work. Transmissible infections were consistently produced only when a black-pigmented *Bacteroides* strain was present in a mixed culture inoculum. The other organisms ('*Bacteroides oralis*', *V. parvula*, anaerobic streptococci, facultatively anaerobic Gram-positive rods) were non-infective and their function appeared to be merely to provide essential growth factors for the black-pigmented *Bacteroides*. Similarly, in studies of bacteria isolated from periodontal pockets, it was

Table 5.8 Bacterial factors implicated in the aetiology of periodontal diseases

Stage of disease	Bacterial factor
Attachment to host tissues	Surface components, e.g. 'adhesins' Surface structures, e.g. fimbriae, fibrils
Multiplication at a susceptible site	Protease production to obtain nutrients Development of food chains Inhibitor production, e.g. bacteriocins
Evasion of host defences	Capsules and slimes PMN-receptor blockers Leucotoxin Immunoglobin-specific proteases Complement-degrading proteases Suppressor T cell induction

Tissue damage (a) direct	Enzymes:
	  'Trypsin-like' protease
	  Collagenase
	  Hyaluronidase
	  Chondroitin sulphatase
	Bone resorbing factors:
	  Lipoteichoic acid
	  Lipopolysaccharide
	  Capsule
	Cytotoxins:
	  Butyric and propionic acids
	  Indole
	  Amines
	  Ammonia
	  Volatile sulphur compounds

(b) indirect	Inflammatory response to plaque antigens Interleukin-1 production and proteinase synthesis in response to plaque antigens

found that the production of protohaeme by *W. recta* stimulated the growth of *B. gingivalis*, while the growth of *W. recta* was itself enhanced by formate produced by *B. melaninogenicus*. Thus, our ability to interpret results from future microbiological studies of periodontal disease would be greatly enhanced if we knew more about the *role* of particular species in the disease process. An organism could still be highly significant in disease

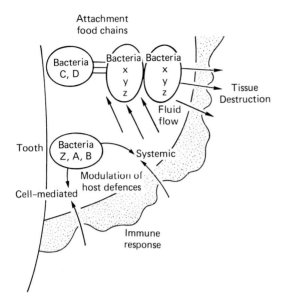

Figure 5.3 Pathogenic synergy in the aetiology of periodontal diseases. Bacteria capable of causing tissue damage directly (e.g. species X, Y and Z) may be dependent on the presence of other cells (e.g. organisms C, D) for essential nutrients or attachment sites, so that they can grow and resist the removal forces provided by the flow of crevicular fluid. Similarly, both of these groups of bacteria may be reliant for their survival on other organisms (Z, A, B) to modulate the host defences. Individual bacteria may have more than one role (e.g. organism Z) in the aetiology of disease

without having the potential to cause tissue destruction directly, while in other pockets, different bacteria could fill identical roles.

The future role of microbiology in the management of periodontal disease

The evidence presented in this chapter has revealed the microflora of plaque associated with the diseases of the periodontium to be complex and that consortia of bacteria appear to be implicated, with many of the involved bacteria being slow-growing and difficult to identify. An important question is to know if any of the above microbiological information can be used by the clinician to, for example, predict susceptible sites or patients, improve treatment or provide a diagnostic aid to assess the success or failure of therapy. So far, it has not proved possible to predict 'at risk' patients or sites although treatment has been influenced by a knowledge of the likely plaque composition at a site. For example, tetracycline, and not metronidazole, is the antibiotic

of choice in LJP patients. Studies are now under way in which microbiology is being used to assess treatment efficacy. In a pilot study of 20 adults with moderate-to-severe periodontitis, the presence of *B. gingivalis*, *B. intermedius*, spirochaetes and motile rods in subgingival plaque has been related to post-treatment disease activity. The black-pigmented *Bacteroides* were identified by indirect immunofluorescence while the spirochaetes and motile rods were detected by phase contrast microscopy. It was found that the presence of *B. gingivalis* and spirochaetes at sites correlated strongly with continued loss of periodontal attachment, yet no associations were found with motile rods or *B. intermedius*. However, these bacteria were not detected at several active lesions and so treatment decisions based solely on the absence of these organisms could result in the omission of necessary therapy. It was concluded that treatment should be continued as long as *B. gingivalis* and spirochaetes could be detected in samples of subgingival plaque.

These studies suggest that, in the future, it may be possible to use the presence of selected key bacteria in plaque as markers of a risk of further tissue breakdown or, possibly, even as predictors of sites at risk of future disease activity. Such bacteria could be detected rapidly using diagnostic kits; the specificity of identification would be assured by the use of appropriate DNA probes or monoclonal antibodies. However, before such a possibility becomes reality, it will be necessary to refine clinical diagnostic methods and to determine the role of a wider range of plaque bacteria in disease.

Further reading

Genco, R. J. and Mergenhagen, S. E. (Editors) (1982) *Host-parasite Interactions in Periodontal Disease.* American Society for Microbiology, Washington DC

Loesche, W. J. and Syed, S. A. (1978) Bacteriology of human experimental gingivitis: effect of plaque and gingivitis score. *Infect. Immun.* **21**, 830–839

Loesche, W. J., Syed, S. A., Laughon, B. E. and Stoll, J. (1982) The bacteriology of acute necrotizing ulcerative gingivitis. *J. Periodontol.* **53**, 223–230

Maiden, M. F. J., Carman, R. J., Curtis, M. A., Gillett, I. R., Griffiths, G. S., Sterne, J. A. C., Wilton, J. M. A. and Johnson, N. W. (1990) Detection of high risk groups and individuals for periodontal diseases: laboratory markers based on the microbiological analysis of subgingival plaque. *J. Clin. Periodontol.* **17**, 1–13.

Marsh, P. D. (1991) Do bacterial markers exist in subgingival plaque for predicting periodontal disease susceptibility? In *Periodontal. Diseases: Markers of Disease Susceptibility and Activity* (Ed. Johnson, N. W.). Cambridge University Press, Cambridge, UK.

Marsh, P. D. and Martin, M. V. (1984) *Oral Microbiology,* 2nd Edition. van Nostrand Reinhold, Wokingham

Moore, L. V. H., Moore, W. E. C., Cato, E. P., Smibert, R. M., Burmeister, J. A., Best, A. M. and Ranney, R. R. (1987) Bacteriology of human gingivitis. *J. Dent. Res,* **66**, 989–995

Moore, W. E. C. (1987) Microbiology of periodontal disease. *J. Periodont. Res.* **22**, 335–341

Moore, W. E. C., Holdeman, L. V., Cato, E. P., Smibert, R. M., Burmeister, J. A. and Ranney, R. R. (1983) Bacteriology of moderate (chronic) periodontitis in mature adult humans. *Infect. Immun.* **42**, 510–515

Slots, J. (1977) Microflora of the healthy gingival sulcus in man. *Scand. J. Dent. Res.* **85**, 247–254

Slots, J. and Genco, R. J. (1984) Black-pigmented *Bacteroides* species, *Capnocytophaga* species and *Actinobacillus actinomycetemcomitans* in human periodontal disease: virulence factors in colonisation, survival and tissue destruction. *J. Dent. Res.* **63**, 412–421

Socransky, S. S., Haffajee, A. D., Smith, G. L. F. and Dzink, J. L. (1987) Difficulties encountered in the search for the etiologic agents of destructive periodontal diseases. *J. Clin. Periodontol.* **14**, 588–593

Theilade, E. (1986) The non-specific theory in microbial etiology of inflammatory periodontal diseases. *J. Clin. Periodontol.* **13**, 905–911

van der Velden, U., van Winkelhoff, A. J., Abbas, F. and de Graaff, J. (1986) The habitat of periodontopathic micro-organisms. *J. Clin. Periodontol.* **13**, 243–248

Zambon, J. J. (1985) *Actinobacillus actinomycetemcomitans* in human periodontal disease. *J. Clin. Periodontol.* **12**, 1–20

6

The epidemiology of periodontal disease

A. Sheiham

Introduction

Epidemiological studies have led to a reappraisal of the extent of the periodontal disease problem, the natural history of the disease and the need for treatment. It has become clear that periodontal disease is less of a public health problem than previously imagined. That is, although many people have gingival inflammation, the probability of such inflammation progressing to severe loss of periodontal attachment and tooth loss, is not great. Tooth loss due to periodontal disease in large populations appears to be relatively uncommon. However, it does appear that the majority of tooth loss due to periodontal disease is experienced by a small group of people within the total population.

The prevalence and severity of periodontal disease

One of the aims of epidemiology is to describe the distribution and size of disease problems in human populations. By providing evidence of the nature and relative size of problems and indications of their importance to the community, objectives for reducing the problems can be established and alternative strategies can be proposed to achieve these objectives.

The prevalence of gingival inflammation is high in most large populations and affects adults and children. These data must be interpreted with caution because the presence of inflammation does not imply the need for treatment, particularly if it is mild inflammation affecting only one or two teeth. The high prevalence levels are a consequence of most epidemiological surveys, which have scored as positive any individual with one or more inflamed gingival sites.

An understanding of the pattern of gingival inflammation in relation to periodontitis can be obtained by examining data from a survey carried out in 1983 in New Zealand by Cutress *et al.* At 15–19 years, 79% were considered to have gingivitis but only 1% had periodontitis. When the data were analysed by the number and percentage of teeth affected, 65% of tooth sites had no inflammation, 34% had gingival inflammation, but only 0.4% of tooth sites showed periodontitis. Of the total population aged between 15 and 44 years, only 2.6% of teeth had periodontal pockets with an average of 1.3 teeth per person.

A reanalysis of existing dental epidemiological data suggests a similar picture to that shown above. Whereas many people have gingival inflammation, only a small percentage of the total population have periodontal pockets and in the majority of persons with pockets only a few teeth are affected per person.

The prevalence and severity of chronic periodontal disease have declined in some industrialized countries in the 1970s. In the USA Douglass *et al.* have shown a substantial downward trend in the prevalence of gingivitis and a decrease in periodontitis among younger adults. Although there were more pockets in the older groups this does not imply greater severity of pocketing. Indeed, there is a case for not treating shallow pockets in people aged over 65 years because the rate of progress of the disease is sufficiently slow to ensure adequate periodontal support for the lifetime of the individual. Similar trends in improvement in periodontal health have been reported in Sweden by Hugoson and Jordan and in England by Sheiham *et al.*

In summary, most of the populations in dentally surveyed industrialized countries appear to have few periodontally diseased teeth and the rate of progress of the disease is slow. A small group are at risk of severe rapidly progressing periodontal destruction but as yet no accurate estimates of the size of this group are available.

In underdeveloped countries the prevalence and severity of periodontal disease has been reported to be high. Yet, despite these high levels of disease, tooth loss due to the disease is uncommon there. For example, Sheiham showed in 1967 that in Nigeria where the prevalence of periodontal pockets is high, persons aged 50 years and older had lost an average of four teeth per person. More recently, in 1984, Ekanayaka has shown a similar situation to prevail in Sri Lanka. These findings indicate that the rate of progression of periodontal disease could be compatible with maintaining sufficient periodontal support to retain many teeth for the lifetime of most individuals. However, an examination of mean data alone gives no idea of the distribution of affected people in the examined population.

The natural history of periodontal disease

The natural history of periodontal disease progression is not as simple as has been formerly suggested. The dominant model of periodontal disease is that of a continual progression from gingivitis to periodontitis, which is accompanied by a loss of attachment and bony support ('the continuous disease model'). Recent evidence has questioned this concept and led to the proposal of other models. 'The episodic burst model' proposed by Socransky differs from 'the continuous disease model' in that some inflamed gingival sites remain free of destructive periodontal disease. Other sites experience a brief burst of destructive disease followed by a period of remission or repair which may be permanent or intermittent. The model suggests that a past history of severe gingivitis or periodontal destruction is not necessarily followed by further destructive activity. This model would explain the inactivity in sites with 'contained gingivitis' and why

in some individuals at some point, stable lesions become converted into slowly, or even rapidly, progressive destructive lesions for unknown reasons. The main finding of the associated studies was the large percentage of periodontal sites which showed no change, plus the finding that rapidly destructive disease can cease without treatment.

A third ('simultaneous burst') model has also been suggested. This describes certain sites remaining free of destructive disease, whilst others have simultaneous bursts of destruction. The main difference between this and the episodic burst model is that most of the destructive periodontal disease takes place within a few years of an individual's life.

Acceptance of any one of these three models will require a change in the concepts of treatment because, even if the continuous progressive loss model is correct, the mean rate of loss of attachment is very slow in most populations. In addition, the fact that the total mean loss of attachment is small in most sites means that in most people any bursts are either relatively small, or that reversal and spontaneous repair occur frequently. If either of the 'burst models' is correct then the indications for aggressive intensive treatment of all periodontal pockets are no longer clear. It is possible that a reduction of plaque could reduce the probability of a further burst, shorten or decrease its intensity or increase the probability of regression.

The causes of periodontal disease

Periodontal disease is strongly associated with dental bacterial plaque but the particular response of the periodontal tissues to the presence of plaque appears to be influenced by ill-defined and poorly understood systemic and local factors. The severity of periodontal disease is greater in groups of people having larger amounts of plaque and calculus thereby demonstrating a biological gradient of disease, equivalent to a dose-response relationship. This dose-response relationship appears to be S-shaped, indicating that there is a level of plaque which is compatible with no progression of periodontal disease. Beyond this level the rate of progression and severity of disease in a population increases with higher levels of plaque. Beyond a certain level, which differs from one population to another, no further increases in severity of periodontal disease occur.

Local factors and periodontal disease

Malocclusion, iatrogenic factors such as overhanging restorations, poorly fitting dentures, crowns and bridges and orthodontic appliances, cigarette smoking and trauma from occlusion have all been implicated as local contributory factors in periodontal disease.

The relationship between malocclusion and periodontal disease is equivocal, for some studies have demonstrated a relationship whereas others have not. The inconclusive findings may in part be due to the frequent use of mean plaque and malocclusion scores for the whole mouth so that individual teeth irregularities have not been analysed rigorously. Malpositioned teeth frequently have more plaque than well-aligned teeth. The degree of malalignment correlates with plaque accumulation and severity of periodontal disease only in subjects with low plaque scores. However, the amount of plaque which accumulates on a group of teeth depends more on the position of the group of teeth in the arch than the presence or absence of malaligned teeth within a group.

There are few restorative procedures that do not present a potential hazard to the periodontal tissues. When restorations are poorly finished and badly positioned they become important secondary aetiological factors in periodontal disease. Dentures and fixed appliances may also be associated with more severe periodontal disease. Where these treatments promote periodontal disease they do so by complicating the removal of plaque and not as a result of mechanical irritation.

Periodontal disease is associated with the use of tobacco in several forms. Smokers generally have more severe periodontal disease than non-smokers but they also have higher plaque and calculus levels than non-smokers.

There is no positive relationship between traumatic occlusion and periodontal disease. This consistent epidemiological finding is supported by experimental data and throws doubt upon the value of occlusal therapy as a basis for periodontal care.

Systemic factors and periodontal disease

There is no epidemiological evidence that systemic factors are a significant factor in the initiation of chronic periodontal disease. Some hormonal, metabolic, immunological, genetic and nutritional variables may modify the progress of the disease (*cf.* Chapter 3). However, at the present time there is insufficient sound epidemiological research to identify the part that systemic factors play in periodontal disease. Most of the reports concerning this problem are based upon small numbers of people and have not used appropriate measurements of periodontal disease. This should not be interpreted as a dismissal of a role for systemic factors in the progress rather than the initiation of periodontal disease, but rather

that the researched information available at present is inadequate.

Other epidemiological variables in periodontal disease

Periodontal disease severity can be shown to vary with age, sex, ethnic group, occupation and socio-economic status. The increase with age may be a result of the cumulative effect of a number of bursts of periodontal destruction or a gradual increase in disease severity over time. The latter could be due to at least two factors. More gingival units become inflamed or the frequency of destructive periodontal lesions increases in a proportion of the dentate population. More people in older age cohorts have destructive disease and the disease affects more teeth in the older person.

In people with established periodontal disease the loss of periodontal attachment does progress, albeit very slowly on average, with increasing age. One long-term study on the natural history of periodontal disease by Löe *et al.* showed that half of the 17-year-old Norwegians in the study had experienced no loss of attachment. If those losing up to 1 mm of attachment are included with those experiencing no loss, then the combined group accounted for 99% of all root surfaces in 17-year-olds. Each age group showed a very slow increase in loss of attachment over a 6-year period. At 37 years and over the mean loss of attachment was 1.66 mm, 46% of surfaces had experienced 0 or 1 mm loss and 46% between 2 or 4 mm loss. The mean annual rate of loss of attachment did not increase significantly with increasing age and ranged from 0.07 mm to 0.11 mm a year. At that average rate of loss, about 6 mm of attachment would be lost by the age of 80 years, although it must be stressed that such mean data cannot account for the individual patient or for site variations.

Clinical research findings indicate that continuous progressive deterioration at established periodontal pockets is not inevitable and that many sites stay the same or even develop spontaneous pocket closure. It is also becoming clear that people with low plaque scores have little loss of attachment, whatever their age, and retain most of their teeth. Moreover, each age group in adulthood is experiencing better periodontal health than their predecessors. This suggests that the higher periodontal disease scores encountered in older people may be a consequence of the cumulative effects of past disease rather than the physical conditions of old age. For these reasons an improvement in the overall periodontal health of older people can be anticipated for the future.

Variations in disease severity between the sexes can be due to physiological or behavioural differences. Women have less severe periodontal disease than men and fewer women have the disease. The sex difference in disease severity can be ascribed to the superior oral cleanliness of women.

Periodontal disease is less severe in people in the higher socio-economic groups and those having more skilled occupations than it is in the poorer and less skilled groups. Oral cleanliness also varies by socio-economic status and occupation, accounting for the better periodontal status in the higher socio-economic groups. Similarly, variations in severity of periodontal disease by the social variables such as sex, ethnic groups and socio-economic status are not found when individuals from these groups are matched for age and level of oral cleanliness. So, although women have less severe periodontal disease than men, when women and men of the same age and oral cleanliness level are compared, no differences in periodontal disease, by gender, are found. This shows therefore that social factors, such as gender, social class and ethnicity, affect oral cleanliness and thereby the severity of periodontal disease.

Public health aspects of periodontal disease

In the scale of important public health problems in industrialized or underdeveloped countries periodontal disease is seldom awarded high priority in the claims upon limited resources. This is because it is not life-threatening nor is it a frequent cause of pain or distress. Furthermore, it is now evident that the traditional view of periodontal disease as a major cause of tooth loss after the age of 35 years has stemmed from the professional recommendation for tooth extraction rather than the effects of the disease process itself. Thus, studies in Finland and Holland have shown that periodontal disease accounted for only 25% of extractions in 41–50-year-olds. This suggests that the contribution of periodontal disease to tooth loss, whilst being important, is much smaller than previously imagined. This is also true for underdeveloped countries where more severe periodontal disease is prevalent. However, these findings are influenced by shorter life expectancies which do not allow sufficient time for periodontal disease to cause significant tooth losses. The foregoing analysis does not mean that the problem of periodontal disease can be dismissed by the clinician or the public dental health worker. There is a great deal that can be done to raise the overall level of periodontal health and to prevent the onset of destructive disease. For the smaller group of the population who have been unable to prevent advancing disease there is the possibility of therapeutic help.

Dental plaque is the prime causative factor of periodontal disease, so that the dominant factor in controlling the disease is oral cleaning behaviour which is influenced by many social and educational variables. One of the most important of these is socialization, which is the process whereby informal knowledge, values, attitudes and routines are transmitted to individuals through social interaction. Young children copy the mouth-cleaning habits of their parents and teachers. In adolescence, brushing teeth becomes an integral part of personal hygiene and grooming behaviour, both of which are influenced by the family and peers. Thus, although the majority of people do clean their teeth regularly, tooth-brushing behaviour is not primarily health-directed but is associated with grooming and personal hygiene. Because tooth cleaning is part of general hygiene behaviour, dental health education programmes directed at improving tooth cleanliness should be incorporated in general health education programmes. This is considered further in Chapter 7.

The measurement of periodontal diseases

In clinical practice a dentist carries out several clinical tests to diagnose the disease and its extent, whereas, for the community, the dental epidemiologist should carry out the minimum number of tests necessary to measure the occurrence and severity of periodontal disease with a degree of accuracy sufficient for the purpose. In epidemiological studies it is often unnecessary to make measurements with the same precision as that required for clinical work, but it is essential that the degree of imprecision can be specified approximately. The most important considerations when choosing a technique for measuring periodontal diseases are that the technique is valid and standardized. Only in this way can results obtained in one study be compared with those obtained in others.

There are four types of epidemiological investigations:

(1) surveys of prevalence, severity and incidence;
(2) longitudinal experimental studies to evaluate the life history of the disease, or prophylactic and/or therapeutic measures in populations;
(3) controlled clinical trials on small well-balanced groups;
(4) surveys to assess periodontal treatment needs.

In all four types of studies an index is used to measure periodontal disease, although different measurements may be required in each. An index is a numerical value describing the relative status of a population on a graduated scale with upper and lower limits, which is designed to permit and

Table 6.1 Parameters assessed

	Type of study			
	Epidemiological surveys	Longitudinal studies	Controlled studies	Treatment needs studies
Plaque	(1) Present or not (2) OHI (S) (3) PI	(1) PI (2) OHI (S)	(1) PI (2) QHT[b] (3) Plaque weight	[a]
Calculus	(1) Calculus present or not (2) OHI (S)	(1) CSI (2) MLC (3) VM	(1) CSI (2) MLC (3) VM	(1) Calculus present or not (2) CPITN
Gingival inflammation	(1) Bleeding present or not (2) GI (3) PBI	(1) GI (2) PBI	(1) Bleeding present or not (2) GI	(1) Bleeding present or not (2) CPITN
Loss of periodontal attachment	(1) Probing depth	(1) Probing depth (2) Probing attachment levels	(1) Probing depth (2) Probing attachment levels	(1) Probing depth (2) CPITN
Tooth mobility	(1) Mobility present or not	(1) Periodontometry	(1) Periodontometry	[a]

PI Plaque Index (Silness and Loe)
OHI (S) Simplified Oral Hygiene Index (Greene and Vermillion)
QHT Quigley, Hein and Turesky plaque index[b]
CSI Calculus Surface Index
MLC Marginal Line Calculus Index
[a] This indicates that the parameter is not useful *per se* for a study of treatment needs
[b] An alternative disclosing solution to basic fuchsin is recommended

VM Volpe Manhold probe method
CPITN Community Periodontal Index of Treatment Needs
GI Gingival Index
PBI Papillary Bleeding Index

facilitate comparison with other populations classified by the same criteria and methods. Each index should ideally possess the following characteristics:

(1) practicality — it should be sufficiently simple and inexpensive to use;
(2) reliability — the index should measure the chosen parameters consistently at different times and under varied conditions;
(3) quantifiability — the index should be amenable to statistical analysis, so that the status of a group can be expressed by a number that corresponds to a relative position on a scale from 0 to the upper limit.
(4) sensitivity — the index should be able to detect reasonably small shifts in the condition;
(5) clarity, simplicity and objectivity — the examiner should be able to remember and apply the clear and unambiguous criteria easily;
(6) acceptability — the use of the index should not be painful or embarrassing to the subject.

There are a number of indexes for measuring periodontal disease and aetiological factors. The periodontal indexes recommended for each type of study are listed in Table 6.1. The choice of the index will depend on the objectives of the study and the ability of the examiners. It is wise to consult a dental epidemiologist about the choice of the appropriate index before embarking on a study.

The Community Periodontal Index of Treatment Needs (CPITN) has attracted much attention recently and has been accepted by the World Health Organization and the International Dental Federation. It has been recommended for use in general dental practice. Whereas the index is an improvement on the existing subjective methods of determining treatment needs it requires considerable refinements. In particular, the treatments suggested for the grades of severity of periodontal disease need to be validated. The index is also claimed to have an important evaluative function for the assessment of improvements in periodontal health.

Further reading

Ainamo, J., Barmes, D., Beagrie, G., Cutress, T. and Martin, J. (1982) Development of the World Health Organization (WHO) Community Index of Treatment Needs (CPITN). *Int. Dent. J.* **32**, 281–291

Axelsson, P. and Lindhe, J. (1974) The effect of a preventive programme on dental plaque, gingivitis and caries in schoolchildren: results after one and two years. *J. Clin. Periodontol.* **1**, 126–138

Cutress, T. W., Hunter, P. B. V. and Hoskins, D. I. H. (1983) *Adult Oral Health in New Zealand 1976–1982*. Dental Research Unit, Medical Research Council of New Zealand, Wellington, NZ

Douglass, C., Gillings, D., Solecito, W. and Gammon, M. (1983) The potential for increase in the periodontal diseases of the aged population. *J. Periodontol.* **32**, 54–57

Ekanayaka, A. (1984) Tooth mortality in plantation workers and residents in Sri Lanka. *Comm. Dent. Oral Epidemiol.* **12**, 128–135

Ennever, J., Sturtzberger, O. P. and Radike, A. W. (1961) The Calculus Surface Index method of scoring clinical calculus studies. *J. Periodontol.* **32**, 54–57

Hugoson, A. and Jordan, T. (1982) Frequency distribution of individuals aged 20–70 years according to severity of periodontal disease. *Comm. Dent. Oral Epidemiol.* **10**, 187–192

Löe, H. (1967) The Gingival Index, The Plaque Index and The Retention Index systems. *J. Periodontol.* **38**, 610–616

Löe, H., Anerud, A., Boysen, H. and Smith, M. (1978) The natural history of periodontal disease in man. *J. Periodontol.* **49**, 607–620

Manhold, J. H., Volpe, A. R., Hazen, S. P., Parker, L. and Adams, S. H. (1965) *In vivo* calculus assessment: Part II. A comparison of scoring techniques. *J. Periodontol.* **36**, 299–309

Muhlemann, H. R. (1951) Periodontometry, a method for measuring tooth mobility. *Oral Med. Oral Path. Oral Surg.* **4**, 1220–1233

Muhlemann, H. R. and Villa, P. (1967) The Marginal Line Calculus Index. *Helv. Odont. Acta* **11**, 175–179

Quigley, G. and Hein, J. (1962) Comparative cleansing efficiency of manual and power brushing. *J. Am. Dent. Assoc.* **65**, 26–29

Schaub, R. H. M. (1984) *Barriers to Effective Periodontal Care*. Rvksuniversiteit Te Groningen, Groningen, Holland

Sheiham, A. (1967) The epidemiology of periodontal disease: studies in Nigerian and British populations. PhD Thesis, University of London

Silness, J. and Löe, H. (1964) Periodontal disease in pregnancy II: Correlation between oral hygiene and periodontal condition. *Acta Odont. Scand.* **22**, 121–135

Socransky, S. S., Haffajee, A. D., Goodson, J. M. and Lindhe, J. (1984) New concepts of destructive periodontal disease. *J. Clin. Periodontol.* **11**, 21–32

Turesky, S., Gilmore, N. D. and Glickman, I. (1970) Reduced plaque formation by the chlormethyl analogue of vitamine C. *J. Periodontol.* **41**, 41–43

7

Guidelines for health education to control dental plaque

A. Sheiham

The principles

Health education and motivation

The control of dental plaque is essential for the prevention and control of periodontal disease. Health education, to improve the effectiveness of oral hygiene, is of fundamental importance because the regular removal of plaque by the individual is the only rational long-term means of controlling dental plaque. Health education has been defined by Green as any combination of learning experiences designed to facilitate voluntary adaptations of behaviour conducive to health. Health education cannot motivate behaviour, in the psychological sense. Motivation is not something done to people but a drive that occurs within the individual. Health education can enhance and appeal to existing motives but cannot initiate them. The existing motives relating to the control of plaque include the desire to be clean, to conform to social norms, be socially and sexually attractive, and only to a lesser degree to improve oral health.

Cleaning behaviour in childhood

An analysis of oral cleaning behaviour shows that young children learn from their experiences and that learning may include the children's cognitive development and the acquisition of new attitudes and behaviours. The prime route by which children learn new behaviour is not through passive absorption but through activity. Therefore, in health education, participation and activities are important in producing behavioural changes. Passive instruction alone will fail to be effective in teaching dental hygiene, so the prevention of periodontal disease requires the establishment of effective oral hygiene practices at an early age. Thus, children learn to brush their teeth by copying their parents and this behaviour can be reinforced by teachers and friends.

Informal and formal health education

Informal health education, whereby empirical knowledge and behaviours are transmitted, is carried out mostly within the family setting and through interaction with the immediate and wider social environment. Formal health education is in turn mediated through formally institutionalized organizations in the education and health systems.

Insufficient attention has been given to the informal health education provided by family members and, in particular, peer groups, who are defined as people sharing common characteristics and interests, and who therefore have strong influences in patterns of behaviour. The success of formal dental health education in improving oral cleanliness can, on the other hand, not be guaranteed. This is borne out by the need to attend for repeated regular scaling and polishing. In this context the mouth is probably unique in respect of the widely practised requirement, as defined by the dentist, for regular examination and treatment.

There are several reasons for the profession's limited success in ensuring long-term effective plaque control. In the first place, dentists use an inappropriate approach to health education which is directed at motivating individuals. The motivational approach is based upon the cognitive learning of the KAB model. This model presumes that information leads to knowledge (K), which leads to attitude (A) change, which in turn leads to the desired changes in behaviour (B). However, little evidence exists to show that the methods implicit in this model are effective in changing oral hygiene practices for significant periods.

Secondly, health education is usually carried out in clinical settings inappropriate for learning. The third shortcoming is that most dental health education methods and programmes are not coordinated with those of general health education. Therefore, general hygiene and grooming should also be stressed in the attempt to improve oral hygiene.

Improving dental health education

Dental health education can be greatly improved by implementing the suggestions put forward by Rayner and Cohen. First and foremost, any approach should recognize and utilize the significance of occupational status and peer identification and belonging to an education, income, age, sex, race or ethnic group. Formal dental health education should optimize salience, pertinence, credibility, habit formation, long-term change and reinforcement. Progress should match observed behaviour with defined objectives and the imitation of other significant persons such as mothers and teachers needs to be stressed. The methods should, furthermore, include community involvement and attempt to change values by showing inconsistencies in currently held values, attitudes or behaviours, and by gaining the attention and support of the mass media. Finally, all the adopted methods should be carefully integrated because planning for behavioural changes necessitates directing several tasks simultaneously and differentially to various target groups.

Objectives and aims of dental health education

The objective of both informal and formal dental health education is to achieve a level of oral cleanliness which is compatible with maintaining a functional, aesthetically acceptable natural dentition for all individuals throughout their lives. The aim is to elicit, to facilitate and to maintain efficient oral hygiene practices. These demand a planned, consistent, integrated series of educational, economic and political strategies based on the following principles.

Firstly, dental health education should be integrated with general health education so that, in addition to all members of the dental team, others such as teachers, health workers, community leaders, professional and cultural leaders, sports people can play a part. Health education must incorporate a number of diverse approaches such as individual instruction, group discussion, behaviour modification, mass media and community organizational methods, because each subpopulation in the community will respond differently to any one given approach. These educational methods must be cumulative and consistent. Thus, there is no best method, for any given combination may be effective for some people but not for others.

Finally, the earlier the intervention in the health career of individuals, the more effective is the result likely to be. In health careers, various agencies and influences impinge on the developing individuals but the influence of primary socialization remains paramount. Community, patient and staff participation in the planning of health education programmes should increase the probability of their success. The objectives should be expressed in terms of behavioural outcomes. Each objective should answer the question 'Who is expected to achieve how much of what by when?' 'Who' refers to the target groups or individuals expected to change. 'What' to the actions to be carried out, 'How much' to the desired reduction of disease and 'When' to the time by which the reduction is to be achieved. Evaluation is needed to assess whether the educators are achieving their aims, whether they are doing so effectively and efficiently and whether their planning methods are sound.

Goals and strategies of periodontal care
Individual and the community

Good clinical practice involves both prevention of disease and care for those with periodontal disease. The dental practitioner by definition concentrates efforts on those attending the practice and in particular on so-called 'high risk' patients. By contrast, the community dental health dentist favours the mass approach seeking to influence whole populations. Each strategy has its distinctive contribution, and each has its costs and limitations.

A high risk strategy is expensive in terms of manpower and time and clearly cannot affect the distribution of disease in the population, so cannot be accepted as a realistic cost effective strategy. Furthermore, although the regular prophylaxis implicit in this strategy has been shown to be effective in the individual, the benefits could be due more to socio-psychological effects than to therapy itself. In addition, Hamp and Johansson have shown that the repetition and reinforcement of oral hygiene in such regimes may have a dampening influence which reduces its effectiveness. Finally, the value of professional prophylaxis and instruction for everyone is questionable, for the high levels of oral hygiene in adults have been attributed by Glavind and co-workers mainly to psychological and feedback methods.

Social and educational strategies directed at groups are more likely to be effective and less costly. With this in mind Sheiham has proposed a strategy which concentrates on community health education, combined with a system of screening to identify those people who have rapidly progressing periodontal disease. The rationale and role for prophylaxis in those with established periodontal disease is discussed further in Chapter 8.

Programme formulation and implementation

When a feasible strategy has been chosen the actual programme can be formulated. Implementation of the programme should focus on community-wide approaches and incorporate the principles mentioned earlier which are integration, diversity of approaches, participation and concentration on behavioural objectives and evaluation. Programmes which integrate oral hygiene demonstrations with general hygiene and provide people with feedback methods for assessing the effectiveness of their attempts to clean their teeth should be implemented. Programmes should be continuous and not limited to a series of short campaigns and to exhortations to brush teeth.

In summary, to be effective the programme requires a variety of approaches which should be channelled through significant members of the community, professional educators and all members of the dental team.

Dental health education in practice

Clinical, behavioural and educational diagnosis

Thus far the general principles of dental health education to improve oral cleanliness in the community have been dealt with. Specific approaches applicable to the individual in practice will now be outlined. The individual case history should establish the background social, psychological, educational and attitudinal characteristics of the patient. This history should ideally precede the clinical examination which is followed by any necessary radiographs. On the basis of these findings an overall diagnosis is made and alternative therapeutic strategies considered. This approach to treatment planning contrasts with that traditionally practised in which a great deal of stress is laid on the clinical diagnosis and relatively little on the behavioural and educational aspects. Without the

latter it is unlikely that the appropriate health education will be instituted.

The systematic identification of the health practices that appear to be causally linked to the clinical periodontal problem diagnosis constitutes the behavioural diagnosis. The establishment of the causes of the identified behaviour is, in turn, called the educational diagnosis. The causes are of three distinct kinds: predisposing, enabling and reinforcing, each of which, according to Green and coworkers, has a different influence on behaviour. Predisposing factors are those such as knowledge, attitudes, beliefs and values. Enabling factors are those that allow a motivation to be realized and include personal skills plus social, financial and physical resources. Reinforcing factors are rewards, incentives and punishments for a behaviour, and which may be social, psychological as well as physical. These influencing factors must be taken into account when planning to change oral hygiene behaviour, and doing otherwise is likely to court failure.

Professional misconceptions

Any approach to improving the effectiveness of oral hygiene must be based upon not only a thorough educational and behavioural diagnosis, as outlined above, but also a revision of the profession's traditional view about the public's attitude towards their teeth. Thus, the public are generally not apathetic about oral hygiene nor are insufficiently motivated to care for their mouths, for most people do clean their teeth daily and many of them attend dentists regularly for check-ups. Indeed, they probably give more attention to their mouths than to much of the rest of their body. This misunderstanding by professionals can be a major barrier to communication and when coupled with the frequently unrealistic and unnecessarily high level of plaque control demanded of the patient lead to an element of fatalism on their part.

Patient history

As part of the history of the patient the following information about knowledge, attitudes, beliefs, values, perceptions and behaviours should be obtained.

Perceived seriousness and perceptions of causation

It is necessary to establish how serious the patient considers the particular periodontal problem and the long-term effects of periodontal disease. These effects should be specified such as gingival recession and longer teeth, appearance of the teeth and mouth, redness of gums, bleeding, bad taste and bad breath, mobility of teeth, spacing and food impaction and tooth loss. It should also be established whether the patient knows that incorrect cleaning methods cause periodontal disease and if not, what he/she considers to be the cause of the disease.

Reasons for toothbrushing

Toothbrushing can be either health-directed or health-related. Health-related behaviours are those behaviours which affect health but are not carried out for health reasons. Toothbrushing is a cleaning habit copied from others. As a grooming behaviour it is also strongly influenced by social and psychological forces so that brushing might be carried out to maintain gum and tooth health or merely as an ingrained ritual. Brushing may be carried out because it makes the mouth feel good or because of a concern about eliminating body and mouth odour.

The methods of oral hygiene being used, including details about oral hygiene implements, should be established. The importance of dietary control for oral health should not be neglected and the patient's intake of sugar and acidic dietary components noted and the appropriate counselling provided.

Perceptions about the benefits of therapy

Most patients use a toothbrush without being aware of the benefits accruing to periodontal health from improved toothbrushing. They may have greater faith in the use of a medicine, mouthwash or the massaging of the gums in achieving gum health. If they do know about dental floss, wood points and single-tufted interspace type brushes it is important to find out how they are used. Knowledge of previous periodontal therapy is invaluable and also of the patients' views of the experience and whether greater hope and emphasis is placed by them upon the therapeutic process rather than on self-care.

Dental goals of the patient

It is unlikely that the patient will be motivated by the same dental goals as the dentist. Patients may be motivated mainly by appearance of the teeth and face, the avoidance of disease, pain or discomfort, the avoidance of dental treatment or the prevention of halitosis. For example, if mouth appearance and health is considered important for their work or for personal relationships this should act as a powerful motivating factor. Their expectations about keeping their teeth for life and their views about the wearing of false teeth should also be elicited.

No patient arrives for periodontal therapy without his own highly individual mix of dental knowledge, attitudes, beliefs, values, perceptions and behaviours. Because the successful outcome of continuing periodontal care depends ultimately upon patient cooperation it is inappropriate to embark on any course of periodontal care without some idea of this personal background.

Behaviour modification

Whatever the existing personal background, it will be necessary to a greater or lesser degree to modify existing oral hygiene behaviour if improvement in periodontal health is to be achieved.

Analysis of behaviour

The oral cleaning behaviours should be carefully analysed to establish which areas and sites are not being cleaned adequately. Next, it is necessary to examine the cleaning technique to determine whether the devices are properly directed against the teeth, that the appropriate force and hand grip of the brush and interdental device are being used. This cleaning behaviour should, for preference, be carried out with the patient standing in front of a mirror using a bathroom-type basin and mirror to create an environment similar to the home.

Periodontal problem identification

Clinical examination should be carried out with the patient holding a large mirror so that he can see where the dentist is probing. This will help to focus his attention on inadequately cleaned areas where there is bleeding, pocketing and plaque retention factors. It is important to explain the meaning of the terms used as the examination progresses.

Selection and demonstration of oral hygiene devices

The appropriate tooth cleaning devices are selected and their value and use discussed with and demonstrated to the patient (*cf.* Chapter 8).

A combination of cleaning demonstration methods can be used, but it is essential that techniques are actually demonstrated in the patient's mouth and with his full participation. This is because the durability of cognitive and behavioural change has been shown to be proportional to the degree of active, as opposed to passive, participation of the learner. Educational material or instruction alone is insufficient, although an instructional pamphlet is useful to reinforce aspects such as the direction of brushing and the angle of the brush head. Film or video recording of efficient cleaning can also be helpful.

Establish a contract

It is important to agree with the patients exactly what they are expected to do, how they are to do it, by when they might achieve agreed targets and the phasing of therapy, including the post-therapeutic maintenance. The roles played by the dental team and the patient should be outlined and the therapy explained. Alternative therapeutic approaches should also be discussed.

A practical regime

Demonstration technique

The actual form of the cleaning regime will depend not only upon the wishes and current practice of each individual operator but also on the capacity of each patient to demonstrate improvement. Ideally, it should involve a phased demonstration in the patient's mouth of the methods of hygiene recommended for him. One view is that the demonstration should if possible be short and concentrate on the problem areas alone, with only one or two altered practices being shown at each visit. Additional devices are therefore only introduced in a phased programme over several appointments. Others favour a more comprehensive approach as described in Chapter 8.

Most people clean their teeth regularly and any method of brushing should be permitted (permissive brushing) if it removes plaque effectively and causes no damage to the tissues. Any existing good behaviours should be the basis for improvement and their use encouraged at other sites of the mouth. It is considered important not to condemn any current method in use as this may lead to alienation, confusion or hostility.

Rewarded reinforcement

The behaviours carried out by patients with periodontal disease should be directed ideally at elimination of the disease and about returning to normality rather than becoming a perpetual patient. In other words, when patients adopt a sick-role they will adhere strictly to the guidelines set down for them to get better. The sooner they leave this role and their dependency upon professionals the better they like it. The health education programme should be devised to take these behaviours into account. Recommended practices should not be very demanding and should include some element of reward or mark of positive progress as described below. The aim is to reinforce behaviours so that ultimately the behaviours become habits. Guidelines should be established to trigger an improvement in the habit if the behaviour is inadequate.

Rewards for improved oral hygiene behaviours include reduction in gingival redness, decrease in the number of bleeding points, less bad taste or halitosis and the emergence of dark subgingival

calculus following gingival shrinkage. Demonstrating these improvements in the mouth and the feedback gained from the recording of these results on clinical records will help to reinforce the good behaviours. In addition the pain-free removal of calculus can be achieved by limiting scaling to only the readily accessible deposits, as advocated in Chapter 11. This, together with the subsequent similarly pain-free removal of residual calculus following a good gingival response, and the use of increased intervals between recalls, can also be a reward for improved behaviour.

Maintenance without professional reinforcement

One of the goals of periodontal care is to achieve an acceptable, functional, natural dentition which can be maintained by the person for his lifetime, independent of, or at least with minimal, professional help. The level of health must be understood by the person, be attainable and demonstrable if the person is to assume this responsibility.

The health education programme for periodontal patients should therefore incorporate methods and concepts which will encourage the maintenance of an adequate level of oral cleanliness without professional reinforcement. That is, the relevance of behaviours, the social acceptability and simplicity of the methods plus their ability to be incorporated into normal daily activities and to be accepted as an essential part of general cleanliness, are fundamental to success. Finally, feedback methods are necessary for the patients to assess the effectiveness of their efforts. Bleeding on brushing or flossing is one such method.

Prevention of periodontal disease

There is much in common between the methods used for the prevention of periodontal disease and the care of patients with established periodontal disease. However, the prevention of periodontal disease requires effective oral hygiene practices from an early age. Every effort should be used to encourage parents to brush their young children's teeth regularly and effectively. It is also important to brush their own teeth in front of the children to encourage and reinforce their children's toothbrushing. Thus, children learn to brush their teeth by copying their parents and this behaviour should be reinforced by teachers and friends. If patients accept the responsibility to instruct others it will help reinforce their own oral hygiene practice and help prevent periodontal disease in their own family members. In addition to accepting this role within their own family, those patients who are teachers, health workers, communicators or belong to different cultural or professional groups can spread the idea of preventing periodontal disease among their contacts. As stated previously, the question of oral cleanliness should be stressed as an integral part of general bodily cleanliness and hygiene.

Do's and don'ts of dental health education

Do make an adequate educational and behavioural diagnosis of the patient and remember that oral hygiene is most frequently carried out for social reasons and not to prevent disease. Furthermore, involve the patient in the clinical diagnosis by demonstrating the problem areas.

Limit the number of new instructions and concepts given to the patient at any one session and be content to make small changes to oral hygiene methods.

Provide the patient with easy signs of progress and give positive reinforcement about the good behaviours performed.

Do not arouse fear in patients by threatening dire consequences of non-compliance or blame them for their oral condition. Similarly, periodontal disease should not be mystified by technical jargon, but at the same time, the patient should not be patronized and appropriate information must be available.

The patient should be given some opportunity to respond and express his views to lessen the chance of pre-judging him and perhaps compromising the result.

Finally, do not start professional cleaning before the patient has demonstrated a good gingival response. To do so may work against a successful outcome which aims at the patient becoming independent of the dentist and capable of maintaining his own periodontal health.

Summary

A realistic aim for a preventive programme is to reduce dental plaque to levels compatible with rates of progression of periodontal disease which will allow functional, aesthetic and socially acceptable dentitions to be maintained throughout life.

Since tooth cleaning is mainly influenced by socialization, and most people do brush their teeth, the objective of health education is to improve the effectiveness of oral hygiene behaviour. However, much dental health education, whether directed at individuals or groups, is based upon incorrect concepts. Where possible the modification of existing oral hygiene practices has a much greater chance of improving effectiveness than attempting radical changes in technique. Oral health should be integrated with programmes dealing with general hygiene and grooming rather than becoming bogged down by technical niceties of cleaning methods. A diversity of approaches with maximal participation by others in the community, should also be encouraged.

Programmes should concentrate on educating significant individuals in the community, educating educators and educating the dental team. Furthermore, a strategy centred solely upon dentist and hygienist is unlikely to be effective in reducing periodontal disease at a community level so that social and educational strategies directed at groups are likely to be more useful.

Finally, programmes should be continuous and low key, refraining from victim-blaming exhortations to clean teeth with devices of questionable usefulness. In the dental practice setting, the health education programme should be based upon a thorough educational and behavioural diagnosis and a phased programme to improve the oral cleanliness behaviours.

Further reading

Axelsson, P. (1978) The effect of plaque control procedures on gingivitis, periodontitis and dental caries. University of Goteborg, Sweden, 1978

Axelsson, P. and Lindhe, J. (1974) The effect of a preventive programme on dental plaque, gingivitis and caries in children: Results after one and two years. *J. Clin. Periodontol.* **1**, 126–138

Axelsson, P. and Lindhe, J. (1981) Effect of controlled oral hygiene procedures on caries and periodontal disease in adults. Results after 6 years. *J. Clin. Periodontol.* **8**, 239–248

Glavind, L. (1977) Effect of monthly professional mechanical tooth cleaning on periodontal health in adults. *J. Clin. Periodontol.* **4**, 100–106

Glavind, L., Zeuner, E. and Attstrom, R. (1981) Oral hygiene instruction of adults by means of a self-instructional manual. *J. Clin. Periodontol.* **8**, 165–176

Green, L. W., Kreuter, M. W., Deeds, S. G. and Partridge, K. B. (1980) *Health Education Planning. A Diagnostic Approach.* Mayfield Publishing Company, Palo Alto

Hamp, S. E. and Johansson, L. A. (1982) Dental prophylaxis for youths in their late teens. 1. Clinical effect of different preventive regimes on oral hygiene, gingivitis and dental caries. *J. Clin. Periodontol.* **9**, 22–34

Rayner, J. F. and Cohen, L. K. (1974) A position on school dental health education. *J. Prev. Dentistry,* **1**, 11–14 and 17–23

Sheiham, A. (1980) Current concepts in health education. In *Efficacy of Treatment Procedures in Periodontics.* (Shanley, D. B., editor). Quintessence, Chicago

8

Plaque control

Introduction

Plaque control is fundamental to the prevention of gingivitis, during treatment of the established disease (gingivitis and periodontitis) and, finally, in the maintenance of health following effective treatment. The variable dentogingival morphology in health and disease, does however demand that the methods used be appropriately modified to cater for these differences. These modifications revolve about the basic regime used for the prevention of gingivitis in the presence of a normal dentogingival morphology. Thus, whatever morphological aberrations are encountered in disease, a comparable superficial relationship always exists between tooth and gingiva. This basic regime is therefore presented here and the necessary modifications in technique only introduced when the morphologic characteristics of disease are described in subsequent chapters.

The principle of plaque control

Plaque control can be achieved by either preventing formation or by removing plaque *in situ*. Topical chemotherapeutic methods (see Chapter 35) are most effective at preventing plaque formation on a clean tooth surface and, at present, mechanical measures are necessary when dealing with formed plaque. Current knowledge dictates that, for the vast majority of patients, these mechanical methods are highly effective and constitute the predominant manner by which disease is both prevented and controlled.

The responsibility for plaque control must rest with the individual patient, when the operator has pointed out the inherent difficulties involved and advised upon the different mechanical methods available. The operator's responsibility also extends to monitoring the efficacy of these efforts. The attainment of gingival health depends very much on a system of professional tutelage represented by the dentist or hygienist. The operator does, however, assume a progressively more active role in plaque control with the advancing levels of disease which are discussed in subsequent chapters. (For a discussion of primary prevention in the community see Chapter 7.)

Whilst individual dexterity is very important, the success of plaque control is, in many instances, more dependent on other less well defined socio-psychological factors. These relate to the patient comprehending the instructions given, translating them into practical actions and, last but not least, being sufficiently well motivated to actually carry them out effectively. Total compliance in plaque control measures is adversely affected by their tedious and time-consuming nature as well as their technical difficulty. In addition, the patients' perceived risk of disease developing is often small, whilst they may not consider the effects of disease to be serious.

The accessibility of plaque

It can be assumed, for practical purposes, that the morphology of the normal dento-epithelial junction is totally accessible for individuals with average levels of dexterity. Access may be impeded by altered gingival morphology, tooth position in the arch or vestibular mucosal variations.

Gingival form

When the gingival margins are well formed and evenly contoured in well-aligned arches and fill the interdental spaces (Figure 8.1 A) plaque removal is straightforward. Cleaning is a little more difficult when the gingival margins are at uneven levels on neighbouring teeth. This may result from different rates of gingival maturation following tooth eruption and from minor tooth malpositioning in the arch, each of which may give the impression of gingival recession (pseudo-recession, *cf.* Chapter 32) at neighbouring units with normal clinical crown heights (Figure 8.1 B,C). Uneven gingival margins develop most commonly from gingival recession, following a combination of traumatic toothbrushing habits and periodontal disease (Figure 8.1 C,D). Gingival hyperplasia of developmental or chronic inflammatory origins may also alter gingival margin positions (Figure 8.1 E). A further consequence of gingival recession in chronic disease is the loss of interdental papillary form and a resulting patency of interdental spaces (Figure 8.1 D,F). Interdental patency is a normal finding with developmental tooth spacing (Figure 8.1 B,E).

Although these altered gingival contours may complicate plaque removal, the patient's failure to recognize their existence is most commonly responsible for ineffective oral hygiene. That is, the minor modifications in cleaning technique necessary to negotiate these sites have simply not been carried out. Once aware of the situation, plaque removal may be improved and gingival health restored. It must also be emphasized that disease develops even in the presence of ideal dentogingival form and in well-aligned arches when cleaning is ineffective (Figure 8.1 G,H).

Other factors

Tooth crowding (*cf.* Chapter 33), shallow facial vestibules and prominent facial or lingual mucosal frena (*cf.* Chapter 21), large and poorly controlled tongues, strong lip reflex activity, a well developed gagging reflex and limited interocclusal opening may each restrict access for plaque control. Individuals with poor manual dexterity, arthritis, or other debilitating conditions present even greater challenges.

Clinical implications

The mere existence of any of the morphological hurdles cited does not mean that gingival inflamma-

tion is inevitable. However, should inflammation develop the operator must point out these potential problem sites and advise on the appropriate cleaning techniques. Thus, even grossly imbricated teeth can be maintained plaque free (Figure 8.1 I). The methods of cleaning where there is marginal gingival unevenness or vestibular tissue interference during cleaning, are described in Chapter 21. An interfering lip or cheek can usually be displaced with the fingers of the other hand while lingual interference (Figure 8.1 K) and a tendency to gagging is best overcome by placing the tip of the tongue just apical to the site being cleaned (Figure 8.1 L).

Frequency of plaque removal

There is no clear evidence about the optimal interval for tooth cleaning but it is related strongly to the susceptibility of the marginal tissue to disease and the effectiveness with which the plaque is removed. Furthermore, it seems likely that regular disruption of the bacterial colony, rather than its total removal, might be all that is necessary. Alternatively, a less frequent absolute removal of plaque might also suffice. Total plaque removal performed once every 48 hours has been shown by one investigation to be consistent with the maintenance of gingival health in young adults. Nevertheless, the traditionally accepted twice-daily cleaning regime would be prudent as a first stage. Then, progressively less frequent cleaning could be attempted provided that gingival health is still being maintained. This would then represent a personal plaque control regime for that individual.

Assessment of efficacy of cleaning
Self-assessment

Self-assessment is considered to be of fundamental importance in plaque control. Most individuals fail to appreciate shortcomings in their cleaning because the small, but significant, residual plaque deposits at the dentogingival junctions cannot be detected either visually or with the tongue. The principle of disclosing this plaque by the selective staining effect of colouring agents on the tooth surface is well established as a simple yet reliable means of self-assessment. An alternative method of judging the efficacy of plaque control by the patient is by the presence or absence of gingival margin inflammation (*cf.* Chapter 10).

Disclosing agents

Numerous proprietary disclosing agents are available both in liquid and tablet form. The red, blue

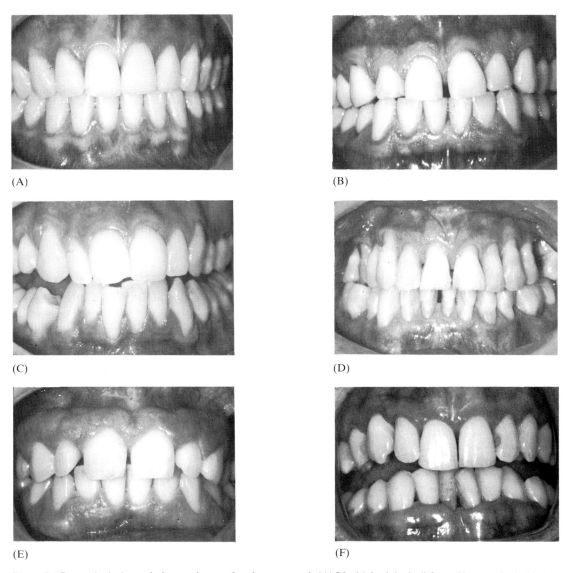

Figure 8.1 Dentogingival morphology and access for plaque control. (A) Ideal (physiological) form. Uneven gingival levels at adjacent teeth associated with (B–D) different rates of gingival maturation, tooth malpositioning and gingival recession, and (E) gingival hyperplasia. Interdental space patency as (B) developmental finding, (D) following gingival recession, and (F) loss of papillary form from recurrent necrotizing ulcerative gingivitis.

and green agents most commonly used are essentially colorants used in food preparations. Food colorants (e.g. Rayners Blue, Rayner-Burgess Ltd, Edmonton, London N18 1TQ, UK) are equally effective and yet cheap. The concentrated solution (2-3 ml dispensed in a teaspoon) is vigorously swished about the mouth then carefully spat out. The mouth is then rinsed thoroughly with water and

the teeth closely examined in a good light. Any plaque will be densely stained.

Disclosing agents are best used after cleaning so that inadequate cleaning can be identified and rectified primarily by trial and error, but where necessary using professional guidance. Stained plaque soon fades so the possibility that staining has been eliminated during further cleaning efforts,

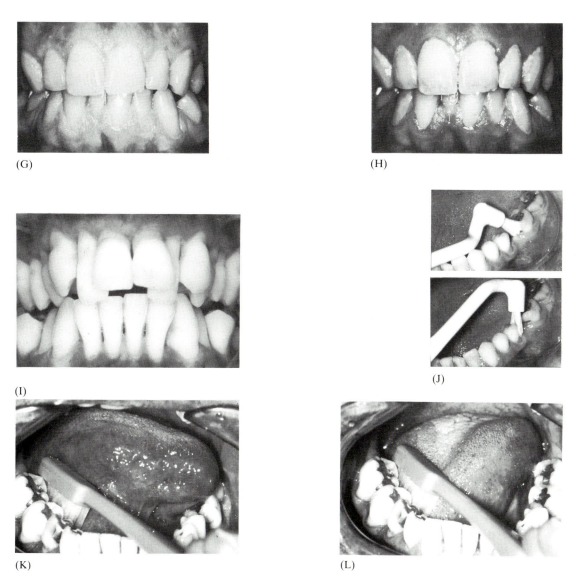

(G) (H)

(I) (J)

(K) (L)

Figure 8.1 (*cont.*) (G and H) Development of gingival inflammation following experimental withdrawal of oral hygiene in presence of ideal form in maxilla and uneven gingival contour in mandible. (I) Gingival health achieved despite gross imbrication. (J) Tilted teeth related to edentulous zone negotiated with modified shaped interspace brush. (K) Tongue displacement to opposite side during brushing at lingual aspect impedes access and may induce gagging. (L) Tip of tongue locates site to be cleaned and when placed just apical to brush head, enhances access, guides bristle and precludes gagging

without total removal of the underlying plaque, should be excluded by restaining.

Mucosal staining inevitably occurs with the use of disclosing agents and persists for some hours, so that it may be unacceptable to some individuals. The embarrassment of temporarily blue tongue, lips and gums by day can be obviated by restricting the exercise to before retiring or alternatively using a less conspicuous red food dye. The latter option does however lack the strong colour contrast, provided by the blue dye, in relation to the adjacent gingival margins and may also mask the redness of gingival inflammation (*cf.* Chapter 10). Another option is a barely visible pale yellow fluorescein disclosing solution which fluoresces a bright yellow when illuminated with a special light (e.g. Broxo test, Broxo Test, Addis Ltd, Hertford, Herts, UK). The system is rather expensive and is therefore mostly reserved for surgery use. There is some merit, in the interests of uniformity of assessment, in using the same agent both clinically and at home.

Indirect vision

The lingual and palatal aspects of the teeth are frequently overlooked by the patient. As a result they are most likely to be cleaned ineffectively, so they need to be checked by the obligatory use of an intra-oral dental mirror. The tendency for misting during use can be stopped by warming the mirror under hot running water. The lack of good illumination, necessary for this intra-oral examination, is easily overcome by fixing a pen-light to the mirror handle with a rubber band or tape. Several proprietary mirror torch combinations are also available.

Mechanical cleaning

The currently available mechanical devices are, when properly used, effective at all tooth surfaces associated with intact dento-epithelial junctions. The exception to this might be at some approximal surfaces occurring in grossly crowded arches. In summary, marginal gingival health can be achieved on grounds of both the reasonable accessibility of the dento-epithelial junctions and efficacy of the available devices.

Ordinary toothbrush

Applications

The brush is suitable for all facial, oral and occlusal surfaces. Distal aspects of last standing teeth and approximal surfaces bounding edentulous zones are not readily cleaned, whilst interproximal tooth surfaces are rarely negotiated.

Brush types

There are innumerable brush-head and handle designs and sizes available; but there is insufficient evidence to clearly commend any particular one. The multi-tufted head with a straight edged trim is most widely accepted at the present time. Nylon filaments are preferred to natural bristle, if only because they are more rigid when within the range of the most popular individual filament diameter size of 0.2–0.3 mm. When using the advocated miniscrub brushing technique to negotiate the gingival sulcus, the nylon filaments of a chosen brush should pass easily into the gingival sulcus and

not become displaced out of position. The choice of brush should always be based on the effectiveness of plaque control in the hands of each individual.

Brushing methods

There can be no one correct method of brushing but rather the appropriate one that in each case removes plaque effectively without damaging either tooth or gingiva. A particular method must be dictated by individual preference and dexterity and the variable dentogingival morphology occurring with different levels of disease. The following descriptions of brushing and other oral hygiene methods will therefore incorporate these morphological variations where necessary. More detailed attention to post-surgical plaque control and that necessitated by variations of furcation morphology will be considered in subsequent chapters. Many brushing methods have been advocated over the years, of which only the two most commonly used, the miniscrub and the roll technique, need be considered here. The miniscrub is advocated for general use, whilst the roll technique is best restricted to situations with knife-edged gingival margins. Most individuals find the miniscrub technique easier especially at less accessible sites and it is certainly more effective in most hands. None of the other brushing techniques offers any special advantages. Finally it should be stressed, when instructing the patient, the emphasis should be on objective rather than technique.

Miniscrub (Figure 8.2)

The bristles are first placed against the teeth pointing in an apical direction. The brush-head is then firmly pressed, splaying the bristles slightly and producing a chisel-like leading edge, which is directed apically into the gingival sulcus. The head is then agitated in a mesio-distal direction with a short scrubbing action so that the bristle tips move no more than a few millimetres. Disruption of the adherent plaque in this way takes some 5–7 seconds. The brush is then moved to the adjacent tooth surfaces and the sequence then repeated, for all facial and oral aspects (Figure 8.3). The occlusal surfaces are scrubbed in a comparable manner.

Roll

The bristles are placed over the gingiva with the most coronally located bristles approximating the dentogingival junction. The brush head is rotated coronally with a rolling sweeping action, each successive row of bristles thus passing over the gingival sulci and the teeth. About five to seven strokes are required for each site before moving on

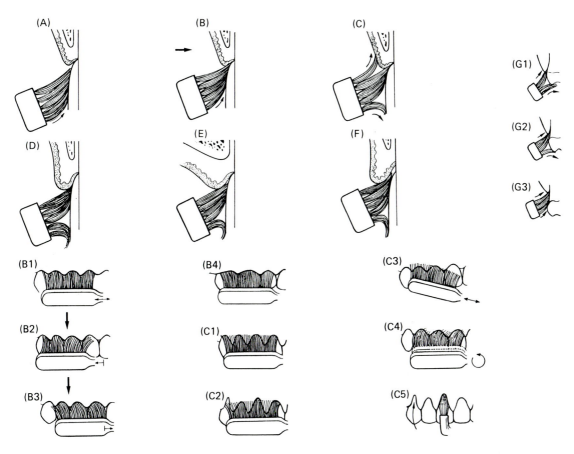

Figure 8.2 Miniscrub technique. (A) Initial brush placement with bristles 45 degrees to tooth and splaying out towards gingival sulcus. (B and B1) 'Leading edge' bristles penetrating sulcus with others flattened against tooth surfaces and passing into embrasure spaces. (B2 and B3) Horizontal miniscrub movement maintaining bristles within sulcus, although some may become displaced (C) over the gingiva and others occlusally. Coronal displacement is dictated by (G1–G3) clinical crown heights and brushing pressure. Apical displacement tends to occur with (C1) physiological gingiva form, (C2) prominent interdental papillae following recession and when, as shown in (C5), a single-tufted brush used with a miniscrub-like action is preferable, or when (C3) an oblique action has been used unwittingly. The rotatory miniscrub (C4) is best avoided, for sulcus penetration can neither be ensured nor maintained. The miniscrub is most effective at (B1 and B4) evenly scalloped marginal tissues, (D and E) thick gingival form, and (F) within pocket spaces

to the next. The technique is illustrated in Figure 8.3.

Gingival cleaning and massage

Attached gingiva does not require separate cleaning, for gingival health can be achieved and maintained quite adequately when using the miniscrub technique. The importance of cleaning of the gingival margins is however more difficult to establish as a separate entity, as it is an inevitable consequence of any effective toothbrushing technique. There appears to be no clinical advantage to gingival massage or stimulation by the toothbrush or by eating fibrous foods (see also Chapter 34 – Restorations, pontic forms and the periodontum).

Automatic brushes

Numerous models are available which may appeal to individuals for several reasons. These include the novelty effect and appeal of mechanical gadgetry plus a conviction of greater efficiency and ease and convenience of usage over manual brushes. They are undoubtedly helpful in cases of limited dexterity and in handicapped patients. Their universally

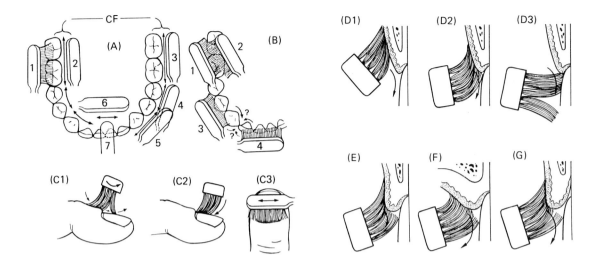

Figure 8.3 Brush-head positioning: (A 1–6) Brush-head aligned along arch form for optimal gingival sulcus penetration and overlapping strokes. Note 'trailing edge' bristles on occlusal surfaces and similar brush positioning (CF) at (A2) lingual aspect and (A3) buccal aspect. (A6) Limited intercanine space may necessitate use of (A7) brush-tip bristles as 'leading edge'. (B1 and 2) Oblique brush-head positioning to be avoided. Incomplete cleaning action (?) when switching from backhand (B3) to forehand (B4) brushing strokes averted by overlapping brushing or supplementary use of single-tufted brush. Use of (C1) roll and (C2 and C3) miniscrub techniques readily demonstrated on thumb nail. Roll technique. (D1) Initial brush placement at 45 degrees to tooth with bristles gently splayed out apically over attached gingiva. (D2) Rotating sweep of successive rows of bristles coronally over gingival margin, into sulcus and then over clinical crown. (D3) Final rotation as flexed bristles straighten out. Technique best suited to ideal physiological form (shown at D) for elsewhere (E and F) flexed bristles pass over and miss gingival sulcus and, more importantly, (G) any pocket space

smaller brush head sizes have an advantage when there is limited mouth opening or restricted access to the posterior teeth. The variations of direction, frequency and amplitude of the mechanical movement of the different types appears insignificant, each resolving into an essentially miniscrub-like action when the brush is applied to the tooth surfaces, as advocated with the ordinary toothbrush above. The torque of the motor is critical as some slow down significantly or stop when the requisite pressure is applied. Furthermore, battery powered models, suffer a gradual loss of torque as the batteries fail which is often not appreciated and results in progressively less pressure being applied, to the detriment of cleaning. The findings of investigations on the comparative efficacy of automatic and manual brushes are equivocal.

Interproximal devices

A wide range of different devices exists, the most widely used being dental floss and wood points, although more recently a number of different sized interproximal brushes have become available. The choice is dictated primarily by tissue morphology, space dimensions and patient preference.

It is not clear at what age specific interproximal plaque control should first be introduced. In young individuals the interdental septal tissues totally occlude interproximal spaces and when the diligent and effective use of the toothbrush alone presumably prevents the development of interdental gingival inflammation. However, where inflammation does occur the use of dental floss becomes necessary. It is not known whether its prophylactic use would avert interdental inflammation in such vulnerable individuals. It also seems unlikely that many would be prepared to use floss in this way when neither the need nor the benefits of doing so can be clearly shown.

Dental floss

This is produced as a thin cord or a flattened tape which may also be impregnated with wax. Comparative studies on the efficacy of plaque removal of waxed and unwaxed varieties have failed to demonstrate significant differences in effectiveness. Waxed floss is easier to use and is less likely to fray and break or catch on minor rough edges or overhangs of restorations. Any such retained snagged strands of floss may be difficult to remove

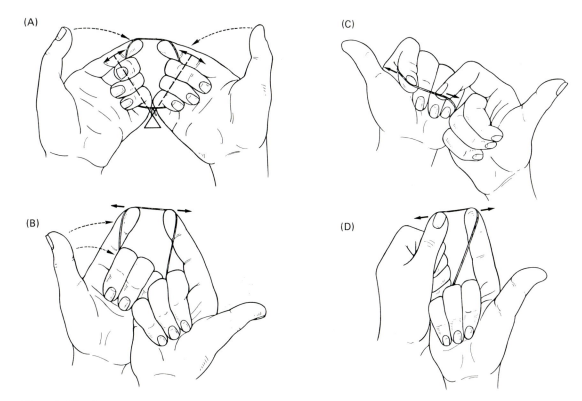

Figure 8.4 Flossing technique. (A) Floss loop passing about fingers of both hands and tension maintained by pulling index fingers apart whilst pivoting on small fingers. Additional support by adopting thumb/index finger grip when flossing anteriorly may impede manipulation posteriorly. (B) Longer reach necessary for left molars achieved by withdrawing all but the straightened right index finger from the loop and shifting the right hand pivot point to the third finger knuckle. Access permitting, added support may be gained from left thumb positioned at the tip or base of the left index finger. The reverse action may be used for the right side of the mouth. (C) From initial position shown at (B) the index fingers are flexed for mandibular anterior and then straightened for more distally placed teeth. (D) Optional left thumb/right index finger grip for maxillary anteriors is derived from an initial left thumb and index finger tip apposition indicated at (B). The index finger is then withdrawn and flexed against the other fingers

by the user. The abrasive portion of Superfloss (Cooper Health Products Ltd, Aylesbury, Bucks HP19 3ED, UK) appears to offer no special advantage in routine interdental cleaning.

Floss must be gripped firmly for precise control and the application of pressure necessary for cleaning. Traditionally a 15–18 inch length of the floss is wound around the first or second fingers of each hand and then pulled taut, by parting the hands. A simpler more effective alternative exists in which an 8–10 inch length is tied into a small loop instead, so that the hands must be held against each other and the required tension of the floss then produced by merely pivoting on the apposing small fingers (Figure 8.4 A). This loop method has several distinct advantages. In the first place, only finger movement is possible so ensuring positive control and little chance of slipping and cutting the tissues.

The floss can also be held taut without simultaneously strangulating the ends of the fingers as with other methods. In addition, the whole circumference of the loop may be used by simply rotating it as sections become frayed. This in turn obviates the need to constantly replace the floss, as with other methods, and so is more conducive to completing the exercise at each interproximal surface rather than giving up in frustration. Finally, the greater difficulties of flossing at the back of the mouth are readily overcome by withdrawing all but the index finger on one hand from the loop and when several combinations of finger, and finger to thumb, positioning are possible for use in different parts of the mouth as shown in Figure 8.4 (B–D).

Less dexterous individuals might prefer floss holders but they are difficult to use for the back teeth where they are most needed. This is because

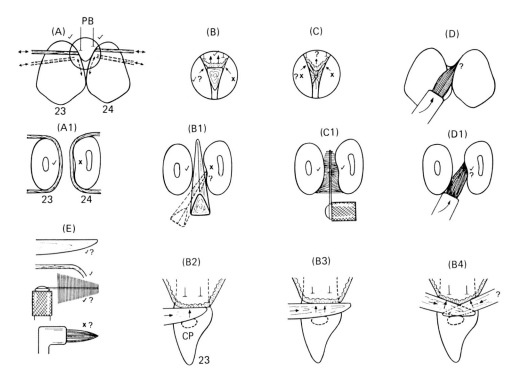

Figure 8.5 Interdental cleaning at shallow pockets depicted at 23 and 24. (A) Dental floss used with a sawing action and negotiating (A1) 23 root surface convexity (indicated by √) but not 24 mesial concavity (X). Adequate subgingival passage of floss to interproximal pocket bases (PB) as shown by (√) permitted by labial and palatal marginal gingival contours. (B, B1–3) Horizontal wood point penetration apical to contact point (CP) compresses interdental tissue resulting in greater but possibly still incomplete (?) subgingival cleaning at convex/flat surfaces. Ineffective at 24 supragingival interproximal concavity although (B1) obliquely directed point might suffice. Note: (B4) Oblique horizontal insertion path is less effective and is also often not feasible from lingual aspects (?). (C and C1) Interproximal brush readily negotiates all supragingival surfaces but produces little tissue compression. Some bristles may pass subgingivally and negotiate convex/flat (?X) but possibly not concave surfaces (X). (D) Access for interspace brush impeded by restricted interproximal dimensions and papillary form (?), but (D1) facilitated at wider spaces by first splaying out bristles against supragingival tooth surface. (E) Summary of efficacy of respective devices at subgingival convex/flat surfaces graded as effective (√), questionable (?) and ineffective (X)

the arms of the basically 'Y' shaped implements are either too flexible or are too short even when rigid enough for effective manipulation. Consequently, in the former the arms flex during use so that the floss bows too easily. This not only complicates cleaning but can snap through and cut into the gingiva when the floss is being passed through tight contact points, which does little to encourage use. The latter more rigid devices have shorter thicker arms which impede access by fouling the teeth and even the gingiva during use.

The method of using floss can be compared to the technique used when polishing shoes with a cloth. The floss is inserted interdentally to pass about each tooth surface in turn, which is then rubbed gently but firmly for several seconds at each level, using a sawing action (Figure 8.5). This action facilitates more precise control of the floss as it is passed as far apically as the gingival attachment allows without actually cutting the tissue, although this does carry the potential risk of tooth surface grooving with over-vigorous use. The alternative purely 'up and down' cleaning movement is more difficult to check apically, is liable to traumatize the attachment and so discourage further cleaning. Efforts to avoid such trauma do, in turn, tend to lead to ineffective cleaning. The depth to which floss is able to pass is also dictated by the facial and oral gingiva contour.

Wood points

These are triangular in cross section to conform to the shape of the interdental spaces and taper to a point. The point is held like a dart between the index finger and thumb, whilst resting the other fingers on the lower jaw. It is inserted gently but firmly into the interdental space apical to the contact point, until it wedges with the base of the triangle against the gingiva at 90 degrees to the long axis of the teeth (Figure 8.5). It is then partially withdrawn and the sequence is repeated four or five times at each space. The tapered structure ensures a progressively tighter fit, the wedging effect against the tooth surfaces not only displaces the plaque but also compresses the interdental tissue which exposes for cleaning the subgingival tooth surfaces (Figure 8.5 B2 and 3).

The several different types of wood point are similar in design, but differ in consistency. The Boots Dental Sticks (Boots plc, Nottingham, Notts, UK) are advocated for most situations, but the equally firm, slim, double-ended Oral B-Sanodent (Cooper Health Products Ltd, Aylesbury, Bucks, UK) points are best suited to small interdental spaces. The similarly shaped plastic points and cocktail-type sticks, that are not triangular in shape and so do not fit the interdental spaces adequately, are not recommended. Rubber points, originally conceived for gingival massage, are also not advocated for interdental plaque control.

Interproximal brushes

There are several different sized straight or tapered bottle type brushes available. Only the very smallest ones are likely to be accommodated in early disease, elsewhere being dictated by the size of the interdental spaces following gingival detachment due to disease. They are inserted interdentally like toothpicks the bristles being compressed by the related teeth (Figure 8.5 C). Some are used with a special handle. The bristles of these brushes tend to wear rapidly, their wire stems bend and break readily and they are quite expensive, so are not advocated for routine interdental cleaning. They are useful at interproximal supragingival root surface concavities but appear of little value subgingivally.

Special brushes

There are a number of single-tufted brushes available, the trade names of which imply, somewhat erroneously, their effectiveness in interdental plaque control. That is, whilst marginally more effective than an ordinary toothbrush used with the miniscrub technique, because of their smaller size and manoeuverability, they are of limited use interdentally in early disease (Figure 8.5 D and E). However with the development of interdental pockets they become very much more useful (see below and Chapters 10, 11 and 18).

The Halex Interspace Brush (Addis Ltd, Hertford, Herts, UK) which has a fairly stiff, natural bristle tapered tuft and the similarly styled but softer nylon filamented Mentadent Interspace Brush (Gibbs Dental Division, London, UK) are recommended. The handles are constructed of a thermoplastic material, allowing the neck of the brush to be bent (Figure 8.6) into different shapes to enhance access to the more difficult areas in the mouth.

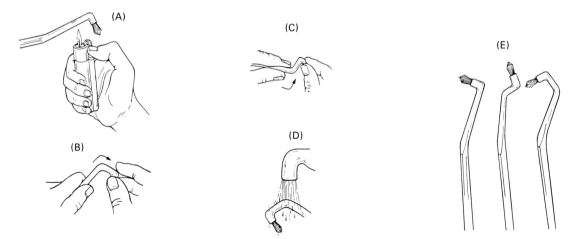

Figure 8.6 Shaping interspace brush. (A) Thermoplastic neck of brush gently heated with gas lighter whilst preferably covering bristles with the fingers to avoid singeing. (B and C) Once softened, brush is bent to required shapes and then (D) chilled under running water. (E) Different shapes. See also Figure 8.1 (J)

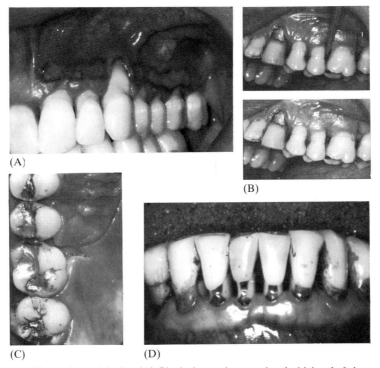

Figure 8.7 Damage caused by mechanical device. (A) Gingival recession associated with band of ulcerated mucosa and extensive loss of cervical enamel and dentine from abrasion and apparently also acidic erosion. Interdental grooving from use of (B) wood point and (C) dental floss. (D) Abrasion of teeth from use of wood points and abrasive dentifrice ([A] reproduced from *Restorative Dentistry,* by permission of A. E. Morgan Publications Ltd)

The brushes are used mainly where there is limited mouth opening, interference from the tongue, at distal aspects of the last standing teeth, lingually inclined and tilted molars, teeth bounding edentulous spaces and at imbricated units. However, as will be seen in subsequent chapters, the main applications of these brushes is for disease at localized pocket sites, large patent interdental spaces and within exposed root surface concavities and furcations.

Irrigation devices

These devices project a pulsating intermittent jet of water through a fine nozzle to remove loosely adherent superficial plaque. Originally conceived for interproximal plaque control, the persistence of firmly adherent plaque means they are of no apparent value in plaque control. They may be of use in subgingival irrigation techniques (see Chapter 35 – Subgingival plaque control).

Dentifrices

A dentifrice makes cleaning more pleasant and leaves the mouth feeling fresh and, as such, is useful for plaque control. Two other benefits are its use for stain removal in some individuals and as a vehicle for the topical application of, for example, fluorides for caries control (as in most currently available toothpastes), dentinal desensitizing agents (as in Sensodyne [Stafford-Miller Ltd, Hatfield, Herts, UK]), and antiseptic agents (as in Corsodyl gel [Imperial Chemical Industries plc, Macclesfield, Cheshire, UK]). There is some evidence that fluoride might also be advantageous to gingival health. Fluoride is also highly effective in controlling sensitivity although some of the stronger flavoured pastes appear to perpetuate this.

Damage caused by mechanical devices

The over-enthusiastic use of any toothbrush could traumatize the gingival margins and lead to gingival recession (Figure 8.7 A) (see Mechanisms of Recession, Chapters 13 and 21). Brushing should therefore be carried out with finesse. Similarly, dental floss and toothpicks might also lacerate and cause interdental gingival recession (Figure 8.7 B,C). However this is unusual in the absence of existing attachment losses and when it does occur should be regarded as advantageous, for any associated pocketing is reduced simultaneously.

Loss of tooth substance following tooth cleaning (Figure 8.7 A,D) appears to be due mainly to dentifrice abrasion than the device used. Acid erosion may also contribute to the decalcification, whilst its softening effect predisposes to greater mechanical abrasion. This acid may be of dietary (citrus fruit, vinegar, carbonated drinks, etc.) or gastric origin via regurgitation (see Chapters 24 and 25). Toothbrushing might, therefore, be prudent before or when some time has passed following an acidic meal, bearing in mind the gradual spontaneous salivary mediated tooth surface recalcification.

Sequence of cleaning

Tooth cleaning is an essentially straightforward exercise, no different from cleaning hands after engine maintenance work. Thus, it is unimportant whether the palms are clean before the spaces between the fingers, or a nail brush or file used to clean about and under the nails. These decisions will simply depend on individual preferences, what happens to work best and in the sequence deemed most suitable. Similarly, as all tooth surfaces must be cleaned, it is up to the patient to do so in whatever manner and sequence that best suits him following appropriate professional advice. Although there is merit in traditional thinking that effective toothbrushing must be mastered before interdental cleaning devices are introduced, this credits the patient with very little common sense and de-emphasizes the importance of interdental cleaning. A set sequence of cleaning, proceeding methodically about the mouth is sensible, but the time devoted to each site is best judged by the patient using trial and error. Ultimately, providing the objectives of cleaning are understood and achieved the logistics are immaterial.

Further reading

Addy, M., Abji, E. G. and Adams, D (1987) Dentine hypersensitivity. The effect *in vitro* of acids and dietary substances on root planed and burred dentine. *J. Clin. Periodontol.* **14**, 274–279

Addy, M. and Dowell, P. (1983) Dentine hypersensitivity – a review. II. Clinical and *in vitro* evaluation of treatment agents. *J. Clin. Periodontol.* **10**, 351–363

Axelsson, P. and Lindhe, J. (1978) Effect of controlled oral hygiene procedures on caries and periodontal disease in adults. *J. Clin. Periodontol.* **5**, 133–151

Baab, D. and Weinstein, P. (1986) Longitudinal evaluation of a self-inspection plaque index in periodontal recall patients. *J. Clin. Periodontol.* **13**, 313–318

Bergenholtz, A. and Brithon, J. (1980) Plaque removal by dental floss or toothpicks. *J. Clin. Periodontol.* **7**, 516–524

Bonfil, J. J., Fourel, J. and Falabregues, R. (1985) The influence of gingival stimulation on recovery from human experimental gingivitis. *J. Clin. Periodontol.* **12**, 828–836

Dowell, P. and Addy, M. (1983) Dentine hypersensitivity – a review. I. Aetiology, symptoms and theories of pain initiation. *J. Clin. Periodontol.* **10**, 341–350

Frandsen, A. (1980) Preventive programs in clinical practice. In *Efficacy of Treatment Procedures in Periodontics,* pp. 79–93 (Shanley D., editor) Quintessence, Chicago

Gillette, W. B. and Van House, R. L. (1980) Ill effects of improper oral hygiene procedures. *J Am. Dent. Ass.* **101**, 476–481

Hansen, F. and Gjermo, P. (1971) The plaque-removing effect of four toothbrushing methods. *Scand. J. Dent. Res.* **79**, 502–506.

Jenkins, W. M. M. (1983) The prevention and control of chronic periodontal disease. In *The Prevention of Dental Disease,* pp. 265–277. (Murray, J. J., editor). Oxford University Press, Oxford

Lindhe, J. and Wićen, P. (1969) The effects on the gingivae of chewing fibrous foods. *J. Periodont. Res.* **4**, 193–201

Smith, B. G. N. and Knight, J. K. (1984) A comparison of pattern of tooth wear with aetiological factors. *Br. Dent. J.* **157**, 16–19

Tan, A. E. S. (1981) Disclosing agents in plaque control: a review. *J. West. Soc. Periodont. Periodont. Abstr.* **29**, 81–86

Part II The treatment of disease

Section I

Disease management

9

The rationale for periodontal therapy

The variable presentation of periodontal disease
The fundamental role of plaque control
The levels of disease and therapeutic regimes
The outcome of gingival therapy

Stages of periodontitis and pocket therapy
Modular treatment planning
The roles of patient and operator in treatment

The variable presentation of periodontal disease

Periodontal disease is the term commonly used to describe the whole range of presentations associated with chronic inflammatory periodontal disease from mild gingivitis to advanced periodontitis. It is possible to find every stage of progress in this disease range within a single mouth (Table 9.1). The essential destructive lesion is not evenly distributed around the mouth or even around individual teeth, so that the tooth site must be regarded as the basic unit of pathology for therapeutic purposes. This means that assessment methods suitable for epidemiological purposes or the treatment needs of groups of people, which have long been used in clinical practice, will not be suitable for treatment planning of the individual.

It is, therefore, necessary to examine all tooth sites for the clinical signs of gingival inflammation such as redness, bleeding, suppuration and swelling.

The latter may be due to either oedema or hyperplasia or both. The loss of attachment, as a measure of the extent of tissue destruction with its concomitant gingival pocketing or recession, should also be noted at each site (Figure 9.1 A–X).

Diagnosis

Gingival inflammation (gingivitis) is frequently distributed widely within a mouth showing varying grades of severity. However, these signs of superficial inflammation cannot be related directly to the deeper underlying connective tissue inflammatory changes (periodontitis) associated with the loss of attachment. Whilst the clinical diagnosis of gingivitis is easy, there is at present no reliable clinical method of diagnosing active and destructive periodontitis. It is true that attachment loss and pocket depth can be measured by probing but the clinician can only interpret this as evidence of past activity. Consequently, it is only possible to establish the active or

Table 9.1

Gingival health
Zero or minor pocketing
Zero or minor recession
Inactive periodontitis
}
(Combined clinical conditions)
{
Marked gingivitis*
Deep pocketing
Marked recession
Active periodontitis

*May be accompanied by gingival hyperplasia (overgrowth)
Combinations of the clinical conditions shown here tend to occur in the same mouth, but may even present about the same tooth.

68

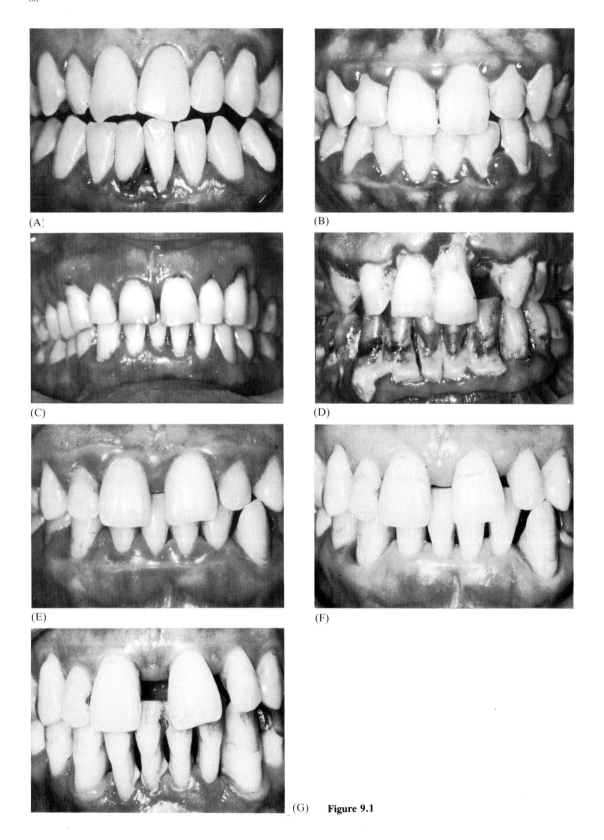

(A)

(B)

(C)

(D)

(E)

(F)

(G)   **Figure 9.1**

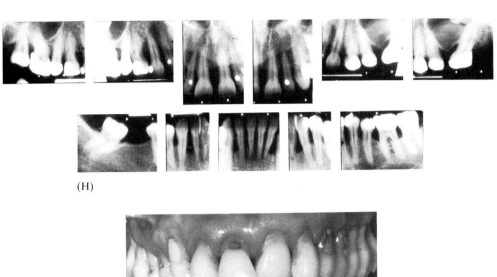

(H)

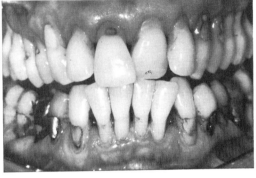

(I)

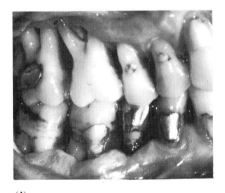

(J)

(K)

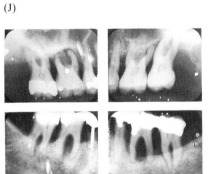

(L)

Figure 9.1 Variable clinical presentation of disease. (A) Isolated sites of marginal inflammation alternating with gingival health. (B) Generalized oedematous/hyperplastic gingivitis. (C) Chronic periodontitis with gingival recession exposing subgingival deposits. (D) Gross deposits of plaque and calculus with obvious signs of disease. (E) Advanced level of disease with obvious inflammation of detached tissues and pathological drifting. (F) Same case after improved plaque control. Note: resolution of inflammation that belies extent of underlying destruction. (G) Same case 3 years later following further deterioration. (H) Radiograph of previous case displaying great variations in pattern of disease. (I, J, K) Extensive periodontal destruction and recession at molar teeth with only modest attachment loss anteriorly. (L) Radiograph of previous case.

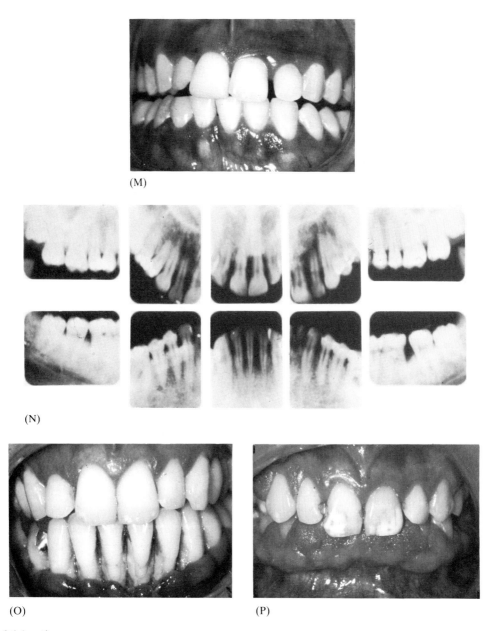

(M)

(N)

(O)   (P)

Figure 9.1 (*cont.*)

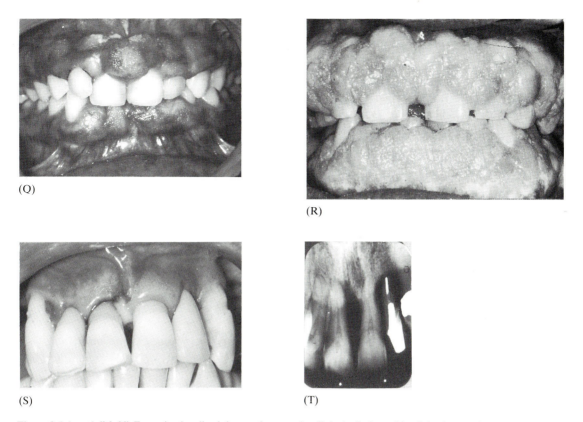

(Q)

(R)

(S)

(T)

Figure 9.1 (*cont.*) (M, N) Extensive localized destruction noted radiologically but with minimal overt signs of disease. (O) Destruction consistent with recurrent ANG at mandibular anterior units alone. (P) Idiopathic gingival hyperplasia in mandible anterior segment alone, and (Q) in both arches. (R) Epanutin hyperplasia. (S) Pus discharging from extensive pocket at 12. Note (T) radiographic findings.

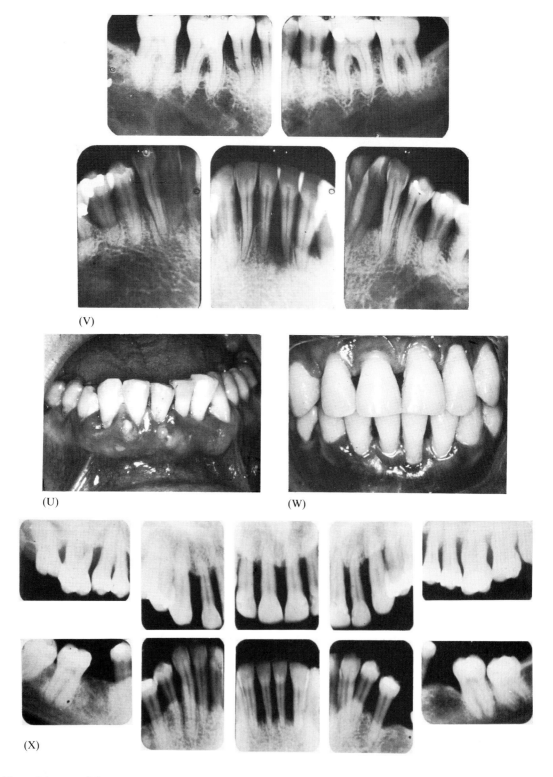

(V)

(U)

(W)

(X)

Figure 9.1 (*cont.*) (U) Multiple abscess mandibular anterior teeth. (V) Radiographs of previous case displaying different levels of disease. (W) Extensive but irregular pattern of destruction in young adult. (X) Radiograph of previous case

passive nature of the lesions by a series of measurements taken at regular intervals over a period of years. Even then the judgement can only be made retrospectively. Contrary to traditional belief, even the signs of inflammation at the dento-epithelial junction at the base of periodontal pockets, such as bleeding on probing or the expression of pus, may not be indicative of active attachment destruction. This is true for any stage of the disease, including that of extensive destruction, so that even in these cases tooth loss can no longer be considered inevitable. However, the risk of further destruction does always exist while these signs of inflammation are present.

Therapeutic implications

The therapeutic implications of this complex clinical picture, might at first sight appear daunting but are in reality quite straightforward. This is because all treatment revolves simply about the control of bacterial plaque although the methods used for gaining this control may need to be modified from site to site. This is necessary to cater for the various topographical changes encountered in disease and may in some instances include altering dentogingival form to facilitate future plaque control measures. Although the tooth site is the location of the destructive lesion and thereby needs careful site by site examination and evaluation, this does not imply that therapeutic considerations should be limited to such areas. So, treatment planning should always be based upon the assessment of the whole mouth, integrating the dental needs of the total individual.

Therapeutic objective

Although, as stated above, bleeding and pus at the dentogingival junction may not be indicative of active destruction they do demonstrate the existence of plaque-induced inflammation and are certainly not signs of health. Accordingly, all treatment of periodontal disease must have as its objective the production and maintenance of uninflamed dento-epithelial junctions, be they located at the bases of gingival sulci or periodontal pockets, regardless of the extent and pattern of destruction, by the control of bacterial plaque. This concept of periodontal therapy, as advocated throughout this text, is quite simple, although technically difficult procedures may sometimes be involved. It challenges the traditional emphasis placed upon the surgical creation of a classic dentogingival form as a therapeutic objective.

The fundamental role of plaque control
A rational approach

The traditional aim of periodontal therapy has been to apply a specific operative exercise to each clinical variation, whereas it is now evident that the most important factor is simply the mechanical control of bacterial plaque, as described in Chapter 8. The problems that have been created for this control of plaque as an aftermath of continuing periodontal breakdown do, however, need to be overcome as part of the treatment plan. It is a fallacy to assume that the re-establishment of a normal dentogingival anatomical relationship by therapy will by itself prevent further disease. This assumption is illogical because the disease is initiated in the presence of a normal dentogingival junction associated with the gingival sulcus. Consequently, whilst the development of the characteristic topographical changes in progressive disease will create difficulties in effective plaque control they will only represent additional obstacles to cleaning. These topographical changes, however complex, should therefore be seen only as secondary factors to the effectiveness of the patient's plaque control and cannot in themselves be held as solely responsible for the persistence of the disease.

It follows from the foregoing explanation that the operative correction of morphological complications to plaque control cannot by itself arrest periodontal disease. It is also axiomatic that the maintenance of periodontal health, following any operative treatment, will depend primarily upon the patient's success in controlling plaque at the healed dento-epithelial junction. Attention will now be paid to topographical changes in disease (Figure 9.2) and how these appropriately designated plaque retention factors will affect plaque control.

Plaque retention factors

These factors can be classified as those that modify the form of the clinical crown and those resulting from progressive periodontal disease and its involvement of the anatomical form of the periodontal supporting tissues and tooth roots, as depicted in Figure 9.2. Any of the above might impede plaque control measures, so are referred to as plaque retention factors (Table 9.2).

The first group consists of ledges or interproximal obstructions formed by calculus, the overhanging margins and deficiencies of restorations, and fixed prostheses adjacent to the gingival margin. The next are periodontal pockets, especially when associated with uneven patterns of destruction, and gingival deformities of hyperplasia (overgrowth) and recession of the gingival margin. Recession may in turn initiate further problems where it causes the gingival margin to approximate to the vestibular sulcus. Finally, there is the group of problems caused by concavities, grooves and furcations of the root surfaces exposed by attachment loss. It should also be appreciated that in some instances tooth imbrication and developmental aberrations of mucogingival

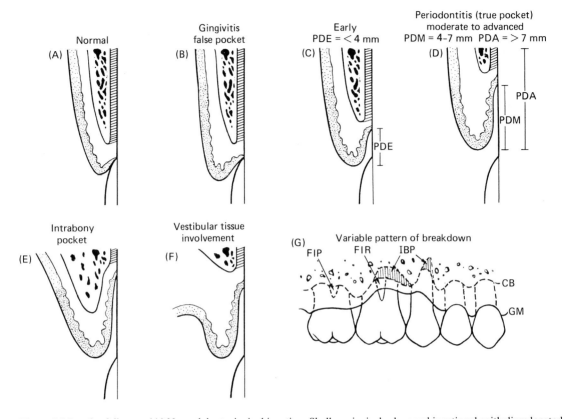

Figure 9.2 Levels of disease. (A) Normal dentogingival junction. Shallow gingival sulcus and junctional epithelium located on enamel. (B) Gingivitis with false pocket. (C) Early periodontitis. Loss of attachment and more apical location of dento-epithelial junction (junctional epithelium) on root surface at pocket base. (D) Moderate to advanced periodontitis. Note progressively greater probing depths in early (PDE), moderate (PDM) and advanced (PDA) levels. (E) Intrabony pocket. (F) Vestibular tissue involvement. (G) Variable pattern of disease. Uneven pattern of gingival recession and of bony resorption. Furcation involvement within pocket space (FIP) and exposed by recession (FIR); gingival margin (GM); crest of bone (CB); intrabony pocket (IBP)

Table 9.2 Plaque retention factors

Factor	Nature of impediment to plaque control
Calculus	Surface roughness, ledges and occluded interproximal spaces
Restorations	Surface roughness, ledges and occluded interproximal spaces
Tooth position	Imbrication and tilting
Root form	Surface concavities and grooves. Furcation involvement
Gingival form	Uneven marginal contour – recession or hyperplasia (overgrowth)
Vestibular form	Prominent frenal insertion, shallow vestibular sulcus and poorly controlled lips, cheeks and tongue
Pockets	Subgingivally located periodontally-involved root surfaces

form, especially prominent frenal insertions, may also represent plaque retention factors. Similarly, removable prostheses may encourage plaque retention.

Each of the above merely serves to frustrate the efforts of the patient to remove bacterial plaque effectively. Moreover, it would be illogical to deal with these factors before the patient has demonstrated the capacity to control the basic cause of the problem, inadequate oral hygiene. Thus, only when the required standard of patient cleaning has been achieved, should attention be directed at any plaque retention factors. Stemming from this is the identification of the respective roles that patient and operator should play in achieving and maintaining periodontal health.

Patient access to plaque

It is of great practical importance to differentiate between those surfaces that are accessible to plaque control by the patient and those that are not (Figure 9.3). It must be accepted at the outset that all those surfaces adjacent to anatomically normal dentogingival junctions are *totally accessible* to the patient. Furthermore, although the presence of light calculus deposits, minor overhangs or deficient margins of fillings, crowded teeth, root surface grooves and concavities contiguous with furcations (as depicted in Figure 10.3), as well as altered gingival and mucogingival form and subgingival root surfaces within shallow pockets will present some difficulties in plaque control, these will in most instances remain *reasonably accessible* to the patient. These minor structural and topographical features can therefore be taken to delineate the responsibility of the patient in treatment.

It is not possible to define clearly situations that are *inaccessible* to the patient and, in turn, the need for professional cleaning. This is because of the great variations that exist in individual patient

dexterity and determination. It must, however, be reiterated that this differentiation need only be considered when optimal plaque control has been achieved at the totally accessible and reasonably accessible sites listed above. Doing otherwise is like running before one can walk.

Professional cleaning

Although the patient's responsibility has been strongly emphasized, there are situations where plaque control can be extremely difficult, if not impossible. For example, tooth surfaces that are heavily encrusted with calculus or are associated with grossly overhanging margins of fillings, and where there is extensive pocketing present, may constitute insurmountable plaque retention factors that demand professional cleaning or other measures to facilitate the patient's future oral hygiene measures. Accordingly, the terms *relative* and *total inaccessibility* are used to separate sites which might be negotiated by the patient from those where there is no possible chance of this. This serves to delineate further the respective roles of patient and operator.

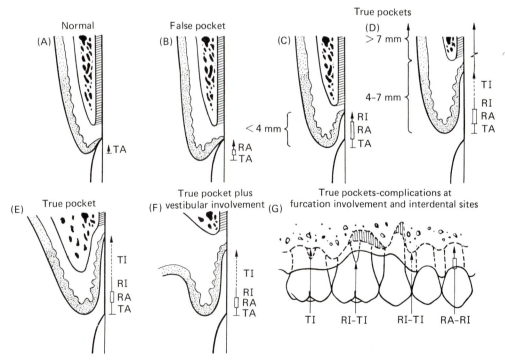

Figure 9.3 Levels of disease and accessibility for oral hygiene. Plaque deposits become progressively less accessible as pocket depths increase but superficial deposits present no difficulties at (A–F). Note: (E) Presence of infrabony component to pocket irrelevant to accessibility. (F) Vestibular tissues may however impede access so limiting depth of accessibility. (G) Added complications to access exist at interproximal sites (compared to facial and oral aspects) and within furcation involvements, but much depends upon individual dexterity. Key to accessibility: TA, totally accessible; RA, reasonably accessible; RI, relatively inaccessible; TI, totally inaccessible

The periodontal pocket constitutes the most significant plaque retention factor in periodontal disease. In most instances, as stated above, all but the most coronally situated subgingival plaque is totally inaccessible to the patient which makes professional cleaning essential. This root surface instrumentation consists of the removal of plaque, calculus and any possibly contaminated root surface material. This is carried out by techniques termed *subgingival debridement, subgingival scaling* and *root planing* respectively. It should be realized that these individual techniques are frequently performed together. In those instances where the root surfaces are not accessible to the operator a surgical approach may be necessary. This, in turn, implies that the principle of the accessibility or otherwise of plaque for the patient is equally applicable to the operator, with respect to root surface instrumentation, and similarly, that an element of individual ability is involved. Surgery is therefore reserved for sites deemed to be totally inaccessible to each individual operator, but it must be stressed that the outcome will only be successful if it facilitates future plaque control by both patient and operator.

The levels of disease and therapeutic regimes

A therapeutic scheme

The foregoing outline represents the basis for the therapeutic scheme, presented in Table 9.3 and Figure 9.4 revolving around the degree of accessibility to plaque at the dento-epithelial junctions. This simple scheme of periodontal care does not attempt to present discrete entities because of the variable pattern of destruction that is encountered at adjacent units, and that some overlapping is accepted as being inevitable. It is intended rather as a guideline for treatment planning in a number of different clinical situations.

The development of the periodontal pocket represents the clinical dividing line between gingivitis and periodontitis. This has important clinical implications because, for all practical purposes, the former stage is reversible and the latter is not. This is reflected in the treatment needs, in that greater professional intervention is demanded in periodontitis than in gingivitis.

Table 9.3 Levels of disease and therapeutic regimes

Disease levels	Gingivitis	Periodontitis			
	All degrees	Early	Moderate	Advanced	Complicated
Pocket depths	Nil/false	< 4 mm	4–7 mm	> 7 mm	Variable**
Regimes	Gingival therapy	Periodontal pocket therapy	Simple pocket surgery	Complex pocket surgery	
Predictability of therapy	Good	Good	Good–Fair		Poor

*Gingivitis may or may not be clinically evident in periodontitis as depicted by broken arrow (– – – →)
**Variable pattern plus furcation, bony and vestibular tissue involvement.
***Gingival therapy applicable to all levels of therapy.
Note overlapping of disease levels and therapeutic regimes as depicted by

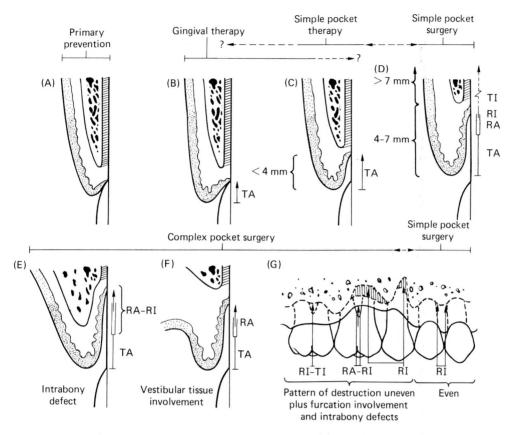

Figure 9.4 Limits of accessibility of subgingival plaque front to instrumentation at different disease levels and the applications of therapeutic regimes. Key as in Figure 9.3. Gingival therapy is applicable to all situations as the first stage of therapy but will, according to the clinical features, need to be supplemented by other operative regimes. Some overlapping (depicted by ←======→) is inevitable between gingival and simple pocket therapy and also between the other regimes shown. Note (E, F and G) added complication of access at intrabony defects, uneven patterns of breakdown, interproximal sites and furcation involvement. These features may thwart surgical objective and are handled by complex pocket surgery

Gingival therapy

In gingivitis, treatment consists of the patient's control of reasonably accessible plaque plus the professional removal of any plaque retention factors. These measures represent gingival therapy. Gingival therapy is also applicable in those situations where root surfaces have become exposed as a result of gingival recession. Gingival therapy does, in addition, constitute the essential first stage of periodontal pocket therapy.

Periodontal pocket therapy

Periodontal pocketing requires additional measures to the above, because plaque within all but shallow pockets is totally inaccessible to the patient and requires professional removal. This subgingival root surface instrumentation is hereafter referred to more specifically as debridement. In addition, any subgingivally located plaque retention factors such as subgingival calculus and root furcations may also require professional attention. These measures constitute periodontal pocket therapy.

Pocket therapy has for treatment planning purposes been subdivided into simple pocket therapy, and simple and complex pocket surgery, based upon the depth of the pockets and their accessibility. However these subdivisions cannot always be demarcated clearly, because the accessibility of the plaque front at the dento-epithelial junction located within the pocket does not depend on depth alone. Equally important is the pattern of attachment loss, the variable root forms encountered and not least, the ability of the operator. Accordingly, plaque associated with non-furcated root surfaces within pockets of less than about 4 mm, as in the early stages of periodontitis, may be regarded as *totally accessible* from the operator's point of view and as such constitutes simple pocket therapy. Management of this level of disease thus merges closely with gingival therapy. Plaque located at the base of pockets having a depth of between about 4 mm and 7 mm in moderate periodontitis will, root form permitting, be judged as *reasonably accessible* to the operator. The treatment of this subdivision will therefore also represent simple pocket therapy. Where, on the other hand, the root morphology associated with these pockets precludes root surface debridement, simple pocket therapy will be inadequate and additional measures to enhance access become necessary.

In pockets of about 7 mm or more, in advanced periodontitis, the plaque front and its related accretions are likely to be *relatively* or even *totally inaccessible* to the operator, regardless of root form. It is this subdivision of disease level, together with situations of adverse root morphology alluded to above, for which surgery might be considered. This surgery is designed to ensure not only efficient root surface instrumentation at operation but more importantly, future plaque control measures. This level of therapy constitutes simple pocket surgery (*cf.* Chapters 15 and 16), although the surgical objectives will, in many instances, be thwarted by the morphological hurdles encountered at operation. Thus, the root morphology may prevent both effective instrumentation, despite the enhanced access and future oral hygiene efforts. Similarly, technical problems arising from the different degrees of attachment loss occurring at adjacent sites, the variable patterns of bone resorption and the proximity of pocket bases to the vestibular sulcus may all preclude simple pocket surgery. The therapeutic measures designed to cope with these morphological complications of disease that char-acterize complicated periodontitis, constitute complex pocket surgery (*cf.* Chapters 18–20).

The outcome of gingival therapy

Gingival response

In all instances, whatever the degree of periodontal destruction, the effective control of the *reasonably accessible* plaque by the patient is paramount and when, combined with any necessary professional cleaning results in healing, referred to as the *gingival response*. This is characterized by gingival shrinkage (gingival recession) with close physical adaptation of the pocket wall to the root surface (pocket closure) (Table 9.4 and Figure 9.5). This tissue adaptation is associated ideally with the development of a long junctional epithelium; that is an epithelial attachment to the tooth which extends along the entire epithelium tooth relationship as depicted in Figure 9.5 (C1 and C3).

Where initial pocketing has been shallow, as in early periodontitis, a cleansible dentogingival junction can be expected from the gingival response. The arrest of disease is therefore predictable (Tables 9.3 and 9.4). In moderate periodontitis, pocket reduction may also come about by pocket closure and gingival recession, although the extent of the latter is unpredictable. The progression of disease is also often halted by the gingival response alone. This form of therapy is then referred to as simple pocket therapy.

Pocket closure and gingival recession may occur even in the more advanced stages of disease, but the outcome of the gingival response depends very much upon the individual operator's skill and diligence in the necessary subgingival root surface instrumentation. The progressively poorer accessibility in advanced periodontitis, and especially in complicated periodontitis, often demands surgical

Table 9.4 Gingival response and levels of disease

	Marginal resolution	Pocket closure	Gingival recession	Predictability of treatment
Gingivits	+	Not applicable		+
Early periodontitis	+	+	+	+
Moderate periodontitis	+	+	+	±
Advanced periodontitis	+	±	+	±
Complicated periodontitis	+	±	+	−

+ and − signify likelihood of positive and negative responses and of levels of predictability

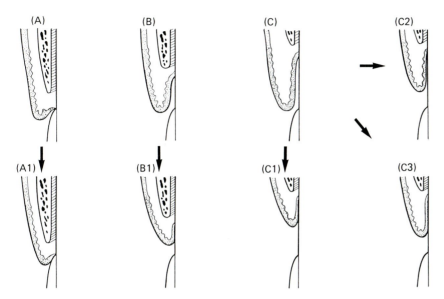

Figure 9.5 Gingival response in gingival and simple pocket therapy. (A) False pocket reverts to (A1) normal dentogingival junction. (B) Pocket with (B1) optimal healing by both gingival recession and pocket closure associated with long junctional epithelium. (C) Deeper pocket sites may also undergo similar healing in conjunction with (C1) marked or only (C3) slight marginal recession, occur by (C2) pocket closure alone or by various combinations of these possibilities

Table 9.5 Periodontal pocket features, surgical methods and predictability

	Simple pockets	*Complex pockets*
Features	Suprabony with even loss of attachment No furcation or vestibular tissue involvement	Intrabony with uneven loss of attachment Furcation and vestibular tissue involvement
	Simple pocket therapy is the essential first stage in all surgical situations, but permits incorporation of complex surgical measures required.	
Surgical method and outcomes	(1) Pocket elimination by apical repositioning or resection Ideal dentogingival form achieved by both methods	As for simple pocket surgery plus additional specific measures Surgical objectives complicated or thwarted by pocket features so that residual pockets and non-cleansible dentogingival form may persist
	(2) Pocket reduction by surgical reattachment. Optimal healing by long junctional epithelium	Some pocket reduction is possible with optimal healing by long junctional epithelium
Predictability	Outcome predictable for pocket elimination alone	Outcome unpredictable

intervention, represented by simple and complex pocket surgery respectively.

Surgical intervention

The need for surgical intervention to facilitate root surface debridement is dependent primarily on the individual operator's skill, although the attitude of the operator, and indeed also the patient, to surgical therapy will inevitably influence treatment planning. The degree of difficulty encountered with respect to debridement is dictated more by the morphological features of the tissues than by the linear depth of the probing attachment loss. This is the basis for associating the level of disease with the different therapeutic regimes depicted in Figure 9.4 and listed in Table 9.3. The various levels of periodontitis are thus handled by simple pocket therapy, simple pocket surgery and complex pocket surgery. The predictability of the treatment is in turn determined by the complexity of the treatment required (Table 9.5).

The traditional use of the terms early, moderate and advanced disease is directly related to *linear amounts* of attachment loss. While these terms do reflect the past history of the disease they are less able to determine the nature of and the outcome of therapy. For example, pocketing at sites traditionally described as having advanced loss of attachment can be successfully and predictably treated at anterior teeth. Elsewhere this is not so, because of the associated more complex root, alveolar and vestibular mucosal morphology. Therefore, such anterior pockets would be amenable to simple pocket surgery as advocated here, whilst posterior pockets of similar depth would require complex pocket surgery. A further disadvantage of treatment planning, based upon linear measurements of attachment loss, can be the difficulties associated with the characteristically uneven pattern of the disease at adjacent sites.

Stages of periodontitis and pocket therapy

For the reasons outlined above, treatment planning is based upon the morphological changes encountered in disease. These changes reflect the influence of the normal anatomical features of the teeth, the supporting tissues and the contiguous osseous and vestibular mucosal tissues on the presentation of the disease and will, in turn, determine the operative treatment requirements. It must be reiterated that some overlapping is inevitable. The periodontal pocket features the appropriate therapeutic measures, their indications and expected outcomes are summarized below (Tables 9.3 and 9.5 and Figure 9.4).

Simple pocket therapy

The subgingival plaque front, situated at the dento-epithelial junction, is accessible to the operator so that the involved root surfaces are amenable to 'closed' or 'blind' debridement. Repair of the pocket occurs by a gingival response represented by tissue shrinkage and adaptation to the root (pocket closure), ideally with the development of a long junctional epithelium as shown in Figure 9.5 (C). Decreased probing depths, reflecting some gingival recession and pocket closure with gains in probing attachment levels, is the expected clinical outcome. Various combinations of these possible outcomes may occur within the same case as represented by Figure 9.5 (C1–C3).

Simple pocket surgery

This is indicated when the subgingival plaque front is inaccessible to the operator and necessitates gaining access by surgical flap reflection for 'open' surgical debridement (Figure 9.6 A) in anticipation of a soft tissue to tooth reunion. This attempted surgical reattachment technique does, at best, achieve some *pocket reduction* brought about by pocket closure with, optimally, a long junctional epithelium plus some gingival recession (Figure 9.6 A) but is unlikely to achieve pocket elimination. Accordingly, it would seem more reasonable to use the opportunity gained by surgical access to attempt *elimination of* the pocket space, in the interests of future plaque control. To achieve this result the gingiva forming the pocket wall can either be surgically repositioned in a more apical direction or resected (Figure 9.6 B and B1). These two alternative surgical techniques represent *pocket elimination*.

In simple pocket surgery no impediments to the surgical sequence of events occur (Table 9.5). A predictable outcome is assured by the totally accessible dentogingival morphology which follows pocket elimination. Surgical reattachment is, in contrast, unpredictable because it depends on the biological closure of the pocket during healing (*cf.* Chapter 29). It must, however, be realized that in many instances of elective pocket elimination surgery, pocket reduction rather than the ideal objective of pocket elimination results. This is due to a failure to achieve the technical objective because of the difficulties associated with the morphological features (see below) encountered at operation (Figure 9.6 C–E and Table 9.5). Consequently, the outcome of much of pocket surgery frequently constitutes a *surgical compromise* of pocket reduction only regardless of surgical technique (see also Chapter 29). This in turn implies that some overlapping of simple pocket and complex pocket surgical regimes is frequently necessary.

Complex pocket surgery

In many situations it will be clear that the pocket elimination objectives of simple pocket surgery will not be possible because of complicating morphological features encountered at operation (Figure 9.6 C–E and Table 9.5). These relate to the complexity of root forms, the uneven pattern of attachment loss and bony resorption and lastly, the proximity of the vestibular mucosal reflection. When these factors do occur additional operative measures are required. These measures constitute complex pocket surgery.

A surgical compromise is often enforced because some or all of the above factors frustrate the objectives outlined for simple pocket surgery. These compromises entail incomplete root surface debridement (especially at root furcations), pocket

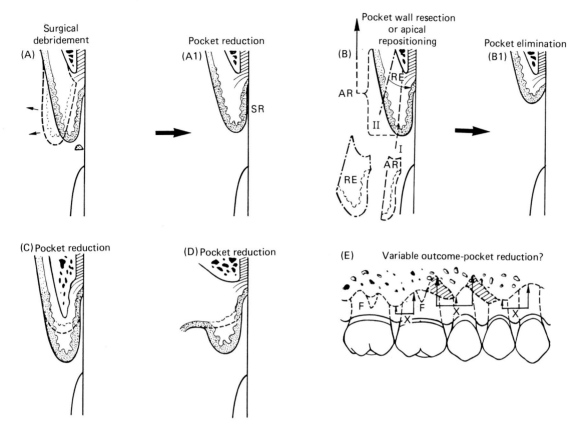

Figure 9.6 (A and B) Simple pocket surgery. (A) 'Open' surgical debridement for (A1) surgical reattachment (SR). Healing is unpredictable by pocket closure (with, ideally, the development of a long junctional epithelium) and some gingival recession. (B) Pocket wall resection (RE) and apical repositioning (AR) incisions with (B1) predictable pocket elimination. Pocket wall tissue is largely preserved in apical repositioning by surgical incision (I) but sacrificed in resection by incision (II). (C–E) Complex pocket surgery. Pocket elimination precluded by (C) intrabony defects and complicated by (D) vestibular tissue involvement, (E) differences in bony levels at adjacent sites (indicated by arrows 'X'), and by furcation involvement (indicated by 'F') which impede debridement and creation of cleansible postsurgical dentogingival morphology. Note optimal (broken lines) postsurgical gingival form shown at (C and D)

reduction rather than elimination and an acceptance of adverse vestibular and furcation morphology, which result in a dentogingival junction that may not be accessible for future plaque control. It follows then that the outcome of complex pocket surgery is difficult to predict.

Modular treatment planning

The evaluation of treatment needs based on morphological changes, may still present some difficulty because of the variable pattern of disease presenting in any one quadrant. Because of this, a single basic approach to treatment, divided into separate modules, is advocated. The first covers the non-surgical gingival response and the second covers surgery.

Gingival response module

The gingival response module is represented by gingival therapy. This is applicable to every clinical situation regardless of the extent or pattern of periodontal breakdown. Thus, although debridement becomes more difficult in periodontal pocket therapy, the measures themselves remain unchanged. The application of this basic gingival response treatment module to gingivitis will be considered first in Chapter 10. This is then followed by its clinical applications to the more complex treatment needs of early, moderate and advanced periodontitis in Chapters 11 and 12.

Surgical module

The surgical module will also be shown to be applicable to all the various situations requiring surgical intervention (*cf.* Chapter 14). This is because the flexibility of simple pocket surgery means that any additional measures, found to be necessary at operation, will be little more than deviations from the predetermined basic procedural sequence. This also means that all clinical cases can be handled essentially in the same way, irrespective of their presentation, so simplifying both treatment planning and treatment itself.

The surgical module will first be described for the management of the simple periodontal pocket, which is distinguished by the pocket base lying coronal to the crest of the alveolar bone (suprabony pocket), in Chapters 15 and 16 followed by a miscellany of surgical considerations in Chapter 17. This basic module is then extended to complex pocket surgery, where and when necessary, to cope with the various morphological situations encountered. These are adverse root furcation morphology (Chapter 18), uneven patterns of attachment loss and the extension of the pocket base apical to the crest of the alveolar bone (intrabony pocket) (Chapter 19), the relationship of the pocket base to the vestibular mucosal folds (Chapter 20) and finally, pockets associated with the mandibular retromolar, maxillary tuberosity and palatal vault mucosal and bony forms (Chapters 16 and 20).

Each of these operative hurdles can be handled as they are encountered at operation and, moreover, as individual surgical exercises incorporated within the basic sequence of simple pocket surgery. However, the attainment of the basic surgical objectives may be thwarted at some sites, thus enforcing a compromise result.

The roles of patient and operator in treatment

The patient and gingival therapy

The gingival response to the patient's effective plaque control is predictable. That is, regardless of the extent of disease, complete resolution of inflammation of the pocket wall *marginal tissue* will occur by the patient's efforts alone, provided the adjacent root surfaces are reasonably accessible. This goal of gingival therapy is paramount in achieving optimal healing following not only subgingival debridement but, more importantly, disease control at persistent pocket sites following periodontal surgery. There are a number of reasons for this.

Firstly, success in all but a few investigations of both non-surgical and surgical treatment methods has been shown to depend primarily upon the maintenance of a high level of supragingival plaque control by the patient. Secondly, it appears that the frequency of any subsequent subgingival debridement, regardless of the initial treatment method, is also dependent upon supragingival plaque levels. This is because subgingival recolonization is more rapid in the presence of poor oral hygiene. Thirdly, the variable pattern and extent of the disease means that sites, which are relatively or even totally inaccessible to the patient, frequently persist following surgical therapy. The proven ability of the patient to negotiate such areas following surgery, based on the efforts demonstrated during gingival therapy, is essential before embarking upon surgery. Whilst frequent compensatory professional cleaning may be possible technically in such cases, the demands made upon professional resources to compensate for the patient's ineffective efforts will preclude its implementation on a community basis.

Finally, it is important to accept that pocket surgery alone cannot ensure plaque control. It follows then that to undertake surgery before the demonstration of efficient plaque control and an optimal gingival response, as outlined above, is to court failure. Similarly, recurrence of the disease, following even successful surgery, cannot be prevented unless the criterion of efficient plaque control by the patient is observed.

The operator and gingival therapy

The creation of the conditions conducive to an optimal gingival response, at all levels of periodontitis, is the function of the operator. This consists primarily of the removal of plaque which is inaccessible to the patient and which, next to patient education and the supervision of plaque control, represents the operator's main task.

In contrast, the surgical techniques designed to facilitate debridement, to correct any residual pockets, alter unfavourable root forms or vestibular morphology must be considered of only secondary importance. The importance of these techniques is related to facilitating the operator's management of sites deemed to be totally inaccessible and, therefore, responsible for persistent plaque retention and in turn, progressive disease. However, recent periodontal research indicates that not all plaque-induced inflammation at pocket-associated dentoepithelial junctions will be accompanied by progressive tissue destruction. Unfortunately, there is no current method of distinguishing between the inactive sites from those that are potentially destructive, although the overall risk of further destruction appears to be greater at inflamed sites. The rationale of therapy in this text is therefore based primarily on the creation and maintenance of plaque-free and uninflamed dento-epithelial junctions at individual sites, regardless of their locations, by gingival therapy to minimize the risk of any future acute episodes.

In summary, the control of bacterial plaque activity by the combined cleaning efforts of patient and operator remains the fundamental objective of therapy and any operative manipulation of dento-gingival form serves only to expedite these plaque control measures. The rationale supporting the role of surgical therapy in plaque removal deserves further examination.

The rationale for surgical intervention

It must be re-emphasized that the results of research have shown that in moderate and even some cases of advanced disease it has been possible to maintain comparable levels of attachment using either surgic-al or non-surgical treatment methods (*cf.* Chapters 28 and 29). However, the bulk of these findings are based on the analysis of mean data relating to treatment of segments rather than individual sites. Such analysis may be misleading because recent concepts about the pattern of disease suggest that it has a site-specific distribution. Furthermore, the clinical parameters used in these investigations have been shown to be unreliable predictors of disease activity (*cf.* Chapters 13, 28 and 29).

There are instances when further loss of attach-ment has occurred following periodontal surgery. This is presumably because the surgical objective, of a cleansible dentogingival junction, has not been achieved in cases of advanced disease, and more especially, when complications are present. The justification for surgery might then be questioned, although the creation of less inaccessible root surfaces for subsequent periodic professional clean-ing could contribute to a reduced rate of attachment loss. On the other hand, creation of cleansible dento-epithelial junctions must remain the fun-damental surgical objective. Where unattainable, the prognosis with regard to subsequent subgingival debridement should be evaluated carefully before intervening surgically. It is also worth considering whether more intensive subgingival debridement, with or without chemotherapeutic measures, could achieve a similar result to the inevitable compromise of pocket reduction surgery. In some instances, even in moderate cases, the disease will continue due to a misconception on the patient's part that surgical treatment constitutes an end in itself. There should be no doubt on the patient's part that any failure to maintain the level of plaque control established

prior to therapy will create a risk of further tissue breakdown.

It follows that the role of the patient is paramount and that non-surgical therapy must take precedence over surgical therapy. Optimal plaque control by the patient at *totally* and *reasonably accessible* sites must be mastered as the essential first stage of any treatment plan. If this cannot be accomplished at these sites then it is unlikely to be achieved elsewhere following pocket surgery. Moreover, it has been shown that increased rates of loss are likely to follow surgical intervention in the presence of, and when followed by, persistent plaque-induced inflammation.

Finally, the ethical demands of using the simplest and least invasive forms of professional interference highlight the essential role of non-surgical therapy. This is reinforced by the limitations of skilled manpower and the high cost of appropriately trained professional expertise. These factors provide an economic reason for limiting such an expensive resource to only those situations where it is essential.

The prevention of recurrent disease

For the vast majority of individuals, recurrent disease can be prevented whenever the dento-epithelial junction is cleansible and is coupled with an effective patient cleaning regime. Patient super-vision at defined periods and professional care appear to be necessary in most cases, although the importance of professional cleaning has been placed in perspective by the maintenance of gingival health in individuals where professional cleaning has been matched against patient cleaning of contralateral sites (*cf.* Chapter 27). Sites which, despite surgical treatment, prove to be inaccessible to oral hygiene methods can be expected to demonstrate persistent signs of inflammation, with or without further losses of attachment. Where attachment loss is apparent, the rate of this progressive breakdown might be retarded by careful periodic professional cleaning. The use of chemotherapeutic measures should also be considered. When, by these aptly described continuation therapy measures, the longevity of the dentition is extended giving a level of disease which can be regarded as tolerable, this could be accepted as a reasonable alternative to attaining absolute periodontal health. Indeed, the objective of *toler-able disease*, rather than *absolute periodontal health*, might prove ultimately to be the objective of choice in most individuals (*cf.* Chapters 26 and 27).

10

The principles of disease management

The marginal gingival lesion
The importance of inflammatory resolution
The accessibility of plaque
The oral hygiene regime

Professional tooth cleaning
The patient's assessment of oral hygiene
The operator's assessment of oral hygiene
The barriers to plaque removal

As stated in the previous chapter, the successful therapy of existing disease and the prevention of further disease consists of controlling dental plaque at the dento-epithelial junction. In early disease, this junction is located at the base of the slightly deepened gingival sulcus and when it is clear that disease control must depend primarily on the patient, for whom professional guidance and support is provided. This relates to attention to plaque retention factors adjacent to the detached marginal tissues and, where necessary, professional cleaning. This, in turn, constitutes gingival therapy, although some overlapping is inevitable in some instances with simple pocket therapy, which is characterized by subgingival debridement at the more apically located dentogingival junctions at the pocket bases. Because this gingival therapy regime is also the essential feature of all periodontal therapy, regardless of the extent of periodontal destruction and the location of the dento-epithelial junction at the pocket bases, the management of early disease serves as a blueprint for all treatment.

The marginal gingival lesion

Plaque and marginal inflammation

Marginal gingivitis is due solely to persistent plaque deposits on the adjacent tooth surface as shown in Figure 10.1 (A–C). It is also known that the presence of marginal inflammation will itself encourage the further development of plaque (cf. Chapter 29 – Post-surgical maintenance) whilst systemic effects, such as pregnancy, will merely alter the nature of the reaction by the gingivae to the plaque. Resolution of this gingival inflammation will occur when plaque is removed and prevented from

reforming. It follows from this that the signs of marginal inflammation, such as redness and bleeding, can be attributed to inadequate plaque control by the patient and in turn, that evaluation of the patient's cleaning efforts can be based upon the clinical status of the marginal gingivae. This evaluation of the patient's cleaning effort is also of fundamental importance in the management of all stages of disease.

Marginal inflammation and attachment loss

The relationship between marginal inflammation and the progressive loss of periodontal attachment in the pathogenesis of the disease is not understood clearly. The classic view of the inevitable progress of disease is also being increasingly questioned. Thus, it is now known that a marginal gingival lesion can persist without any loss of attachment, and that even established areas of periodontal destruction may persist for years without progressing further. On the other hand, in those instances where destruction does progress, the exact sites at which this occurs can neither be predicted nor the rate of resultant loss of attachment established. This destruction could, in some instances, be so slow that a tolerable level of disease is maintained for the individual's life span, yet in others be quite rapid. Unfortunately, it is not at present possible to distinguish, in the short term, the sites of slow deterioration from others where the lesion is progressing at a more rapid rate (cf. Chapter 28 – Probing and disease progression).

The many different stages of the disease encountered within the same mouth bear evidence to the unpredictability of the reaction of the periodontium to the presence of plaque as shown in Figure 9.1. The clinician is unable, even in retrospect, to determine exactly how any particular presentation

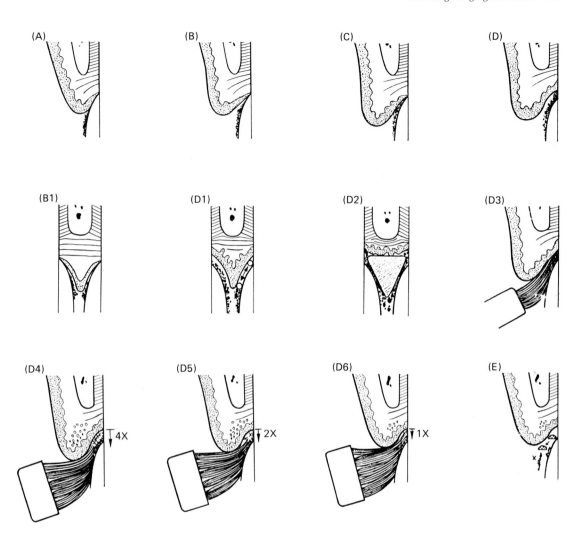

Figure 10.1 The dentogingival form and plaque accessibility. (A) Normal sulcus with totally accessible supragingival plaque. (B) Slight gingival swelling and detachment of coronal part of junctional epithelium with onset of gingivitis – note (B1) corresponding interdental lesion. (C) Further swelling with epithelial proliferation and development of rete ridges but no attachment loss (false pocket). Associated 'subgingival' plaque still accessible. (D and D1) Loss of attachment and apical proliferation of junctional epithelium (true pocket). Subgingival plaque is reasonably accessible to (D1) dental floss and (D2) wood point at interdental sites and elsewhere to (D3) interspace or (D4) ordinary toothbrush when bristles splayed out subgingivally. (D4–D6) Gingival response to phased removal of only reasonably accessible plaque denoted by (4X–1X) in the presence of calculus deposits. Note: progressive inflammatory resolution and gingival shrinkage with gradual reduction of pocket depth, which facilitates (E) professional cleaning

has occurred. The variable clinical presentation of disease is presumably due to different times of onset and differing rates of breakdown. These may, in turn, be due to inconsistent levels of plaque control, changes in the types of bacteria or their pathogenicity, variable local interactions between organisms and defence factors, or changes in systemic defence factors that allow existing combinations of bacteria

to become locally destructive. Similarly, the altered local environment associated with gingival swelling and the false pocketing it causes, may tilt the balance between microbiota and host and lead to the loss of attachment. The resulting true pocket then constitutes a plaque retention factor and, unless overcome, the disease may continue. The need for the professional management of the root surface by subgingival debridement does, at this stage, represent the link between gingival therapy and simple pocket therapy.

The importance of inflammatory resolution

Therapeutic axioms

Whatever factors do underly the distribution of sites undergoing destruction or the rate at which this destruction proceeds, there are four fundamental practical considerations. The first of these is that persistent marginal inflammation is due to the patient's failure to control plaque. The next is that destruction will not progress in the absence of plaque at the dento-epithelial junction, be this located at the base of the gingival sulcus or a periodontal pocket. The third is that subgingival bacterial colonization from the outset, and following debridement, is dependent upon the supragingival plaque levels. The last is, as destruction of the periodontium continues progressively greater obstacles to the patient's efforts in control of plaque develop. It is, therefore, essential to strive for optimal plaque control by the patient and marginal tissue inflammatory resolution at all sites, as the primary clinical objective in all therapy.

Therapeutic rationale

The initial clinical objective of achieving inflammatory resolution of the marginal gingivae may be construed as over-treatment. This charge can however be readily refuted because only the simplest means of achieving plaque control, at reasonably accessible dento-epithelial junctions within pathologically deepened sites, are demanded for any situation. The patient should merely aim, by normal cleaning methods described in Chapter 8, to achieve the basic objective of routine tooth cleaning, that is clean teeth. Such an optimal cleaning regime is moreover not harmful to patients and only commits them to a greater expenditure of time and effort in home care.

The relevance of professional cleaning in any therapeutic regime must be put in perspective. Thus, while it has been shown that marginal gingival health can be maintained by a regime of optimal oral hygiene and frequent professional cleaning, one study has demonstrated that attending simply for professional supervision, without any professional cleaning, was sufficient for the maintenance of health. The need for, and frequency of, professional cleaning should, therefore, be established according to individual requirements related to the accessibility of plaque and should not become a periodic routine (*cf.* Chapter 29 – Post-surgical maintenance). Moreover, the economics of current clinical practice and the limited manpower, in most communities, does also mean that any professionally mediated periodontal care system could only be offered to relatively few people. Yet, even in these few cases, the responsibility for plaque control must still rest ultimately with the patient. It is this factor therefore that must remain the most important component in effective periodontal care. The accessibility of the tooth surfaces to plaque control measures can now be considered.

The accessibility of plaque

Ideal dentogingival form

Most individuals will have possessed dentogingival junctions with a normal morphology before disease commenced (Figure 10.1 A). Despite this, and the reasonable assumption that totally unimpeded access existed for cleaning at the outset, disease does occur as shown in Figure 8.1 (G and H) and Figure 10.1 (B and B1). The inescapable conclusion must be that a normal dentogingival relationship will not in itself preclude the initial onset of disease and that the patient's failure with oral hygiene must be held solely responsible for the occurrence of disease (*cf.* Chapter 29).

Dentogingival form in early disease

The minor morphological changes of early disease should present no difficulties to routine cleaning measures in individuals with average manual dexterity (Figure 10.1 C and D). Thus, the offending plaque is located on the tooth surfaces immediately adjacent to the gingival margins and within the shallow subgingival spaces, created by swollen gingivae (false pockets) (Figure 10.1 C) or the development of true pockets where minimal detachment has occurred (Figure 10.1 D). These sites are therefore deemed to be reasonably accessible as shown in Figure 10.1 (D1–D6). This has fundamental implications in the management of all disease, for where oral hygiene is not improved, disease will persist even without the development of inaccessible sites with the progression of disease, as depicted in Figure 10.2.

Relatively and totally inaccessible plaque

Any effort made by the operator to improve accessibility at sites which are difficult to clean would, at best, have only limited and short-lived benefit in those who have not already mastered plaque control at reasonably accessible sites. It should also be clear that efforts devoted by both patient and operator in controlling the plaque front,

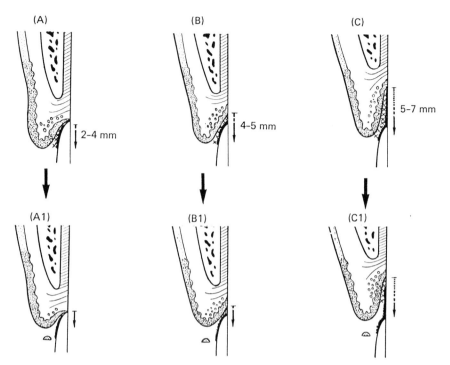

Figure 10.2 Accessibility of plaque front to oral hygiene measures and phased therapy. (A) Plaque (×××) reasonably accessible (———→) in gingivitis. (B) Relatively inaccessible (– – – –→) in early periondontis. (C) Totally inaccessible (--------→) in moderate periodontitis. Removal of reasonably accessible plaque followed by (A1–C1) gingival response facilitates subgingival instrumentation. Note: tissue shrinkage following instrumentation to only reasonably accessible depths renders plaque front progressively more accessible to subsequent cleaning (phased professional cleaning)

before its downgrowth has rendered it inaccessible to routine oral hygiene measures, will prevent many of the problems subsequently encountered in periodontal therapy. This does, however, not mean that the bacterial plaque front at these deeper subgingivally located root surfaces will inevitably be inaccessible to all patients. The conscientious, dexterous individual will often succeed in subgingival cleaning and should be encouraged to attempt to do so at these relatively inaccessible sites although, as shown in Figure 10.2, there will be areas that are inaccessible to even these high performers.

Sites where the plaque front is totally inaccessible to the patient require specific professional attention which is dealt with in subsequent chapters (simple pocket therapy). Although the need for this professional intervention will vary from site to site and from one patient to the other and that as a result, gingival therapy and simple pocket therapy will often overlap (see Figure 9.4 and Figure 10.2 (B and C)), the initial objective in the management of all levels of disease still remains the same. That is the resolution of marginal inflammation by the

control of the reasonably accessible plaque by the patient. The clinician must therefore ensure that the patient understands the problems of cleaning and knows how to cope with them (see below). The effects of these plaque control efforts are then monitored by the response of the gingival tissues. The associated gingival shrinkage as shown in Figure 10.1 (E) and Figure 10.2 (A1–C1), results in improved access for professional cleaning of subgingival deposits of residual plaque and of calculus. This forms the basis for the phased professional cleaning advocated.

The oral hygiene regime

The techniques in early disease are no different from those used for preventing disease in the presence of physiological or an uninflamed altered dentogingival form (*cf.* Chapter 8). The patient need merely adapt them to the minor morphological changes that have developed, as shown in Figure 10.1 (D). These technical modifications have already been referred to in Chapter 8, but are briefly reiterated here.

Brushing technique

The toothbrush bristles will need to be more splayed out in order to penetrate into the deeper gingival sulci or pockets (Figure 10.1 D4). Where the disease is unevenly distributed a single tufted brush is preferable (Figure 10.1 D3), for it can be more readily introduced into the most involved sites. Over-eager vigour is unnecessary for plaque removal and may even be counter-productive, by scratching the inflamed gingivae which might in turn inhibit subsequent cleaning.

Interdental cleaning

The detached interdental papillae allow a greater area of approximal tooth surface to be exposed to plaque growth and so necessitate more diligent interdental cleaning. Consequently, the interdental cleaning devices such as dental floss, interspace and interproximal brushes and wood points must be manipulated more carefully to engage these relatively inaccessible subgingival surfaces as shown previously in Figure 8.6 and in Figure10.1 (D1 and D2). Suitable techniques should be chosen and adapted as necessary and their efficiency judged on the basis of individual achievement. Any difficult sites should be identified and their cleaning demonstrated to the satisfaction of the patient, so that the simplest route to effective plaque control for each individual can be selected.

Scheduling professional supervision

The appropriate cleaning techniques are demonstrated at the initial appointment. Once these have been grasped by the patient a review appointment is made. Sufficient time must then be allowed for the patient to learn to clean efficiently and also for some inflammatory resolution to take place, by the gingival response as depicted in Figure 10.1 (D4–D6). An initial interval of about 4–6 weeks is considered reasonable for this, but as oral hygiene is deemed to be a self-learning process the patient's view on this, and subsequent time intervals, must also be sought. Flexibility is essential for both operator and patient to find a regime that suits them both. For example, some clinicians advocate weekly intervals between appointments, for closer supervision of the patient's efforts and more importantly it seems, for regular professional tooth cleaning. The role of professional cleaning can now be examined.

Professional tooth cleaning

Routine scaling and polishing

It has become a convention for patients attending a periodic dental review to expect to have their teeth scaled and polished. This probably stems from a widespread professional acceptance of routine scaling and polishing. However, the rationale for this is by no means clear. Many studies have demonstrated the clinical benefits of regular professional cleaning but without establishing why this is effective. This is probably due to the difficulty in distinguishing between the removal of calculus and the removal of plaque. The feeling of well-being derived from professional cleaning might also be important for some people and certainly the motivational effect of the visit alone has already been the subject of comment (*cf.* Chapter 7).

It must be assumed that provided all plaque is removed during professional cleaning some benefit must accrue even if the effect may be short-lived. However, it is questionable if the type of professional cleaning commonly carried out is effective. This is presumably a reflection of the short time taken to carry out the procedure as well as a lack of appreciation of the problems encountered. It might therefore be helpful to examine the clinical importance of calculus before considering further the role of professional tooth cleaning.

The relevance of calculus

Calculus is a feature of only secondary importance in periodontal disease. The importance of calculus lies in its comparative roughness, which may complicate or even prevent the complete removal of plaque by both patient and operator. Plaque is undoubtedly the primary instigator and will accumulate on any tooth surface whether calculus is present or not. Furthermore, it is possible to achieve a favourable gingival response with calculus still present (*cf.* Chapter 28 – The assessment of adequate debridement). In addition, patients who do not clean effectively will, despite regular professional cleaning, present with further deposits of calculus. Whereas, those who do clean effectively between review appointments will have no calculus. Finally, although some patients appear to have a greater propensity to form calculus than others, there is no indication that it will form in the absence of plaque. Residual islands of calculus which remain behind following incomplete professional cleaning may, however, promote the development of further calculus (see also Chapter 28).

The sequence of professional cleaning

At the initial appointment instruction in oral hygiene is the major consideration. Emphasis must therefore be placed on the importance of the removal of plaque, as opposed to calculus. Furthermore, although removal of calculus (scaling) at this stage will inevitably also be accompanied by the simultaneous removal of any superimposed or adjacent uncalcified plaque, it is advocated only where the deposits are so extensive that they totally block access to the interdental spaces, or prevent reasonable access to the necks of the teeth (see Figure 9.1 D).

There are several potential disadvantages to carrying out the traditionally practised professional cleaning, scaling and polishing at the initial diagnostic visit. First and foremost, it de-emphasizes the importance of the patient's own role in cleaning. Secondly, it reinforces the long established dependency of the patient on professional care for the purpose of maintaining gingival health. Thirdly, it should be evident that professional care is not the solution to periodontal health for, if it were, patients who had been attending routinely in the past would not present with persistent disease. Fourthly, it is possible that patients, apprehensive about the impending scaling, may not give sufficient attention to the advice about oral hygiene. In addition, this advice might be regarded simply as a chairside ploy to allay fear of the 'real' treatment of scaling, that is to follow. Finally, scaling can be quite difficult to carry out at the initial visit in individuals with marked gingival inflammation and tenderness and, more especially, when pocketing is also present. This scaling may even discourage further attendance in some cases. These arguments form the basis of the phased therapy advocated for both gingival and simple pocket therapy, as depicted in Figure 10.2.

As much of the instrumentation in professional cleaning in the management of disease is directed at subgingival bacterial plaque, and although both plaque and any calcified accretions may be removed, the term subgingival debridement, introduced in Chapter 9, is preferable to that of the more traditional and imprecise use of the term subgingival scaling. This terminology also describes the subgingival professional cleaning procedure more clearly with respect to its objective of plaque control.

The advantages of phased therapy

The principle of delaying instrumentation here in gingival therapy, but more especially in simple pocket therapy, until subsequent visits (as will be shown later) has yet to be substantiated by objective studies. The adoption of such a regime of phased therapy is therefore a matter of professional judgement. The possible risks involved in any delay in resolving subgingival inflammation caused by this approach must not be discounted but should, however, also be put in perspective. Thus, in the vast majority of cases the delay could hardly be relevant when related to the existing history of the disease, whilst the practical advantages of deferring instrumentation soon become apparent to the clinician as treatment proceeds (*cf.* Chapter 13 – Gingival response).

Subgingival debridement becomes much easier as a result of the gingival response to the initial improved cleaning efforts of the patient. The gradually reduced amount of inflammation means that the gingivae become less tender, making subgingival professional cleaning more acceptable for the patient, while the associated shrinkage of the gingival margins provides easier access to subgingival deposits as shown in Figure 10.2 (A1–C1). There is also a reduction in the amount of bleeding that occurs during instrumentation which might otherwise obscure operator vision and thus complicate the exercise.

Finally, where the exposed dentinal surfaces are sensitive to instrumentation, this will gradually decrease with time and so further justify delaying professional cleaning. The sum total effect of the gingival response is that a difficult task is made much easier.

In summary, while the establishment of plaque and calculus-free dento-epithelial junctions, at deepened gingival sulci and pockets, at the earliest possible time following diagnosis is theoretically an ideal objective, it is often impractical. In addition, the effects of intentionally delaying subgingival cleaning, as advocated here, should be weighed against the common professional practice of ineffective subgingival instrumentation because of technical difficulties, being accepted by default.

The patient's assessment of oral hygiene

Self-examination

In view of the importance of the dominant role of the patient in treatment and that of self-learning advocated here, the patient's ability to assess his own cleaning effort is considered crucial. The traditional direct method of evaluating cleaning, by the use of disclosing agents, is described in Chapter 8. This requires no further comment save to reiterate that any problem of reduced visibility within the mouth can be overcome with practice, especially if a pen-light is used in conjunction with the obligatory dental mirror.

Once a patient, seeking periodontal health, is convinced of the importance of homecare in treatment, concern is aroused to ensure that this is properly carried out and more importantly that the expected healing does actually follow. This self-interest may therefore be utilized by extending the principle of self-examination, with respect to the use of a disclosing agent, to the marginal tissues as well.

Plaque and gingival inflammation relationships

Bleeding or mild gingival tenderness during tooth cleaning is considered by many patients to be quite normal. This assumption is incorrect and the importance of interpreting these signs instead as positive indicators of inflammation as a result of inadequate oral hygiene, must be stressed. Conversely, that resolution of these signs represents a reliable indirect indicator of the efficacy of plaque control.

The direct relationship between inflammation and bacterial plaque on the teeth, is most readily demonstrated to the patient, by scraping away with a probe some of the plaque from one small area of a tooth adjacent to marginal inflammation. Plaque that may initially be invisible to a patient, accumulates on the probe and can then be seen readily. This visual impact can be reinforced by applying a small amount of disclosing solution to just this tooth, demonstrating the presence of staining on only the adjacent uninstrumented parts of the tooth surface. This small demonstration may also serve concurrently as a convenient introduction, in some instances, to the use of disclosing agents.

Recognition of marginal inflammation

The marginal gingivae can be examined by the patient who has been taught to recognize the signs of redness and swelling that signify gingival inflammation. These simple visual signs of inflammation should be no more difficult to recognize than those associated with a pimple on the face. Marginal inflammation can also be detected by the finding of gingival bleeding, with or without tenderness, during cleaning. The patient can be persuaded quite readily, that this bleeding is not normal, by attempting and failing to provoke bleeding by forceful brushing at any obviously healthy site.

On the other hand, gingival pain and bleeding can be provoked by traumatic abrasion of the gingivae. Such lesions simply reflect the patient's lack of finesse or over-enthusiastic use of the toothbrush or other cleaning aids. Faulty brushing is often associated with the presence of abrasion grooves at the necks of some teeth, together with marginal gingival recession (see Figure 8.7). Bleeding and tenderness associated with trauma can be distinguished from that associated with plaque by the site at which bleeding occurs. The former arises from an ulcerated gingival surface, whilst the latter comes from within the inflamed gingival sulcus. (For other causes of bleeding see Chapter 25 Acute conditions.)

Detection of subgingival inflammation

When resolution of marginal gingival inflammation occurs, marked by a disappearance of redness from the gingival margin and an absence of bleeding during cleaning, the borderline between health and disease within the gingival pocket can be more difficult to judge. The disclosing agent is unhelpful here, because it only reveals the presence of supragingival plaque. Persistent subgingival inflammation may however be detected quite readily by the patient, by simply directing the bristles of a single tufted brush, more firmly than usual into the gingival pocket and provoking bleeding.

The choice of assessment methods

Clinical experience indicates that most interested patients have little difficulty in identifying marginal inflammation or even subgingival inflammation. The visual signs sought by the patient are in effect no different from those used by the clinician to diagnose disease, and more importantly and logically, to monitor its subsequent progress in response to treatment. Some patients might be reluctant to use this particular method and prefer to use disclosing agents instead. Indeed, some might choose to do nothing and to simply assume that an effective oral hygiene is being practised, whilst awaiting the operator's judgement at recall visits.

Ultimately it does not matter which method of self-assessment is used by the patient, provided that the correct information is obtained. A method should therefore be selected that is best suited to the individual preferences and abilities of the patient.

The operator's assessment of oral hygiene

Direct and indirect assessment

The patient's performance of oral hygiene can be assessed both directly and indirectly. For the former, the plaque is detected by either passing a probe about the neck of every tooth in the arch or by the use of a disclosing agent. Probing is tedious and time consuming, whilst the routine use of disclosing dyes at review appointments is not without its disadvantages. Firstly, most disclosing agents also stain the gingivae, thus masking their true colour and obscuring any visual assessment of the inflammatory status. Secondly, patients might clean uncharacteristically well before the appointment if they know a dye is to be used, or on the other hand, not clean as well as usual, because of some upset in their daily routine. Finally, mucosal staining by the dyes may persist for some hours and so possibly be resented by the patient. This last embarrassment could, however, be avoided by the use of a fluorescent dye.

The 'indirect' method of assessment is preferred because the inflammatory state of the marginal gingivae is quite unequivocal in determining the effectiveness of the patient's cleaning efforts. At this stage the operator functions as a physician concerned primarily with the clinical signs of disease.

Furthermore, as the initial diagnosis is based on such parameters it is logical that the effects of therapy should also be assessed in a similar fashion. However advanced the disease, the 'indirect' method of assessing plaque control remains valid.

Interpretation of assessment

The presence of marginal redness, with or without bleeding on blunt probing (with a 'Williams' periodontal probe, *cf.* Chapter 13) is usually due simply to faulty oral hygiene. This and other reasons for the persistence of bacterial plaque are discussed below together with the appropriate corrective measures.

The status of the marginal gingivae at the affected site is first compared with that at another site which is readily accessible for cleaning and at which no signs of inflammation would be expected. The buccal aspects of the upper incisors might be representative of such an area. If this area is also inflamed it is difficult to avoid the conclusion of faulty oral hygiene. The fault may be due to the basic mechanics of brushing, a lack of understanding or even concern about the problem. It may also merely be due to poor manual dexterity. Each of these possibilities should be considered and the true reason established by elimination.

When marginal inflammation is observed only at isolated sites it should first be assumed that there is a problem of accessibility. The manner of cleaning is first observed and followed by questioning to reveal any other possible factors. The cause can usually be established if the operator merely takes the time to observe the patient's cleaning technique. Where the cleaning technique is shown to be at fault, appropriate advice is given. A modification to the existing technique may be sufficient or an alternative technique may be needed.

Where the cleaning technique of the patient cannot be faulted, a search should be made for some factor inhibiting effective plaque removal. This could be a plaque retention factor (Figure 10.3) such as calculus or an overhanging restoration margin, a morphological feature of the tooth surface, or the soft tissue morphology related to the site, impeding access for cleaning. These various factors are briefly reviewed below, but their management will not be considered until the following chapter.

The barriers to plaque removal
Surface features of the tooth

The normally smooth glossy surface of a tooth (Figure 10.3 A) is readily cleaned, whilst the

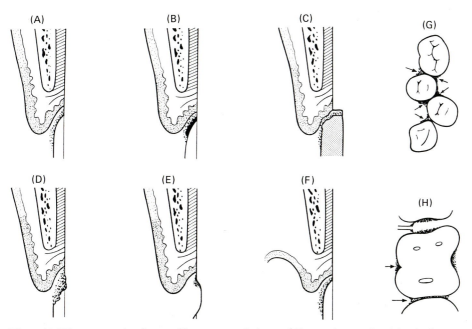

Figure 10.3 Plaque retention factors. Plaque accumulation on (A) smooth enamel and dentine/cementum surfaces within shallow pockets, (B) subgingival calculus, (C) restoration margin excess or deficiency. Plaque associated with (D) carious lesion, (E) abrasion cavity margin, (F) shallow vestibular sulcus, (G) imbricated teeth, and (H) root surface concavities/grooves, especially at approximal surfaces and closely related adjacent root surfaces

presence of a rough or uneven surface must be considered difficult and so represents the most basic of the plaque retention factors. This should therefore be excluded before moving further.

Calculus represents a rough surface which may impede removal of plaque, because of its form and site of deposition (Figure 10.3 B). This is also true of the excess margin and deficiencies found on fillings and crowns (Figure 10.3 C). Surface defects caused by concavities and grooves of the natural shape of the anatomical crown or of roots exposed by gingival recession/abrasion (Figure 10.3 E and H) and by caries (Figure 10.3 D) may also be plaque retention factors. In addition, the relationships of adjacent teeth, where these are imbricated or otherwise malaligned (Figure 10.3 G), may impede access.

Dentine sensitivity

Dentinal sensitivity is commonly caused by toothbrush abrasion and root surfaces exposed by gingival recession. Acid erosion may also be present to complicate the situation, as may caries, as additional causes of cervical sensitivity (*cf.* Chapter 25). All or any of these factors can make it difficult for the patient to remove plaque efficiently from the cervical margin of the tooth.

Soft tissue problems

Soft tissue can also interfere with efficient control of plaque because of morphology or physiology. The former occurs with such factors as changes of marginal gingival form brought about by disease (Figure 10.3 A), or a prominent mucosal frenal insertion or a shallow vestibular sulcus (Figure 10.3 F). The latter are such factors as a hypersensitive gag reflex, a hyperactive tongue or a strong reflex lip activity.

Each of the above create potential obstacles to effective cleaning that need to be identified by questioning and observation. It is better to start with the most obvious possibility and progress by elimination to the other factors. The patient must then be advised and convinced to his own satisfaction of the problem, which can then be corrected.

Differential diagnosis

Finally, although the signs of persistent inflammation of the gingivae can, for all practical purposes, be attributed to the presence of plaque, the possibility of another condition should not be overlooked. For example, erosive lichen planus, which is not uncommon, might masquerade as periodontal disease, as might localized gingival redness and ulceration associated with toothbrush trauma (*cf.* Chapter 25).

11

The technique of disease management

I.   Gingival therapy

It should be clear from the foregoing text that there is really no fundamental difference between treating early disease or preventing the onset of disease. The key to both is access to, and control of, plaque at the dentogingival junctions by the patient. The operator's function in early disease is to help, where necessary, the suitably instructed patient, by improved oral hygiene technique, to gain access to these sites. In early disease, this consists mainly of removing any plaque retention factors, of which calculus is the most ubiquitous. It must be reiterated that any such calculus removal without optimal supragingival plaque control will achieve no lasting results. The technical management of these plaque retention factors is now considered.

Calculus deposits

The difficulties of scaling

The attachment of calculus to subgingival root surfaces can be very tenacious, making its removal extremely difficult. The confined nature of the pocket space obviously complicates scaling and increases the potential hazard of trauma to the soft tissues. In addition, the dentine is often sensitive to instrumentation. With these difficulties, plus the painstaking nature of the operation, it is hardly

surprising that scaling is frequently carried out ineffectively and is popular with neither patient nor operator. It must also be stressed that while the removal of plaque retentive calculus is the prime consideration here, such efforts will inevitably remove the associated non-calcified bacterial plaque. Similarly, as any professional removal of subgingival plaque will use the same instruments, most if not all the associated calculus will also be removed in the process. Those parts of the following discussion, relating to subgingival calculus removal, can therefore not be divorced from that of subgingival plaque removal, with which it is clinically so inseparably linked but more precisely defined as subgingival debridement.

Instrument types

There are numerous patterns of scalers, curettes and hoes available for scaling, each of which has presumably been the favourite of someone at some time. Choice is therefore subjective and the recommendation of Hawe–Neos scalers (Hawe–Neos Dental Dr H. v. Weissenfluh AG, CH-6925 Gentilino, Switzerland; supplied by Glover Dental Supplies Ltd, Lancaster Road, Shrewsbury SY1 3NF, Shropshire, UK), Goldman–Fox curettes (Goldman–Fox Hu-Friedy Manufacturing Co. Inc., Chicago, IL, USA) and hoes (Figure 11.1), Gracey periodontal finishing curettes (Gracy

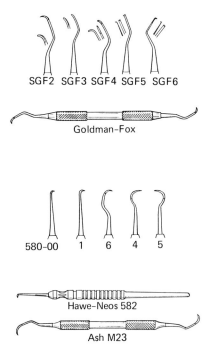

Figure 11.1 Instruments. Goldman–Fox curettes (SGF 2, SGF 3, SGF 4) and hoes (SGF 5 and SGF 6). Note SGF 2 is a 'special curette' with only one cutting edge while SGF 3 and SGF 4 are 'universal' with two cutting edges. Hawe–Neos scaler No. 580 with removable tips. '00', miniature sickle; '1', small sickle; '4', left sickle; '5', right sickle; '6', straight sickle. Ash M 23 scaler

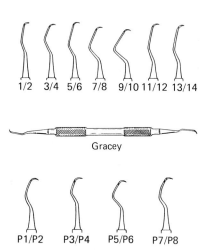

Figure 11.2 Instruments. Gracey periodontal finishing curettes (1/2–13/14). Gracey prophylactic instruments (curettes) with heavier shanks (P1/P2–P7/P8). All Gracey curettes have only one cutting edge. Note 7/8, 11/12 and 13/14 constitute an effective 'short' set

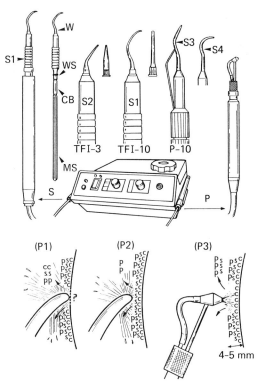

Figure 11.3 Cavi-jet dental prophylaxis unit incorporates ultrasonic scaling (S) and air abrasive polishing (Prophy-Jet) (P) modes. Cavitron insert (SI) showing TFI-10 insert tip, water outlet (W) for preheated water (from cooling the hand-piece) to the activated tip, collar with water seal (WS), connecting body (CB) which transmits motion from magnetostrictive stack (MS) to insert tip. Enlarged views of TFI-3 (S2) and TFI-10 (S1) inserts and the original P-10 (S3) design type P-10 with external water tube. The temper of the P-10 tip allows tip curvature to be modified for improved access to certain sites. Tip has been straightened slightly at S3 for deep lingual and palatal pockets at anterior teeth and curved more (S4) for distal surfaces of posterior teeth and retroclined incisors. Cavi-Ultrasonic mode (P1) for removal of plaque (PP), calculus (CC) and staining (SS) by a combination of mechanical oscillation of the tip and cavitational implosive effect of the spray. (P2) Plaque removal alone by cavitation effect. (P3) Prophy-Jet insert used 4–5 mm from tooth surface for removal of plaque and staining

Hu-Friedy Manufacturing Co. Inc., Chicago, IL, USA) and prophylactic curettes (Figure 11.2) and the Cavitron ultrasonic scaler (Cavitron Dentsply International Inc., York, PA, USA) with the newer designed thru-flow TFI-3 and TFI-10 inserts or the original P3 and P10 insert design (Figure 11.3) is a matter of personal choice. The Ash M23 scaler (Ash Instrument Division, Dentsply Ltd, Gloucester GL1 5SG, UK) is also very useful, being very similar in design and rigidity to that of the Hawe–Neos No. 4 and 5 inserts.

The instruments recommended above can be used for all levels of disease, although some are better suited than others. Thus, the delicately sized blades of the Gracey periodontal finishing curettes are especially useful at deep localized pockets, while the shorter and slightly heavier shanks of their prophylactic counterparts are more suitable during pocket surgery. Similarly, the Goldman–Fox curettes are preferred for surgical use. Their short, comparatively heavy, blades are also ideally suited to heavy deposits and tenaciously adherent subgingival calculus in deep pockets that are not accessible to the Hawe–Neos scalers. Hoes are also used in such situations. All but the Hawe–Neos scalers, the tips of which are replaceable by the operator, are available as double-ended instruments and these are recommended.

The ultrasonic devices operate by generating 25 000 microscopically small mechanical strokes per second at the insert tip. The activated tip when applied to the tooth will, in conjunction with the cavitational implosive effects of the water coolant, dislodge calculus and other accretions as shown in Figure 11.3 (P1). The latter cavitational effect will also remove plaque but not staining or calculus (Figure 11.3 P2). Supragingival staining and plaque is also removed readily by the air-abrasive devices (Figure 11.3 P3) (see also Chapter 28).

Instrumentation

It is not the intention of this text to describe in detail the technique of root surface instrumentation and which particular instrument to use at each tooth surface or the way in which it should be manipulated. Clinical training under careful supervision is essential for this, there being no substitute for practical 'hands on' experience with access to a phantom head as the first stage. The principles of instrumentation are, however, covered below and in Figures. 11.4 and 11.5. It must be realized that whilst gingival therapy alone is under consideration here, these underlying principles are also applicable to simple pocket therapy and simple and complex pocket surgery. The additional technical problems peculiar to more advanced levels of disease, and in particular those of root furcation morphology, are considered in subsequent chapters.

Instrument manipulation

When using the hand instruments it is essential to have a firm comfortable grip on the handle, a stable finger rest on adjacent teeth and to use precise controlled movements (Figure 11.4). Any inadvertent slip of the instrument could lacerate the soft tissues. The two-finger (thumb and first finger) pen-grip (Figure 11.4 B) is recommended for greater precision and control, whereby the second finger is

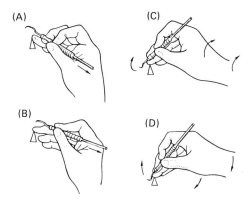

Figure 11.4 Instrument grasp and working strokes. In all instances firm support must be maintained on a tooth represented here by a pivot. (A) Linear stroke executed by resting on the third finger and flexing all three grasping digits towards the palm pulling the instrument (Hawe–Neos 580-6 shown) along its long axis. (B) Linear stroke using the optional two-finger (pen) grip and resting on the second finger. Other working strokes vary only in the direction of instrumentation action at different sites. (C) Lateral hand rotation stroke (Hawe–Neos 580-4 shown) using the third finger as the fulcrum and with the hand and forearm and rotated as a unit. (D) Wrist drop stroke pivoting on the third finger as the fulcrum

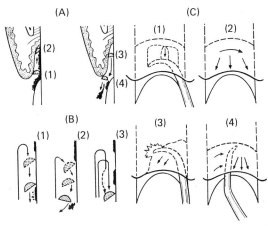

Figure 11.5 Instrumentation technique. Using curette (A1) initial apically directed 'exploratory' stroke to (A2) the appropriate depth judged by tissue resistance and limits of reasonable accessibility. (A3 - A4) Coronally directed 'working' stroke to remove accretions using a (B1) linear or (B2) rotating action, whilst ensuring complete (B3) vertical, and (C1) lateral overlapping. Non-overlapping may also occur when the blade is not maintained in firm even contact with the root as shown by the broken line at (B3). (C) Instrumentation paths may be (1) vertical, (2) oblique or even (3) horizontal direction but when extreme care is required, especially at (C3) sites with uneven pocket depths to avoid laceration of the dento-epithelial junction. (C4) Cavitron TFI-10 tip with optional directions of subgingival instrumentation necessitating use of the side of the tip with a 'sweeping' action and only light pressure

used as the main fixed rest around which all movements are made. The rest of the hand is kept comparatively still during instrumentation giving greater finesse to the exercise. However, digital fatigue soon results. A similar action is used with the three-finger grip (Figure 11.4 A) in which the third finger provides the fixed rest and makes greater instrumentation pressure possible. In contrast, the working strokes with the three-finger grip may also involve the whole hand pivoting about the third and fourth fingers (Figure 11.4 C and D). Even greater force can then be exerted and less fatigue results, so this method may be preferred by some operators. The different instrument grasps and working strokes for the three finger and two finger grips respectively are shown in Figure 11.4.

Patient discomfort will be minimized if the smallest possible instrument is used to achieve any specific task. This is especially important during subgingival scaling with hand instruments, to avoid undue displacement of the related soft tissues (Figure 11.5). Less tissue displacement is required during ultrasonic scaling as the activated instrument tip need only make contact with subgingival deposits. This advantage is however partly offset by the greater dentinal sensitivity usually experienced with ultrasonic instrumentation.

Complete overlapping of instrumentation strokes is absolutely critical (Figure 11.5 B and C) for effective subgingival plaque removal. This is because plaque cannot be detected (like subgingival calculus) by the feel of the instrumented surface.

Non-overlapping instrumentation (Figure 11.5 B) and plaque retention will result in more rapid bacterial recolonization (see below and Chapter 28 – The significance of residual pockets). No such problems exist supragingivally, where calculus is visible and plaque can be disclosed. A more complete tooth surface instrumentation is likely with ultrasonic devices if only because of their greater ease of use (*cf.* Chapter 28). For this reason, coronal tooth surface staining is also most readily removed with ultrasonic tips, although the air abrasive polishing devices (Figure 11.3) are particularly helpful at unevenly worn surfaces and at adjacent tooth surfaces. The latter are, however, less selective in their removal of accretion or tooth tissue.

Instrument care

It is stressed that hand instruments can only be used effectively when sharp. Sharpening instruments is essentially a practical skill, becoming better with practice, and learning from books alone is inadequate. The principles however are covered in Figure 11.6.

Accessibility of calculus

Supragingival calculus is totally accessible to the operator and requires no special attention here. Those deposits located adjacent to the inflamed gingival margins and within shallow pockets, present

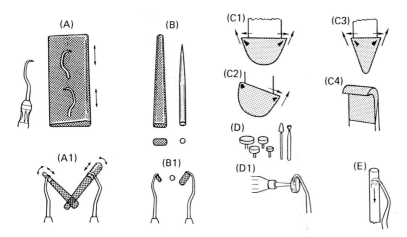

Figure 11.6 Sharpening hand instruments. (A and B) Hand-held wedge-shaped and tapered conical Hu-Friedy oil stones of various grits (e.g. medium India, fine Arkansas) or (D) mounted composition stones are advocated. The technique shown below (A2, B1 and D1) using the appropriately shaped stone. (C1) Universal curettes and (C3) scalers have two cutting edges so may be sharpened (arrowed) on either the face of the blade, the sides of the blade, or on both aspects. (C2) Gracey type curettes with single cutting edges are sharpened on only one side. (C4) Hoes with tungsten tips are best returned to the manufacturer for sharpening or tip replacement. (E) Instrument sharpness is checked by applying the blade at a working angle to a smooth plastic rod or the surface of the fingernail. A sharp edge will gouge out the surface with minimal pressure

in early disease, are in turn reasonably accessible to the operator and should also present no difficulties. These limits represent the extent of gingival therapy. The removal of calculus deposits from within deeper pockets is described under 'Simple pocket therapy'.

The presence of marked inflammation of the gingivae with its accompanying swelling, bleeding and tenderness can complicate the removal of any related calculus by causing the patient pain and obscuring vision during instrumentation. As discussed previously, this complication may be avoided by obtaining partial resolution of the inflammation prior to any professional cleaning. Moreover, unless patient cooperation in oral hygiene can be gained, there is little therapeutic advantage in continuing the scaling regime (*cf.* Chapter 26).

Gingival inflammation and phased instrumentation

Only those deposits readily accessible to the operator are removed in the first instance (*cf.* Periodontal pocket therapy). In addition, patient discomfort can also be minimized by limiting the extent of subgingival instrumentation undertaken at any one appointment. The gingival shrinkage resulting from the gradually improving plaque control means that any residual deposits will be located more superficially, and so make them more accessible at subsequent visits.

Apprehensive patients and those with a low threshold of pain may make instrumentation well nigh impossible. Even the gentler action of the ultrasonic scaler may not be tolerated because of its vibration and high frequency sound. Although local anaesthesia can be used, it skirts the real problem of patient confidence. These situations are best managed by concentrating solely on the patient's control of plaque until it reaches a level at which the benefits of gingival inflammatory resolution become obvious to them. The deposits of calculus can then be removed in stages always ensuring that minimal discomfort is caused. Sensitive dentine may however still require the use of local anaesthesia. There is no universal rule for managing these problems and each case must be treated on its individual merits.

Residual calculus detection

The traditional systematic examination of each tooth with a fine calculus probe is designed to detect any residual deposits of calculus. The fine hook at the end of the probe tip is thus used to locate areas of surface roughness. This 'direct' method of assessment is however not recommended, for it is rather tedious and must be performed both before and immediately after scaling has been carried out and at successive appointments. It is better to delay

any assessment until the subsequent review appointment when residual calculus (and the associated subgingival plaque) may be detected 'indirectly'. This is determined by the signs of persistent gingival inflammation detected by bleeding on blunt probing, or by the bluish discoloration of the overlying marginal gingiva caused by areas of subgingival calculus. Whenever such deposits are suspected they are located with and then removed by the appropriate hand instrument or ultrasonic tip. Although the latter lacks the tactile sensitivity of hand instruments to detect residual calculus, this is of little practical importance. This is because debridement is necessary at such sites regardless of the actual presence of subgingival calculus. Thus, bacterial plaque is of primary importance and the demonstration of subgingival calculus simply confirms that plaque is also present. The clinical significance of this is considered further under 'Simple pocket therapy'. With this option of phased instrumentation, the need for subgingival instrumentation is determined indirectly by the clinical signs related to the presence of deposits. It need therefore be carried out only in the affected sites, which further simplifies treatment.

Supragingival staining

Polishing technique

It is traditional practice to polish the teeth with a fluoridated prophylaxis paste after scaling. This is to remove offending stains (see below) plus any invisible residual plaque as a result of non-overlapping instrumentation within the gingival sulci or shallow pockets. Polishing cups are preferred to avoid abrading the gingivae with rotary brushes. Neither are suitable for the approximal surfaces, at which additional methods, such as the Dentatus 'Eva' (Dentatus Eva System, Dentatus, Hagersten, Sweden) plastic tips (see Figure 11.8 D), manual interproximal spiral brushes or even dental floss are required.

Significance of polishing

The therapeutic rationale for polishing is questionable, for not only is specific interproximal polishing frequently overlooked, presumably reflecting its unimportance clinically, but also none of the methods above are effective beyond a subgingival depth of about 2–3 mm, without traumatizing the gingiva. Also, all those sites that are accessible for such professional polishing are equally accessible to routine oral hygiene measures. Thus, it appears that, beyond the removal of unacceptable staining, the incidental benefit of topical fluoride applications and, possibly, patient motivation, tooth polishing achieves little more than efficient home care. This requires further investigation.

Tooth staining

The presence of extrinsic tooth staining has no significance for gingival health but its removal may provide a powerful motivational incentive for the patient. The introduction of devices such as Cavi-Jet (Figure 11.3) for stain removal have made the procedure quicker and easier, but their potential for damage to hard and soft tissue presents an additional hazard (*cf.* Chapter 28).

Overhanging margins of restorations

Detection

The existence of a restoration overhang is often detected on routine radiographic examination, or clinically by a localized area of inflammation persisting in relation to its cervical margin, whilst adjacent marginal gingival sites appear healthy. Similarly, when bleeding experienced during routine oral hygiene measures is restricted to only such sites. The effects are seen most clearly at subgingival margins of individual porcelain jacket crowns (Figure 11.7 A and B), at grossly overhanging margins of amalgam restorations (Figure 11.7 C) and where approximal cervical overhangs either catch and break dental floss or even prevent the use of any interdental cleaning devices. These findings mean that the patient is usually the best detector of such iatrogenic factors. Indeed, until encountered by the patient, any overhang is of little practical importance because it suggests that routine cleaning at the site will not have been practised. Correction of these restoration margins can well be delayed until the patient has actually complained of difficulties in cleaning. Deferring operative intervention is further warranted by the difficulty sometimes experienced in rectifying the restorations especially when porcelain or cast metal is involved (see below). In addition, practical experience indicates that, where technical difficuulties have precluded modification of any such restorations, the eventual outcome is often no different from sites elsewhere in the mouth, at which comparable margins of easily reduced amalgam restorations have been dealt with. This implies that an adequate gingival response may still accrue from improved plaque control measures, even if they are not optimal. The inherent potential for gingival recession (*cf.* Chapter 13) is critical to the outcome in these situations, because the receding gingival margin will frequently expose the previously inaccessible edges to the restoration.

Site management options

The gingival response

In the first instance, each site is cleaned as well as possible with the Cavitron TFI-10 tip. Specific advice is then given about cleaning with a single tufted brush or where appropriate, dental floss, wood sticks or interproximal brushes. The initial effects of this regime are reviewed after 4–6 weeks. Some resolution of inflammation, accompanied by gingival shrinkage, should have occurred by this stage but if necessary, longer time periods are permitted in the interests of further simplifying any subsequent corrective measures (see below). In some instances, the offending margin of the restoration might even become exposed totally and so no longer impede effective oral hygiene, as shown for example in Figure 11.7 (G–I).

Restoration trimming or replacement

The defective restoration margin may either be trimmed down or the restoration replaced. The choice of options depends primarily on the indication for replacement on other grounds and secondarily, on the technical difficulties involved. Aesthetic implications and not least economic factors must also be considered. The cost is especially relevant for cast-metal and porcelain restorations. Whatever the decision, the initial aim will be to obtain an optimal gingival response before carrying out any corrective measures.

Replacement of the offending restoration, if necessary, is best delayed, with or without any intermediate minor corrective modifications to the margins, until progressive inflammatory resolution has substantially improved the gingival state. Existing modified restorations can often be used as perfectly acceptable 'temporaries', which are cosmetically and functionally agreeable, until the completion of periodontal therapy as shown in Figure 11.7 (O and P). This will serve to avoid any technical, functional, cosmetic or economic problems encountered by fitting provisional restorations instead, pending the outcome of the associated periodontal therapy. Other considerations such as pulpal integrity may, however, overrule this. The ultimate objective is that gingival inflammation should not impede the placement of good quality permanent restorations. In some instances surgical exposure of the restoration margins is necessary (*cf.* Chapter 24).

Trimming technique

Trimming away excess metal with high or low speed burs needs some care to achieve the required reduction without causing damage to adjacent structures. This is especially true of approximal

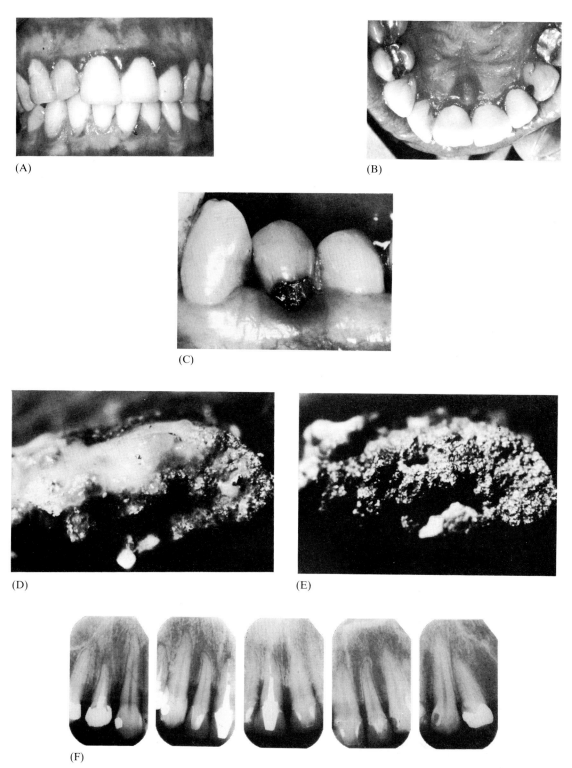

Figure 11.7 Plaque retentive restorations. (A, B) Obvious localized gingival inflammation about poorly fitting crowns at 11, 21, 22. (C) Marginal inflammation localized to site of defective amalgam restoration. Amalgam removed showing (D) plaque laden and (E) cleaned roughened surface. (F) Initial radiographic findings of patient shown at (G).

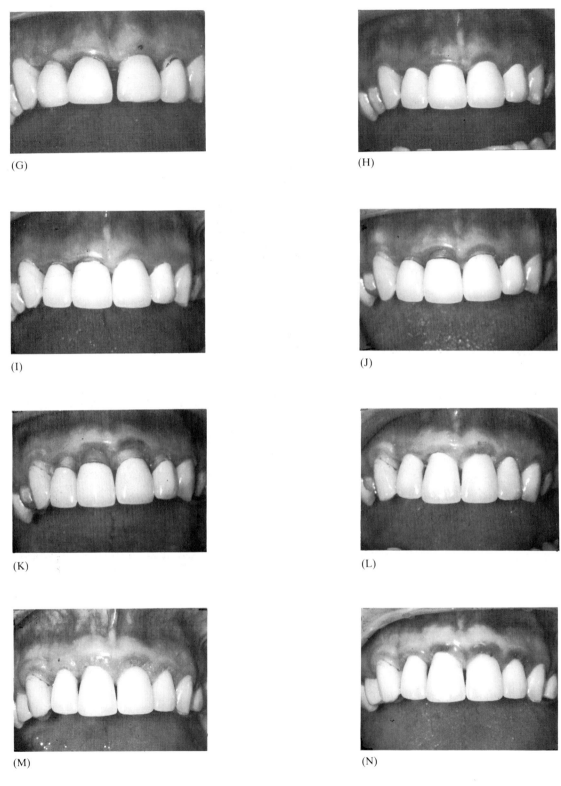

(G)

(H)

(I)

(J)

(K)

(L)

(M)

(N)

Figure 11.7 (*cont.*)

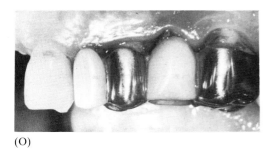

(O)

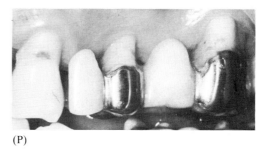

(P)

Figure 11.7 (*cont.*) (G) Note pathological drifting and gingival recession exposing poor crown margins. (H) Crown replacement on aesthetic grounds by referring dentist 4 months later. Further recession ensued, once again exposing margins which are also defective, as shown after intervals of (I) 12 months and (J) 18 months. (K) Residual pocketing then surgically eliminated and further moderately well fitting crowns to just within the gingival sulcus provided (L) 6 months postoperatively. Presentation a further (M) 36 months and (N) 42 months later. Inflammatory gingival hyperplasia developing at 21, 22, in particular, of iatrogenic origin. Adult on (O) presentation and (P) 18 months following restoration modifications in anticipation of replacement bridge. Note gingival inflammatory resolution and recession (O and P reproduced from *Dental Update*, by permission of Update-Siebert Publications Ltd)

aspects of porcelain and cast metal restorations as depicted in Figure 11.8 (G). In the latter, there is a tendency for the bur to become snagged against and to run off the metallic surface being trimmed to the detriment of adjacent structures. Local anaesthesia is rarely necessary and is indeed best avoided, for this imposes greater operator care lest pain be caused by contact with, and in turn, the risk of inadvertent damage to gingival or dentinal surfaces.

Multibladed finishing burs or fine grade diamond points are suitable for trimming all types of restorative material (Figure 11.8). Enamel chisels, push scalers or ultrasonic devices will only be effective for removing poorly condensed and other minor amalgam ledges. The latter is however quite effective in dealing with minor excesses of composite restorations, although the risk of dislodging the entire restoration does always exist. The Dentatus Eva metal tip is useful for removing interproximal amalgam overhangs especially in confined interproximal spaces, where burs would damage adjacent teeth. The flat side of the insert, with its diamond coating abrasive, is placed against the restoration excess and the vibratory movement used to polish it down towards the tooth surface (Figure 11.8 B1 and B2).

Complete removal of any restoration excess may require several attempts at successive appointments as gingival resolution gradually proceeds and makes the task easier. The creation of highly polished margins is unnecessary, for smooth surfaces, that will not impede the cleaning action of oral hygiene devices, are quite sufficient (see Chapter 34 – The correction of defective restorations).

Patient awareness and consent

It is essential to keep the patient informed of decisions taken with regard to the modification of defective restorations, especially when this may affect appearance (see Figure 11.7 P) or patient comfort. For example, revealing the gold at the buccal margin of an anterior bonded crown, without prior agreement, could lead to resentment. Recontouring a plaque retentive bridge pontic could lead to food trapping at a previously apparently satisfactory prosthesis (see Figure 18.10 K). Consequently, the patient must participate in any decision with full knowledge of the consequences for and against any proposed modification. However, when faced with a dilemma, a great deal can be achieved by delaying operative intervention by instituting the best possible plaque control measures and awaiting optimal gingival resolution before making any decisions. Adopting this approach, the defects become more apparent with gingival shrinkage and the patient can appreciate the problem more readily. Furthermore, in some instances the resulting supragingival location of the plaque retention is no longer a threat and the situation becomes acceptable without modification.

Malaligned teeth

Therapeutic options

Access to approximal surfaces is made difficult, but seldom impossible, by malpositioned teeth. However these sites do tend to become blocked more easily

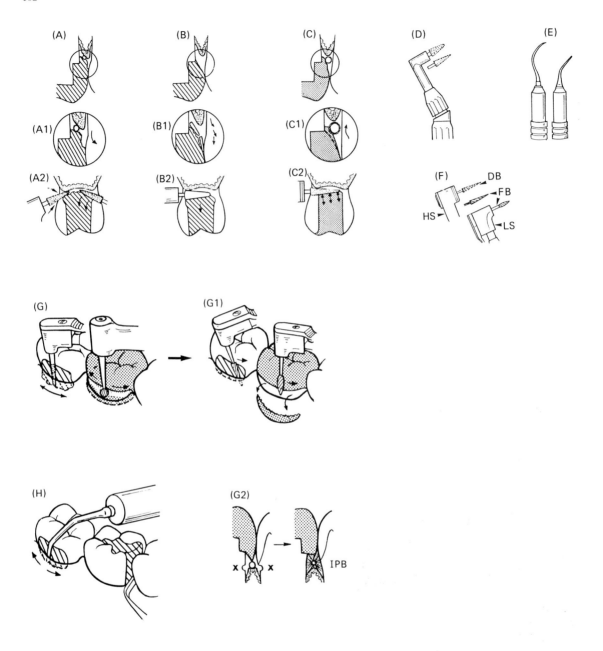

Figure 11.8 Trimming subgingival overhanging restoration margins. (A–A2) Gross edge of amalgam first reduced with (F) low speed (LS) diamond bur (DB) working coronally. (B–B2) Residual roughness smoothed down with (D) Dentatus Eva system diamond tip. (C–C2) Gold edge reduced with (F) low or high speed (HS) diamond bur (DB) and then finishing burs (FB) working corono-apically. Note: different shaped (D) metal Eva tips. Different sized, colour coded plastic tips are also available for use with polishing paste on interproximal surfaces. (E) Cavitron (TFI-3 and TFI-10) inserts may also be used to correct amalgam (H), and composite restorations. (G) Amalgam edge at 47 trimmed with low speed diamond bur then smoothed down with finishing bur (G1), while gold crown at 46 best corrected by first cutting through metal with high speed bur just coronal to gingiva to isolate offending margin. (G1) Edge removed and new margin created smoothed down. (G2) The associated interproximal overhanging gold edge is reduced with a fine tapered diamond bur taking care not to notch teeth (shown as 'X'). Risk of damage also avoided by accepting residual ledge related to contact point. Note use of interproximal brush (IPB) for subsequent plaque control. (I) Radiograph overhanging interproximal margin. (J) Dentatus Eva Tip. (K) Probe caught under overhang. Trimmed with (L) Eva Tip and/or (M) fine diamond bur

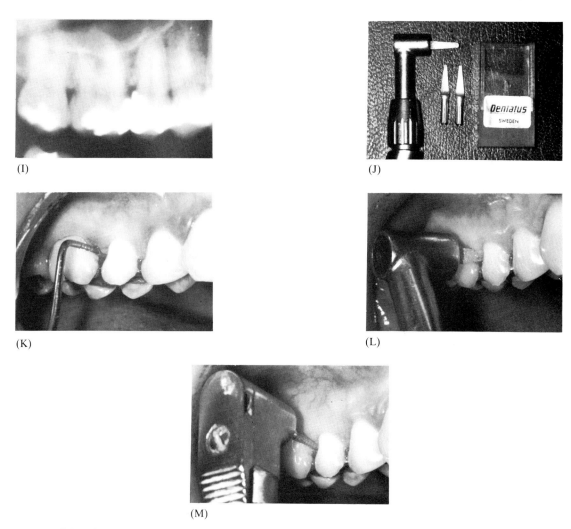

(I)

(J)

(K)

(L)

(M)

Figure 11.8 (*cont.*)

by calculus which may necessitate more frequent scaling to permit cleaning by the patient. Tooth position should only be incriminated in the persistence of marginal inflammation when this inflammation is restricted to such suspected sites alone.

Correction of the position of imbricated or tilted teeth, by orthodontic means, to facilitate oral hygiene measures is a possible solution but one that is frequently discarded for economic reasons. In addition, many patients faced with the prospect of lengthy and socially unacceptable orthodontic treatment, demonstrate previously hidden talents for effective cleaning (see Figure 8.1 I). The simple expedient of extracting one offending tooth, might also be considered in some cases, but only when there is no doubt about the stability of the post-extraction result.

Whenever orthodontic treatment is contemplated it should be realized that tooth alignment cannot by itself ensure periodontal health, for disease exists in many well aligned arches due to ineffective cleaning alone. Similarly, the deleterious influence of imbrication on the rate of disease progression at the teeth in question and upon neighbouring teeth must be established. It is also necessary to weigh the advantages of realigning the teeth against the likely future prognosis of the dentition. Unfortunately neither of these requirements are easily accomplished.

Periodontal tissue changes

Mucogingival form

In cases of early disease there may be difficulties of access to plaque, at the dento-epithelial junction, caused by soft tissue morphology. This can be due to uneven contour of the gingival margin as a result of gingival hyperplasia or recession, or to the existence of prominent frenal insertions or shallow vestibular mucosal form (*cf.* Chapter 21). The interference of these soft tissue factors in plaque control can usually be overcome by identifying the problem to the patients (see Figure 12.1) and improving their technique, by advice and demonstration. It may also be necessary in cases of gingival recession to overcome an unexpressed fear that efficient cleaning will lead to further recession. In those few instances where marginal inflammation does persist, having resolved elsewhere in the arch, surgical intervention should be discussed with the patient (*cf.* Chapter 21). This proposition may, even at such a late stage, be countered by a new found enthusiasm for efficient cleaning!

Factors in more advanced disease

All of the aspects of the gingival therapy regime discussed thus far are equally applicable to those situations with more advanced periodontal breakdown. However, some technical modifications, coupled with additional measures, are necessary to cope with the altered dento-epithelial relationships

associated with the greater losses of attachment experienced. These morphological changes merely represent further and greater plaque retention factors, related in turn to the depths of the periodontal pockets, the complex shapes of the roots involved and the proximity of the vestibular sulcus. Consequently, while the commonly encountered presence of differing levels of disease within the same mouth does create greater difficulties for subgingival debridement, it does not require any fundamental change in the approach to treatment. The progressively more complicated treatment measures are catered for by 'Simple pocket therapy', and by 'Simple pocket surgery' and 'Complex pocket surgery', which will be dealt with in subsequent chapters.

II.   Simple pocket therapy
The problem of the periodontal pocket
The nature of the problem

As periodontal disease advances by the loss of attachment a pocket develops with an outer soft

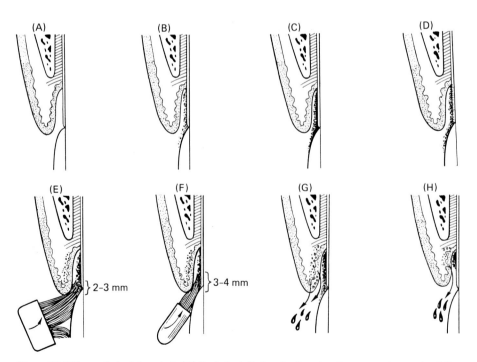

Figure 11.9 The periodontal pocket. (A) Periodontally involved root surface cementum and soft tissue pocket wall with dento-epithelial junction located at pocket base. (B) Bacterial plaque on root surface. (C) Calculus and superficial layer of plaque. (D) Possible cementum contamination from bacterial plaque. (E) Subgingival penetration (2–3 mm) with ordinary toothbrush. (F) Deeper penetration (3–4 mm) possible with interspace brush. (G) Bleeding occurs initially from both marginal gingival and subgingival sources. (H) Following effective brushing marginal inflammation resolves and only subgingival bleeding persists. Note relationship of tissue inflammation to residual subgingival plaque

tissue wall formed by the detached gingiva, and an inner hard tissue wall formed by the 'periodontally-involved' root surface (Figure 11.9 A). In addition to the well-established noxious effects of bacterial plaque and its calcified root surface accretions upon the soft tissues, there is a belief that the cementum itself becomes contaminated (Figure 11.9 B–D). Together, these result in a state of biological incompatibility between the tissues and, in consequence, persistent pocketing.

The periodontal pocket represents a plaque retention factor which impedes but does not necessarily prevent plaque control. Oral hygiene techniques described for gingival therapy must therefore be adapted to reach as far as possible into the subgingival pocket spaces. Clearly, there is a limit to the extent of this accessibility, when compensatory professional cleaning of the remaining, inaccessible, root surfaces becomes necessary.

Subgingival professional cleaning

The professional removal of subgingival plaque and calculus is similar to that of their supragingival counterparts, but is more difficult to carry out. An even greater technical problem will arise when attempting to identify the possible presence of any allegedly contaminated cementum and of actually removing it by root planing. Thus, although technically similar to subgingival scaling and plaque removal, the removal of root surface cementum is even more difficult to ensure. For each type of instrumentation, described collectively as subgingival professional cleaning, the periodontally involved root surfaces must be negotiated blindly. In addition, this difficulty is compounded by the topographical problems associated with the characteristically uneven pattern of breakdown and the increasingly more complex root forms exposed by advancing disease. In addition, there is an inability to establish when professional cleaning has been satisfactorily completed.

Assessment difficulties

The success of 'blind' subgingival professional cleaning can only really be determined retrospectively. This can be assumed when the clinical signs of healing and repair (the gingival response) develop within the soft tissue wall of the pocket. When, on the other hand, healing does not occur at this stage or following further careful subgingival instrumentation, surgical intervention for 'open' surgical professional cleaning is indicated. The operator may also consider 'open' surgical cleaning when access for instrumentation is inadequate due to more advanced levels of disease.

Treatment rationale

The fundamental problem of the pocket is accessibility to the plaque front at the dento-epithelial junction located at the base of the pocket. The roles of patient and clinician in gaining this access will now be examined in more detail. This will be considered in conjunction with the clinical problems arising from dealing with subgingival plaque and its effects upon the two components of the periodontal pocket. These aspects are summarized in Table 11.1.

The patient's role in subgingival plaque control

Accessibility of plaque

The oral hygiene measures in simple pocket therapy are no different from those applied in gingival therapy as described in Chapter 8. However, the measures include the need to extend further subgingivally and cater for the root morphological changes encountered with greater periodontal destruction. The degree to which the patient can gain access to the subgingival root surfaces will vary according to the dexterity and diligence of the individual and the position of the site within the mouth. Generally, it would be unrealistic to expect the patient to remove with a toothbrush, subgingival plaque located at depths of greater than about 2–3 mm (Figure 11.9 E and 11.10 A,B). At interproximal pocket sites however, dental floss can be passed as far apically as the contour of the facial and oral gingival contours allow, but is only effective in the absence of root surface concavities (Figure 11.11 A). Interproximal pockets may also be negotiated with an interspace brush (Figure 11.10 C–E and 11.11 B–D), the bristles having first been pressed firmly against the crown of the tooth, splayed out and then passed apically into the pocket space. Some patients may be able to reach as far as 3–4 mm subgingivally at anterior and other readily accessible tooth sites when using the interspace brush as depicted in Figure 11.9 (F).

The interproximal brush appears to be of limited value within interproximal pockets (Figure 11.11 E,F) (see also Figure 18.5 H), despite its established efficacy supragingivally especially where root surface concavities are present, and within gingival sulci (see Figure 8.5). The misinterpretation of this latter facility of interproximal brushes, coupled with the benefits of comparative ease of use, has led to their widespread recommendation as exclusive interdental cleaning devices in the presence of pocketing. The limitations of these brushes in such situations must be stressed to the patient and other more effective techniques demonstrated. In all

Table 11.1 The problems of the pocket

Root surface	Nature of involvement and identification of possible features	Plaque Calculus Surface contamination Penetrating contamination?
	Surface topography	Cemental micro-roughness Resorption lacunae Instrument scoring/gouging
	Root morphology	Tapering root contours Surface concavities/grooves Furcation features
	Instrumentation	Non-overlapping strokes Variable levels of plaque front/ dento-epithelial junctions
Pocket wall	Operator vision	Confined space for instrument insertion and manipulation

	Operator access	Limited displacement of tissues
		    possible during
		    instrumentation

		Variable attachment levels
		Risk of trauma with further attachment loss
	Patient discomfort	Inaccessible plaque front

Assessment efficacy of debridement	Root surface features	Plaque not identifiable
		Roughness only suggestive of
		    inadequate debridement
		Clean/unclean surfaces are non-
		    differentiable
		Burnished calculus, cementum
		    and dentine are similar

	Gingival response	Absence of bleeding/suppuration Pocket closure with/without long junctional epithelium Gingival recession
	Microbial sampling Crevicular fluid constituents	Feasibility questionable *See* Part III

instances, subgingival cleaning may be complicated by plaque retention factors such as subgingival calculus, root furcation involvement or the close approximation of adjacent tooth surfaces.

Assessment of cleaning

Although subgingival plaque cannot be seen by the patient, it is certain that if residual plaque can be disclosed adjacent to the gingival margin following cleaning, then subgingival plaque is still present. The reverse situation is, however, not true, so the indirect method of assessing retrospectively the subgingival tissue inflammatory status is necessary. Where bleeding can be elicited by the subgingival penetration of toothbrush bristles or the passage of dental floss, then subgingival plaque is undoubtedly still present (Figure 11.9 G). This method of assessment will however only be valid in the absence of marginal gingival inflammation (Fig 11.9 H). It also depends upon the implicit assumption that a relationship exists between the precise location of plaque on the tooth surface and that of the

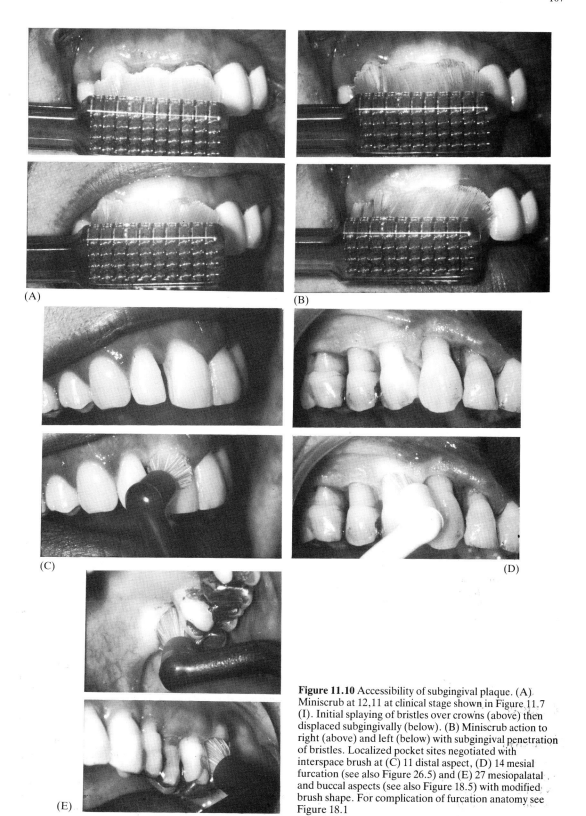

Figure 11.10 Accessibility of subgingival plaque. (A) Miniscrub at 12,11 at clinical stage shown in Figure 11.7 (I). Initial splaying of bristles over crowns (above) then displaced subgingivally (below). (B) Miniscrub action to right (above) and left (below) with subgingival penetration of bristles. Localized pocket sites negotiated with interspace brush at (C) 11 distal aspect, (D) 14 mesial furcation (see also Figure 26.5) and (E) 27 mesiopalatal and buccal aspects (see also Figure 18.5) with modified brush shape. For complication of furcation anatomy see Figure 18.1

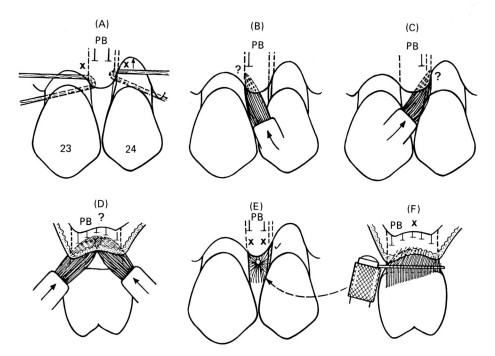

Figure 11.11 Interproximal cleaning in simple pocket therapy. (A) Access of floss to 23 pocket base (PB) impeded (as shown by 'X') by marginal gingival contour. Greater recession at 24 will allow floss to pass sufficiently apically (arrow) but mesial root surface concavity remains inaccessible 'X'. (B) Incomplete subgingival penetration ('?') by interspace brush likely at 23, because of brush-head impaction against the teeth, the confined interdental space and prominence of the gingival septum and limited bristle length. (C) Interspace brush passing into 24 mesial concavity but not necessarily to pocket base. (D) Buccopalatal view of 24 mesial surface. The associated interdental soft tissue crater and subgingival root surface concavity may be (?) negotiated by the bi-directional angulated use of interspace brush. Interproximal brush is highly effective within (E) supragingival root surface concavities and (F) soft tissue craters but much less so within (E and F) interproximal pocket spaces, as at 23 and subgingival concavities, as at 24

inflammatory reaction within the adjacent soft tissues. It follows from the latter that marginal gingival inflammation should not be attributed to deeply placed subgingival plaque and that resolution of marginal inflammation is possible even in the presence of this inaccessible plaque. This is of great practical importance in the treatment regime advocated.

The operator's role in subgingival plaque control

Initial clinical assessment

The first priority is to ensure that the patient controls all reasonably accessible plaque, for until this has been achieved there is little merit in trying to control the deeper subgingival plaque. Total resolution of the signs of marginal gingival inflammation thus becomes the initial objective in treating any stage of periodontal disease. When this stage has been reached the detection of bleeding from subgingival sites examined with a blunt probe, indicates persistent subgingival inflammation. The patient's attention is then directed to cleaning as far as possible into these relatively inaccessible subgingival regions, as shown for example in Figure 11.10 (C–E). If this is successful then the bleeding, in response to blunt probing, will disappear and indicate that inflammatory resolution has occurred at the dento-epithelial junction located at the base of the pocket.

If subgingival bleeding persists (as depicted in Figure 11.12 A), in spite of optimal cleaning efforts by the patient, it can be assumed that the subgingival plaque is totally inaccessible to the patient. Professional cleaning must then be carried out (Figure 11.12 B). It must be reiterated that

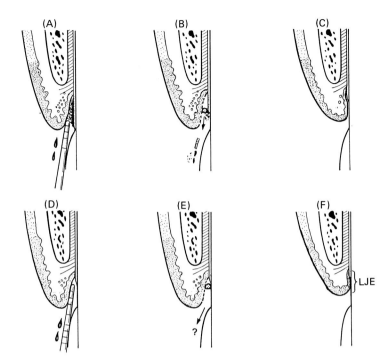

Figure 11.12 Subgingival instrumentation. (A) Subgingival plaque, calculus and 'contaminated' cementum. Note location of residual inflammatory cell infiltrate in the tissue following removal of reasonably accessible plaque, and production of bleeding on subgingival probing. (B) Instrumentation removes plaque, calculus and usually also some cementum (or dentine in absence of cementum) but it is not possible to judge clinically what remains. Note pocket wall tissue may be inadvertently traumatized – see also (E). (C) Pocket closure with gingival shrinkage and adaptation to root surface. (D) Persistent pocket with bleeding on probing despite extensive subgingival root surface instrumentation necessitates (E) further debridement although the nature of the material removed cannot be judged clinically. (F) Optimal healing with further shrinkage and complete pocket closure with development of a long junctional epithelium (LJE)

individuals who fail to demonstrate optimal removal of reasonably accessible plaque will derive only limited benefit from this subgingival instrumentation. This is because, whilst bacterial recolonization of the subgingival region stems from both residual subgingival and supragingival plaque sources, it will occur much more rapidly in the presence of inadequate supragingival plaque control. It is also seldom practical to compensate for such patient shortcomings by increasing the frequency of professional care. Similarly, unless there is optimal plaque control, any attempted surgical correction of such plaque retentive dentogingival relationships will be followed by recurrent disease.

Subgingival professional cleaning

The object of subgingival root surface instrumentation is to remove plaque that is inaccessible to the patient, plaque retentive subgingival calculus and any possibly contaminated cementum. This ensures that the hard and the soft tissue walls of the pocket will become compatible with each other. This is currently achieved by mechanical means, using hand instruments and ultrasonic scalers, although future developments of plaque control by chemical means may make this an effective alternative (*cf.* Part III).

The mechanical cleaning of subgingival root surfaces is essentially no different from cleaning supragingival surfaces, but is complicated by additional difficulties (see Table 11.1). These are due to the limited access, the complex shapes of the pockets coupled with the variable degrees of attachment loss associated with the soft tissue pocket wall on the one hand, and the root surface topography and overall root morphology on the other. The lack of direct visibility and limitations of tactile examination mean that it is also difficult, if not impossible, at the time of instrumentation to judge when the technical objectives have been achieved. Thus, while the finding of subgingival root surface roughness is usually due to deposits of calculus, any clinical assessment of root smoothness is fairly subjective and, moreover, does not necessarily mean an absence of calculus. In addition, no way exists of differentiating clinically at the time, between plaque free and plaque-laden subgingival root surfaces, or between root surface cementum and dentine. It is also impossible to assess any risk of further loss of attachment being sustained inadvertently from over-instrumentation (see also Chapter 29 – Clinical implications). Each of these clinical problems will be examined further as a separate entity.

Instrumentation and root form

Instrument design

The roots exposed by the loss of attachment present difficulties in instrumentation because of their variable root contours. The difficulty caused by even the simplest of root shapes to instrumentation is readily demonstrated by attempting to remove a coating of nail varnish applied to the root of an extracted tooth held in the fingers. This reveals how difficult it is not only to match the shape of the cutting edge of the chosen instrument to the variable shape of the root, but also to ensure that the entire root surface is covered by the adequate overlapping of instrumentation strokes. This overlapping must be ensured both concentrically about the root surface and vertically along the length of the diseased root, as shown in Figure 11.5. These problems are all too familiar when attempting to remove supragingival tobacco staining with hand instruments. A technically analogous situation is that of renovating a table with curved tapering legs. The flat table top presents few technical difficulties. However, the variable contour of the table legs means that the chosen scrapers will frequently not scrape away the tarnished surface to an even depth and tend instead to gouge out, unevenly, parts of the surface at some sites, while missing others completely.

The problem of fitting the shape of the cutting edge of hand instruments to the tapering shapes of the roots is compounded by the complexities of root surface morphology (see Figure 18.1 A–F). These relate to the surface concavities and grooves of both individual roots and those formed by the root furcations, the confined interradicular spaces where the roots diverge and, not least, uneven levels of attachment loss at adjacent surfaces of the root. The problems encountered at closely related roots of neighbouring teeth must also not be overlooked.

The numerous scalers and curettes available and their uses have already been described and require little further comment. Suffice it to say that the

ultrasonic scaler is probably the easiest to use and therefore the most effective for subgingival instrumentation. This is endorsed by the ease with which it removes supragingival calculus and staining compared with hand instruments and thereby, the facility with which complete overlapping ultrasonic instrumentation may be achieved. Ultrasonic tips have also been shown to be most effective within root furcations, the specific management of which is considered further in Chapter 18 (*cf.* Chapter 30 – The efficacy of therapy).

Instrumentation objectives

The different clinical objectives of subgingival scaling (removal of clinically obvious subgingival calculus), subgingival debridement (removal of subgingival plaque and any residual flecks of calculus) and of root planing (removal of possibly contaminated cementum) warrants their separate consideration. However, in practice these techniques are commonly carried out together even though this may not have been the original intention. Thus, the removal of subgingival calculus, by scaling, is accompanied inevitably by the simultaneous removal of any attached and adjacent plaque and possibly also, albeit only incidentally, some or even all the underlying cementum (Figure 11.12 B). Whereas, the attempted intentional removal of root surface cementum, by root planing, cannot fail to remove also any overlying calculus and bacterial plaque. It is only when, in the absence of clinically detectable deposits of subgingival calculus, the removal of subgingival plaque alone is intended by the gentle superficial use of hand instruments or ultrasonic devices, namely subgingival debridement, that significant amounts of underlying tooth substance are not removed (*cf.* Chapter 28 – Instrumentation for debridement).

Subgingival scaling and debridement

The finding of roughened subgingival root surfaces should be assumed initially to be due to calculus. Subgingival instrumentation then aims to achieve surface smoothness if only to ensure that no bacterial plaque, inevitably associated with this subgingival calculus, remains. The importance of this objective must, however, be kept in perspective, for although persistent root surface roughness does, for practical purposes, signify incomplete instrumentation, the opposite finding of root smoothness does not exclude the presence of residual bacterial plaque and possibly even burnished calculus. Consequently, where the root surfaces appear smooth at the outset, it has to be assumed that only plaque is present, for it is impossible to identify burnished calculus. The operator is then obliged to carry out as methodical a cleaning as possible of all subgingival root surfaces, using a carefully executed pattern of cleaning that ensures overlapping of instrumentation and then trust that all the plaque has been removed. As a practical guideline, this pattern of debridement should be equivalent to that necessary to remove supragingival tobacco-type staining. Furthermore, whether hand instruments or ultrasonic scalers are used for this debridement depends on operator and patient preferences, for they have been shown to be equally effective in both clinical and laboratory investigations (*cf.* Chapter 28). Where debridement has been carried out effectively pocket closure will occur (Figure 11.12 C) (see below).

Root planing

The need for root planing is based traditionally upon the claimed contamination of the cementum by bacterial products (see Chapter 28 – Nature of the roof surface). Root planing is therefore designed to remove contaminated root surface material be it cementum, as is normally assumed, or dentine. It is deemed to be necessary when subgingival inflammation persists despite previous careful subgingival debridement and the creation of smooth root surfaces as depicted in Figure 11.12 (D). However, this inflammation could equally be due to residual subgingival plaque thereby necessitating further debridement alone. Unfortunately, this possibility is neither readily confirmed nor refuted, for subgingival plaque cannot be detected by any reliable means (Figure 11.12 E). Indeed, even surgically exposing the root surface and staining it with a disclosing agent is not wholly reliable (see Chapter 28 – The assessment of adequate debridement). That subgingival plaque itself, rather than contamination by bacterial products of the root surface cementum (and possibly also dentine), is responsible for persistent subgingival inflammation, is supported by the technical difficulties of ensuring the total removal of root surface substance itself, let alone that of the elimination of plaque as described above. There is, in addition, the questionable validity of the traditional concept of cemental contamination, in the light of recent research findings (see Chapter 28).

The reasons for the retention of subgingival plaque following debridement or indeed attempted root planing, are reiterated and expanded upon here. Firstly, instrumentation strokes may not have overlapped adequately or the instrument cutting edge or Cavitron tip not have been maintained in even contact with the tooth surface so skipping over areas of plaque (see Figure 11.5). Secondly, minor surface irregularities of the root surface, which cannot be detected by probing, are passed over during instrumentation and the associated bacterial plaque is left undisturbed (Figure 11.13) (*cf.*

Chapter 28). These topographical variations may be either normally present, associated with cementum resorption lacunae, islands of smoothly burnished calculus, or even be the result of instrumentation, grooving the tooth surface. Finally, root surface concavities and grooves related to root furcations (see Figure 11.10 and Figure 11.13) could be responsible, but these should be anticipated and readily recognized as such, so need be considered no further here.

It must be appreciated that the removal of root surface cementum by root planing would, in the circumstances cited above, not only result in the elimination of any surface features that might harbour plaque and as such constitute a rationale for root planing, but in the process would also remove any superficial plaque that might be present. Disregarding any incidental cementum removal during previous root surface instrumentation as depicted at Figure 11.12 (D), the intention at this stage would be to carry out the operation of removing contaminated root surface substance (cementum/dentine) as a deliberate exercise. It is performed with the same hand instruments used for debridement and in the same manner, although ultrasonic devices are apparently not as effective in removing tooth substance (see Chapter 28). Root planing therefore represents simply an extension of debridement that attempts to remove underlying tooth material as well. Where subgingival instrumentation has been effective and a high standard of plaque control by the patient is maintained, optimal healing with a long junctional epithelium may accrue (Figure 11.12 F).

Rationale for debridement

The nature of both periodontally involved and root planed surfaces has been clarified by recent investigations (see Chapter 28). In the first place, the extent of the claimed contamination of the root surface cementum appears to have been overestimated because, for example, the bulk of bacterial endotoxin which has been strongly incriminated in disease, can be removed by simple plaque removal techniques alone. Secondly, it is possible to remove all cementum by root planing with hand instruments *in vitro* and to establish this with some confidence, by the absence of staining following application of a disclosing agent. This is, however, not readily achieved clinically. Thirdly, it is at present not possible to distinguish between apparently contaminated and uncontaminated cementum or indeed even the state of underlying dentine. This implies that clinical investigation findings in support of root planing on the basis of the actual removal of root surface cementum cannot be substantiated. Fourthly, the comparable clinical findings following both surgical and non-surgical root surface instrumentation, coupled with the widely claimed difficulties of carrying out an effective blind instrumentation, suggest that a less extensive surface instrumentation without any attempted removal of cementum will suffice. This has been endorsed by recent laboratory investigations of the removal of bacterial endotoxin by very conservative regimes of both hand and ultrasonic instrumentation (see Chapter 28 – Difficulties of subgingival instrumentation). Lastly, the total removal of cementum appears to offer no clinical advantage over efficient debridement alone. For these reasons, the intentional removal of root surface cementum would seem to be unnecessary and is not recommended as a routine exercise. In conclusion, its use should be restricted to those sites at which it is suspected that minor root surface roughness exists which may harbour residual bacteria and cause a persistent subgingival inflammation.

Instrumentation and the pocket wall

Technical difficulties

The soft tissue wall lies over the root surfaces like a drawn curtain. This not only obscures the roots from the operator's sight precluding any visual assessment of the adequacy of instrumentation but, more importantly, creates problems of access and soft tissue traumatization (see Table 11.1). The problems of access are primarily associated with the depths of the pockets, but are compounded by variations of pocket depth at adjacent surfaces (Figure 11.13 A). In addition, instrument insertion and manipulation can be very difficult within the confined pocket spaces, as at localized pocket sites and where partial inflammatory resolution and pocket closure impedes instrumental displacement of the soft tissue pocket wall (Figure 11.13 B,D). The crowns of the teeth may also complicate instrumentation by their contacts with the instrument shanks impeding manipulation at deeper pocket sites (Figure 11.13 D,E). In some instances this may prevent instrument penetration to the required operating depth (Figure 11.13 E,F). This latter difficulty is most commonly encountered at the lingual and palatal aspects of retroclined anterior teeth, at the palatal roots of maxillary molar and at the distal aspects of last standing molars.

There can be no predefined limit of pocket depth beyond which access for debridement is deemed impossible (see Chapter 28 – Difficulties of subgingival debridement). Access does depend to a large extent on individual operator attitude and skill on the one hand and patient acceptance of therapy on the other. This is considered further in the following chapters.

Tissue trauma

Logically, subgingival cleaning should extend only as far as the base of the pocket. The depth of instrumentation is judged carefully at each site by the resistance created by the soft tissues. The risk of instrumentation trauma which might in turn cause attachment loss is well documented, although this is paradoxically most likely to occur at the shallowest pocket sites (see Chapter 29 – Clinical implications).

Damage is also likely where uneven depths of pocketing exist about any single tooth, because the instrument tip is liable to penetrate the attachment at adjacent shallower sites, while its cutting edge is being directed more apically elsewhere, as shown in Figure 11.5 (C). Access to such sites is thereby impeded and results in incomplete instrumentation (Figure 11.13 A,B). This particular difficulty is most easily overcome by the use of ultrasonic devices (Figure 11.13 C), because the shape of the recommended Cavitron TFI-10 tip facilitates instrumentation with a gentle periodontal probing-like action, while at the same time carefully sounding out the undulating contour of the dento-epithelial junction.

The inadvertent removal of soft tissue from the pocket wall, 'inadvertent curettage' may also occur during subgingival instrumentation as shown in Figure 11.12 (B). The extent of this soft tissue trauma will, however, be small where only those surfaces that are reasonably accessible to the operator are tackled initially, and local anaesthesia is avoided, so that the warning signs of imminent trauma are not masked. Soft tissue trauma is, on the other hand, virtually inevitable at deeper pockets (>6–8 mm) and those with complex root forms. As a result of this, local anaesthesia is often considered necessary. Finally, it must be stressed that the intentional removal of the soft tissue from the pocket wall by gingival curettage is unwarranted. Curettage not only fails to enhance the clinical effects of careful root surface cleaning alone (see Chapter 29 – Tissue curettage), but causes needless post-instrumentation pain and may result in further loss of attachment.

Local anaesthesia for debridement

The rationale for the routine use of local anaesthesia for subgingival debridement is contentious and appears to stem from the now well established use and acceptance of anaesthesia by the patient for restorative dentistry. That this should also apply to the potentially painful subgingival root surface debridement might therefore not seem unreasonable. However, the potential risk of inadvertent damage to the attachment does always exist and should not be overlooked in treatment planning. Local anaesthesia is usually required where the root

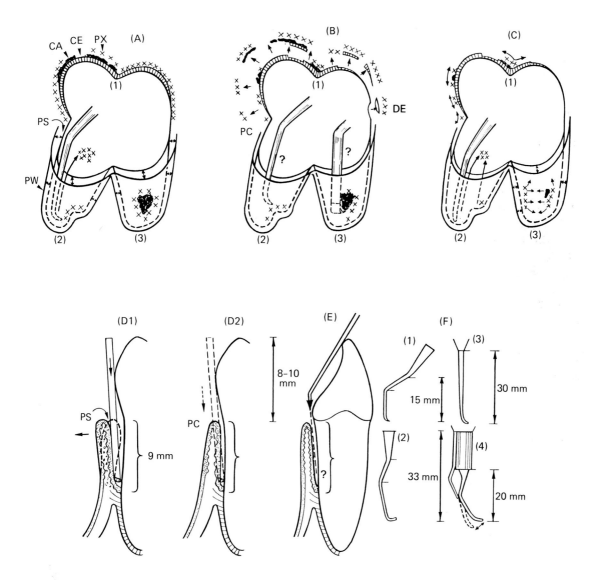

Figure 11.13 Subgingival instrumentation and the pocket wall. Diagrammatic representation of pocket space at molar tooth. (A1) Root surface cementum (CE) with variable distribution of deposits of calculus (CA) and plaque (PX). (A2 and 3) Pocket space (PS) (arrowed) associated with inflamed swollen pocket wall tissue (PW), permits tissue displacement during insertion and manipulation of fine curette for effective instrumentation to dento-epithelial junction. See also (D1) which depicts debridement with curette to depth of 9 mm. Note residual plaque from possible non-overlapping strokes or that related to (B2) uneven pocket base and (B3) calculus deposit. (B1) Various combinations of plaque, calculus, cementum and even dentine (DE) may be removed but this cannot be judged clinically. Detection of calculus deposits does however indicate incomplete instrumentation and residual plaque. (B2 and 3, D2) Pocket closure (PC) following instrumentation resists tissue displacement. This coupled with tapering root forms and (D2 and E) coronal tooth contours complicates access to residual deeper deposits. Use of (B2) fine curette and (B3) hoe not wholly successful (?) but access may still be possible with (C1) Cavitron modified (P-10) tip. (E) Access to, say, 9 mm deep lingual and palatal pockets anteriorly, by any hand instrument, impeded by limited instrument dimensions as shown at (F1–5): (1) Goldman–Fox curette SGF6, (2) SGF11/12; (3) Hawe–Neos 580-00; (4) Cavitron P-10 with modified tip (ghosted). Instrument shanks likely to engage the incisal or occlusal surface represented at (E) whenever the level of instrumentation is more than about 15 mm apical to this. The Hawe–Neos scaler (00) is most suitable provided access is not impeded by opposing teeth. Note: angulation of many maxillary molar palatal roots to their coronal surfaces will also impede subgingival debridement. (C1 and 3) Bacterial recolonization in direction of arrows from residual plaque, associated with opening up of pocket space as recurrent inflammation develops

surfaces are ultrasensitive to instrumentation, although some individuals may still prefer to tolerate this during the relatively short debridement times than sustain the prolonged after-effects of anaesthesia. Accordingly, the need for anaesthesia will depend as much on individual patient requirements as on operator objectives and each situation is managed as such.

Phased debridement and continuous assessment

The difficulties of debridement encountered in pocket therapy can be circumvented, to a great extent, by implementing the phased instrumentation approach adopted for gingival therapy and which will be dealt with in greater detail in the next chapter. Thus, having established an optimal level of supragingival plaque control by the patient, as determined by resolution of the signs of marginal tissue inflammation (see Figure 12.2 A), only those root surface deposits that are reasonably accessible to the operator are removed at the first instrumentation appointment. The remaining deeper deposits are then removed at subsequent appointments at about 4–6-week intervals, by which time progressive subgingival inflammatory resolution will have resulted in tissue shrinkage and reduced tenderness. This sequential approach not only simplifies further subgingival instrumentation but, it must be stressed, also limits this need to only those sites which exhibit bleeding, as determined by a site-by-site examination of the subgingival tissues by probing (see Figure 12.2 A and D), or by the expression of pus (see Figure 12.2 B). Furthermore, it must be re-emphasized that over this continuous assessment period there can be no relaxation of the patient's plaque control which is essential for an optimal gingival response.

The principle of reasonable accessibility advocated in phased debridement will, in the hands of careful operators, ultimately allow pockets of initial depths of up to about 7 mm to be instrumented with minimal patient discomfort (see Figure 12.2 C). Accordingly, local anaesthesia is rarely required and then usually only at the less accessible parts of the mouth and within molar furcations, and more obviously, at persistent deeper sites, where pocket closure complicates access (see Figure 12.2 E) or if dentinal sensitivity is encountered. In the latter, further instrumentation is preferably delayed, for this sensitivity usually resolves following improved home care, coupled with the daily use of fluoride toothpastes and mouth rinses (e.g. Fluorigard Weekly, Colgate-Palmolive, London, W1, UK) between appointments.

In summary, a definite sequence of procedures is advocated for this technically exacting, yet paradoxically imprecise, exercise. Subgingival instrumenta-

tion is restricted initially to only reasonably accessible surfaces. A satisfactory gingival response is then gained before instrumentation is extended sequentially to deeper levels and ultimately to the pocket bases. Furthermore this subgingival instrumentation is only carried out at sites where subgingival bleeding persists in the presence of good oral hygiene.

Quadrant instrumentation

The phased instrumentation regime is considered superior to the more traditional quadrant approach, where total debridement of the subgingival root surface is attempted, using shorter time intervals between visits. In the latter method, the patient's discomfort is increased inevitably and often necessitates the use of local anaesthesia. This might in turn increase the risk of inadvertent trauma to the dento-epithelium junctions with possible loss of attachment (*cf.* Chapter 29). A further disadvantage of this quadrant approach is that it seems to have invoked a greater dependency upon the need for surgical access depicted at Figure 12.2 (F). This is because of the demands made for an immediate thorough instrumentation stemming from the long-standing, yet unsubstantiated, belief in the need to remove 'contaminated' cementum, with its attendant technical difficulties. In addition, the extent to which the obscuring soft tissue pocket wall does actually impede effective subgingival instrumentation would seem to be questioned by the frequently comparable clinical outcomes of both 'blind' debridement and the 'open' surgical approaches (see Chapter 28 – Introduction).

Post-instrumentation assessment

Residual plaque

Any assessment of the efficacy of subgingival debridement can only be based upon the post-instrumentation gingival response, as there is no reliable method of doing this at the time of instrumentation, even with the benefits of surgical access, (*cf.* Chapters 28 and 29). While it is not yet clear what component of subgingival instrumentation actually achieves the inflammatory resolution, it does appear that removal of subgingival plaque is paramount. Conversely, where in the presence of a high standard of supragingival plaque control, subgingival inflammation persists following debridement, it should be assumed that residual plaque is primarily responsible. Residual plaque will occur in islands on the root surface where instrumentation overlapping has been incomplete because of poor debridement technique, or where plaque has not been negotiated within root surface irregularities.

These residual deposits contribute to a more rapid recolonization of the subgingival root surface (Figure 11.13 C) than by bacterial downgrowth from supragingival sources alone (see Chapter 28 – The significance of residual pockets). The subgingival inflammation, detected at periodic review appointments, may be the result of recurring inflammation from bacterial recolonization at partially disrupted bacterial foci or, alternatively, inflammation due to an episodic noxious effect upon the tissues of persistent totally undisturbed subgingival flora. The difference is however of little practical importance, for in either event further debridement is necessary.

Where, despite conscientious operator efforts and optimal supragingival plaque control, subgingival bleeding still persists then surgical procedures may be necessary. These are designed not only to gain access for improved root surface debridement (see Figure 12.2 F), but more importantly, to ensure future accessibility for plaque control by effecting surgical pocket reduction if not elimination (see also Chapter 14). In practice, the decision to intervene surgically is unfortunately dominated by individual operator priorities and patient attitudes to treatment rather than any reproducibly measurable parameters. For this reason, assessment of the effects of blind instrumentation is necessary over long periods of time before committing any patient to surgical therapy. Periodic assessment of the dento-epithelial junctions is also essential following any surgical measures and so underlies the treatment of all levels of disease. The practical implications of this continuous assessment regime are considered in the next chapter.

12

Continuous assessment in gingival and simple pocket therapy

The principles of continuous assessment

The therapeutic sequence

The typically variable pattern of gingival inflammation and attachment loss, normally encountered in an individual presenting for periodontal treatment, means that a combination of therapeutic measures comprising gingival therapy and simple pocket therapy, as described in the previous chapter, and possibly also even pocket surgery, to be described later, may be required. Although each of these measures becomes progressively more complex with respect to oral hygiene and operative techniques, the concept underlying treatment remains simply that of plaque control.

The treatment sequence will be, first and foremost, plaque control by the patient, followed by the removal of any plaque retention factors and where necessary, periodic professional cleaning at sites that are inaccessible to oral hygiene measures. In following this sequence, sufficient time must be allowed for tissue healing (the gingival response) to occur. Treatment needs are determined by constantly assessing the inflammatory status of the tissues at each site (continuous assessment).

The resolution of inflammation

The continuous assessment approach advocated revolves about the basic biological principle that an inflammatory reaction will resolve when its cause is removed. The nature of the gingival response is dealt with in the latter part of this and in the next chapter. The incidence of bleeding in response to subgingival probing decreases and pocket closure takes place in conjunction with gingival recession. Although this healing potential is normally predictable, the differing degrees of destruction sustained, and the corresponding difficulties of access to the advancing plaque front, means that the rate and extent of healing might vary from site to site and indeed also from one patient to the next. Accordingly, no predetermined time limits can be imposed on this phase of therapy.

Periodic re-evaluation

Detailed clinical re-evaluation, including subgingival bleeding points, pocket depths and probing attachment levels, should be carried out at about 9–12 monthly intervals. This is to ascertain the need for any further treatment measures. The findings may vary considerably from site to site. Where periodontal health is found, be it from the outset or following inflammatory resolution, maintenance care only is required. Sites with persistent *marginal gingival* inflammation indicate the patient's failure to remove reasonably accessible plaque and are dealt with accordingly.

The finding of persistent *subgingival* inflammation, demonstrated by bleeding on gentle probing to the pocket base, suggests plaque retention factors. This demands more careful subgingival debridement or, in some instances, even surgical intervention to render such sites more accessible to current, but more importantly future, plaque control measures.

The treatment sequence recommended for the typical patient presenting with periodontal disease will now be reviewed. The nature of the gingival response and the clinical dilemma as to whether to persevere with non-surgical debridement or to intervene surgically, will then be considered.

The initial appointment

Patient consultation

The nature of the disease is explained and the extent of its involvement demonstrated to the patient.

When marginal gingival inflammation is fairly generalized (e.g. Figure 9.1 B), this is noted in only general terms in the clinical record and an improved overall oral hygiene regime then demonstrated. When, in contrast gingival inflammation is interspersed with marginal tissue health (e.g. Figure 9.1 A) or where inflammation is restricted only to isolated sites, its distribution is recorded on the clinical chart (Figure 12.1 A). An appropriate copy of this chart (Figure 12.1 B) is then provided for

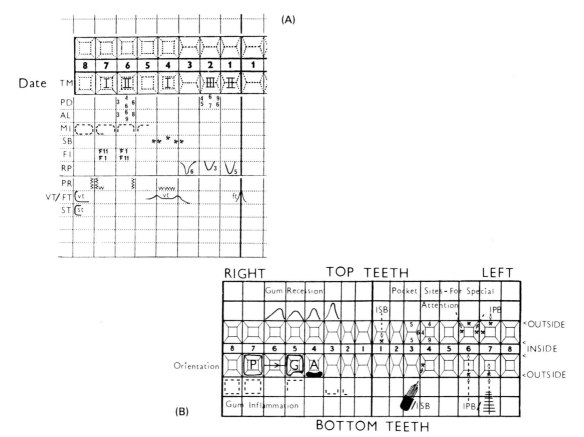

Figure 12.1 (A) Mandibular right segment of clinical chart shown as used to record tooth mobility (TM) as Grade I–III then in successive lines below 1–9 as follows: (1) pocket depths (PD) and (2) attachment levels (AL) measurements with option of recording at six sites per tooth as at 42; sites of (3) marginal inflammation (MI) by a red line and (4) subgingival bleeding on probing (SB) with 'X'; (5) furcation involvement (FI) by Grade I–III at furcation entrance; (6) recession pattern (RP) by drawing in actual marginal contour – linear extent may also be recorded (see also chart puncturing method Figure 21.9 C); (7) plaque retentive restoration margin (PR) by serrated line; (8) vestibular tissue (VT), frenal insertion (FT) interference with oral hygiene measures; (9) pericoronal pocketing associated with variations of soft tissue (ST) form, e.g. retromolar/maxillary tuberosity tissue. This method of charting permits total flexibility of individual operator preferences and recordings at subsequent periodic assessments. (B) Clinical chart for patient reference. The particular manner in which sites requiring more specific supra- and subgingival oral hygiene efforts are depicted on the copy chart is optional. Actual pocket depth measurements may be more instructive than merely depicting sites with an 'X' as shown. Marginal inflammation may be represented by a red line, sites at which specific brushes must be used and direction of insertion denoted by symbols or letters, e.g. IPB (interproximal brush) and ISB (interspace brush). The location of clearly identifiable teeth by virtue of porcelain crown (P), gold inlay (G) and isolated amalgam restoration (A), gingival margin recession outlines as at 16–13, tilted tooth positioning (arrow at 47), etc. may be marked on the chart with appropriately coloured outline shapes to facilitate localization by the patient. Note optional charting method in Figure 3.3

reference by the patient during homecare and more specific advice in plaque control given.

Probing assessment

The measurement of neither pocket depths nor attachment levels is considered to be important at this stage. In any case, the efforts to do so are usually precluded by gingival tenderness and will do little to enhance patient–operator relations! A fairly cursory probing and charting is carried out instead, to provide an overall view of the pattern and extent of periodontal breakdown and to confirm any radiographic findings (see Chapter 3). Where the patient presents atypically, with no clinical signs of gingival inflammation but clinical probing and radiographs reveal loss of attachment, the location of subgingival bleeding sites together with pocket probing depths and probing attachment levels should be recorded (Figure 12.1 A). The reason for this is that, unlike other patients, where at this stage treatment is being directed at the *marginal gingival* lesion, the treatment requirements are dictated by the consequences of persistent *subgingival* inflammation. This particular phase of therapy is considered later (see Detection of subgingival inflammation).

The appropriate cleaning devices and techniques

The operator must ensure that the appropriate cleaning devices are available and used in an effective fashion. In essence, the bristles of the toothbrush should be seen to actually negotiate the required subgingival tooth surfaces and dental floss observed to pass sufficiently apically. The interspace brush is especially useful at localized pocket sites as well as at interproximal pockets, where wood points and interproximal brushes may have certain limitations (see Figure 11.11).

Plaque retention factors

Only those gross deposits of calculus that totally occlude interproximal spaces or prevent the patient's reasonable access to the necks of the teeth (see Figure 9.1 D) are removed at this stage. Similarly, only overhanging restoration margins that give cause for complaint should be modified. The patient is finally reassured of the clinical improvement that can be expected following better home care alone and a review appointment is made for 4–6 weeks' time. This will allow sufficient time for cleaning techniques to be improved and for gingival inflammation to subside.

The second appointment

Marginal tissue inflammatory status

Examination is best carried out after drying the tissues with high volume aspiration to allow the minor differences between marginal tissue health and slight inflammation to be distinguished. A good source of light and a clean, clear, front surface dental mirror (for indirect vision) are also essential.

The inflamed gingivae will be found to have become less reddened and swollen and display a reduced tendency to bleed on gentle probing. While marginal gingival health will have developed at some areas, residual inflammation at others may simply reflect a transitional phase in healing and require further time for total inflammatory resolution. Nevertheless, it is prudent to check the patient's cleaning methods at such sites and where necessary to advise accordingly. The patient must be informed of the progress overall and be encouraged to persevere with his efforts.

In some instances, little or no improvement in the marginal gingival inflammation is noted and is associated with obvious deposits of plaque. Poor home care is implicated and the reasons for this should be established. The patient's understanding of the problem and interest in resolving it should be reassessed tactfully. Also, oral hygiene instructions should always be repeated, for these may possibly not have been explained properly earlier; perhaps too much information was given at the time, or perhaps the patient may have been too apprehensive to grasp the details.

Plaque and plaque retention factors

The gingival shrinkage accentuates the presence of any supragingival deposits of calculus and more importantly, will often expose the coronal aspects of any subgingival deposits (e.g. Figure 9.1 C). The marginal gingivae might appear more inflamed at these sites, suggesting plaque retention and, in turn, the need for scaling. Similarly, the finding of localized marginal inflammation related to a restoration may indicate plaque retention and should be dealt with as necessary.

Only those deposits of supragingival calculus, together with the reasonably accessible subgingival calculus that actual impede plaque removal by the patient, need to be removed at this stage. However, any unsightly calculus or extrinsic staining could also be removed in the interests of patient motivation. Conversely, staining that does not show should be ignored at this stage, for it is likely to recur until an effective oral hygiene regime is maintained. The deeper, less accessible, subgingival deposits are also best left alone for these will not impede the patient's cleaning and are much more difficult to remove at this early stage.

Professional cleaning

Supragingival professional cleaning is carried out methodically at all teeth in conjunction with subgingival debridement within the limits of *reasonable accessibility* to the operator, at any pocket sites. Ultrasonic devices will be found to be most convenient at this stage and should be followed, where necessary, by polishing with rubber polishing cups and paste. The application of a disclosing solution to check the efficacy of professional cleaning is prudent, although it could be dispensed with when confidence is gained from previous experience. A review is arranged after an interval of a further 4–6 weeks.

The third appointment

Persistent marginal inflammation

Resolution of marginal gingival inflammation will have occurred at the majority of sites where good oral hygiene has been practised consistently. Persistent inflammation must therefore be attributed to ineffective plaque removal by the patient and the reasons for this should be sought. When located at *relatively inaccessible* parts of the mouth a fault in cleaning technique is most likely. The methods actually used at these sites are reviewed and corrected as necessary. Elsewhere, and more especially when marginal inflammation is irregularly distributed, a plaque retentive factor should be suspected. Any residual deposits of subgingival calculus, or a defective restoration margin thus incriminated, are dealt with. Where a root surface concavity or groove, an uneven marginal gingival contour or adverse vestibular tissue morphology proves to be responsible, the patient's cleaning methods at the site should be checked. Further advice is then given and the effects assessed at the next appointment. Giving the patient a chart (Figure 12.1 B) to indicate the precise location and the nature of any plaque retention factor and which particular oral hygiene device to be used, can be most helpful at this stage.

Detection of subgingival inflammation

Once the marginal gingival inflammation in any area has been controlled by the patient's routine cleaning efforts, then the presence of any subgingival inflammation can be identified and attended to. This therapeutic sequence is critical to successful clinical examination to distinguish between the clinical signs of bleeding on probing, stemming from inflamed marginal gingivae, and that from inflamed subgingival sites, associated with the periodontal pocket. The true source of bleeding can only be reliably ascertained by first eliminating the former possibility of marginal inflammation, as shown in Figure 11.9 (G and H).

A methodical examination of the subgingival tissues using a periodontal probe is carried out. The finding of bleeding on blunt probing within any pocket in the absence of marginal inflammation (Figure 12.2 A) or the expression of pus, by digital pressure against the pocket wall (Figure 12.2 B), is indicative of subgingival inflammation and must be attributed to residual subgingival plaque. The location of these inflamed subgingival sites is recorded on the clinical chart, an appropriate copy of this charting is provided for the patient's use during home care and specific advice in subgingival cleaning is given.

Where subgingival inflammation cannot be detected by probing to the base of any pocket, it can be assumed that subgingival plaque is either not present or is not provoking inflammation at that time. The possibility must, however, also be considered that this absence of the clinically detectable signs of inflammation may only represent a transient phase of remission of disease activity. This is a common phenomenon during the course of any chronic inflammatory condition. It is therefore prudent, at least at this stage and when pocket closure has not occurred, to carry out a prophylactic debridement to disrupt any inactive subgingival flora at such pocket sites in conjunction with subgingival debridement elsewhere.

Subgingival debridement

Fine scalers, hoes and curettes, or a fine pointed ultrasonic tip (especially a modified slightly straightened P10 insert) may be used (Figure 12.2 C). The most effective and methodical subgingival debridement, within the limits of *reasonable accessibility*, is carried out. For this, the instrumentation extends as far apically as patient tolerance allows, without local anaesthesia. It is realized that in some instances dentinal sensitivity or individual patient or operator preferences may dictate otherwise. Supragingival polishing is carried out as the final step, if only in the interests of patient motivation. Then, depending on the features of the case and the patient's wishes, the next review appointment is made for about 2 months later.

Successive appointments

Re-evaluation

Resolution of all signs of marginal gingival and shallow subgingival tissue inflammation, indicative of the operator's control of reasonably accessible plaque, will be achieved by about the fourth or fifth

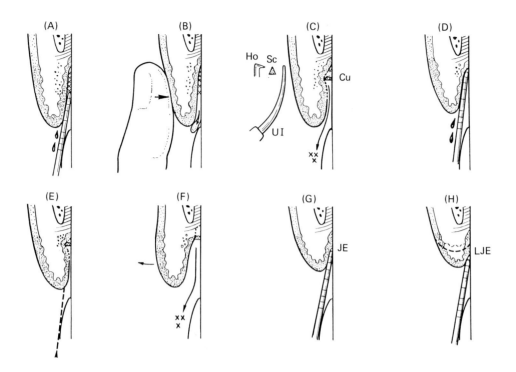

Figure 12.2 Continuous assessment. (A) Resolution of marginal inflammation following debridement at initially reasonably accessible sites. Bleeding on probing from residual inflammation associated with relatively to totally inaccessible remaining plaque. (B) Expression of pus by digital pressure against pocket wall. (C) Debridement to new limits of accessibility possible by previous gingival response using appropriate instruments (hoe [Ho], scaler [Sc], ultrasonic TFI–10 or P10 modified tips [UI] or curette [Cu]). Note: displacement of pocket wall tissue by instrument tip. (D) Gingival recession and pocket closure despite residual subgingival plaque at dento-epithelial junction manifested by bleeding on probing. (E) Access to the plaque front for both diagnostic probing and further debridement may be difficult. This is because of pocket closure and coronal tooth form interfering with instrument insertion (arrowed broken line) and manipulation. Debridement is also likely to result in an inadvertent soft tissue trauma. Local anaesthesia may then be required in some instances. (F) Sites considered totally inaccessible even with local anaesthesia may require surgical flap reflection to facilitate effective debridement. (G) Reduced probing depths following further debridement (be it blind or open) result from a combination of gingival recession, pocket closure and development of a longer junctional epithelium. (H) Further reduction in probing depth associated with long junctional epithelium or more gingival recession (represented by ghosted outline)

appointment in individuals willing to clean effectively (Figure 12.2 D). Where this is not the case, further oral hygiene advice and encouragement coupled with a compensatory professional cleaning is indicated.

At each assessment appointment, the presence of persistent disease due to residual subgingival plaque is sought by the methodical probing to the depth of each pocket (Figure 12.2 D). Any subgingival bleeding elicited will tend to be rather irregularly distributed in both arches. These sites are recorded, the patient is advised of the progress and with the aid of an updated chart, more careful subgingival cleaning with a single tufted brush, is emphasized.

Debridement difficulties

The necessary debridement to the pocket bases at the residual diseased sites will be facilitated by the reduced tissue sensitivity associated with inflammatory resolution, and the greater accessibility of the plaque front as a result of gingival recession. On the other hand, instrument insertion and manipulation may be restricted by the firmer pocket wall tissues and further impeded by prominent coronal tooth contours (see Figure 12.2 E). Local anaesthesia may therefore be required at some sites. Where however, despite anaesthesia, access for debridement is considered inadequate, or where the risk of unnecessary stretching and traumatizing of the tissue with the instrument shanks exists, surgical flap reflection to provide the necessary access may be indicated (Figure 12.2 F) (*cf.* Chapters 13 and 28). The case is reviewed after a further period of some months, when each of the vulnerable sites recorded previously is re-examined for any improvements and treated accordingly. In this way, a progressively reduced number of subgingival sites exhibiting bleeding will be found at successive appointments. This will be associated with the gradual development of pocket closure and reduced probing depths (Figure 12.2 G and H).

Probing levels

The recording of probing pocket depths and attachment levels may be carried out at the commencement of treatment, but it is considered preferable to delay detailed clinical examination until a significant improvement in subgingival inflammation has been achieved. This is primarily because of the difficulties experienced in recording true pocket depths and attachment levels in the presence of marginal and subgingival inflammation. The patient's discomfort caused by this probing has already been commented upon. Moreover, as gingival recession and pocket closure with a corresponding reduction in pocket depths, can be anticipated in the vast majority of cases, confirmation by physical measurements appears superfluous. Finally, the comparative unimportance of these measurements until this stage is reached, is placed into perspective by the fact that resolution of *marginal gingival* inflammation is the primary objective, and only then that of *subgingival* inflammation. Bleeding on probing remains a simple and reliable method of assessing this, although its long-term implications are less clear, as will be discussed in the next chapter and in Chapter 28 – Assessment of the need for surgical access.

Significance of delayed subgingival debridement

The benefits of delaying subgingival debridement to the plaque front, at the base of deep pockets, until resolution of inflammation of the marginal pocket wall tissue has been achieved was discussed in previous chapters, but warrants re-emphasizing here. In the first place, subgingival recolonization following subgingival debridement is inevitable in the presence of ineffective supragingival plaque control. It is, therefore, both reasonable and logical that supragingival plaque control should be established before any other steps are taken. Secondly, any attempt to compensate for the patient's failure by more frequent professional cleaning is rarely feasible in clinical practice. Thirdly, the inherent

difficulties of subgingival instrumentation to the bases of deep pockets are complicated by the presence of inflammation of the marginal parts of the pocket wall. The free bleeding which results obscures vision and may increase the likelihood of inadvertent minor trauma and pain to the marginal tissues which, in turn, precludes further instrumentation. These problems can be minimized by simply deferring this component of subgingival instrumentation until marginal inflammation, in response to the removal of reasonably accessible subgingival plaque, has subsided. The alternative use of local anaesthesia to permit more extensive debridement to be undertaken, may not be acceptable to all patients and may even lead to an inadvertent further loss of attachment (*cf.* Chapter 29 – Clinical implications). Lastly, it appears that temporarily delaying subgingival instrumentation deeply to the plaque front has no significant detrimental effect on attachment levels.

In summary, phased instrumentation makes an already difficult task of treatment easier for both patient and operator, with little or no risk to the patient. The elective delay in therapy will also be put in true perspective by the fact that this provisional neglect of subgingival plaque may ultimately be little different from what frequently occurs in traditional clinical practice. That is, the deepest deposits are likely to be retained anyway, albeit unintentionally, because of the widely claimed difficulties of carrying out a totally effective subgingival debridement. Indeed, the recent increased emphasis on the need for surgical access for such debridement reinforces this possibility.

The clinical outcome

Variable findings

The ultimate objective of the continuous assessment regime is the resolution of the clinically detectable signs of subgingival inflammation at all sites. However, the variable pattern of breakdown and different rates of healing encountered, in any one patient, means that resolution may take many months to effect and, in many instances, not be accomplished at all.

Furthermore, some sites may display signs of subgingival inflammation at some assessment appointments but not at others. Each of these possibilities may present in the same case. Finally, some individuals undergoing periodontal care may still present with persistent signs of marginal inflammation (see below).

Optimal healing

Where subgingival inflammatory resolution is achieved and maintained over several successive appointments, the arrest of disease by the gingival response and the establishment of periodontal health can be assumed. This optimal healing response, as depicted in Figure 12.2 (H), is most likely at situations where initially shallow pockets existed or where significant degrees of gingival recession plus pocket closure have occurred. These sites should therefore be reviewed at about 4–6-monthly intervals to ensure that health is maintained (*cf.* Chapter 27).

Persistent marginal gingival inflammation

There is a group of patients, referred to above, who demonstrate persistent or periodic phases of marginal gingival inflammation in some areas, despite the claimed homecare and the operator's efforts. These individuals, having failed to control reasonably accessible plaque, should not simply be dismissed as being uninterested or uncooperative. These charges can hardly be legitimately levelled at those who have attended so regularly. The fault might instead lie with the operator and the inappropriate plaque control methods being advised. Ineffective management of the relationship between patient and dentist, or a failure to understand the psychosocial factors in health and disease that are peculiar to that patient, may also have played a part (*cf.* Chapters 7 and 26).

Periodic recall for further motivation and professional cleaning is best continued for these individuals for a few years at least, in an effort to achieve marginal inflammatory resolution and, of more significance, possibly retard the rates of any ongoing attachment loss. Unfortunately, the relationship between the presence or indeed extent of marginal tissue inflammation and the loss of periodontal attachment is at present not known. In some instances, little or no destruction occurs so that the presence of the disease becomes tolerable and of minimal clinical significance, although the risk of further breakdown might exist.

In other situations, the periodontal destruction may only occur at a relatively slow net rate, apparently consistent with the retention of a functional dentition for the individual's natural lifespan. Once again, tolerable levels of periodontal disease will have prevailed but this can only be determined retrospectively, because of the lack of reliable prognostic indicators of disease activity.

Finally, some situations might demonstrate significant rates of deterioration and tooth loss over a period of some years. These are considered further in Chapter 26. It is therefore not possible to distinguish currently between sites of tolerable disease levels and those at which more rapid, and thus potentially significant, attachment losses occur. Some indication might be gained from previous disease activity and the age of the individual, but this cannot be regarded as a reliable prognostic indicator. The temptation to carry out anything other than subgingival debridement, for example surgical therapy, should be avoided in these cases for it would be of limited benefit and might even result in greater losses of attachment (*cf.* Chapter 29 – Post-surgical maintenance).

Persistent subgingival inflammation

Where the signs of subgingival inflammation are detected consistently, whilst the marginal tissues remain uninflamed, the existence of persistent disease due to previously inaccessible plaque is assumed. Nevertheless, even at this stage more careful debridement, if necessary under local anaesthesia, and even greater emphasis on the patient's subgingival cleaning efforts could be rewarded by inflammatory resolution. This will be achieved by either a more complete overlapping of debridement strokes or the removal of plaque associated with previously undetected calculus or other minor root surface irregularities.

The operator will not know whether this ultimate success has been the result of the additional root surface debridement or the removal of tooth substance by root planing. This is not of academic interest alone, as there are fundamental practical implications here for the management of such sites. Thus, if more complete debridement alone would suffice, the deliberate removal of tooth substance would be unnecessary and possibly even damaging. On the other hand, where an obvious plaque retention feature, such as a root furcation has been involved, inflammatory resolution presumably reflects the appropriate disruption of the harboured bacterial colony. This is most likely to be achieved when ultrasonic instruments have been used. Such a response is often only transient, for the root morphology predisposes to bacterial recolonization and the signs of inflammation tend to recur. These sites must therefore be carefully recorded and observed closely at subsequent review appointments.

Where the signs of disease still persist, or occur intermittently, the risk of further attachment loss must be assumed. Periodontal surgery to render these sites accessible to instrumentation (Figure 12.2 F) and, more importantly, future plaque control measures should then be considered. When presented with this option some patients develop new skills in negotiating sites previously thought to be inaccessible! The operator might, under these circumstances, be similarly persuaded and become capable of more careful and effective subgingival debridement. The choice of treatment in any one case will therefore depend on the clinical features, the dexterity and willingness of the operator and the patient's attitude to surgical treatment.

Surgical intervention

Some situations will impede debridement and so demand ultimately the creation of access by the surgical reflection of the soft tissue pocket wall. These are deep isolated pockets, uneven pocket depth sites and the furcation involvements of posterior teeth. The reparative response to this more effective surgical debridement does often result in some pocket reduction (Figure 12.2 G), which will facilitate subsequent cleaning. However the outcome is not predictable, so the option of extending this *surgical access* to attempted *pocket elimination* instead, or possibly even only an elective limited pocket reduction to facilitate future debridement, should not be discounted (*cf.* Chapter 29 – Clinical implications). On the other hand, it should also be realized that in many of the situations cited above, the ultimate outcome of pocket reduction and pocket elimination surgery is not very different. This is because of progressive gingival recession in the former and the operative difficulties of achieving pocket elimination, plus the tendency for coronal tissue proliferation, particularly interdentally, in the latter leading to the reformation of significant probeable pocket depths (*cf.* Chapters 14 and 15 and Chapter 29 – Clinical implications).

The dilemma of surgical versus non-surgical debridement

The management of the comparatively small residual number of sites that are totally inaccessible to routine debridement is considered in the subsequent chapters. The technical difficulties involved, plus the commensurate attention given to detail, means that surgical therapy commands a *disproportionately large* part of this text. This apparent emphasis upon surgical therapy must not be misinterpreted as downgrading the importance of subgingival debridement considered thus far. It is also stressed that no definitive evidence has yet been produced to determine the treatment of choice, whether this be further 'blind' or 'open' surgical debridement (each of which is invariably followed by some pocket reduction), limited pocket reduction surgery or elective pocket elimination surgery. Consequently, the manner in which these sites are handled by individual operators will be influenced very much by personal preferences of patient and operator. Whatever the chosen option, the onus must rest upon the operator to explain to the patient all the available options and the reasons for the particular treatment method adopted.

The method advocated in this text, in keeping with the continuous assessment philosophy, is the use of the *most conservative* subgingival debridement measures, consistent with achieving and maintaining subgingival inflammatory resolution.

Then where surgery is deemed necessary, the creation of the best possible access for future debridement is attempted, to minimize the need for any further possible surgical intervention.

The risks of retained inaccessible plaque

Where removal of the deepest level of subgingival plaque is delayed, as advocated in the phased debridement regime, the risk of further attachment losses must be accepted. Indeed, the very existence of the more extensive breakdown at such sites in the first place, would tend to support this *a priori* possibility. Any potential hazard to the remaining reduced periodontal support in any one situation must therefore be reconciled with this treatment approach.

Pattern of attachment losses

The chances of a significant deterioration occurring during the phased 2–3-monthly assessment periods of this gingival response regime are extremely small. This assumption is supported by clinical investigations (*cf.* Chapter 28 – Assessment of the need for surgical access) in which a very small incidence and extent of attachment losses have been observed, following traditional subgingival instrumentation, despite the likely retention of residual plaque in many instances. Indeed, even in untreated populations, significant losses have been reported only at isolated sites in comparatively few individuals. Finally, clinical experience of the continuous assessment regime in periodontal practice endorses this possibility. Thus, where marginal pocket wall tissue health is being maintained, only a very small number of isolated sites in a few individuals might actually deteriorate over the period of attempting to resolve the deeper subgingival inflammation by phased debridement.

Prediction of deterioration

It is, at present, impossible to tell which sites will deteriorate, because phases of destruction appear to occur randomly at different locations and at different times. However, in some individuals the possibility of a rapidly advancing periodontitis will exist (*cf.* Chapters 4 and 5). This is usually characterized by localized sites of severe destruction within an otherwise apparently healthy mouth and is readily identified by the radiographic appearance. As these few sites might be more vulnerable to further rapid breakdown, careful debridement should be carried out to the pocket bases at the earliest opportunity. This usually necessitates the use of local anaesthesia when, paradoxically, the risk of further attachment losses from inadvertent trauma from instrumentation is greatest. The supplementary use of antibiotic therapy might also be considered (*cf.* Chapter 35).

Disturbance of microbial activity

Loss of attachment prior to clinical diagnosis of disease will have occurred in the presence of an established supragingival and subgingival microbial flora. The phased removal of the supragingival and reasonably accessible subgingival components, by the patient and operator respectively, might well influence the pathogenic potential of the remaining deeper plaque thus limiting further destruction of the host tissues. This possibility is supported by the relationship demonstrated between supragingival plaque levels and subgingival recolonization following instrumentation (*cf.* Chapter 28 – Assessment of the need for surgical access), and by the comparable clinical attachment levels maintained following non-surgical and surgical debridement techniques, bearing in mind the widely claimed difficulties of carrying out the former blind method.

Feasibility of traditional therapy

As the sites at risk cannot be identified, traditional therapy would demand that all subgingival surfaces in all individuals would require thorough instrumentation. The feasibility of such a regime must be questioned. In the first place, the acknowledged technical difficulties accompanying such 'blind' instrumentation will mean that debridement would be incomplete in many instances, if only by default. Secondly, the cost in relation to benefit of such a policy being applied in general practice will preclude this. Finally, any attempt to carry out more effective root surface instrumentation by surgical means instead would be even less feasible (*cf.* Chapter 28, Access for root surface debridement).

Consequently, the management of only the reasonably accessible plaque within all pocket sites as an initial procedure, followed by more selective progressively deeper debridement at residual diseased sites, would seem to be a reasonable and biologically sound practical compromise for both patient and operator. Furthermore, while the ultimate effects of such a conservative regime have yet to be assessed in any controlled investigation, the outcome is likely to be little different from that accomplished by more traditional non-surgical instrumentation therapy. Finally, it is only in those very few instances where unacceptable levels of disease persist, in spite of the conscientious application of the continuous assessment regime, that surgical measures may be required.

13

The gingival response to plaque control

The gingival response refers to the reparative tissue changes that follow plaque removal by the patient and root surface debridement by the operator. With resolution of inflammation, the gingival pocket wall tissues shrink and remodel, becoming closely adapted to the tooth surfaces. The tissue findings and clinical implications are considered here.

Tissue findings

Influence of disease levels

Although inflammatory resolution in the gingiva is essentially the same as inflammatory resolution in other tissues, the unique nature of the dentogingival junction will greatly influence the ultimate tissue form following healing. Thus, where no loss of attachment has occurred the hyperaemic, oedematous marginal tissues revert to normal (Figure 13.1 A); whereas, in established disease, despite the comparable pattern of healing, the progressively more extensive destruction sustained will preclude the recreation of normal dento-epithelial form (Figure 13.1 B,C). The more advanced the level of disease, the more improbable is the re-establishment of a dento-epithelial form consistent with effective plaque control.

Instrumentation trauma

The inflamed and ulcerated pocket lining epithelium is prone to trauma during subgingival cleaning by the patient but this is even more likely to occur with root surface instrumentation. In the latter, carried out by either hand instruments or ultrasonic devices, the pocket lining and even some of the pocket wall

tissue may be removed inadvertently (Figure 13.1 D). The bleeding from the traumatized tissue provides some benefit by flushing out residual detached debris from the pocket space. A gingival inflammatory exudate persists for some hours after arrest of this bleeding and the development of a clot. This flow of exudate tends to remove any non-attached organisms and other fine debris (Figure 13.1 E,F). (See also Chapter 29 – Tissue curettage.)

Inflammation resolution

Healing of the inflamed gingivae proceeds with a progressive reduction in exudate, tissue oedema and cellular infiltrate. The pocket lining and junctional epithelial remnants and the gingival oral epithelium then proliferate rapidly under the surface clot (Figure 13.1 F) to re-epithelialize the wounded and ulcerated pocket wall and form a new lining epithelium. The gingival connective tissue organization is associated with a progressive increase in collagen density having the net clinical effect of tissue shrinkage and tight 'cuff-like' adaptation about the roots (see below).

Pocket epithelium changes

With effective debridement, the residual epithelium, and that which proliferates during healing becomes closely adapted to the root. The resulting attachment is effected by a junctional epithelium which forms the dento-epithelial junction. Where this junction is longer than that normally existing in health it is referred to as a long junctional epithelium (Figure 13.1 G). During healing the characteristically thickened hyperplastic state of the

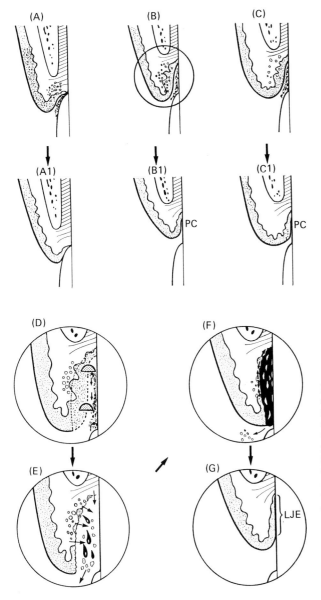

Figure 13.1 Gingival response to plaque control. (A) Gingivitis with no attachment loss reverts to (A1) normal dentogingival junction. (B) Periodontitis with pocketing responds by (B1) gingival recession and pocket closure. (C and C1) Similar healing at thicker hyperplastic tissue sites but with minimal recession. (D) Inadvertent removal of pocket lining tissue and possible disruption of dento-epithelial junction. (E) Gingival haemorrhage flushes out residual debris. (F) Blood clot formation and removal of fine debris by exudate. Pocket wall re-epithelialization commencing. (G) Optimal healing with shallow sulcus and long junctional epithelium (LJE)

existing pocket lining epithelium, with its numerous rete ridges, gradually reverts to the thin epithelium and relatively straight epithelial–connective tissue junction observed in the normal junctional epithelium. However, where the pocket epithelium has been removed during debridement, its replacement tends to be thin as depicted in Figure 13.1 (G).

The speed of wound re-epithelialization outpaces, and therefore virtually precludes, the development of a new connective tissue attachment. Even the optimal outcome of healing via a long junctional epithelium cannot be ensured and is indeed not often achieved. Instead the epithelium lying coronal to the dento-epithelial junction usually becomes closely related to, rather than joined to, the root surface (Figure 13.1 B1 and C1). This relationship, which characterizes pocket closure, permits the passage of a thin probe between the healed epithelium and tooth, whereas in situations with a long junctional epithelium (Figure 13.1 G), penetration and cleavage of the epithelium occurs (see also Figure 2.2). In this context, it must be realized that there has been very little histological documentation of periodontal healing in humans due to the difficulties in obtaining suitable research material.

Accordingly, the reasons for the usual but unpredictable clinical outcome of a close gingival adaptation to the tooth, rather than development of a long junctional epithelium, remain unclear and require further investigation. Similarly, the vulnerability of pocket closure to recurrent plaque-induced disease has not been established, although it has been shown, in the animal experimental model, that a long junctional epithelium is no more vulnerable than a normal dento-epithelial junction elsewhere (*cf.* Chapter 29 – Tissue curettage).

Connective tissue changes

The epithelial changes are accompanied by shrinkage of the pocket wall tissue corium associated with an increase in the gingival collagen, resulting in clinical pocket closure. The degree of shrinkage is influenced by the extent of the preceding inflammatory oedema and in part the tissue morphology. Swollen oedematous tissue thus tends to undergo greater shrinkage and remodelling than fibrous tissue, whilst an inherently thin gingival pocket wall displays greater marginal tissue shrinkage (recession) than elsewhere (Figure 13.1 B1 and C1).

Gingival recession

One hypothesis explaining the development of gingival recession stems from the characteristic proliferation of the pocket epithelium associated with gingival connective tissue inflammation. The resulting pocket epithelial rete ridges extend towards those of the gingival epithelium and in thin gingival tissue an approximation is virtually inevitable (Figure 13.2 A). This merger of epithelial layers, at the expense of gingival connective tissue, is followed by subsidence of the epithelial surface which manifests clinically as recession (Figure 13.2 D). A comparable sequence operates during tooth eruption, when the reduced enamel epithelium merges with the oral epithelium (Figure 13.2 E). When, in contrast, the gingiva forming the pocket wall is thick, the more substantial connective tissue corium remains between the pocket and gingival epithelial layers and the pocket persists instead (Figure 13.2 F).

There are two further hypothetical mechanisms of gingival recession. In one, the radius of the connective tissue inflammatory infiltrate is proportionately greater in thin gingival tissue (Figure 13.2 A), possibly compromising the integrity of the overlying gingival oral epithelium, resulting in recession (see also Chapters 4 and 32 – Aetiology of recession). In the other, the patient traumatizes the

marginal gingivae with over-enthusiastic toothbrushing. These traumatic lesions will be comparatively deep when located within thin detached tissue and may extend close to the pocket epithelium (Figure 13.2 B), possibly even perforating the pocket wall (Figure 13.2 C). In the former, the epithelial proliferation during healing leads to an epithelial merger and gingival recession; while in the latter, epithelialization of the perforation from both its oral and radicular aspects results in a mucosal fenestration with subsequent loss of the coronally located detached tissue. The development of gingival clefts in periodontal disease may be explained in this way. (See also 'traumatic' gingival recession and Deep incisor overbites in Chapter 21.) Similar traumatic lesions within thick tissue will have little effect on overall marginal tissue integrity (Figure 13.2 F–H).

Clinical effects

Site variations

The gingival response depends on a combination of the extent of periodontal destruction, the rate of repair and the gingival morphology. Thus, there will be variation from site to site in the same mouth and from patient to patient. The inflamed swollen, detached tissues become progressively paler in colour, firmer in consistency and undergo shrinkage so adapting more closely to the teeth. At the same time, gingival tenderness and bleeding experienced on tooth cleaning and during instrumentation, gradually diminish. Pocket closure and gingival recession are cardinal clinical signs of a favourable gingival response and must be regarded as being advantageous because the associated pocketing is reduced. Access for plaque control is improved and the likelihood of inflammatory resolution at the formerly deeper subgingival sites is enhanced. Finally, where any looseness of the teeth has occurred, this too diminishes.

Gingival tissue shrinkage

Shrinkage may occur both concentrically and longitudinally about the tooth. This results in reduced pocket depths by a closer adaptation of the gingiva about the tooth (pocket closure) and a reduction in the amount of detached tissue present (gingival recession). The latter is manifested as a progressive elongation of the clinical crown as shown in Figure 13.3. Pocket closure and gingival recession may operate independently or together in the reduction of pocketing and considerable inter-patient and intra-individual variations may be encountered (see also Figure 9.5). Localized pocket sites tend to become reduced, mainly by gingival adaptation with minimal marginal recession, whilst

128

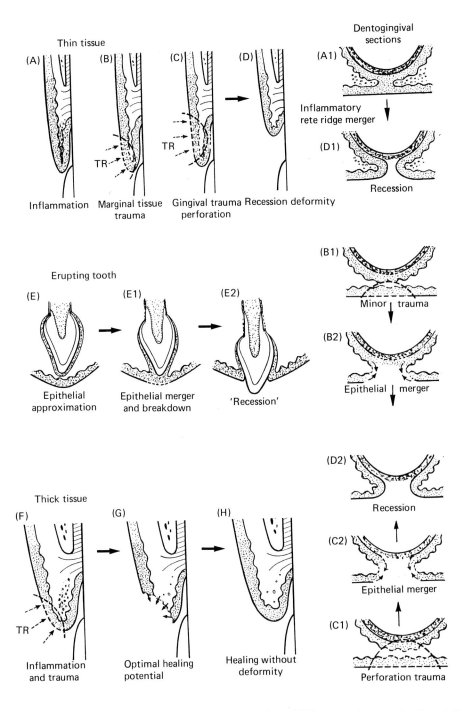

Figure 13.2 Mechanisms of gingival recession in disease. (A and F) Pocket wall connective tissue inflammatory cell infiltrate is proportionally greater in thin (A) than thick (F) tissue sites. Associated approximation and merger of pocket and gingival epithelial rete ridges at (A1) thin sites with subsidence of epithelium and development of (D and D1) gingival recession. Note: (E–E2) Sequence of epithelial breakdown occurring with tooth eruption. The extent of tissue damage sustained from gingival trauma (TR) is proportionally greater in thin (B and B1) than in thick (F) tissue sites with (C and C1) possibility of gingival tissue perforation. In the former, healing at (B2 and C2) thin tissue sites associated with pocket and gingival tissue epithelial proliferation and merger resulting in (D and D2) deformity of marginal recession. Healing of relatively shallow lesion at (G) effects (H) total repair with no recession

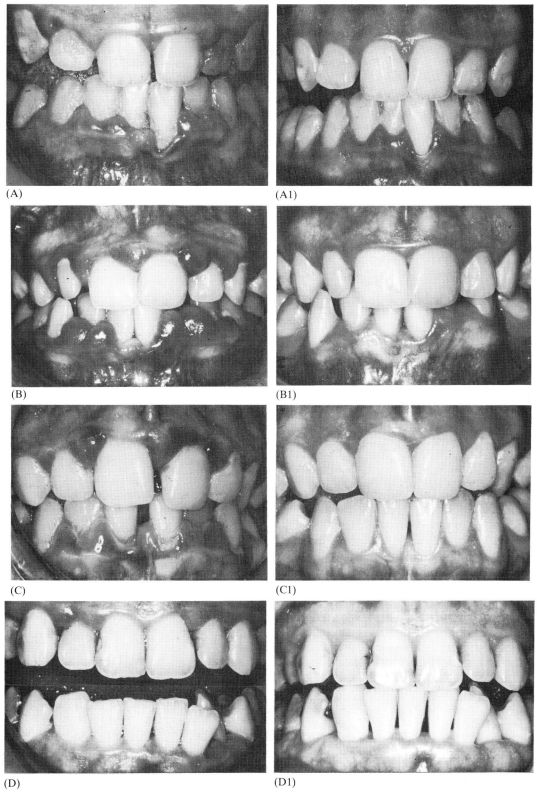

(A) (A1)

(B) (B1)

(C) (C1)

(D) (D1)

Figure 13.3

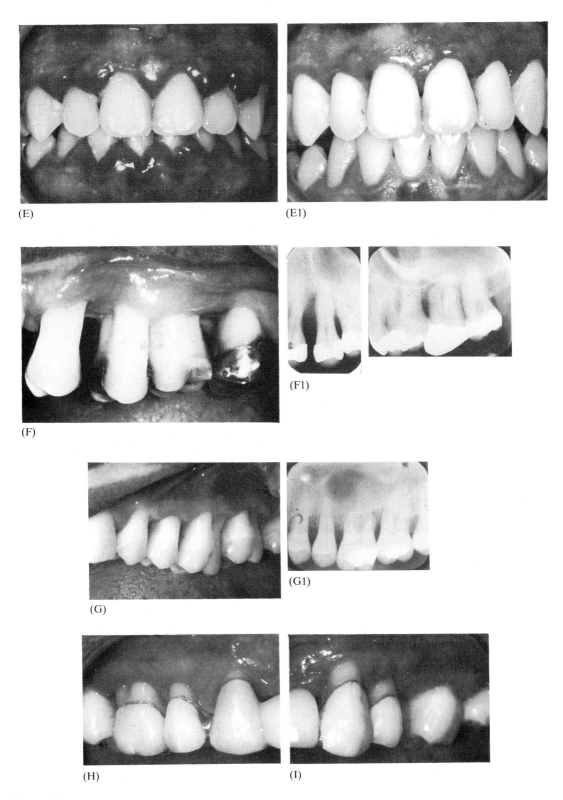

(E)

(E1)

(F)

(F1)

(G)

(G1)

(H)

(I)

Figure 13.3

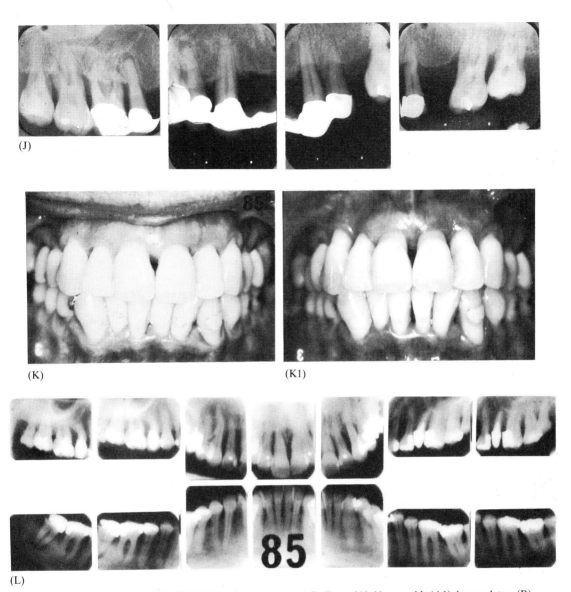

Figure 13.3 Gingival response. (A–E) Initial and post treatment findings. (A) 11-year-old. (A1) 4 years later. (B) 13-year-old. (B1) 2 years later. (C) 16-year-old. (C1) 3 years later. (D) 21-year-old. (D1) 2 years later. (E) 27-year-old. (E1) 1 year later. (F–I) Post-gingival response findings. (F) 34-year-old. (F1) Radiographs. (G) 40-year-old. (G1) Radiograph. (H and I) 43-year-old – coronal reconstruction fitted 4 years previously. (J) Radiographs. (K) 55-year-old. (K1) 3 years later. (L) radiograph on presentation (by courtesy of Dr S. Nyman). (E and E1 reproduced from *Dental Update*, by permission of Update-Siebert Publications Ltd)

areas with more generalized pocketing will display greater amounts of marginal recession. The influence of tissue morphology on the pattern of gingival recession and tissue remodelling has already been referred to. On the other hand, in some situations only minimal reductions of probing depths are achieved in spite of obvious inflammatory resolution. Pocket closure is therefore incomplete in these sites and little marginal recession will have occurred.

It is possible, in most instances, to estimate how much marginal gingival shrinkage is likely to occur from observing a combination of the morphology of the tissues, the degree of existing gingival recession and the patient's age. These factors then determine the *recession potential* for each case. Thus, in subjects with a strong recession potential, minor pocketing will be self-correcting and deeper pockets reduced significantly by the gingival response to subgingival debridement. Conversely, where a weak potential exists, there is little improvement in probing depths due to marginal recession, but pocket closure with a tight gingival adaptation or optimally a long junctional epithelium may still occur. This potential will also be applicable to the ultimate outcome of elective pocket reduction surgery (see Chapter 14).

The series of clinical cases involving individuals of different ages shown in Figure 13.3 (see also Figures 11.7 G–J, O and P; 21.8 A–D; 21.11 M–O; 23.1 G–I and 26.3 C), demonstrate the clinical changes that have occurred by the gingival response over various periods of time. The gingival remodelling observed tends to be more apparent in adolescents, because of the marked differences between clinical and anatomical crown sizes occurring with delayed passive eruption. In addition, there exists in adolescents a tendency for the development of a marked gingival oedematous and hyperplastic tissue reaction to plaque, which results in a false pocketing which is reversible. Each of these factors not only makes the clinical crowns appear even shorter on presentation but also contribute to the recession observed following therapy. Although the shrinkage in such instances appears clinically to be due to gingival recession, this is not strictly true, for root surface exposure does not ensue (*cf.* Pseudo-recession, Chapters 21 and 32).

Probing depths

The development of pocket closure and gingival recession are associated with decreasing clinical probing depths, while progressive periodontal breakdown would be indicated by increasing depths. However, this apparently simple assessment technique is fraught with difficulties. These relate to the recording of actual levels of periodontal destruction and the interpretation of the finding with respect to existing and future disease activity. These important issues are therefore considered more closely below.

Bleeding and suppuration

Bleeding, provoked by blunt subgingival probing, can reasonably be attributed to breaches in the pocket lining epithelium. These breaches could be due to trauma from probing causing tears in the thin friable epithelium or to the pre-existence of frank ulceration. This bleeding is indicative of subgingival inflammation and together with the expression of pus, is suggestive of tissue breakdown (see Figure 12.12 A and B). However, it is impossible to establish whether a progressively destructive lesion exists or this indicates a transient more active phase in a non-destructive chronic inflammatory cycle. Similarly, the absence of these clinical signs might suggest either a cyclical period of remission of

disease activity unrelated to therapy, the transient effect of recent debridement or that the progress of disease has actually been arrested. The clinical interpretation of these signs is often complicated further by the inconsistencies detected from one appointment to the next (see also Chapter 28 – Assessment of the need for surgical access).

The pattern of the clinical findings over long periods of time may on the other hand, be more significant and so warrant continuous assessment. Where there is a consistent absence of any signs of inflammation, periodontal health can be assumed. Where these signs occur inconsistently, a state of controlled disease may exist, in which an unstable truce between the host and the microorganisms is being maintained. Only when bleeding on probing and the expression of pus are consistently noted at the same site should progressive disease be suspected and especially when accompanied by increased probing depths.

Tooth mobility

Increased tooth mobility should be expected both in the presence of inflammation and following the loss of attachment in established disease. This is because increasing mobility in disease reflects, first and foremost, altered levels of pocket wall tissue inflammation (*cf.* Chapters 23 and 33 – Hypermobility and periodontal healing). Conversely, with inflammatory resolution in the gingival response, tooth mobility will gradually decrease which corroborates the clinical findings. The use of tooth mobility in clinical assessment is, at this stage therefore, best simply limited to its secondary confirmatory role. The finding of increased mobility in the absence of subgingival inflammation may also reflect occlusal overloading or periapical disease. The clinical implications of mobility are dealt with in Chapters 23 and 33.

Periodontal probing
Probing objectives

Periodontal probing is the most informative of the available diagnostic and evaluation methods. Thus apart from its use in recording pocket probing depths (PPD) and probing attachment levels (PAL), as examined in Chapter 4, it is indispensible in the detection of subgingival inflammation as described in Chapters 11 and 12. However, it must be reiterated that each of these have certain shortcomings and limitations, with none greater than the inability to determine future destructive disease activity (*cf.* Chapter 28 – Probing and disease progression). The various types of probes in use are shown in Figure 13.4. The Williams type has been found to be most suitable for routine clinical use.

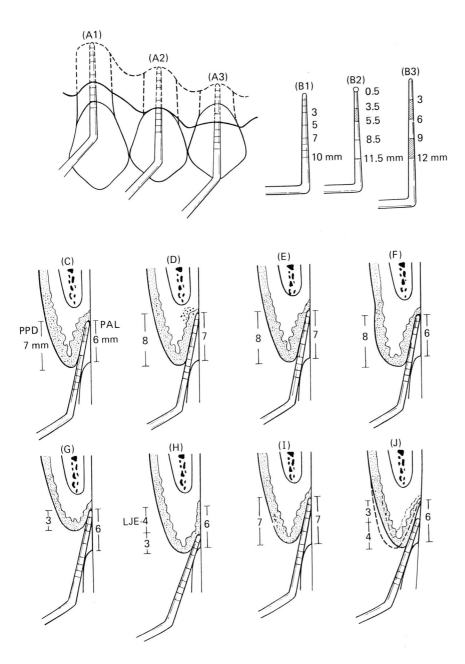

Figure 13.4 Interpretation of probing. Probing pocket depth (PPD) measured from gingival margin to pocket base. Probing attachment level (PAL) from cemento-enamel junction to pocket base. (A1–A3) PPD = 6 mm but PAL differs because of varying attachment losses and gingival margin positions. (A1) PAL = 9 mm less 3 mm recession. (A2) PAL and PPD = 6 mm (A3) PAL = 3 mm plus 3 mm gingival hyperplasia. Other variations shown in (C–J). (C) PAL = 6 mm and PPD = 7 mm. (D) Further probe penetration associated with increased inflammation at pocket base PAL = 7 mm and PPD = 8 mm. (E) Further loss of attachment PAL = 7 mm and PPD = 8 mm. (F) Gingival swelling PAL = 6 mm but PPD = 8 mm. (G) Recession and (H) development of long junctional epithelium (LJE) so that PAL = 6 mm and PPD = 3 mm. (I) Further loss of attachment PAL = 7 mm but concurrent gingival recession PPD = 7 mm. (J) Partial pocket closure and coronal tooth contour impeding probe insertion PAL = 6 mm and PPD = 4 mm. The initially inflamed tissue (ghosted) permitted deflection by probe for accurate probing measurements. (B1–B3) Periodontal probe types shown with graduations (B1) Williams, (B2) WHO 621 and (B3) Prima PX colour coded. Probe depicted in (A and C–J) is Goldman–Fox/Williams DE pattern.

Interpretation of probing depths

The distance from the gingival margin to the point reached by the tip of the periodontal probe denotes the *pocket probing depth* (PPD). While the PPD also gives an indication of the amount of destruction sustained, determined by the *probing attachment level* (PAL), this will only be accurately represented when the gingival margin coincides with the cemento-enamel junction as shown in Figure 13.4 (A2). Elsewhere, under- or over-estimated attachment levels are obtained (Figure 13.4 A1 and A3). Probing pocket depths may be helpful to some clinicians in treatment planning to assess the difficulties of access likely to be encountered during the subsequent plaque control and subgingival debridement measures. This facility is not required when phased debridement is practised.

The limitations and disadvantages of pocket probing depths at the initial examination, in the presence of tender inflamed tissues, has already been a matter of comment. Suffice it to add that any such attempted recordings will inevitably constitute an inaccurate baseline for subsequent measurements. Furthermore, as pocket reductions are to be expected following subgingival instrumentation efforts, evidence thereof produced by probing merely serves to confirm that already clinically obvious to the operator. This probing is therefore wasteful of valuable clinical time whilst causing unnecessary patient discomfort. In addition, the lack of detailed information regarding the pattern of periodontal destruction, as provided by any attempted careful periodontal probing of attachment levels, is of little practical importance in the early stages of treatment. Finally, the findings from routine radiographic examination (*cf.* Chapter 3) are quite adequate for overall diagnostic and treatment planning purposes at this stage.

Probing is best delayed until some inflammatory resolution has been achieved, when changes recorded have greater clinical relevance. Even then, pocket probing depths are of limited value in assessing the progress of therapy. In the first place, although reduced measurements do indicate shallower pockets they cannot differentiate between marginal recession and pocket closure (Figure 13.4 G and H) and may even be associated with concurrent losses of attachment (see below).

Secondly, an increased pocket depth could mean either further attachment loss or a coronal movement of the marginal gingiva due to gingival swelling (Figure 13.4 E and F). There might also simply be a transiently increased subgingival inflammation, allowing the probe tip to penetrate beyond the apical termination of the dento-epithelial junction thus giving an over-estimation of true probing depth (Figure 13.4 D). Then, as inflammation subsides, the associated deposition of new collagen in the tissues resists probe penetration and results in a reduced recording. For this reason, successive probing measurements might differ by as much as 2 mm for the same attachment levels, according to the state of the tissues (*cf.* Chapter 4).

Thirdly, when pocket depth measurements remain unchanged this demonstrates either just that, or that similar degrees of attachment loss and marginal recession have occurred concurrently (Figure 13.4 I). Finally, it must be reiterated that none of these recorded changes are reliable indicators of future disease activity.

The difficulties of interpretation of probing depths must also be viewed in the light of the purely technical problems encountered when recording probing attachment levels, relating to coronal reference points, and the manipulation of the probe within the pocket spaces. These are considered next.

Probing reference points

The gingival margin is a convenient but unsuitable reference point for both measuring attachment levels, as shown in Figure 13.4 (A), and more importantly recording any changes to these levels. The latter is because of possible gingival shrinkage as part of the gingival response and the difficulties of accurately measuring this marginal recession in turn (*cf.* Chapter 4 and 21), because of the lack of convenient fixed reference points. The gradual development of gingival recession in the gingival response to plaque control is nevertheless easily detectable, if not measurable, by root surface exposure, the interproximal spaces becoming patent and by the increasing distances between any restoration margins and the gingival margins.

The use of the cemento-enamel junction as a coronal reference point is also impractical because it can be difficult to locate. A convenient restoration may be used for fixed reference but restorations may themselves be changed. The provision of an individually made occlusal overlay (see Figure 21.9), as used in clinical research, is probably the most accurate and reliable occlusal reference point method but is much too costly and impractical for routine use. No simple yet accurate method therefore exists. In addition, whatever reference points are used, problems of visual parallax exists when reading off the probe graduations towards the back of the mouth, and especially when indirect vision is necessary which affects the accuracy of measurements.

Probe manipulation

The accurate determination of the connective tissue attachment level at the base of the pocket is complicated by the technical difficulties of probe manipulation. Thus, allowing for the effects of possible inflammation at the pocket base, the problem also exists of maintaining reproducible probing forces and paths of probing from one review appointment to the next. The former cannot be ensured, although with experience each operator will presumably develop a reasonably consistent technique. The operator's individual enthusiasm, or perhaps reluctance, for detecting any change might sometimes also influence the findings. For example, there may be a temptation to probe firmly during pre-surgical treatment planning, yet more gently following surgery. This probably forms the basis for the cynical remarks made by students about probing before and after surgery! The patient's tolerance of pocket probing might also vary from time to time and so possibly interfere with accurate recordings. The use of local anaesthesia would overcome this but is generally impractical for routine use. Standardized electronic probing devices, as used in many controlled clinical investigations, will resolve this difficulty but they are, as yet, not readily available commercially.

One other difficulty experienced relates to inserting a periodontal probe to the base of the pocket when resolution of marginal inflammation causes the detached tissues to tighten concentrically about the neck of the tooth. The reason for this is that the previous path taken by the probe, allowed by the readily deflected oedematous tissue becomes progressively less negotiable as pocket closure ensues (Figure 13.4 J). This difficulty is aggravated by bulky coronal tooth contours. Comparable difficulties experienced during subgingival instrumentation have been considered earlier (see Figure 11.13).

Probing re-evaluation

It must be concluded that the apparently simple exercise of measuring pocket depths by probing and then assessing attachment levels is inexact. Additionally, the margin of error in probing reproducibility is liable to be greater than the very small differences encountered at any one site. Because of the invariably very slow progression of attachment loss, even if a true loss of attachment could be measured, it may take some years to occur. An even more important consideration is that this knowledge may not have any bearing upon future findings (*cf.* Chapters 28 and 29). It is not that attachment loss cannot be appreciated clinically it is just that incremental measures should not be endowed with spurious accuracy, especially when 'measured' over short periods of time. Consequently, once all superficial signs of gingival inflammation have resolved, it is necessary to monitor the subgingival inflammatory status at each site very carefully in conjunction with further debridement and continued optimal oral hygiene. When clinical improve-

ment at the dento-epithelial junction is still not achieved and more importantly, an impression of a progressive loss of attachment gained, surgical intervention should be considered in order to render such sites accessible to plaque control.

The role of pocket surgery

Basic indication for surgery

The fundamental indication for periodontal pocket surgery is when progressive loss of attachment can be demonstrated unequivocally and attributed to inaccessible subgingival plaque. The clinical implications present the operator with a considerable clinical dilemma. Thus, the mere existence of a pocket does not in itself justify surgical intervention, nor can there be any depth of pocketing which automatically necessitates surgery. Instead, the principal concern is whether plaque control is actually being prevented at any particular site, bearing in mind that this will vary considerably according to tooth, patient and not least the operator. Furthermore, it must not only be established that progressive disease is actually occurring but, more importantly, that the rate of deterioration will threaten the dentition.

Clinical dilemma

The detection of progressive disease remains the major difficulty. The chances of measuring true differences in probing attachment levels at any one site over a period of, say, 1 year, are small in view of the very slow rates of disease progress encountered in the vast majority of instances. Consequently, continual assessment over a period of several years, rather than the traditional time span of months, would seem to be necessary. Even with this information about previous attachment losses, further destruction cannot be assumed.

Neither the natural course of the disease nor that following subgingival debridement therapy have been demonstrated with sufficient clarity to permit any reliable prognostic conclusions. More importantly, it has been shown that individuals with established disease who achieved a high standard of oral hygiene, displayed insignificant mean differences in attachment levels between segments treated by 'blind' subgingival debridement alone and 'open' surgical debridement (*cf.* Chapter 24 – Evaluation of modified Widman flap type technique). The operator is therefore presented with a considerable quandary in deciding whether or not to use surgery. Several other factors need also to be considered in resolving this clinical dilemma.

Surgical access or future plaque control

Periodontal pocket surgery may be regarded as having two objectives. First, to gain access to hitherto inaccessible root surfaces in order to allow adequate debridement at operation. Second, to facilitate future plaque control measures by recreating preferably a normal dentogingival form but, where not possible, at least a more readily negotiable form. The first implies that healing following surgical debridement will rectify the pre-existing morphological plaque retention barriers that necessitated surgical intervention and thereby allow routine professional cleaning to be practised and more importantly, obviate the need for further surgery. Unless this can be ensured, the operator has a responsibility to eliminate or at least reduce, in the interests of future plaque control, the morphological features that necessitated surgical access.

The second surgical objective on the other hand, makes the tacit assumption that only a morphological situation, totally accessible to the patient, will suffice for future periodontal health. This appears not to be so, for clinical investigations have demonstrated essentially comparable results regardless of the type of pocket surgery (pocket reduction or pocket elimination) undertaken (see Chapter 29 – Evaluation of different surgical methods). The unexpected finding with respect to pocket probing depths may however be explained by the technical difficulties experienced in ensuring post-surgical flap stabilization and, more importantly, achieving the intended surgical pocket elimination. These may arise because of the frequently uneven levels of periodontal destruction encountered at adjacent sites and the presence of bony defects thwarting this surgical objective. Similarly, this might also have accounted for the observation of unpredictable degrees of post-surgical gingival recession at some sites and coronal proliferation of the marginal tissues at others. In essence therefore, it is not only difficult to judge when to intervene surgically but also which is the best of the different possible surgical techniques to employ. Optimal pocket reduction, if not pocket elimination to facilitate future plaque control efforts, is recommended in this text. This implies that the principle of surgical flap reflection, for the express purpose of gaining improved access for root surface debridement at operation, cannot be endorsed.

It should be clear that surgery in itself, is unable to eradicate disease and its potential is essentially limited to dealing with the consequences of disease. It is also incumbent that where the intended correction of dentogingival morphology is likely to be thwarted on technical grounds, the resulting surgical compromise will have justified surgical intervention. That is, where a surgical compromise is likely to be enforced, might not the same outcome have accrued over further periods of time from more conscientious subgingival debridement alone. However, weighed against this are the potential penalties of further attachment loss by delaying surgery in anticipation of the possible control of disease by conservative measures.

Few of these issues can be resolved here. The reasons for this, coupled with their clinical significance, will be more fully appreciated when the chapters on Simple and Complex pocket therapy have been read and understood.

Psychological and economic considerations

These important aspects of pocket surgery must not be overlooked. Thus, the comparative costs of surgical treatment must be measured against those of a non-surgical approach in terms of effort, time, money and, not least, comfort for both patient and operator. Furthermore, whilst surgery might represent little more than a technical exercise for the operator it could mean very much more, physically, emotionally and even perhaps financially, to the patient. The decision to operate should therefore never be taken lightly and all the implications should be clearly explained to the patient. Ultimately, should any doubt exist about the wisdom of surgical intervention there should be no hesitation in seeking a second opinion.

A pragmatic approach to pocket surgery

Choosing a test area

It is recommended, in the first instance, that a single representative area be selected as a surgical test area. This is designed on the one hand, to assess the likely response to periodontal surgery of the periodontal tissues elsewhere, and on the other, the acceptability of such complex treatment to the patient. Accordingly, the test area should as far as possible incorporate different pocket types for that particular individual. For convenience, this surgical field should extend over an anterior or posterior segment of the arch, involving about five teeth. Pocket elimination surgery is then carried out and, where achieved, a successful surgical outcome can be anticipated. Where this can be shown to be successful and periodontal health then maintained for 6 months, further surgery can, with the patient's agreement, then be performed elsewhere in the mouth with some confidence as to the likely outcome.

It is usually only in areas presenting with moderate disease that a predictable surgical result of a totally cleansible dentogingival morphology is achieved. This is effected by simple pocket surgery, and with patient cooperation, future periodontal health is virtually ensured. Elsewhere, the variable and complex pattern of breakdown encountered, frequently precludes surgical pocket elimination. This means that a less predictable surgical compromise of pocket reduction and the possibility of persistent disease must be accepted instead.

Post-surgical evaluation

Unfortunately, the findings of post-surgical evaluations are seldom straightforward. In the first place, probeable pocket depths are frequently encountered even where pocket elimination had apparently been achieved at the time of operation. Furthermore, bleeding on probing can often be still detected following the healing of sites at which surgical pocket elimination has not been possible. This, in turn, creates a further dilemma, for subgingival bleeding would have been used as one of the clinical criteria in support of the test area surgery. This delicate situation has been handled by the flippant assertion in the student clinic that the finding of bleeding is an indication for surgery, but when encountered after surgery, can be readily controlled by non-surgical means. Fortunately, some pocket reduction will have been achieved in most instances, so improving access for this post-surgical subgingival debridement. Elsewhere, the operator is confronted once again with the same clinical problem that existed before surgery and upon which the decision to operate was based. Finally, it is impossible to judge with any certainty whether further attachment loss will occur at any of these sites, although the risk of this happening presumably does still exist (*cf.* Chapter 27 – Maintenance).

The basis of complex pocket surgery

Those situations which invariably thwart the attainment of surgical objectives of simple pocket surgery and, as a result, lead to persistent disease, fall into three categories. The first relates to the involvement of root furcations. The second to uneven patterns of breakdown at adjacent diseased sites and more especially where the pocket bases lie within bony defects. The last situation is concerned with the involvement of vestibular tissue morphology. Each of these factors preclude successful simple pocket surgery and must be dealt with by complex pocket therapy, but in which it must be stressed treatment compromises must be frequently accepted. Further consideration is given to these problems in subsequent chapters.

Other indications for surgery

The importance of the existence of *progressive disease* at any specific pocket, as the fundamental

indication for periodontal pocket surgery has already been stressed. In addition, the difficulties of actually identifying such disease activity and of the ensuing clinical dilemma when similar clinical signs persist after pocket surgery, have also been considered. However, there are other rather more clearly identified and readily resolved circumstances in which surgical intervention might also be considered. These are as follows:

(1) The surgical elimination of gingival pockets and deformities to expedite restorative therapy. In some instances the removal of even sound supporting tissues might be necessary to expose the margins of tooth preparations, particularly following cusp fractures or tooth wear.
(2) The correction of poor appearance associated with, on the one hand, gingival overgrowth as in drug-induced or developmental hyperplasia or, on the other hand, with localized gingival recession.
(3) The drainage of an acute lateral periodontal abscess. The elective reduction of the pockets at such sites to minimize the risk of recurrent abscesses might also be considered.

Each of these special indications will be dealt with later.

A total perspective of surgical therapy

Although the importance of the individual affected site has been emphasized frequently in treatment planning, the condition of the dentition as an entity and the welfare of the patient as a whole must be borne in mind continually. These necessitate the careful consideration of several fundamental issues.

(1) whether the rate of periodontal destruction in the absence of surgery is likely to cause loss of dentition, or significant parts of it, during the patient's lifetime;
(2) the significance of such partial or total tooth loss in terms of the patient's function, comfort or emotions;
(3) the risk of the dentition being threatened by caries at such a level that necessitates elective tooth extractions because of unmanageable technical problems;
(4) the economic implications arising from the various facets of therapy.

Each of these issues emphasizes the importance of carefully reconciling the various aspects of dental treatment with the patient's required or perceived needs. It can also not simply be assumed that the patient possesses the same set of values in respect of dental therapy as the operator. A great deal of time and effort can be saved and, more importantly, patient discomfort minimized if the true situation is ascertained before embarking upon surgery. If periodontal treatment is phased, as advised in the previous chapters, these matters should become self-evident.

Section II

Surgical therapy

14

The essential basis of pocket surgery

Introduction

The periodontal pocket represents a morphologic deformity, comprised of the detached gingiva and the root surface. The essential problem of the pocket is that the detached gingiva precludes plaque removal and surgery aims to overcome this. The possible technical solutions are either to reflect the pocket wall to permit root surface instrumentation and then to seal the gingiva against the tooth to prevent further plaque accumulation, or remove the detached tissue to eliminate the pocket space and so expose the formerly inaccessible roots for plaque control. These three surgical methods can be likened to eliminating the space between a long shirt sleeve and one's forearm by tightening the sleeve about the forearm (surgical reattachment), cutting off the sleeve at the level of the elbow (resection), or sliding the sleeve up so that the cuff edge lies at the elbow (apical repositioning) (Figure 14.1).

The surgical options

The first option implies that the detached gingiva becomes reattached to the previously diseased root

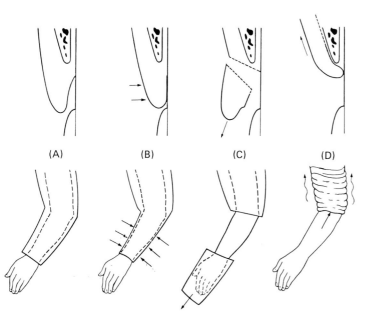

(A)   (B)   (C)   (D)

Figure 14.1 Diagrammatic representation of pocket surgery methods. (A) Pocket space represented by part of sleeve about forearm. (B) Surgical reattachment by tightening sleeve. (C) Resection by cutting sleeve away. (D) Apical repositioning by pulling up sleeve. Note: while rumpling effect represented over upper arm does not occur clinically, any tissue fold being dissipated into the loose vestibular tissues, it does clearly demonstrate the contra-indication of apical repositioning in the palate

surface, and is described as surgical reattachment. The other option can be achieved in two ways. Firstly, by cutting away the detached gingiva by a process of surgical resection. Resection is traditionally, but less precisely, referred to as gingivectomy. Secondly, the tissue forming the pocket wall is displaced in an apical direction, so that its margin lies against the tooth at the level of the former pocket base thereby eliminating the pocket space. This is described as apical repositioning. Together these three surgical options form the basis of simple pocket surgery.

Clinical applications

In both moderate and advanced periodontitis the simple pocket can be surgically corrected in a straightforward and predictable fashion by simple pocket surgery. In contrast, in complicated periodontitis the complex pockets characterized by variable morphological features of the roots, uneven pattern of attachment loss and bony resorption and vestibular anatomical implications, represent additional operative components and are more difficult to correct. Nevertheless, simple pocket surgery remains applicable to all situations, because the specific measures required for the complex morphological features encountered can be readily incorporated into the basic surgical sequence.

The practical implications are that the operator can concentrate on the simple pocket surgical exercise without being distracted by the possibility of any complex pocket features arising, until they are actually encountered during operation, and when they can be dealt with on their own merits, as supplementary technical exercises. The facility to integrate the differing needs of complex pocket surgery into a single surgical regime revolving about simple pocket surgery thus greatly simplifies surgical pocket treatment. The principles of simple pocket surgery must, therefore, be considered first.

Simple pocket surgery

The surgical options of surgical reattachment and apical repositioning each conserve the tissue forming the pocket wall whilst that of resection sacrifices and discards most of this tissue. This aside, the differences between the techniques depend upon comparatively minor technical details. The principles are dealt with in this chapter followed by the technical details in subsequent chapters.

Surgical reattachment

Ideal healing

This technique would seem to be the treatment of choice, because it aims to reproduce the pre-diseased state by the detached gingival tissue becoming attached once again to the root surface by the development of a new periodontal ligament coupled with a junctional epithelium forming the healed dentogingival junction (Figure 14.2 E). This ideal result of healing is referred to as 'new attachment', because new cementum and periodontal ligament fibres forms.

Note: The term 'reattachment' is reserved for healing of a surgically reflected mucosal flap to initially intact supracrestal fibres and occurs in most instances as shown in Figure 14.2 (E–H), whilst 'surgical reattachment' refers to the operative technique under consideration here.

The periodontal pocket appears to be maintained by a combination of subgingival bacterial plaque and any contaminating effects upon the root surface and by the epithelialized pocket lining (Figure 14.2 A). Once plaque has been removed and the root surface decontaminated by mechanical debridement and the gingival connective tissue, exposed by removal of the pocket lining (Figure 14.2 B), closely adapted to the root (Figure 14.2 D), healing should theoretically result in the development of a new periodontal ligament (Figure 14.2 E). This new attachment does however rarely come about although this may develop to a minimal extent as shown in Figure 14.2 (G). Usually, pocket closure alone occurs coronal to the healed junctional epithelial attachment (Figure 14.2 G). In some cases this pocket closure is more optimally associated with the development of a long junctional epithelium (Figure 14.2 F).

The barriers to new attachment

New attachment might be thwarted by a number of possible factors. These include, most importantly, the lack of the appropriate tissue cells capable of forming new cementum, inadequate root surface debridement, pocket wall inflammation, poor pocket wall adaptation to the root and a persistent or rapidly reforming pocket lining epithelium. Each of these are considered briefly here, but see Chapter 31 – The role of bone in new attachment.

The tissue cell types

Contrary to expectation neither gingival connective tissue nor bony cells are capable of forming a new attachment (see Chapter 31 – The role of bone in new attachment). This can apparently be achieved by periodontal ligament cells alone, having proliferated from their base and migrated coronally over the formerly diseased root surface. This occurs in competition with the reparative activities of the adjacent bone and periosteum, the gingival connective tissue and the epithelium derived from the gingival margin and any residual pocket lining. The nature of the healing is therefore dictated by the cell

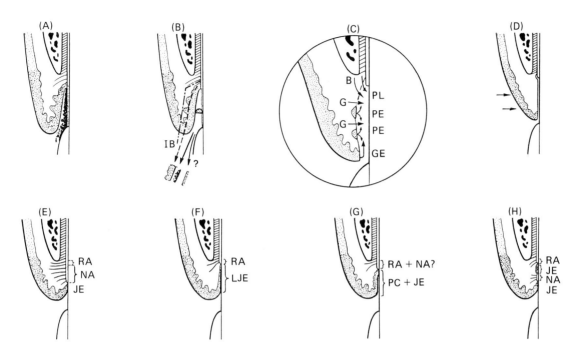

Figure 14.2 Possible outcomes of surgical reattachment. (A) Pocket with subgingival plaque, calculus and suspected cemental contamination. (B) Subgingival instrumentation comprised of debridement plus root planing for elimination of contaminated or possibly even all (?) cementum and inadvertent removal of some pocket epithelium, none of which can be judged clinically. Note inverse bevel (IB) excision of pocket lining. (C) Potential for wound repopulation from gingival margin (GE) and pocket lining (PE) epithelium; gingival (G) and bony (B) connective tissue and periodontal ligament (PL). (D) Following surgical excision of pocket lining, soft tissue closely adapted to root surface. (E) Reattachment (RA) to remaining supracrestal fibres plus new attachment (NA) via new cementum and periodontal ligament. Note: development of physiological junctional epithelium (JE) occurs in all instances. (F) Total re-epithelialization with an optimal development of long junctional epithelium (LJE). (G) More usual healing by pocket closure (PC) coronal to JE. (H) JE associated with NA within epithelial window

types that repopulate the wound (Figure 14.2 C). The apparent advantage of the periodontal ligament cells being closely related to the root from the outset is virtually nullified by the rapid re-epithelialization of the wound as shown in Figure 14.2 (F). However the findings of recent experimental methods of favouring periodontal ligament cell activity by 'guided tissue regeneration' (see Figure 14.3 C1) are encouraging (see Chapter 31 – Preferential repopulation investigations).

The influence of gingival and osseous connective tissues in healing is unclear. Thus animal model investigations reveal that even where epithelium has been excluded and the gingival tissue adapted close to the root surfaces, the gingival fibres invariably only become orientated parallel to the root surface without forming a new attachment. Small discontinuities or 'windows' in the re-epithelialized wound surface, within which gingival connective tissue associated with some cementum formation on the root surface new attachment, have however been

observed (Figure 14.2 H). There is, on the other hand, some experimental evidence that gingival connective tissue might lead to root surface resorption. Osteogenic reparative activity is less promising, for even in the unlikely event of coronal proliferation over the root surface, root resorption and ankylosis ensue. This potential complication is academic here, but assumes considerable importance in complex surgical therapy. (See Chapter 19 and Chapter 31 – Intrabony defect healing and bone grafting.)

Inadequate debridement

Even though the root surfaces are surgically exposed to permit proper debridement, complete removal of the contaminated root surface material cannot be ensured (see Chapter 28 – The assessment of adequate debridement). Similarly, it is difficult to establish to what extent any such inadequate instrumentation has been responsible for failure to achieve new attachment.

Inflamed pocket tissue and tissue approximation

The influence of gingival connective tissue inflammation *per se* and of the possible presence of microorganisms within the tissues on surgical healing is not clear. The removal of such inflamed and/or infected tissue and its implications are considered in Chapter 29 – Tissue curettage.

Close adaptation of the gingiva against the root surfaces is only feasible at the facial and oral aspects (Figure 14.3 C). Interproximally, tissue adaptation is complicated by the difficulties of tissue manipulation in such a confined space, the virtual destruction of the interdental gingival tissue septum by any attempted removal of the pocket epithelium from both its mesial and distal surfaces (Figure 14.3 E and F) and the tendency for any remaining interdental tissue to necrose (Figure 14.3 G). (See also Chapter 17.)

Pocket epithelium

The complete removal of the epithelialized pocket lining and inhibition of epithelial proliferation from the marginal tissues' oral epithelium apically over the detached connective tissues is indicated. Neither is readily accomplished. (See also Chapter 29 – Tissue curettage – removal of epithelium.) The former is complicated by its irregular epithelial rete ridge structure, the inability to judge whether it has been achieved and the vulnerability of the pocket wall to inadvertent perforation during soft tissue curettage. These difficulties at the facial and oral surfaces are best overcome by excising the epithelium by sharp dissection (Figure 14.3 A and B). This is carried out preferably as the initial stage of operation or once the pocket wall tissue has been surgically reflected. The difficulties of doing so interdentally are readily apparent from Figure 14.3 (E).

No practical way exists of preventing the epithelial downgrowth from the oral epithelium, the rate of which has been estimated at about 1 mm per day. Consequently at pockets of moderate depth (5–7 mm) a reparative re-epithelialization develops within a week, so precluding connective tissue attachment. Residual islands of pocket wall epithelium result in more rapid re-epithelialization than by oral epithelial downgrowth alone as shown in Figure 14.2 (C). A new epithelial attachment to the tooth (junctional epithelium) forms at the former pocket base within 7–10 days.

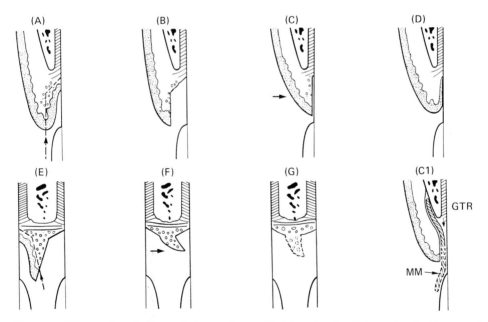

Figure 14.3 Tissue adaptation in surgical reattachment. Excision of pocket lining and underlying granulation tissue at (A) facial or oral aspect (E) interdentally with (B and F), exposure of pocket wall connective tissue. Close adaptation feasible at (C) but not at (F) which shows attempted adaptation of residual interdental connective tissue to one root surface with (G) possible tissue necrosis. (D) Optimal healing with long junctional epithelium. Note: (C1) principle of guided tissue regeneration (GTR) in which millipore filter or synthetic tissue membrane (MM) is placed between tooth and surgical flap. Filter may protrude coronal to flap, as shown by broken outline form, or be trimmed so as to be completely enclosed. (See Part III)

The benefits of removing the epithelialized pocket lining must be questioned, for it not only reforms rapidly and the main aim of the surgical reattachment, a new connective tissue attachment, is so rarely achieved. Similarly its relevance to the development of a long junctional epithelium (Figure 14.2 F) or of pocket closure alone (Figure 14.2 G), which is the more usual surgical outcome is not clear (see also Chapter 29 – Tissue curettage). On the other hand, the removal of both epithelium and connective tissue will be shown to be of some importance in apical repositioning, a surgical method with which surgical reattachment has much in common. These tissues are in turn removed automatically in pocket wall resection.

The likely outcome of surgical reattachment

A new connective tissue attachment will at best form at the base of the former pocket and possibly at any epithelial discontinuities within the re-epithelialized pocket wall (Figure 14.2 H). However, the epithelium invariably proliferates apically to the base of the former pocket to form a junctional epithelium. Where this is coupled with the absence of probeable depths, optimal healing by a long junctional epithelium may be assumed to exist and will be associated with uninflamed connective tissues (Figure 14.2 F). More commonly however, the coronally related gingival tissue becomes only closely apposed to the root representing pocket closure with little or no connective tissue infiltrate (Figure 14.2 G). This in turn permits probing to the coronal limit of the junctional epithelium of this deepened gingival sulcus. On the other hand, the pocket might persist with an associated connective tissue inflammatory infiltrate. This variable healing has, however, not been shown in humans if only because of the obvious difficulties of obtaining histological material.

The role of surgical reattachment

The clinical applications appear to be limited, because pocket closure appears to be the most frequent outcome and therefore little different from that achieved following optimal plaque control and an effective 'blind' subgingival instrumentation alone (see Chapter 28 – Surgical access for debridement). Moreover, the technique is most commonly recommended (on the grounds of post-surgical aesthetics) at the front of the mouth at which difficulties in the alternative of 'blind' subgingival debridement are least experienced. On the other hand, surgical reattachment frequently represents a mandatory compromise where the variable pattern of breakdown encountered precludes the intended surgical pocket elimination. The role of surgical reattachment (and the essentially comparable modified Widman flap and the Kirkland flap techniques) for gaining access for root surface debridement is considered in Chapter 28 – Difficulties of subgingival instrumentation.

Apical repositioning

Common surgical pathway

The surgical sequence is technically identical to that of surgical reattachment, until their courses diverge at the penultimate surgical stage. This common pathway revolves about two major features. Firstly, the inner epithelial lining of the pocket wall is removed and discarded, and secondly, the outer keratinized surface is conserved and utilized in the subsequent management of the pocket. Although the latter feature is, by definition, the essential prerequisite for apical repositioning, the reasons for the removal of lining epithelium might not be immediately apparent.

The basis of apical repositioning

The pocket is corrected by the bodily displacement of the pocket wall tissue (detached gingiva) in an apical direction. This necessitates the detachment of the tissue at the base of the pocket wall from the gingival fibre apparatus at the crestal bone and the reflection of the remaining attached gingiva from the alveolar bone (Figure 14.4 A and B). The contiguous alveolar mucosa, located beyond the mucogingival junction, must also be reflected for it too must be displaced during apical repositioning. Finally, the pocket wall tissue must be separated where necessary from the neighbouring intact gingiva by the appropriate relieving incisions (see Chapter 16). The reflected tissue constitutes the surgical flap (Figure 14.4 B). *Note*: The Kirkland flap referred to above is represented by such a surgical flap reflected via a crevicular type incision.

The surgical flap tissue is displaced bodily over the alveolar bone in an apical direction until its coronal edge just covers the crestal bone (Figure 14.4 C and G). This relationship of gingiva to tooth and bone should ideally be dimensionally comparable to that of the normal dentogingival junction so that, in effect, when healing occurs with the tissues in this position the pocket is eliminated. The extent of surgical flap displacement is dictated simply by the position of the crestal bone. This is revealed by the flap reflection, so presurgical charting of the pocket depths is not critical to this technique. This is also true for surgical reattachment because the pocket wall tissue is merely adapted to the root surfaces. Pocket charting is however helpful for future reference purposes.

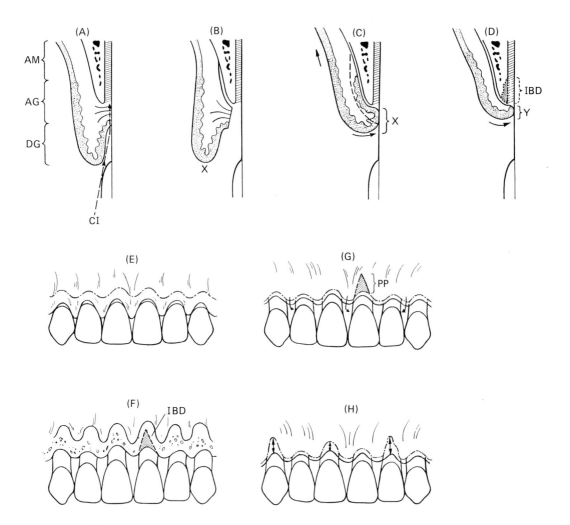

Figure 14.4 Apical repositioning. (A) Crevicular incision (CI) for flap reflection. This represents the Kirkland flap. This surgical flap is comprised of detached gingiva (DG), and any remaining attached gingiva (AG) from the supracrestal attachment and bone and the contiguous alveolar mucosa (AM) from alveolar bone. (B) Surgical flap reflected. (C) Flap apically repositioned. Note: pocket lining epithelium overlying bone and tissue thickness (X) precludes optimal pocket elimination and complicates flap adaptation. Overcome by surgical tissue reduction incision (broken line). (D) Incision removes pocket epithelium, produces thinner flap (Y) and ensures flap margin coaptation to crestal bone. Note: intrabony defect (IBD) depicted by hatched area precludes flap adaptation within defect. (E) Crestal bony contour ghosted under mucosa and (F) revealed by flap reflection. (G) Flap margin and ghosted crestal bony contour well matched for optimal pocket elimination apart from a persistent pocket (PP) site at 21 intrabony defect. Note: scalloped papillary form of flap 'blunted' by tissue adaptation interproximally (arrowed). (H) Uneven marginal bony contour at 13, 11, 22 produces crestal bone/flap margin contour inconsistencies. This results in soft tissue excess (arrowed) and so also precludes pocket elimination

The surgical flap

The inner aspect of the surgical flap is formed coronally by the detached gingival connective tissue and the pocket epithelium of the former pocket wall and, apically, partly by the surgically reflected gingival and alveolar mucosal connective tissues (Figure 14.4 B). This means that following apical repositioning, the latter flap connective tissue will rest upon alveolar bone (Figure 14.4 C), and healing will occur readily. The coronal epithelialized flap tissue will in turn lie about the necks of the teeth and over crestal and alveolar bone, by the amount dictated by the initial pocket depth. This means that flap derived from, say, a 7-mm pocket would have an equivalent amount of about 5 mm of pocket epithelium related to the bone (Figure 14.4 C). The significance of this and of the often thickened fibrous structure of the surgical flap in healing must be examined.

Interposition of epithelium between flap connective tissue and bone is likely to delay healing and so the epithelium is best removed. Doing so is, as in the surgical reattachment technique, not without its difficulties. Epithelium may be curetted away or excised by sharp dissection, either at this stage or before surgical flap reflection. In each instance, the latter option is simpler. Some reduction in the thickness of the pocket wall occurs whenever epithelialized pocket lining tissue is removed. This incidental thinning is advantageous where the pocket wall has been thickened and fibrosed, because it is easier to adapt a thin apically repositioned flap closely to the tooth and crestal bone at completion of operation as shown in Figure 14.4 D and G). Together these also ensure more rapid healing and a more favourable dentogingival form (see below).

Flap margin and crestal bone inconsistencies

The crestal bone contour is frequently uneven because of the various degrees of attachment loss. As a result the normally even scalloped contour of the surgical flap margin will not conform to that of the crestal bone and as shown in Figure 14.4 (H), the intended close relationship at completion of operation will not be possible. Thus, in sites with greater loss, the flap margin will lie too far coronal to the crestal bone and as such represent a flap tissue 'excess' that is more consistent with surgical reattachment. This excess must be corrected by selectively displacing the appropriate part(s) of the flap as far apically as the tissue flexibility allows and where necessary by making appropriate relieving incisions. Bone denudation at less involved neighbouring units should however always be avoided. Tissue excess could be dealt with by a localized surgical reattachment instead or tissue resection, although this can be difficult to do on movable flap tissue. Various combinations of these methods may have to be resorted to (see below).

Irregularly shaped bony depressions or craters (bony defects) might also be encountered about the necks of teeth. As the pocket bases lie within the bone at these intrabony pockets difficulty will be experienced in adapting the soft tissue flap margin about the tooth and crestal bone (Figure 14.4 D and G). The management of these problems are dealt with under 'Complex pocket surgery.'

The stabilization of the apically repositioned tissue

The blood clot between flap and bone virtually glues the flap into position (Figure 14.5 B). Sutures are also used to hold the flap about the teeth. The flap is however liable to be displaced postoperatively by the normal jaw and facial movements, shifting further apically or back coronally towards its presurgical position. The former results in bone exposure (see Figure 15.12) and considerable postoperative pain. The latter results in a surgical reattachment relationship as shown in Figure 14.5 (D) and so defeats the surgical objective. Coronal tissue relapse is prevented by applying a periodontal dressing material which sets hard, having adhered to the teeth (Figure 14.5 B). The sutures and dressing are usually removed after 1 week when the tissues have healed sufficiently.

The similarities to surgical reattachment

The surgical reattachment and apical repositioning techniques can, for practical purposes, be regarded as being the same, but for the final positioning of the surgical flap. The flap is replaced into its presurgical position for attempted new attachment in the one, while in the other is reflected further from the bone and apically repositioned. This facility simplifies pocket surgery for either method could be used as the findings dictate at the time of operation. The management of flap margin/bone contour inconsistencies in particular exemplifies this. The clinical applications of the techniques do however differ slightly, in that surgical reattachment may be attempted in any situation, while apical repositioning is limited by mucogingival and bony anatomical considerations (see below).

A further, albeit unintentional, similarity between the techniques is the tendency postoperatively for a slight coronal relapse of the marginal tissues following apical repositioning and an apical displacement at intended surgical reattachment sites. While the latter gingival recession may, in part, be explained by tissue shrinkage, the technical difficulties of ensuring not only the precise surgical positioning of either flap but also their retention during healing appears to be more critical (see Figure 15.18). As a result the ultimate outcome of the two surgical methods might not be that different at sites with initially moderate (5–7 mm) pocket depths as depicted in Figure 14.5 (D). The interpretation of any comparative surgical method studies must keep this possibility in mind. (See also Chapter 17 – Outcomes of different surgical options.)

The anatomical limitations of apical repositioning

When a flap is apically repositioned a heaped-up fold of tissue might be expected, as when, for example, pulling up shirt sleeves before washing one's hands. No such fold does occur because the

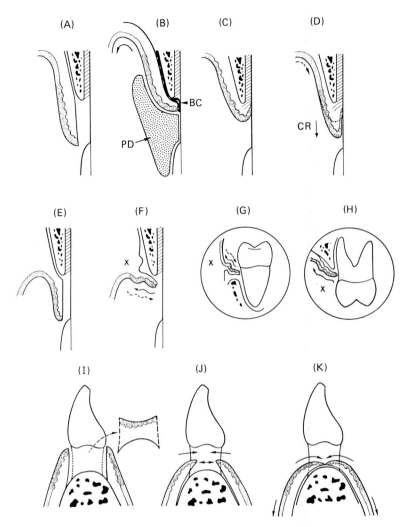

Figure 14.5 Flap stabilization. (A) Surgical flap in surgical reattachment relationship prior to apical repositioning. (B) Vestibular tissues readily permit flap repositioning. Flap supported by blood clot (BC) and periodontal dressing (PD). (C) Ideal healing. (D) Coronal relapse (CR) of apically repositioned flap. This will result in comparable outcome to inadvertent apical displacement and shrinkage of tissue following attempted surgical reattachment. (E) Shallow vestibular tissue form (F) thwarts apical repositioning (depicted by X). Similar difficulty at (G) external oblique ridge and (H) in palate. (I) Interdental septal pocket tissue isolated by labial and lingual surgical flap preparation and removed. (J) Flap stabilization for surgical reattachment results inevitably in interdental cratering. (K) Apical repositioning allows optimal papillary flap adaptation with pocket elimination and labiolingual dimensions permitting (as at mandibular incisors) complete coverage of interdental bone

excess tissue is dissipated within the contiguous loose facial or lingual vestibular mucosa (Figure 14.5 B). Ideally apical repositioning also requires that the contiguous mucogingival complex lies in a similar plane to that of the long axis of the tooth, so that the flap can be displaced in an apical direction. Where, however, the plane of this mucosa (Figure 14.5 E) and that of its underlying bone (Figure 14.5 G), upon which the mucosal form often depends, lie at

an obtuse angle to the tooth, difficulties arise. The surgical flap can then, in effect, only be displaced laterally (Figure 14.5 F and G). This displacement is, in turn, strongly counteracted by the vestibular tissues which push the flap back to its former position. Apical repositioning is therefore often impossible in the presence of a shallow vestibular mucosal sulcus. Similar difficulties arise at the root of the zygomatic arch, the external oblique ridge and the retromolar regions of the mandible and maxilla. In addition, in the palate the firmly bound nature of the mucosa precludes dissipation of any excess tissue and would instead result in a mucosal ridge (Figure 14.5 H). Apical repositioning is therefore obviously not attempted out in the palate. These problem sites are considered separately under 'Complex pocket surgery'.

Interdental pocket management

This presents some difficulties (Figure 14.5 I–K). As in surgical reattachment the dimensions and inaccessibility of the interdental gingival septal tissues virtually preclude the creation of interdental surgical flaps. The isolation and removal of the interdental soft tissues is therefore frequently the only practical alternative. Fortunately, this happens automatically as the facial and oral interdental papillae, which constitute the major bulk of any interdental pocket wall, are incorporated into the surgical flaps created at the facial and oral aspects (Figure 14.5 I). Removal of the septal tissue pocket wall does essentially represent tissue resection as depicted in Figure 14.5 (I) (see also below).

The subsequent management of the papillary flaps depends on that of the contiguous facial and oral flaps. Where these are apically repositioned, so too will be the marginal scalloped papillary peaks. The interdental papillary peaks are then adapted into the interproximal spaces and over the interdental bony septa (Figure 14.5 K). The relationship of papillary flap margins to bone will then be similar to that at the facial and oral flap margins and the pocketing eliminated. On the other hand, where surgical reattachment is being attempted at the facial and oral aspects the papillary peaks will result inevitably in interdental soft tissue cratering (Figure 14.5 J) and preclude the desired healing.

Complete interdental bone coverage is usually only achieved anteriorly as shown in Figure 14.5 K but not at the wider (buccolingual) posterior teeth (see Figure 15.11). This is because the proportionately greater tissue loss sustained by the removal of the wider interdental gingival septal tissue is inadequately compensated for by the displacement of the facial and oral papillary tissue into the interproximal spaces. In addition, the wider (mesiodistal) dimensions of the interproximal spaces at the level of the crestal bone compared to that at the crest of the interdental soft tissue papillae, means that some mucosal deficiency mesiodistally is also inevitable following apical repositioning. This deficiency is exacerbated by interdental root surface concavities (see Chapter 18). It should also be evident that this deficiency would further compromise any attempted surgical reattachment.

In conclusion, co-existing interdental pocketing is dealt with almost incidentally during the surgical management of the associated pockets at the facial and oral aspects. Isolated interdental pockets are in turn handled similarly by conserving the related interdental papillae as in the surgical reattachment/apical repositioning technique, removing the septal pocket tissue and then adapting the papillae into the interproximal spaces as depicted in Figure 14.5 (J and K). This particular technique forms the essential basis of the pocket resection technique that is advocated, and will be shown to be applicable also to pockets related to edentulous areas, the retromolar regions and the maxillary tuberosity. The practical implications of this are that a *single surgical approach* to all pocketing has evolved.

Resection

The resection technique appears the simplest of the surgical options, because the detached gingiva forming the soft tissue pocket wall is simply cut away as shown in Figure 14.6. The gingivectomy technique is, however, rather complicated with respect to presurgical charting, determining the appropriate resection line and the technical difficulties of tissue resection.

The presurgical charting

A careful and detailed presurgical charting of the pocket depths is necessary, for otherwise the operator would not know how much tissue to cut away. Some knowledge of the likely depths and distribution of the pockets will however have been gained from previous assessments. The variable pattern of disease in any surgical field means that pocket measurement and recording results in a complex array of numbers on a dental chart. These must then be translated into a clear mental image of the extent of pocketing at each site and then referred back to the surgical field. The levels of the respective pocket bases must then be marked on the gingiva to indicate the appropriate line of the resecting incision. Determing the appropriate angulation of this incision will be complicated by the irregularly aligned location points not only at adjacent teeth but also at individual teeth.

The marking of the pocket bases

Pocket marking forceps may be used to mark the levels of the pocket bases on the gingival surface. The straight beak is passed to the pocket base, and the other, directed at right angles, punctures the outer keratinized surface of the pocket wall (Figure 14.6 A), producing a bleeding point corresponding to the level of the pocket base.

The graduated pocket marking probe may be used instead (Figure 14.6 B). Having noted the pocket depth, the probe is withdrawn, placed in a similar

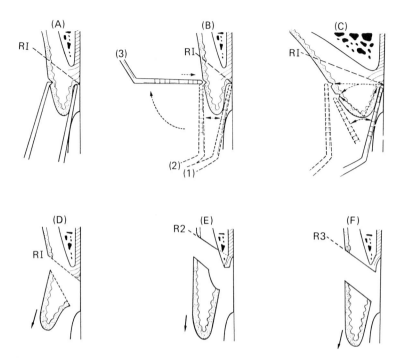

Figure 14.6 Pocket depth marking for resection technique. (A) Pocket marking forceps at pocket base. Note: resection incision (RI) line. (B) Stages (1)–(3) in use of graduated probe at thin tissue. (C) Difficulty in aligning probing depth markings with gingival margin at thick tissue. (C and D) Resection incision (R1) produces larger wound at thick tissue than at thin tissue sites. Note that suprabony pockets are effectively resected. (E) Resection incision (R2) fails to eliminate intrabony component of pocket and results in bone exposure. (F) Incision (R3) avoids bony denudation but is equally ineffective as (R2)

vertical position against the outer surface of the pocket wall, rotated about its tip through a 90° arc, so that it points towards the tooth at the level of the pocket base and the gingiva punctured.

Where the pocket wall tissue is thick and slopes away at an obtuse angle, it is more difficult to judge what point will correspond to the pocket base as shown in Figure 14.6 (C). Thus, when the probe is held against the sloping gingival surface, as described above, the pocket will appear too shallow whereas if it is held away from the gingival surface to maintain its vertical posture, the relevant graduation mark can only be lined up visually. Similar difficulties also arise with pocket marking forceps.

Whatever method is used, the marking sequence is repeated at each pocket measurement site. Ideally, six points are used for each tooth, namely the mesial and distal line angles and the mid axial points of each of the facial and oral aspects. The row of bleeding points is then used to establish the level of the resecting incision.

The incision line

The level and angulation of the resecting incision depends on the thickness and surface plane of the gingiva forming the pocket wall. It is always commenced coronal to the puncture points and slopes coronally towards the pocket base, aiming simultaneously at pocket elimination and the creation of a gingival form condusive to future cleaning. This is easily judged when the pocket wall is thin and so lies almost parallel to the long axis of the tooth (Figure 14.6 B). This is not so where the tissue is thick as in the palate and when, as shown in Figure 14.6 (C), the incision must be made rather more apically instead.

Operative problems

These relate to gingival form, uneven pocket depths, presence of bony defects, limited gingival dimensions and postoperative discomfort.

Tissue form

Gingival form and uneven pocket depth resection are readily accommodated at thin pocket wall sites. A favourable gingival contour results almost automatically so requires minimal embellishment. Resecting thick tissue, as in the palate, is more difficult. Firstly, a greater amount of tissue needs to be traversed by the comparatively short blade of the gingivectomy knife, so that its hub soon becomes impacted into the tissues and its cutting action impeded. Secondly, the tough palatal mucosa soon dulls the cutting edge of the blade necessitating replacement. The inconvenience of doing so may make the operator persevere with a blunt, and so ineffective, blade which further complicates the exercise. Thirdly, having removed the resected tissue the resulting wound surface must usually be shaped further to ensure a healed contour consistent with effective oral hygiene. Fourthly, efforts to embellish this are hindered by the poor access, copious bleeding and the palatal tissue toughness. These difficulties are compounded by uneven pocket depths and when incomplete pocket elimination often results.

Bony defects

Where the existence of a bony defect is not identified at the outset, resection of an apparent suprabony soft tissue pocket wall will result in bony denudation at completion of operation (Figure 14.6 E). This bone does granulate over during healing but not without considerable postoperative pain and some loss of periodontal attachment. The latter constitutes a classic example of adding insult to injury! Should, however, the bony defects be detected by the initial probing, the intrabony component of the pocket cannot be eliminated by soft tissue resection alone (Figure 14.6 F). The management of bone defects is considered under 'Complex pocket surgery'.

Gingival dimensions

The limited gingival dimensions apart from obviously the palate, ranging from about 2–6 mm (Figure 14.7) means that when pockets exceeding these limits are resected, no keratinized tissue will remain. Although the traditionally held clinical and functional benefits of keratinized tissue may be questioned by the findings that marginal tissue health can be maintained in its absence, and the susceptibility to recurrent disease at sites devoid of such tissue is no different from that of a normal dentogingival junction (see also Chapter 21 and Chapter 32 – Gingival dimensions and plaque-induced disease), keratinized tissue is best conserved. The practical implications are that resection is best avoided at the

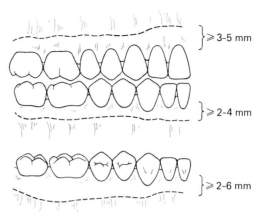

Figure 14.7 Approximate ranges of gingival dimensions at facial aspects of both arches and lingually in mandible

facial aspects in both arches and at the lingual aspect of the mandible, whilst in the palate, bony morphology permitting, resection is the treatment of choice.

Postoperative symptoms

Patient discomfort postoperatively is greatly influenced by the extent of the raw gingivectomy wound surface. This is, of course, primarily dependent upon the tissue morphology as shown in Figure 14.6 (B and C). Thus, at thin tissue only a narrow wound results which heals rapidly and so is less painful than the very much wider wound occurring in the usually thick palatal tissue. The wound is protected from any incidental trauma by the application of an occlusive type periodontal dressing. Healing occurs by a gradual process of re-epithelialization.

Resolving the difficulties

The above problems can be avoided by observing the following rules.

(1) Resection is avoided whenever doubt exists about the resulting gingival dimensions.
(2) The amount of thick pocket wall tissue to be cut away is not based upon the presurgical probing measurements. Instead, a surgical flap comprised of pocket wall tissue is reflected via a crevicular incision (Figure 14.8 A) to expose the involved root surfaces, crestal bone and to reveal the thickness of the tissue (Figure 14.8 B). The amount of tissue to be resected to eliminate the pockets at each part of the surgical field is then established *in situ*, and is based primarily on the position of the crest of the bone. This, in turn, obviates the problems of presurgical pocket charting and assessment and

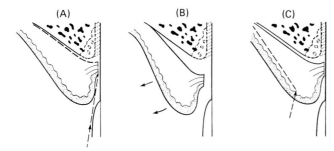

Figure 14.8 Determining resection incision in palate. (A) Initial crevicular type incision to (B) reflect pocket wall and (C) facilitate resection. Existence of any intrabony pockets (ghosted) may be identified *in situ*

so greatly simplifies treatment planning therapy. A record of the existing attachment levels is however helpful for future reference purposes.

(3) Where total pocket resection is precluded by intrabony pockets, other surgical options are adopted but these should still be preceded by the initial surgical reflection of the pocket wall tissue.

(4) An alternative method of resecting the pocket without creating raw surfaces is used (Figure 14.8 C). This resection incision used is very similar to that for conserving the pocket wall tissue in the surgical reattachment/apical repositioning techniques, and so further simplifies surgical treatment.

In conclusion, although the resection method advocated (as described in Chapter 16) is in itself technically more difficult than the conventional gingivectomy, treatment overall is simpler. This is because it is more predictable, the surgical needs can be assessed during operation and any unexpected findings readily catered for.

Summary

Surgical panacea

The many features that the three surgical methods have in common facilitate the use of a single approach for the management of all soft tissue pockets. This represents simple pocket surgery and will be shown in subsequent chapters to accommodate readily any morphological difficulties encountered with various degrees of breakdown. In addition, the treatment measures of complex pocket surgery are, where necessary, simply incorporated. This is in contrast to the traditionally taught, confusing array of different surgical techniques designed to cater for each of the different clinical presentations of pockets present in any one surgical field.

Surgical options

Simple pocket surgery either conserves or discards the tissues forming the soft tissue pocket wall, and as such constitutes the only major division in the surgical ranks. In the former, apical repositioning is preferably carried out but the option of surgical reattachment is always retained. In the latter, the tissue is resected, but only at the penultimate stage of operation, whilst retaining the option of reverting, if necessary, to surgical reattachment, or even apical repositioning in appropriate situations.

The surgical reattachment and apical repositioning techniques are essentially the same, for each conserves the outer keratinized tissue of the pocket wall to form the surgical flap, having initially separated the inner pocket lining epithelium from the pocket wall by sharp dissection (see below – Inverse bevel incision). This surgical excision has the incidental advantage of simultaneously reducing the facio-oral thickness of the soft tissues, but can incorporate any greater degree of pocket wall thinning (filleting) required to simplify subsequent flap management and ensure a more favourable healed gingival form.

Following surgical flap preparation, the remaining soft tissue wedge about the necks of the teeth (and so referred to as the cervical wedge) is removed, to reveal the underlying root surfaces and bone for the necessary instrumentation. The common surgical pathway diverges at this stage. Firstly, the extent of supracrestal root surface debridement necessary is greater for surgical reattachment than for apical repositioning. Secondly, in the one, the surgical flap is merely replaced back up against the tooth for an attempted new attachment, and the other is detached further and then repositioned apically to eliminate the pocket. Finally, although flap stabilization by suturing is common to both methods, a periodontal dressing is also necessary to ensure the apically repositioned flap does not slide back coronally.

The remaining method, resection, cuts away and discards the entire soft tissue pocket wall including the pocket lining. The initial surgical incision is therefore related to the base of the pocket rather than the gingival margin as when conserving tissue. The technical difficulties in assessing the correct siting of this resection incision because of tissue thickness, uneven pocket depths or intrabony defects are obviated by simply altering the sequence of the surgical stages. The pocket tissue is therefore first reflected to permit an *in situ* evaluation of the amount of tissue to be resected. The remaining surgical objectives are then fulfilled as above.

Importance of surgical sequence

Each of the surgical stages must be carried out in the sequence given and completed in its entirety before starting the next. Rigid adherence to this orderly surgical sequence not only overcomes many of the technical difficulties experienced in periodontal surgery, but also allows the operator's undivided attention to be devoted to one single technical problem at a time.

Clinical applications

Apical repositioning is best used at the facial aspects of the maxilla and mandible, and lingually in the mandible, at which the keratinized gingival dimensions might otherwise be compromised (see Figure 14.7). Resection is therefore primarily indicated in the palate, but also where a particularly wide band of keratinized gingival tissue exists. Surgical reattachment is least likely to be used as a definitive surgical method. It is instead held in reserve to cater for difficulties encountered in eliminating pockets at sites with uneven patterns of disease and used more as a surgical compromise. The common surgical pathway adopted permits this option in all sites, and at any time up to the penultimate stage of operation.

Any interdental pocket associated with pocketing elsewhere is automatically incorporated into and eliminated by the surgery carried out at these other sites. Isolated interdental pockets are, in turn,

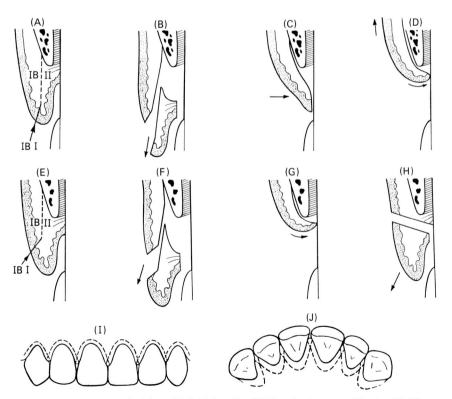

Figure 14.9 Inverse bevel incision. (A) Initial outline (IB I) and subsequent filletting (IB II) components of incision to conserve pocket wall tissue. (B) Surgical flap completed and cervical wedge tissue removal. (C) Surgical flap adaptation for surgical reattachment and pocket reduction. (D) Flap apical repositioning with margin just covering crestal bone. (E) Incision for pocket wall resection. (F) Cervical wedge removal. (G) Flap adaptation over crestal bone for pocket elimination as in (D). (H) External bevel resection shown for comparison. (I) Contour of outline incisions to conserve pocket wall tissue as at labial aspects of 13–23, and (J) resect tissue as in palate

managed by a minor modification of the technique used for conserving pocket wall tissue. Pockets at tooth surfaces adjacent to edentulous areas and at the maxillary tuberosity and retromolar tissues are handled in a similar fashion.

The inverse bevel incision

Technical components

The creation of the surgical flap is necessary in all instances and so requires some dissection of the soft tissue pocket wall (Figure 14.9). The nature of the incision advocated for this is examined here before the operative details of the surgical techniques themselves are described in the following chapters.

The incision used is the inverse bevel incision, so called by virtue of the direction of its plane of cut being the reverse of, or opposite to that of the conventional external bevel gingivectomy incision shown in Figure 14.9 (H). The incision is thus directed in an apical direction. The level at which the incision commences depends on whether the pocket wall tissue is being conserved or sacrificed as shown in Figure 14.9 (A and I and E and J)

respectively. The angulation of the incision is dictated by the extent of thinning (and so referred to as filletting) of the pocket wall required.

There are two separate components to the inverse bevel incision. The initial shallow positional/outlining component and the secondary deeper excisional/filletting component (Figure 14.9 A and E). The former ensures that the pocket wall tissue is conserved or resected as required and that the appropriate marginal contour of the surgical flap is achieved. The latter component is designed to excise the epithelialized pocket lining from the pocket wall and where necessary create the appropriately thinned surgical flap by a progressive filletting dissection.

The surgical flap has ideally a knife-edged scalloped margin and is of even thickness (Figure 14.9 B and F). This ensures optimal soft tissue coverage of the crestal bone and close adaptation of the flap to the necks of the teeth at completion of operation (Figure 14.9 D and G). Success of surgery is therefore very much dependent upon the precision with which the inverse bevel incision is carried out. The technical details of the surgical techniques to conserve and to resect pocket wall tissue are described in Chapters 15 and 16 respectively.

15

Simple pocket surgery:
I Soft tissue conservation technique

Flap preparation
Flap reflection
Cervical wedge management
Management of periodontally involved root surfaces
Management of bone

Flap management
Flap stabilization
Periodontal flap suturing
The periodontal dressing
Clinical case presentations

The technique for conserving pocket wall tissue is described first. This is because it is applicable to most sites in the mouth and so is most commonly used. It is also conceptually and technically simpler than the technique for the resection of tissue. Moreover, many of the features of the basic resection technique and its applications to different clinical situations are derived from that for conserving tissue.

Flap preparation

The surgical objectives

The initial outline (Figure 15.1 A and A1) and the following excisional (filletting) (Figure 15.1 B) components of the inverse bevel incision, split the soft tissue pocket wall into an outer gingival surgical flap layer and an inner epithelialized pocket lining cervical wedge layer (Figure 15.1 C). The ideal incision passes through the pocket wall connective tissue and contacts the bone just apical to its crest. The inner surface of the surgical flap is comprised of connective tissue, although where the epithelial rete ridge proliferation extends deeply into the connective tissues (Figure 15.1 E) some epithelium is inevitably incorporated (Figure 15.1 F). However, this can not be established at operation, and any such epithelial inclusions appear to be of minimal importance (see also Part III – Subgingival curettage). The base of the flap is created by blunt dissection, thereby incorporating periosteum and, in turn, exposing bone. Only a narrow (2 mm) horizontal zone of alveolar bone is exposed between the reflected flap bases and the apical edge of the cervical wedge tissue (Figure 15.1 C and C1). This not only isolates and facilitates the removal of this tissue wedge, but also provides access for subsequent root surface and bony instrumentation (Figure 15.1 D) (see also Figures 15.17 and 15.18).

The outline incision

This is a shallow incision, about 2 mm deep which should run within 1–2 mm of the gingival margin following its scalloped contour and with the blade directed apically (Figure 15.1 A and A1). This ensures that an optimal amount of keratinized tissue is conserved. The blade angulation, being almost parallel to the long axis of the tooth, results in a knife edged surgical flap margin. The scalloped contour also ensures optimal mucosal coverage of crestal bone at the conclusion of the operation. A less scalloped, or even a straight incision (whether by accident or design for technical ease) will result in interdental bony denudation, as shown in Figure 15.1 (H and I) and greater postoperative discomfort. A carefully and precisely executed outline incision will also be found to simplify subsequent flap preparation whereas a failure to do so invariably complicates this.

Practical hints and precautions

(1) The keratinized gingival surface can only be efficiently incised with a sharp blade. This should be replaced once the keen cutting edge has been lost. Failure to do so means that more

155

156

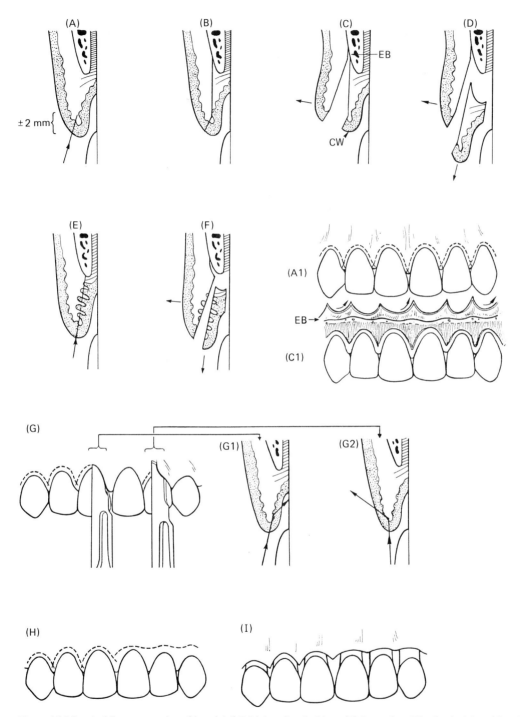

Figure 15.1 Surgical flap preparation. (A and A1) Initial outline incision. (B) Secondary filletting incision. (C and C1) Surgical flap reflection to reveal cervical wedge (CW) and interposed exposed bone (EB). (D) Cervical wedge tissue removed. (E and F) Combination of inappropriate angulation of filletting incision and prominent epithelial rete ridges retains some epithelium within surgical flap. Note at (A1) overlapping outline incisions and at (C1) narrow track of exposed bone (EB) between reflected flap and cervical wedge tissue. (G and G1) Show outline incision slipping into pocket space creating crevicular type incision. (G and G2) Show incision slipping externally and lacerating gingiva. (H and I) Contouring effects of scalloped versus linear outline incisions

pressure is needed to compensate for the less effective cutting action, and when the blade is most likely to slip, so compromising the proposed flap tissue as shown in Figure 15.1 (G). Any blade that needs such pressure should be discarded for this sharp dissection, although it could be retained for subsequent less critical dissection elsewhere.

(2) A Swann Morton No. 15 scalpel blade is used mainly for the surgical incisions, although the No. 12 may be easier to use at the back of the mouth and at the lingual aspects as shown in Figure 15.2.

(3) A series of individual incisions, rather than one continuous incision, is made about each tooth included within the surgical flap. These cross each other close to the peaks of the interdental papillae (Figure 15.1 A1 and Figure 15.2). The outline incision is converted into a crevicular incision at sites with normal dentogingival junctions that are included in the surgical field (Figure 15.2 A, A1 and A3). Similarly, where an exaggerated scalloped gingival contour exists resulting in narrow interdental papillae, the outline incision is best converted at the tooth line angles into a crevicular incision (Figure 15.2 A and C). This avoids creating even narrower papillary peaks to the surgical flap margin which are liable to ischaemic necrosis. This outline incision conversion technique is also indicated in

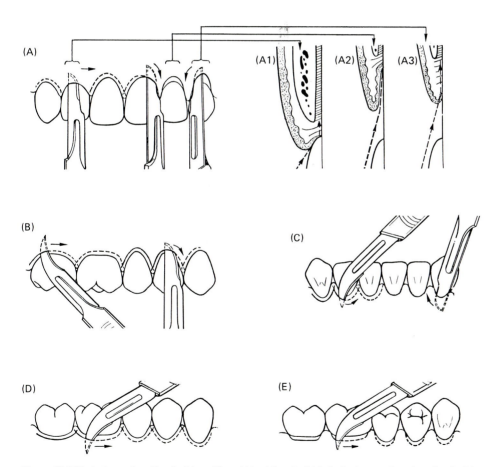

Figure 15.2 Variations of outline incision. Use of No. 15 scalpel blade for inverse bevel outline incisions at accessible sites anteriorly and No. 13 blade elsewhere. Note optional direction of outline incision according to operator preference and convenience. (A–D) Individual outline incisions overlap at papillae creating a scalloped surgical flap margin. Where preservation of existing papillary form as at (A), or where an exaggerated contour is required, as at (E), the outline incisions are converted, at the tooth line angles, to crevicular type incisions instead. Crevicular incisions are also advocated at (A2) thin pocket tissue, (C) poorly accessible sites and when sites with (A1) normal dentogingival junctions or (A3) suspected bony dehiscences must be incorporated within any surgical field

the posterior quadrants, as shown in Figure 15.2 (E) and Figure 15.5 to ensure optimal post-surgical coverage of the interdental bone. Finally, crevicular incisions are preferably used at the outset at sites where the thin pocket wall tissue is shown in Figure 15.2 (A2) and where the limited access, especially lingually (Figure 15.2 C), complicates the making of an outline incision.

(4) The incisions must be directed at the appropriate angle to produce a knife-edged flap margin, not placed too close to the gingival margin and the flat edge of the blade must be constantly aligned with the outer surface of the undulating pocket wall tissue. These steps will avoid the blade slipping and passing into the pocket space to produce either an unintentional crevicular incision or more importantly emerging through the tissue surface (Figure 15.1 G). The latter is euphemistically referred to as a 'relieving incision'! It can be difficult to restart the outline incision once the tissue has become so detached or lacerated in this way, and then to redirect and maintain the subsequent filletting dissection within the pocket wall connective tissue.

(5) The incisions are commenced at the most convenient part of the surgical field and in the sequential direction that best suits the operator (Figure 15.2). Finally, if the blade is sharp and proper finger rests are ensured the incision can be maintained at the appropriate depth and with little likelihood of errors.

Excisional (filletting) incision

The outline incision is deepened progressively by further sharp dissection down to crestal bone to create the surgical flap (Figure 15.3). A filletting-like action is used; this is a lateral slicing movement as when thin slices of fish or meat are being cut. The excisional part of the description refers to the simultaneous excision of the pocket lining epithelium. The incision passes about 2 mm deep to and parallel with the outer surface of the pocket wall. The aim is to produce a surgical flap of a fairly even physiological thickness. The blade angulation must therefore be altered as necessary as shown in Figure 15.3 (A, B and E) to cater for the differing tissue thicknesses encountered.

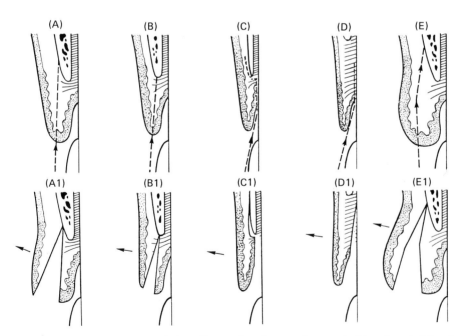

Figure 15.3 Filletting incision technique. Preparation of appropriate evenly thinned surgical flap, by the inverse bevel incision being made at an even depth below gingival surface regardless of (A, B and E) different pocket wall tissue thicknesses encountered. The plane of dissection thus passes more closely to tooth the thinner the tissue, so that crevicular type incision is necessary where, as in (C and D), pocket wall tissue is already of physiological thickness. Note different contact levels of incisions on bone dependent upon varying pocket wall tissue thicknesses at (A, B, C and E). (D) Presence of bony dehiscence apical to pocket base means incision may not engage bone. Surgical flap reflection reveals cervical wedge tissue at (A1, B1 and E1) but root surface at (C1 and D1)

Where existing pocket wall tissue already has acceptable physiological thickness (Figure 15.3 C) it need not be reduced. The creation of a surgical flap then becomes the major objective and, because of difficulties encountered excising the pocket lining epithelium from this thickness of tissue, it is retained. A crevicular type incision within the pocket space is, as stated above, then made from the outset. Normally, excision of the pocket lining can be assumed where the blade is constantly en-sheathed within pocket wall tissue during its filletting action. This blade positioning can be judged readily from the feeling transmitted through the instrument. A scratching sensation means that the blade has either passed into the pocket space and is touching the tooth or has reached the crestal bone. The latter indicates that flap dissection is nearing completion.

The incision should ideally encounter bone just apical to its crest but this will be determined ultimately by the degree of tissue reduction required as shown in Figure 15.3 (A, B and E). Where a long

supracrestal attachment exists apical to the dento-epithelial junction, namely a bony dehiscence, filletting need extend only sufficiently for flap reflection purposes (Figure 15.3 D and D1). Similarly where crevicular incisions have been made at intact dentogingival junction sites within the surgical field these too should simply pass down to the crestal bone as shown in Figure 15.2 (A1) or in the presence of an extensive dehiscence, as far as necessary for flap reflection (Figure 15.3 D and D1).

Practical hints and precautions

(1) Filletting dissection may be commenced at any convenient point within the outlining incision. The mid-axial points are the easiest, because at this point the gingival surface plane is most closely aligned to the long axis of the tooth. This in turn means that the apically directed filletting action of the blade is not impeded by the crowns of the teeth (Figure 15.4 A). Dissection is then

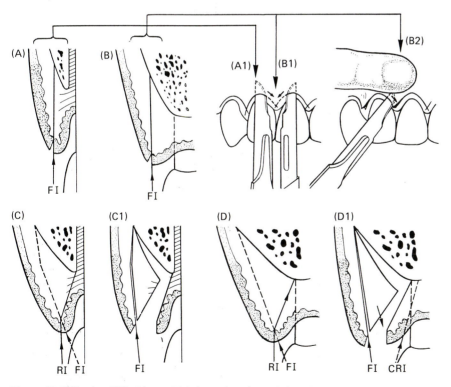

Figure 15.4 Filletting difficulties at thick tissue sites. (A and B) Unimpeded access for incisions (FI) at 'thin' (A) mid-axial and (B) interdental papillary aspects which are aligned in long axis of teeth. Note (A1 and B1) papillary dissection directed from each side towards apex of papilla using (B2) digital support. (C and D) Obtuse angle of the surface of 'thick' (C) mid-axial and (D) interdental papillary pocket wall tissue means filletting incision (FI) will be obstructed by tooth crown. Problem overcome by initial mid-axial and papillary inverse bevel 'relieving' incisions (RI) or alternatively papillary crevicular 'relieving' incision (CRI) shown at (D1) extended to bone. (C1 and D1) Pocket wall tissue can then be deflected into a vertical position for filletting and removal of cervical wedge

extended mesially or distally towards the interdental papillae which are filletted with a cutting action that is directed coronally from their bases (Figure 15.4 A1 and B1). This dissection is most readily carried out where the surface plane of the papillae is also close to the vertical (Figure 15.4 B). The surgical margin peaks, created by the outline incision, can then be easily everted with the flat side on the No. 15 blade and the triangular cross-section of the papilla thus revealed, trimmed down without any coronal interference as shown in Figure 15.4 (B1). In this way, the papillary tissue filletting will have been performed with the blade being used simultaneously as an elevator and a scalpel. It is helpful to support the papilla digitally at this stage (Figure 15.4 B2).

(2) In contrast, difficulties arise at sites with bulky gingival tissue form (Figure 15.4 C) and where the interdental papillae are receded and flattened (Figure 15.4 D), for the gingival surface then lies at a more obtuse angle to the related coronal tooth surfaces. This, in turn, means that when attempting to reduce the associated thicker structure of the pocket wall tissue the teeth will obstruct the required filletting action of the scalpel, because it is impossible to maintain the flat side of the blade parallel to the gingival surface at the mid-axial parts of the tissue (Figure 15.4 C) and even more so interdentally (Figure 15.4 D). In the latter, the limited embrasure space further impedes scalpel manipulation. Indeed, efforts to fillet the papillae whilst located in this position will result in an inadvertent mesiodistal linear resection of the papilla instead, as shown in Figure 15.5 (D).

The difficulties of papillary dissection are best overcome by extending the papillary outline incision (Figure 15.4 D) or, where applicable, the papillary crevicular incisions as shown in Figure 15.4 (D1) and 15.5 (A), down to the interdental bone. The papilla may then be reflected into a more accessible vertical position with the flat side of the No. 15 blade used as an elevator and its inner aspect dissected away by the coronally directed cutting edge of the blade (Figure 15.4 D1 and Figure 15.5 A and B). Digital support of the papilla is again helpful in such instances (Figure 15.5 B). The difficulties at the mid-axial points are, in turn, overcome in a similar fashion having extended the outline incision to the crestal bone (Figure 15.4 C and C1). In addition, this part of the filletting dissection is preferably delayed until completion of that at the adjacent papillae (Figure 15.5 C) so that the tissue can be more easily deflected away from the teeth during filletting with a coronally directed action. The principle of flap reflection prior to filletting is also used in the palate as described in Chapter 16.

It must be re-emphasized that the success of the dissection technique at thick tissues sites depends upon the use of sharp blades and adequate support being provided during the papillary tissue dissection. This is ensured by papillary filletting always being carried out first whilst still supported apically by attachment to bone and mesially and distally by the contiguous gingiva. Furthermore the papillae are also only reflected sufficiently to allow for filletting so maintaining optimal underlying support from the bony attachment. Any unintentional excessive reflection at this stage will remove this support, although this may be compensated for by digital support for the, then mobile, flap. With practice, both reflection and filletting can

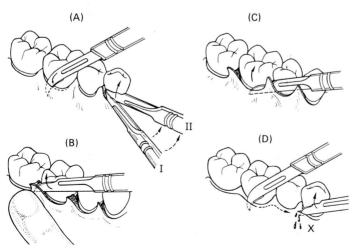

Figure 15.5 Filletting thick tissue and flattened interdental papillae. (A) The mid-axial outline incision (No. 13 blade), passes as crevicular 'relieving' incision into the pocket spaces at the tooth line angles and extends down to bone. No. 15 blade then used for (I) papillary tissue detachment and elevation from bone prior to (II) coronally directed filletting. (B) Papillae deflected into vertical posture showing actual filletting 47/46, completion at 45/44 and still thickened papillae at 46/45. Note: papillary laceration (D) at 'X' when filletting attempted whilst tissue still attached to interdental bone. (C) Thinned papillae deflected to allow deflection of buccal tissue into similar vertical position for mid-axial tissue filletting. (D) Alternative linear incision

be carried out simultaneously, especially when supported externally with the first finger of the other hand as shown at Figure 15.5 (B). It must be realized that the above technical difficulties could be avoided by using a linear outline incision instead, for no interference from the coronal tooth surfaces then occurs (Figure 15.5 D). However, the greater operator convenience that accrues would be at the expense of optimal post-surgical mucosal coverage of the bone, and a resultant greater postoperative discomfort, so it is not advocated.

(3) The use of papillary crevicular incisions (Figure 15.5 A), ensures that the entire papillary surface is conserved for optimal postoperative coverage of the interdental bone. The retained pocket lining epithelium then incorporated in the mesial and distal edges of the reflected tissue will be dissected away during filletting of each papilla (Figure 15.5 B). This technique constitutes the basis of the surgical management of pocketing present at the palatal and edentulous sites and also cases of gingival hyperplasia, to be described in Chapter 16. The uniformity of the approach to surgery being presented here is thus reinforced.

(4) Care must always be taken during filletting not to depart from the track of the outline incision and so inadvertently slice through the outer surface of the gingiva, or to perforate the flap (Figure 15.6 D). The former has already been described as a 'relieving incision', but the latter is more aptly termed 'button holing'. These surgical indiscretions are most likely when the pocket wall tissue is thin (Figure 15.6 A), the surface contour uneven as in a gingival hyperplasia (Figure 15.6 B), and particularly when the underlying alveolar bone form is uneven (Figure 15.6 C). Perforations and lacerations frequently lead to painful postoperative mucosal ulceration with possible total loss of the adjacent tissue (Figure 15.6 D1). (See also Figure 15.21 and 15.22 and Chapter 17.) These complications can be avoided by a more careful technique of simultaneous flap tissue filletting and reflection (Figure 15.6 E and E1).

(5) The apical extent of the filletting incision and the point at which blunt dissection is commenced is dictated primarily by the position of the crest of the bone. This is readily detected at operation by the alteration of the underlying hard tissue contour at the dento-alveolar junction. When pocketing is of similar depth throughout the surgical field sharp dissection extends to an even depth, before reflecting the apical mucoperiosteal component of the surgical flap by blunt dissection. In contrast, where the pocket depths vary, as shown in Figure 15.7 (A), this blunt dissection should be extended

more apically at some sites than at others. This is to ensure adequate flap reflection subsequently and the total isolation of the flap from the cervical wedge tissue. This, in turn, means that a greater amount of bone will inevitably become exposed at the shallower pocket sites as depicted in Figure 15.7 (A3 and B). Bony involvement can however be minimized at these sites by extending the sharp (split thickness) dissection as necessary to preserve the overlying periosteum (Figure 15.7 A2 and B). The flexibility of the technique allows the operator the facility of either option. Although the potentially less traumatic split thickness dissection would seem to be preferable, the benefits appear to be clinically unimportant for insignificant differences in healing have been reported (see Part III). It is only where a bony dehiscence is suspected as shown in Figure 15.7 (A4), that a split thickness flap is advocated to minimize the risk of damaging the supracrestal attachment.

Flap reflection

The flap is reflected from the cervical wedge tissue and bone using a fine periosteal elevator (Hu-Friedy (Chicago, IL, USA) Oh 1 No. 10). An envelope type opening is produced and usually suffices but relieving incisions are made where necessary. The applications and types of relieving incisions used are described in Chapter 17. Flap reflection exposes the narrow horizontal track of bone apical to the cervical wedge of soft tissue (Figure 15.8 A and C). This will provide adequate access for subsequent measures and isolates the flap from the cervical wedge tissue still attached to bone and the necks of the teeth. The surgical flap is deflected out of the way whilst the tissue wedge, the root surfaces and the bone are dealt with.

Cervical wedge management

The inner aspect of the cervical wedge is comprised coronally of epithelialized pocket lining and apically the supracrestal attachment at the base of the former pocket. Its outer surface, visible to the operator, is formed by gingival connective tissue. The overall size of the cervical wedge depends on the depth of the pocket and thickness of the pocket wall and represents the soft tissue remaining *in situ* following preparation of an appropriately thinned flap. This tissue presents as an irregularly shaped soft tissue band about the facial and oral aspects of each tooth in the surgical field and joined by the contiguous interdental septal soft tissues (Figure 15.8 E). For descriptive purposes here it will be assumed that interdental pocketing is also present.

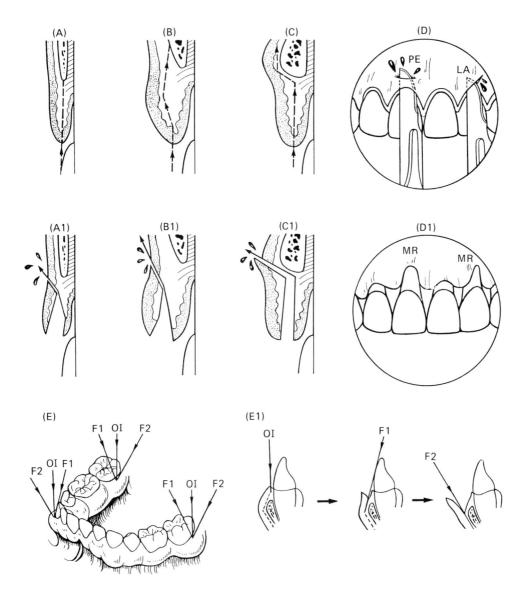

Figure 15.6 Pocket wall laceration and perforation risk greatest during intended filletting (broken lines) at (A) thin tissue and at uneven (B) gingival and (C) bony form. (A1, B1 and C1) Perforations. (D) Perforation (PE) and laceration (LA) likely to lead to (D1) marginal tissue recession (MR). (E) Appropriate directions of outline incision (OI) and subsequent stages of filletting incisions (F1 and F2) with simultaneous flap reflection. (E1) Individual stages shown at 43. Note: diagram at (E) depicts patient shown in Figure 15.21 (G)

The management of situations without interdental pocketing and of isolated interdental pockets will be dealt with later.

The cervical wedge interdental septal tissue complex represents unwanted tissue that is to be removed and discarded (Figure 15.8 B and E). This can usually be scraped away from about the teeth and underlying bone, with heavy curettes or scalers (Figure 15.8 F). Where, however, the tissue is tough and firmly attached it can be gripped with tissue forceps and cut away under tension using a scalpel (Figure 15.8 G). The last, and most difficult, option is surgical excision designed to preserve the supracrestal attachment (Figure 15.8 H). In this method, a horizontal incision is first made just coronal to the crestal bone and then another

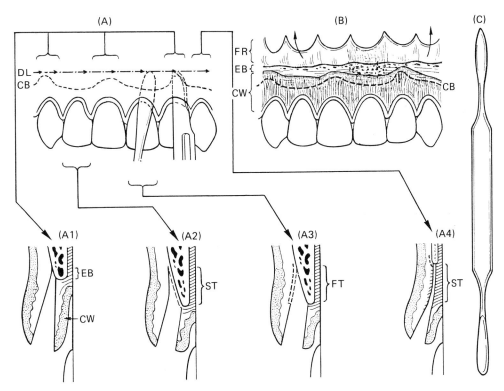

Figure 15.7 Apical extent of flap preparation. (A and A1) Flap filletting dissection extends just apical to crest of bone (CB). (B) Blunt dissection using (C) Hu-Friedy Oh 1 No. 10 Elevator exposes a narrow track of bone (EB) to completely isolate cervical wedge (CW) and facilitate optimal flap reflection (FR). (A1 and A2) Uneven bone levels at adjacent sites [broken line at (A)] necessitates further (A2) sharp split-thickness (ST) or (A3) blunt full-thickness dissection (FT) at less involved sites to an even level of dissection (DL) related to deepest pocket sites. (A4) Split-thickness flap at bony dehiscence

vertically within the pocket space. The thus detached tissue is then carefully curetted away (see Chapter 29 – The modified Widman flap).

Practical hints and precautions

(1) The supracrestal and transeptal fibre apparatus incorporated into the cervical wedge should ideally be retained. This is, however, difficult to carry out within embrasure spaces and interproximally, and even more so when uneven pocket depths and bony defects are present. Fortunately the effects of both the retention and removal of these intact supracrestal fibres appear to be clinically similar (see also Chapter 29). Accordingly, it is expedient to curette away the cervical wedge tissue *in toto*. Any resultant residual small tissue tags could be disregarded although,

when located interproximally, this tissue is frequently responsible for a marked proliferative tissue overgrowth during healing. This tissue may in turn impede post-surgical plaque control measures and is itself prone to trauma from cleaning devices, which may perpetutate the overgrowth and establish a vicious circle. (See also Chapter 17.)

(2) The curetting action required to remove the cervical wedge tissue is no different from that of root surface debridement. Experience gained in mastering this under other circumstances pays dividends, for the removal of this frequently tough and stubbornly adherent tissue can sometimes be very taxing indeed. Ultrasonic scaling devices are also effective especially when used firmly against tooth or bone at inaccessible sites; no detrimental effects appear to be sustained. (See also Chapter 19 and Chapter 31 – Bone resection techniques.)

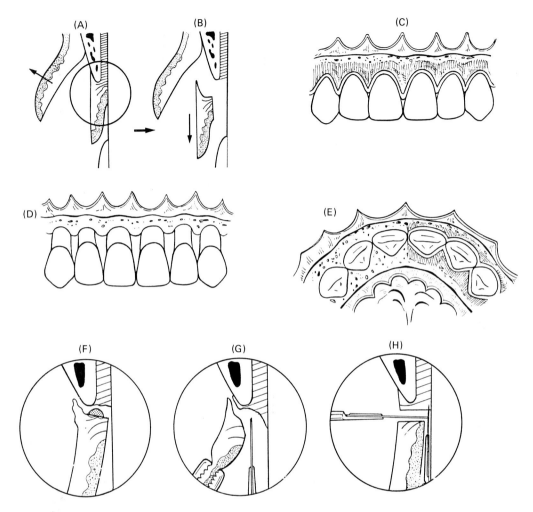

Figure 15.8 Flap reflection. (A and C) Reflected flap and cervical wedge with interposed narrow band of bone. (B and D) Removal of cervical wedge tissue exposes bone. (E) Occlusal view showing exposed bone (left) and contiguity of labial, interdental and palatal cervical wedge tissue (right). Cervical wedge removal options: (F) curette; (G) gripping tissue with forceps and cutting away with scalpel; or (H) sharp dissection to preserve supracrestal attachment

Management of periodontally involved root surfaces

The 'contaminated' root surfaces (Figure 15.9 A) are prepared to receive the surgical flap by being rendered biologically compatible with the soft tissues. This is achieved by the necessary root surface debridement as described in Chapter 11. Ultrasonics are advocated and offers the additional benefits of the flushing effect of the cooling water spray to maintain a clear surgical field. It simplifies this difficult and time consuming exercise.

Debridement need be performed only at surfaces due to form part of the healed dento-epithelial junction. Consequently, this involves only the 2–3 mm of the root surface extending coronal to the crestal bone when apical repositioning is intended (Figure 15.9 B). Surfaces coronal to this have no influence on the dento-epithelial junction. In contrast, when surgical reattachment is being attempted the entire root surface involved must be instrumented (Figure 15.9 C). The more extensive debridement necessary here constitutes but a minor extension of the thus far common surgical pathway

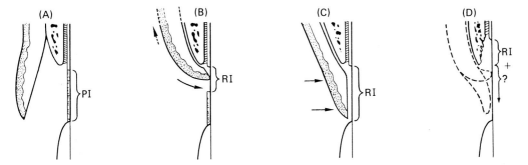

Figure 15.9 Root surface management. (A) Periodontally involved (PI) root surface. This is represented diagrammatically here as 'contaminated' cementum and requisite management by cementum removal, although neither situation can be judged reliably at operation. Root instrumentation (RI) necessary (B) just coronal to crestal bone in apical repositioning, (C) along entire surgical flap related supracrestal surface in surgical reattachment, and (D) within any intrabony defect plus (?) suprabony surfaces according to surgical flap requirements

shared by the surgical reattachment and apical repositioning techniques.

Where any pocket base is apical to the level of the crest of the bone (i.e. an intrabony pocket exists) root surface debridement within these bone defects is also necessary as shown in Figure 15.9 (D). The practical difficulties and clinical implications rank as complex pocket surgery (see Chapter 19).

Practical hints and precautions

(1) The coronal extent of root surface instrumentation is of some practical importance both at operation and postoperatively. Thus, debridement of supragingival root surfaces needlessly prolongs operating time and detracts from wholly effective efforts elsewhere. Furthermore, such instrumentation may lead to dentinal sensitivity and so impede subsequent oral hygiene and professional cleaning efforts.
(2) The routine application of a disclosing agent (like 2% gentian violet) to the root surfaces to assess the efficacy of instrumentation is prudent where any doubt exists, although the significance of residual stained material has yet to be clearly established. (See Chapter 28 – The assessment of adequate debridement.)
(3) Root furcation involvement frequently prevents effective debridement. This problem also qualifies as complex pocket surgery (see Chapter 18).

Management of bone

The crest of the bone is an important surgical landmark for it does, for practical purposes, represent the base of the pocket and the level at which, in apical repositioning, the surgical flap margin is placed (Figure 15.9 B) to ensure an optimal healed dentogingival junction. In contrast, when reattachment is the aim, neither the location nor overall contour of the crest of the bone is relevant for the flap is merely adapted to its presurgical position (Figure 15.9 C). In either event, the bone itself does not demand any specific attention in simple pocket surgery.

In most surgical fields the bone contour is likely to be uneven with the possible additional complications of the presence of bony craters. These bone contour aberrations will inevitably complicate flap margin placement during apically repositioning so is dealt with below under flap management. Bony craters may sometimes also impede access for debridement as will be described under 'Complex pocket surgery'. Suffice it to say here that any specific measures necessary can be readily incorporated into the simple pocket surgical sequence already embarked upon.

Practical hints and precautions

Unnecessary exposure of bone must be avoided and the overlying mucosa reflected only sufficiently to provide reasonable access for root surface instrumentation. Bone exposure should also be limited to the shortest possible time and the bone always kept moist during operation. This is most easily ensured by leaving the surgical flap loosely draped over bone until access is required. Furthermore, the overlying 'protective' layer of blood should be retained until vision is actually impeded. Elsewhere liberal saline irrigation should be used. Prolonged bone exposure and desiccation predisposes to greater postoperative pain. (See also Chapter 19.)

Flap management

The paths of the surgical reattachment and apical repositioning techniques diverge at this stage, so are considered separately.

Surgical reattachment

The objective is biological reunion of the flap tissue to the teeth. The flap is gently but firmly adapted about the root surfaces and then supported in this position (Figure 15.10 A and B). The scalloped surgical marginal contour of the flap ensures close adaptation at both the facial and oral aspects of the teeth (Figure 15.10 C). However, the extent of flap adaptation interdentally is determined by the contour of the flap margin papillary peaks in relation to the facio-oral and mesiodistal dimensions of the interproximal spaces. The limited facio-oral dimensions of the anterior teeth may allow approximation of the opposing flap tissue peaks and their adaptation to the adjacent tooth surfaces. This is, however, likely to be incomplete, as shown in Figure 15.11 (A and C) and moreover results in post-surgical interdental soft tissue cratering with some bony denudation between the papillary peaks.

These discrepancies will be even greater at the wider posterior teeth (Figure 15.11 B).

In contrast, where apical repositioning (or indeed resection) is carried out as described below, the facial and lingual flap positioning over crestal bone means that the papillary components can be closely adapted to the interdental bone and thereby avoid soft tissue cratering, if not bony denudation (Figure 15.11 A–C). The clinical significance of interdental bony denudation and the methods of minimizing this are considered below, under Interdental pocket management (Chapter 16) and in Complex pocket surgery.

The blood coagulum will initially 'glue' the flap to the root surfaces and the bone. Sutures are, however, best inserted to support the flap and minimize any chances of its subsequent displacement which might interfere with optimal healing. The application of a periodontal dressing should also be considered but only when imperfect flap adaptation is evident. The technical details of post-surgical stabilization are dealt with in the next section. The possible outcome of surgical reattachment are depicted in Figure 15.10 (D and E) and having been dealt with in Chapter 14 need not be considered further here. (See also Figure 15.18.)

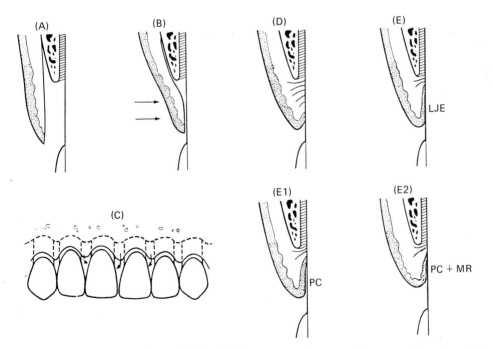

Figure 15.10 Surgical reattachment. (A) Surgical flap (B) adapted to root surface. (C) Scalloped marginal peaks extend (arrowed) into the interproximal spaces. (D) Ideal biological healing by new attachment. (E) Optimal practical healing via long junctional epithelium (LJE) (E1). Pocket closure (PC) associated with (E2) subsequent marginal tissue recession (MR) most likely outcome

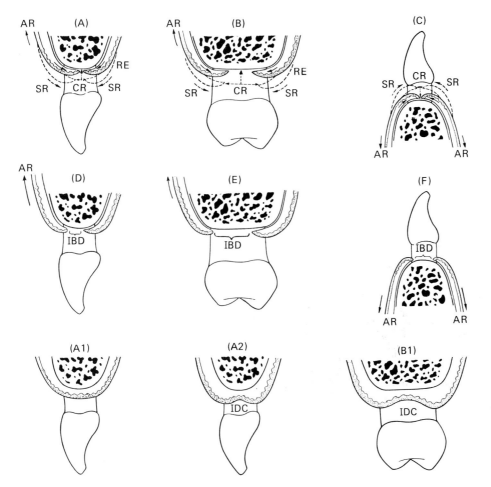

Figure 15.11 Surgical flap papillary tissue management. (A) Tissue peaks coapt over interdental bone in apical repositioning (AR) and resection (RE) but not in surgical reattachment (SR, ghosted lines) when cratering (CR) results (ghosted arrows). Note also interdental bony denudation between tissue peaks; this is more extensive at (B) molars but often avoided at (C) lower incisors. (A1) Ideal healed interdental tissue form following (AR/RE) but (A2) persistent interdental cratering (IDC) following (SR) especially at (B1) molars. (D and E) Interdental bone denudation (IBD) increased with greater degrees of (AR) or when carried out (F) at both flaps

Apical repositioning

The surgical flap is displaced apically so that its margin just covers the crestal bone (Figure 15.12 A–C). This tissue displacement requires further elevation and reflection of the surgical flap and its contiguous, more apically related, mucosa from the alveolar bone. This is most easily achieved by blunt dissection and so incorporates the periosteum (Figure 15.12 A). Dissection must extend beyond the mucogingival junction and vestibular mucosal fold for the tissue would otherwise become bunched upon itself following apical repositioning (Figure 15.12 B). The mucogingival surgical flap complex thus becomes totally isolated from bone, like a curtain suspended from the vestibular mucosal fold. The flap is repositioned apically so that its margin just covers the crest of the bone (Figure 15.12 C and C1), the flap tissue 'excess' being dissipated within the contiguous loose vestibular mucosal fold. The extent of apical repositioning should reflect the initial pocket depth at each site. The flap is adapted into position about the necks of the teeth, the intervening blood coagulum bonding the tissues into place as shown in Figure 14.5 B. Nevertheless, suturing is necessary followed by more critically, a periodontal dressing (Figure 15.12 C) to prevent coronal movement relapse.

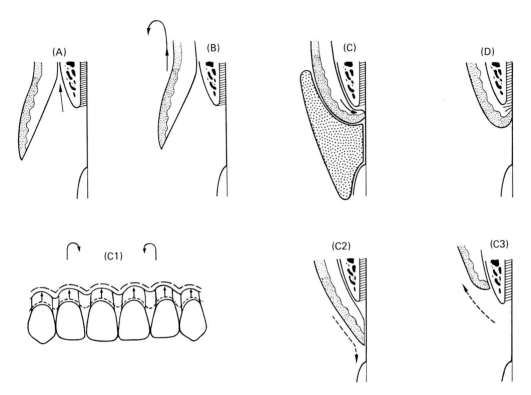

Figure 15.12 Apical repositioning. (A) Blunt dissection to free surgical flap for (B) displacement apically. (C and C1) Flap margin adapted over crestal bone and supported by periodontal dressing. (D) Optimal healing. Post-surgical flap displacement (C2) coronally resulting in surgical reattachment relationship and (C3) apically with bony denudation

The interdental bony denudation tends to be greater than in surgical reattachment, although this does depend on the degree of the displacement of the flap margins from each other during apical repositioning as shown in Figure 15.11 (A–F). Denudation is obviously greatest when both flaps have been apically repositioned as in the mandible (Figure 15.11 F). Bony denudation can, however, be minimized by anticipating the problem and utilizing alternative outline incisions. Thus, the crevicular type incisions of the Kirkland flap provide slightly greater interproximal bony coverage (Figure 15.13 B and B1) than the inverse bevel incision (Figure 15.13 A and A1). The exaggerated scalloped incision of the modified Widman flap provides greatest coverage (Figure 15.13 C and C1) and may even allow total approximation of the papillary edges. The latter is however technically difficult and frequently not feasible because of the limited amount of keratinized mucosa available following gingival recession. (See also Figures 15.17 and 15.20.)

Practical hints and precautions

Inconsistencies encountered between the contours of the bone and surgical flap (Figure 15.14 B) will frequently make it difficult to position the flap margin so that it just covers the crestal bone. Minor discrepancies may be accommodated by the inherent tissue flexibility allowing small differing amounts of displacement to be carried out at adjacent sites (Figure 15.14 C), producing the required flap margin bony relationships as depicted at Figure 15.14 (G1). The remaining larger discrepancies may be handled in several ways:

(1) The flap margin is positioned to cover the most coronally located crestal bone levels and elsewhere the tissue is displaced as far apically as the tissue flexibility permits, accepting a compromise surgical reattachment relationship (Figure 15.14 C and G4). Apart from the additional, more coronally located, root surface instrumentation required, the essential prerequisites for optimal surgical reattachment will

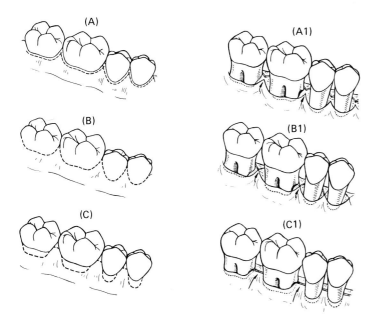

Figure 15.13 Flap incisions and interproximal mucosal coverage following flap apical repositioning. (A and A1) Inverse bevel incision. (B and B1) Kirkland flap crevicular type incision. (C and C1) Modified Widman flap incision. Mucosal deficiencies greater at (A1) than (B1) but are minimized by exaggerated scalloped flap contour at (C1). Mesiodistal deficiencies at (A1 and B1) accentuated by root surface concavities at first molar

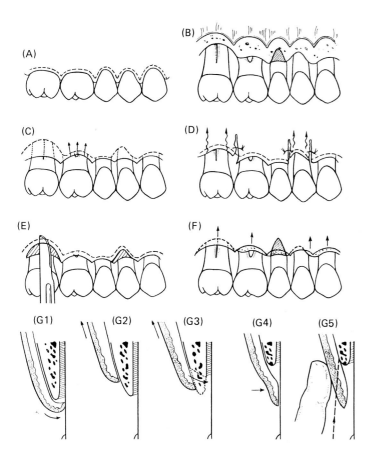

Figure 15.14 Options for management of inconsistencies between flap margins and bone. (A) Surgical flap contour differs from (B) crestal bony form. Note intrabony defect at 15 and furcation involvement at 16. (C) Optimal flap margin to bone relationship (see G1) following apical repositioning at 13 and 15 crest of bone, achieved at 16 by mucosal tissue flexibility allowing (arrowed) correction of minor discrepancies between 16 and 15. Surgical reattachment relationship accepted at 17 and 14 (G4). (D) Relieving incisions for further selective apical repositioning at 17 and 14 with retaining interrupted sutures. (E) 'Excess' flap tissue resected using digital support (G5) to level of bone at 17 and 14. (F) Apical repositioning to satisfy optimal relationship at 17 and 14 causes bony crestal denudation at least involved sites 16, 15 and 13 (G2). Further option (G3) of resection of denuded part of non-supporting intrabony pocket wall at 15 to ensure mucosal coverage

have already been satisfied at these more severely involved sites, making this a reasonable practical option.

(2) Vertical relieving incisions bounding the most involved sites are made to permit the resulting miniflaps to be selectively repositioned apically as required (Figure 15.14 D). The small mucosal fold produced at the base of such flaps is of no practical consequence. The insertion of interrupted sutures, limits coronal tissue relapse.

(3) The 'excess' flap tissue at the most involved sites is trimmed away as necessary by a further inverse bevel incision (Figure 15.14 E). This can be quite difficult to do on a thin movable flap, but is facilitated by digital support (Figure 15.14 G5). (See also Chapter 17.)

(4) Optimal flap positioning is effected at the most involved sites with associated bony denudation at the least severely involved sites (Figure 15.14 F and G2). This option is not recommended but might be considered where bone exposure will be limited to a few small areas. Although this exposed bone soon granulates over with a new mucosa, considerable postoperative pain is experienced and an irreversible loss of attachment might be sustained. On the other hand, where this exposed bone is non-supporting bone, i.e. associated with an intrabony pocket, it could be chiselled away to the appropriate level of the flap (Figure 15.14 G3) to ensure postoperative mucosal coverage. The management and response of bone to surgical techniques is considered in Chapter 19.

In conclusion, as the intended correction of the deepest pocket by apical repositioning is frequently not possible and bony exposure is not recommended, a combination of the first three options, as dictated by the variable features of each case, should be resorted to. A surgical compromise of a reattachment relationship is frequently imposed. Similar compromises will however also be found to be unavoidable in many other situations involving not only bony defects, as outlined above, but also root furcation and vestibular tissue morphology. Each of these qualify for complex pocket surgery, to be dealt with in subsequent chapters. Together these operative difficulties are in part responsible for the frequently comparable pocket reductions achieved by the different surgical techniques. (See Chapter 17 – Miscellaneous surgical considerations and Chapter 29 – Evaluation of different surgical methods.)

Flap stabilization

The rationale

The flap is stabilized by sutures and where necessary the application of a periodontal dressing. Effective flap stabilization is critical following apical repositioning for the tissue is liable to slide back coronally to its presurgical position (Figure 15.12 C2). Further apical displacement, leading to bone exposure (Figure 15.12 C3), may also occur, but usually only as a result of poor suturing and dressing technique. In this context, an unintended apical displacement may sometimes also occur during surgical reattachment. This then produces the effect of poorly controlled apical repositioning, thereby contributing to the frequently comparable outcomes of pocket surgery.

Postoperative failure

Flap displacement may come about for several reasons. Firstly, and most commonly, there is inadequate flap preparation. A flap that is too thick, is of uneven thickness, or has poorly scalloped margins cannot be properly adapted into position; this operative handicap is often compounded by an inconsistent bony form so aggravating the situation. Secondly, when the periodontal dressing used is too stiff (see below), the flap is likely to be displaced when the material is applied. Thirdly, a poorly applied dressing is readily dislodged by the normal functional movements and so predisposes to flap displacement; in addition any sutures embedded within this dressing will inevitably (and painfully!) displace the flap. Finally, the onset of bleeding postoperatively may lift up and displace the flap.

Periodontal flap suturing

Two basic suturing techniques, the interrupted and continuous suture are used (Figure 15.15). The former is described first, to show its technical shortcomings and the reasons for recommended use of the continuous suture in most instances. (See also Figures 15.19 and 15.20.)

Interrupted suture

This consists of a single loop of thread passing through the opposing facial and oral flap margin papillary peaks via the interdental space (Figure 15.15 A). When pulled tight the flap margins are drawn under similar tension towards each other. The suture is then tied off at the facial aspect, because it is easier for the operator and the knot less likely to irritate the patient's tongue. Interrupted suturing is best suited to isolated interdental pockets, where the opposing flaps are equally firmly coapted about the teeth as in rare instances of elective surgical reattachment (Figure 15.19 I and J), where resection technique is carried out at both aspects of the teeth and, finally, for relieving incisions as shown in Figure 15.14 (D).

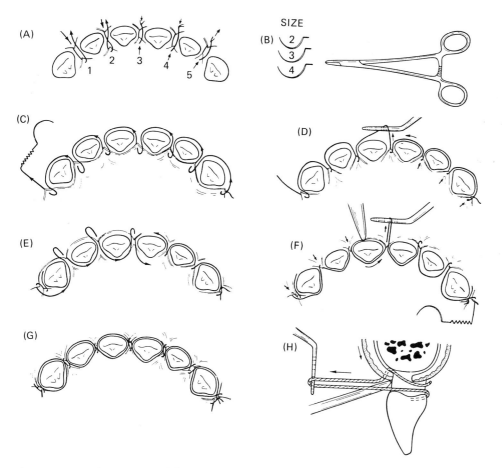

Figure 15.15 Suturing technique. (A) Interrupted suture. Optional paths of insertion (1) 'U' shaped, (2) 'Figure of 8'. Apposing surgical flaps (3) equally firmly and (4) loosely supported. (5) Unequal tension required for buccal apical repositioning and palatal resection not satisfied. (B) Suture needles and Halsey type needle holder. (C) Continuous suture knotted at 23 distopalatal aspect is looped about 23 and through the 22/23 interdental space and then through the related palatal papilla. Sequence repeated to 13 distopalatal papilla. (D) Suture tension adjustment from buccal aspect pulling palatal flap into position. (E) Suture sequence repeated at buccal flap commencing at 13 distobuccal papilla. At conclusion (F) and (H) suture tension adjustment with probe whilst supporting the flap margin with an elevator. Note different but optional points of adjustment in (D) and (F). (G) Suture completed and tied off at starting point

The apically repositioned flap is, in contrast, less easily supported by interrupted sutures. There are two reasons for this. Firstly, it is difficult to hold the movable apically displaced flap in its correct position whilst at the same time pulling up the suture to the appropriate tension and then tying it off. The suture thus often tends to be either too tight, pulling the flap margin back coronally or too slack, leading to bony denudation, and once knotted, the tension cannot be readjusted so requiring replacement of the suture. This difficulty is compounded when different degrees of apical repositioning are re-

quired at adjacent units. Secondly, any post-surgical displacement of an opposing flap will affect the apically repositioned flap in a see-saw fashion. Such flaps are therefore preferably sutured independently about the immobile necks of the related teeth. This is achieved by and forms the basis of the continuous suture.

Continuous suture

This commences at either palatal or buccal aspect at the most accessible extremity of the surgical field.

The suture is inserted and knotted at this selected flap margin papillary peak, in this case the distopalatal aspect of the cuspid as shown in Figure 15.15 (C). The suture is then threaded through the related interdental space, passed around the buccal aspect of the tooth and back palatally through the next interdental space. It is then inserted into the second palatal peak, passed back through the same interdental space, looped around the neck of the next tooth and the sequence repeated for each unit in the surgical field.

The initial objective is to suspend the flap loosely about the teeth (see also Figure 15.19 C). This then allows the flap to be positioned as required, which in this case is firmly about the necks of the teeth following pocket resection, and the suture tension adjusted like pulling up boot laces. A periodontal probe is passed under the suture where it loops around the second tooth in the surgical field and the thread pulled gently outwards creating a small loop as the slack is taken up (Figure 15.15 D). This is repeated at each successive unit producing a progressively larger loop of thread (see also Figure 15.19 D), that is finally taken up at the free needle end. The appropriate tension ensures flap coaptation and prevents flap margin displacement from the teeth.

The suture, having passed from the last palatal papillary peak and through the related interdental space, is inserted into the opposing buccal papillary peak (Figure 15.15 E). It then passes back again through the same interdental space, loops about the palatal aspect of the tooth and continues buccally through the next interdental space, and so on, returning to the starting point. The appropriate positioning of the apically repositioned buccal flap and the associated adjustment of the suture tension, is expedited by placing the end of the periosteal elevator against the tooth at the flap margin as shown in Figure 15.15 (F and H). This prevents the flap from being pulled too far coronally during the adjustment of the suture. The suture is tied off to the knot made initially (Figure 15.15 G).

The continuous suture technique, whilst initially appearing rather complicated, is rather easier to do than to describe and is simpler than the interrupted suture, over which it has several advantages. Firstly, it facilitates more precise flap positioning because the suture tension, upon which flap support is so dependent, can be so easily and reversibly adjusted. Moreover, this can be achieved as an entirely separate exercise that is not complicated by the necessary knotting of interrupted sutures. Secondly, each flap is dealt with independently so they cannot pull against one another and possibly displace them from their intended positions. Finally, as only a single knot is necessary, at the outset and on completion of suturing, it reduces operating time and is less irritating for the patient postoperatively.

Practical hints and precautions

(1) Fine needle holders (e.g. Halsey) are advocated (Figure 15.15 B). These lock and grip the needle firmly in any position and are easily manipulated in different parts of the mouth. Fine braided silk suture thread (e.g. Ethicon W577, Johnstone & Johnstone, Slough, Bucks, UK) with a reverse cutting atraumatic needle (3/0) is recommended. In some instances smaller (2/0) or larger (4/0) needles may be preferred (Figure 15.15 B).

(2) The suture needle is best inserted about 2–3 mm from the surgical flap margin to ensure that the thread does not tear and 'pull through' the tissue. Careful tissue handling will also avoid this. The needle is most easily inserted from the outer keratinized aspect (see also Figure 15.20 L). In addition, the flap tissue can, in this way, be simultaneously pressed against and supported by the teeth bounding the related embrasure space, whilst the needle is inserted. Then having penetrated the tissue, the needle can often be passed directly through the interdental space by a continuation of the initial thrust and its emerging point grasped with the needle holder and pulled through. There is no advantage to inserting the needle from the inner connective tissue surface of the flap. This is not only more complicated and time consuming but is also more traumatic because of the need to grip and, in effect, pinch the tissues with tissue forceps. On the other hand, should any needle having passed in between the teeth, happen to penetrate at an appropriate level the inner surface of the papillary peak to be sutured next it should simply be passed through this tissue as it is. The outer surface of this flap is then best supported digitally immediately adjacent to the point at which the needle emerges.

(3) Where the tooth contact points permit, it is often quicker to pass the suture thread interdentally as though using dental floss for interdental cleaning. Care must, however, be taken particularly when interproximal restorations are present not to snap the thread. Such breakages do only constitute an inconvenience and are readily coped with (see below).

(4) Tissue blanching must be avoided when adjusting the suture tension for it means that the suture has been pulled too tight. This could lead to papillary necrosis, the consequences of which are considered in Chapter 17. The suture tension is therefore always carefully checked, and readjusted as necessary.

(5) The continuous suture may be used in all instances and whatever the surgical objective. However, the loops about the teeth should preferably not become interposed between flap

and tooth (see Figure 15.19 E) lest it interferes with healing, and when interrupted suturing might be considered instead. On the other hand, the relatively short period that any such suture is left in position is unlikely to be of clinical significance.

(6) Where bleeding occurs during the suturing, this is stemmed by applying digital pressure on a moist gauze swab over the area. Haemostasis is essential for proper flap adaptation. This must be ensured upon completion of suturing, before any dressing is applied and the patient discharged.

The modified continuous suture

A modification of the continuous suture permitting both flaps to be sutured concurrently as an alternative to interrupted sutures is described and shown in Figure 15.16 (A and B). Other localized applications of the continuous suture are described and illustrated in Chapter 16. The principle of tying off the modified suture upon completion, as shown in Figure 15.16 (C–E), is used to deal with breakages of any continuous suture thread (Figure 15.16 D–G). Breakages usually occur from fraying against the edges of interproximal restorations or when the thread has been imprudently passed through tight interdental contacts.

The periodontal dressing

The potentially protective function of a dressing stems from the era of the conventional external bevel gingivectomy and the resultant open wounds; this is not applicable to the surgical approach advocated, whilst the frequently denuded interproximal bone gains some protection from any postoperative trauma by its cloistered position. The

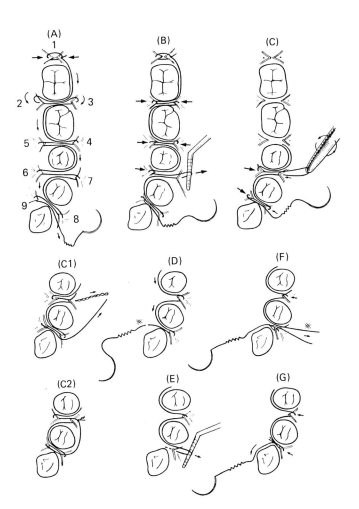

Figure 15.16 Modified continuous suture. (A) Commencement as (1) interrupted suture at one extremity of surgical field followed by continuous suture (in sequence of 2–9) at alternating pairs of papillae at opposing aspects of each tooth to end of surgical field. (B) Suture tension adjustment at each successive papillary loop commencing at site (3). (C) Knotting effected by maintaining a 2-cm long suture loop at (7) and (C1) twisting it into a spiral with the needle holder. The tension is then adjusted at (8) and (9) whilst supporting this spiralled thread to which (C2) the needle end of the thread is finally tied. Note: a spiralled loop may instead be created at 8. Breakage of any continuous suture as depicted at (D) 33/34 dealt with in similar manner. (E) Broken thread withdrawn from 33/34 buccal papilla at which (F) new continuous suture is commenced leaving long suture 'tail' after knotting. (G) Tension distal to 34 adjusted and broken end tied to new suture tail. Continuous suture then proceeded with as before

periodontal dressing also provides support. This is critical to the apically repositioned flap which must be supported in its appropriate position during healing. The success of the dressing here depends upon its firm adherence to the teeth and its bulk to maintain the displacement of the mucogingival tissue complex and to prevent its coronal movement; that is the dressing is intended only to hold the tissue in place, and not to displace it actively. The dressing is therefore applied only once bleeding has been controlled and the flap fixed into place by the blood clot.

The teeth are first dried off with high volume aspiration, to ensure that the Coe-pak (Coe Laboratories Inc., Chicago, IL, USA) dressing material recommended sticks properly. In fact the difficulty in getting the material to stick to moist surfaces, is advantageous with respect to the operator's moistened (or alternatively lubricated with petroleum jelly) fingers and the patient's lips. Special care must be exercised with moustaches and beards!

A very soft mix of the material is advocated, for it sticks better and requires minimal digital pressure during its application. When used in a stiffer state, greater digital pressure is necessary and can lead to both unintentional flap displacement and recurrent bleeding. The latter, then, not only impedes dressing fixation but may also displace the flap even further.

Practical hints and precautions

(1) The material is mixed with a narrow metal spatula, with which it is applied directly to the dry tooth surface flap margin junctions, immediately after mixing and whilst still in its, initially, very sticky soft state. The material is spread evenly along the surgical field with the spatula and then gently smoothed down as soon as possible, with a well lubricated finger. This ensures that the material flows in between the teeth for optimal flap support and added mechanical anchorage. The sticky nature of Coe-Pak and the difficulties of simultaneously displacing the tongue, lips or cheeks lest the material contacts and sticks to them as well, during its application, coupled with its relatively fast setting time means that only four to five units can be dressed at one time. Larger fields, therefore, require several mixes but the operator soon learns, by trial and error, to master the material's peculiar handling properties and to use it accordingly.

(2) The displaced vestibular mucosa is 'muscle trimmed' (as when taking a full denture impression) following the initial digital moulding and whilst the Coe-pak is still setting. This ensures that the material is not over-extended or too bulky. Failure to do so may lead to subsequent displacement of the dressing, and so possibly also the underlying flap, by the normal functional movements. The excess material is readily moulded coronally over the teeth and then carved away with a suitable instrument (e.g. Cumine scaler). This is designed to satisfy aesthetics and avoid interference from the occlusion. Smeared adherent remnants of Coe-pak on the teeth are readily wiped away with a solvent, like Codent Orange Solvent (Codent (UK) Ltd, Hull, UK) used on a cotton wool roll.

(3) Postoperative discomfort appears greater when periodontal dressings are used, although it is not clear whether this is due to the dressing itself or the complexity of the surgery necessitating its use. Dressings are therefore restricted to where postoperative flap support and retention is critical as in apical repositioning and, as will be shown in the next chapter, pocket resection in flat palates.

(4) Before discharging the patient the surgical field must be checked to ensure haemostasis. The mouth is then thoroughly irrigated and freshened up with a warm, air and water syringe, because effective mouth rinsing can often be difficult because of the effects of local anaesthesia. The details of the postoperative instructions, effects and aftercare are given in Chapter 17.

Clinical case presentations

The clinical surgical sequences of conserving pocket wall tissue for apical repositioning on the one hand and surgical reattachment on the other, are shown in Figure 15.17 and Figure 15.18 respectively. The surgical correction of minor pocketing present prior to the replacement of aesthetically displeasing crowns, using a combination of apical repositioning and tissue resection and also demonstrating further the appropriate suturing technique, is shown in Figures 15.19 and 15.20. The management of thick mucosa is, in turn, shown in Figures 15.21 and 15.22.

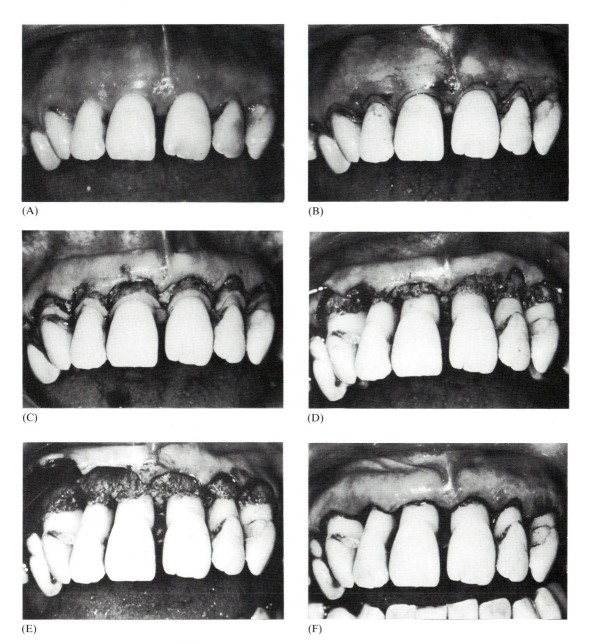

Figure 15.17 Apical repositioning. (A) Presurgical presentation of 35-year-old woman in anticipation of orthodontic realignment and occlusal reconstruction. (B) Outline incision. (C) Surgical flap filletted and cervical wedge isolated. (D) Cervical wedge removed. (E) Flap elevation for apical repositioning. (F) Flap margin just covering crest of bone.

176

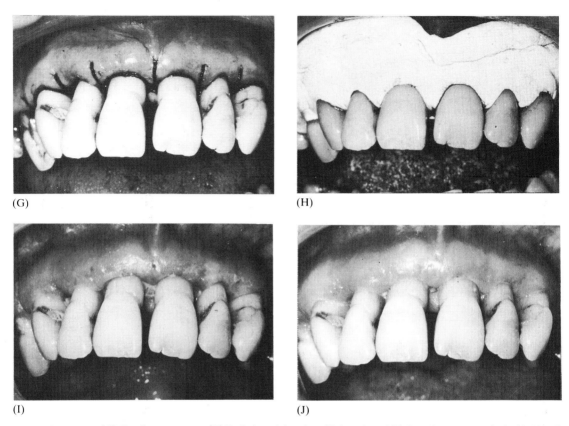

Figure 15.17 (*cont.*) (G) Continuous suture. (H) Periodontal dressing. (I) 1 week and (J) 4 weeks postoperatively (A, E and G reproduced from *Dental Update*, by permission of Update-Siebert Publications Ltd)

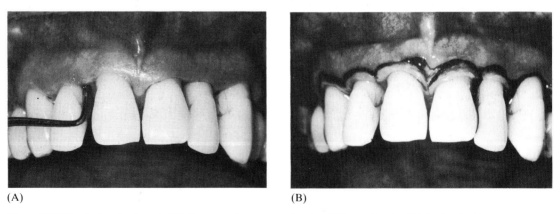

Figure 15.18 Surgical reattachment. (A) Pre-operative presentation in middle-aged male. (B) Outline incision.

177

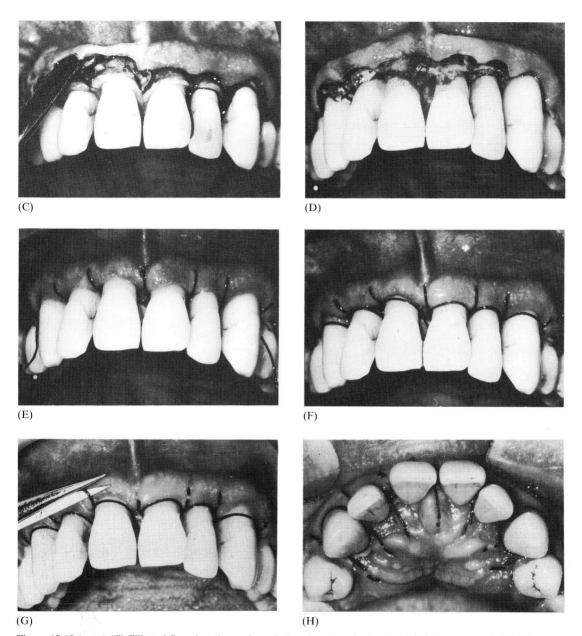

(C) (D) (E) (F) (G) (H)

Figure 15.18 (*cont.*) (C) Filletted flap elevation and cervical wedge tissue isolated and (D) then removed. (E) Flap coaptation with appropriately tensioned labial continuous suture. (F) Suturing completed. (G) 1 week postoperative. Suture being cut through at each interdental papilla buccally and (H) palatally.

178

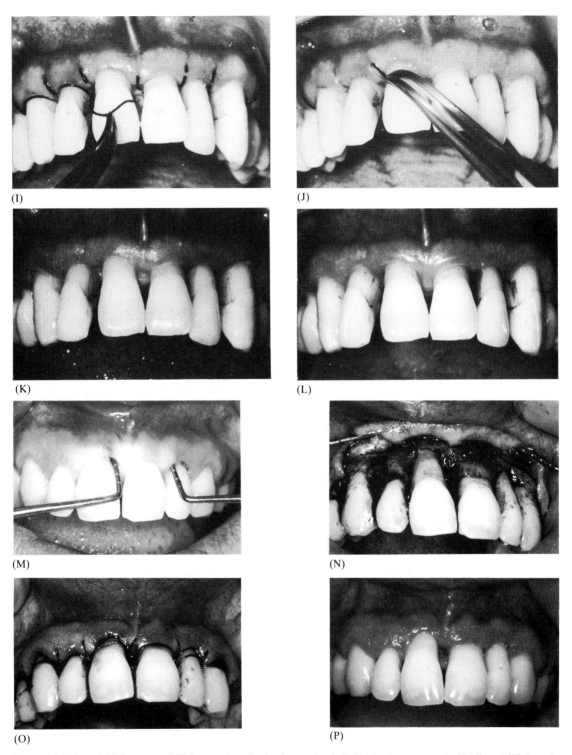

Figure 15.18 (*cont.*) (I) Correct and (J) incorrect methods of removing individual suture segments. Healing at (K) 2 weeks and (L) 3 months. Note marginal tissue recession compared with (A). (M) Uneven probing depths in young adult precludes pocket elimination. (N) Flap margin and crestal bony inconsistencies. (O) Flap adaptation and suturing for surgical reattachment relationship imposed at 11 and 22. (P) Obvious recession at 2-week healing

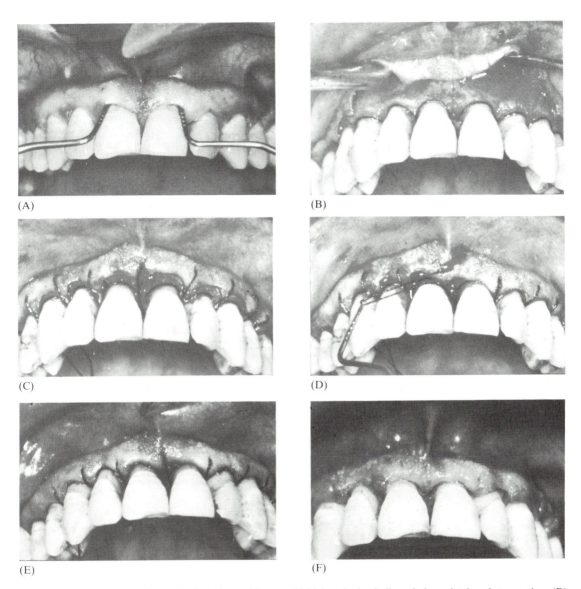

Figure 15.19 Suturing technique. (A) Apical repositioning of labial pocketing indicated plus palatal pocket resection. (B) Palatal flap suturing commenced at 14/13 continuous suture loops shown about teeth. (C) Labial flap loosely sutured. (D) Suture tension adjustment commencing at 23/24. (E) Suturing completed and tied off at 14/13 palatal aspect. Suture loop interposition between tooth and flap as at 13, 11, 21, 23 should be avoided. (F) 1 week postoperative.

180

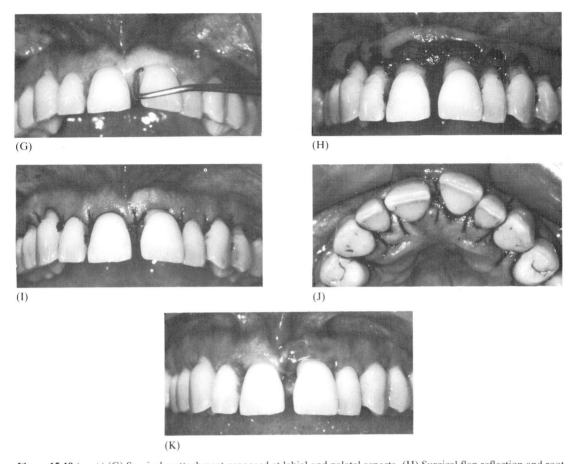

(G)　　　　　　　　　(H)

(I)　　　　　　　　　(J)

(K)

Figure 15.19 (*cont.*) (G) Surgical reattachment proposed at labial and palatal aspects. (H) Surgical flap reflection and root surface debridement completed. (I) Interrupted sutures. (J) Palatal view with equal flap tensioning and labially located knots to minimize irritation to tongue. (K) 1 week postoperative (H and I reproduced from *Dental Update*, by permission of Update-Siebert Publications Ltd)

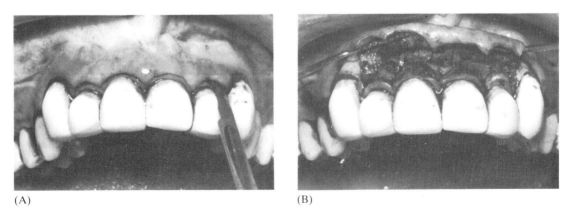

(A)　　　　　　　　　(B)

Figure 15.20 Pre-restorative pocket surgery in 28-year-old woman. (A) Commencement of filletting incision. (B) Surgical flap reflection and exposure cervical wedge – note level of reflection related to 13 and 23.

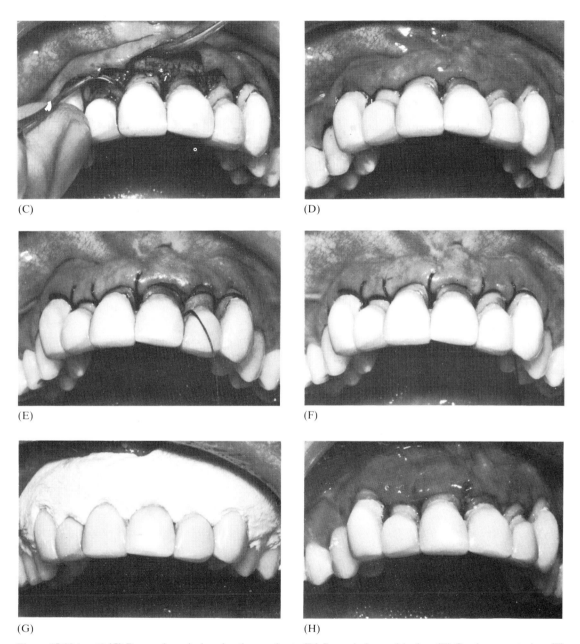

Figure 15.20 (*cont.*) (C) Removal cervical wedge tissue prior to (D) flap apical repositioning. (E) Continuous suturing. (F) Suture tension adjusted and tied off distopalatal to 23. (G) Periodontal dressing critical. (H) 1 week postoperative.

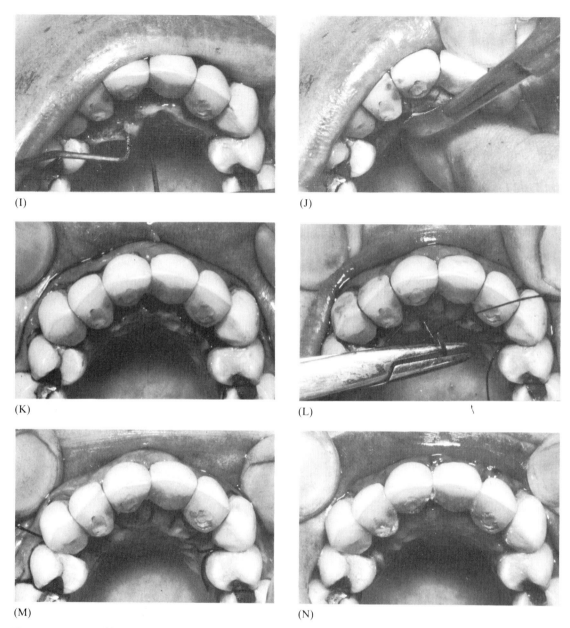

Figure 15.20 (*cont.*) (I) Palatal mucoperiosteal flap reflection for indirect tissue resection. (J) Outline incision No. 12 blade – note digital support. (K) Surgical flap preparation completed. (L) Continuous suturing commenced 23 distopalatal papilla. Note suture insertion from mucosal surface aspect. (M) Palatal suturing completed and flap coaptation. Suturing then proceeds at 13 distobuccal papilla. (N) 1 week postoperative.

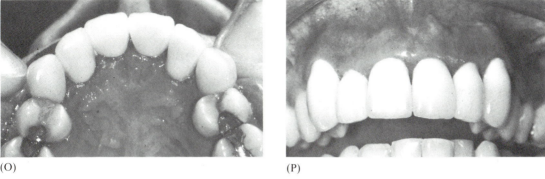

(O)   (P)

Figure 15.20 (*cont.*) (O) and (P) Crowns fitted at 4 months

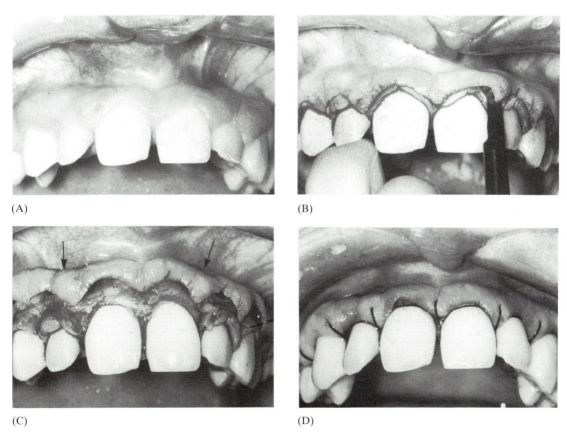

(A)   (B)

(C)   (D)

Figure 15.21 (A) Aesthetically unacceptable gingival hyperplasia in 18-year-old woman. (B) Conservative outline incision but minor tissue resection at 12 for optimal marginal contour. (C) Filletting of unevenly thickened tissue. Complication of inadvertent mucosal perforations (arrowed) at 12 and 22 mucogingival junctions. (D) Continuous suture. Note: marginal tissue puckering at 11 due to ineffective outline incision and mucosal displacement from perforation.

184

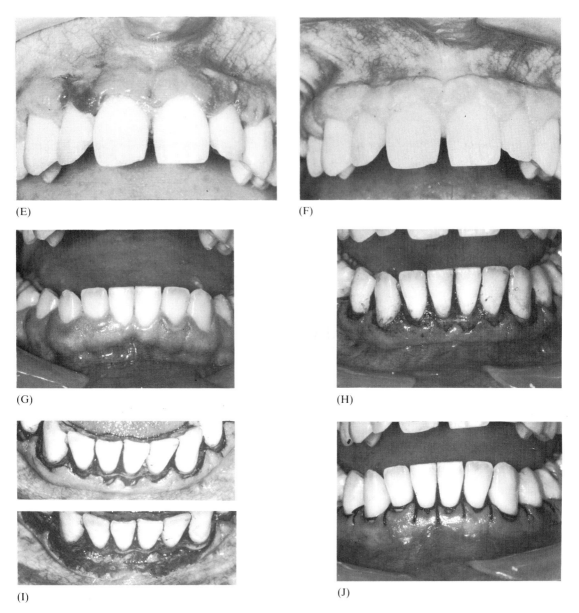

(E)

(F)

(G)

(H)

(I)

(J)

Figure 15.21 (*cont.*) (E) 1 week postoperative – slight mucosal ulceration in relation to perforation wounds but (F) with no residual deformity at 4 weeks. (G) Mandibular presentation with bony prominence especially at 44, 43. (H) Surgical flap reflection and apical displacement. (I) Composite of mucosal and bony form. (J) Flap continuous suture. (See also Figure 15.6)

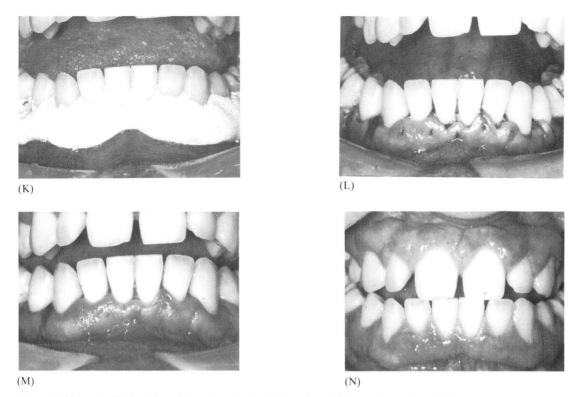

(K)   (L)

(M)   (N)

Figure 15.21 (*cont.*) (K) Periodontal dressing critical. (L) 1 week and (M) 4 week healing. (N) Some recurrence of tissue hyperplasia after 2 years

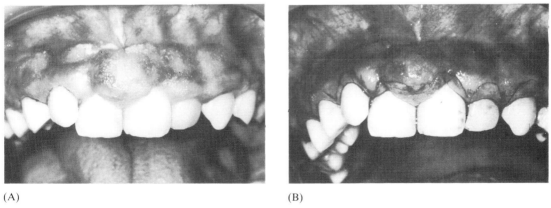

(A)   (B)

Figure 15.22 Cosmetic correction of developmental gingival fibromatosis in 21-year-old woman. (A) Initial presentation. (B) Outline incision – uneven papillary enlargement at 11, 21 complicated dissection.

186

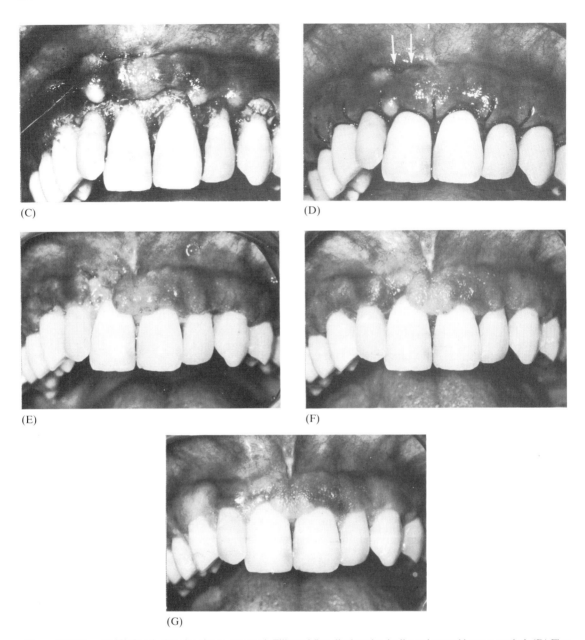

(C)

(D)

(E)

(F)

(G)

Figure 15.22 (*cont.*) (C) Cervical wedge tissue removed. Filletted flap displaced apically and crestal bone revealed. (D) Flap sutured. Note inadvertent mucosal perforation (arrowed) associated with tissue contour changes at 12, 11 mucogingival junction. (E) 1 week postoperative. Flap ulceration coronal to fenestration site and partial relapse coronally to 21, 22, 23 despite use of periodontal dressing. (F) 2 week and (G) 3 month healing. Patient declined further surgical embellishment

16

Simple pocket surgery:
II Soft tissue resection technique

Direct and indirect resection

The surgical technique for pocket resection is very similar to that used when conserving tissue in surgical reattachment, but with the essential difference of the position of the outline incision which determines the amount of soft tissue to be resected. This incision is therefore related to the crest of the alveolar bone which, in the *direct resection* technique, must be established by probing. However, in many instances the inherent morphology of the tissues associated with the pocket complicates this assessment and when an altered surgical sequence is indicated. In this surgical option, referred to as the *indirect resection* technique, a mucoperiosteal flap is first reflected to allow both mucosal and bony form to be assessed *in situ*. This method is also applicable to situations where the varying degrees of soft tissue pocketing and of bony involvement would complicate the performance of the direct resection method.

Influence of tissue morphology on the surgical options

There are two morphologic situations characterized by thin or thick tissue for which the direct and indirect resection techniques respectively are conveniently applied. The features of these situations and their influence on technique must therefore be examined.

Thin tissue

The gingival tissue forming the pocket wall is thin in a facio-oral plane. Its surface and that of the underlying alveolar bone are almost parallel to the long axis of the tooth (Figure 16.1 A). Little difficulty then arises in judging the position of the crest of the bone, by pocket probing and probing horizontally through the pocket wall (Figure 16.1 E). In this way the appropriate location of the resection line is readily established. Similarly, the surgical flap is readily prepared (Figure 16.1 A1 and A2) and on completion of the subsequent surgical stages, the flap margin has only to be translocated along approximately the same horizontal plane to be adapted to the bone, prior to suturing (Figure 16.1 A3). Consequently, the direct inverse bevel resection of thin tissue is a comparatively simple and predictable surgical exercise.

Thick tissue

This is represented by two situations, although these most frequently coexist. In one the gingiva itself is thick, as in a fibrous gingival hyperplasia (Figure 16.1 B) and as shown in Figure 9.1 (P–R). In the other, the alveolar bone surface and its overlying gingiva are at an obtuse angle to the long axis of the teeth, as in shallow vaulted palates and so giving the superficial appearances of thick gingiva (Figure 16.1 C and D). In neither situation is the position of the crest of the bone easily established by probing,

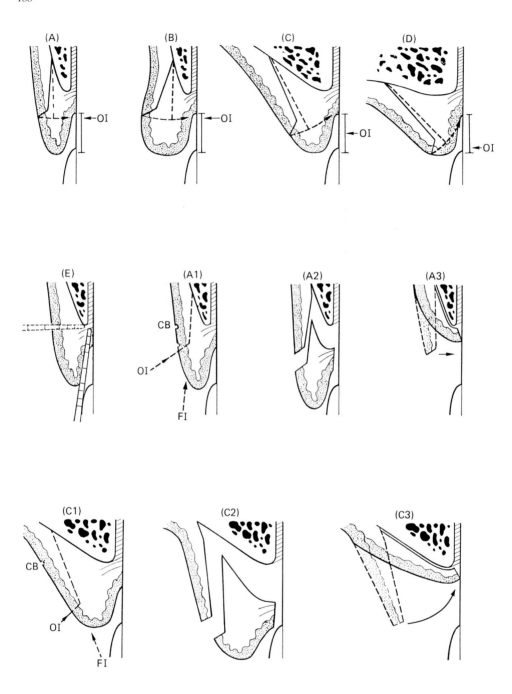

Figure 16.1 Tissue morphology and the inverse bevel incisions. (A) 'Thin' and (B–D) 'thick' pocket walls associated with equal pocket depths. 'Thick' tissue sites represented by (B) hyperplastic gingiva, (C) anatomically thick gingiva and (D) underlying bone. Note similar location of outline incisions (OI) at (A) and (B), but (C and D) progressively more coronally located the thicker the tissue; different arcs of rotation necessary for surgical flap adaptation. (E) Probing of crest of bone critical to determination of appropriate outline incision. This is readily accomplished at (A1) thin tissue but is complicated by (C1) thick tissue form. Similarly, filletting incision (FI) runs almost parallel to tooth surface at (A1) and presents no difficulty, but at (C1) thick tissue is at obtuse angle so is impeded by crown of tooth. (A2 and C2) Surgical flap completion and removal of cervical wedge. Note larger and more broadly based wedge at thick tissue. Flap margin adaptation by (A3) translocation along horizontal plane but (C3) tissue rotation apically necessitating longer flap

whilst in the latter in particular, the point on the gingival surface that would correspond to the crest of the bone is difficult to visualize (Figure 16.1 C1). This is in turn due partly to the larger amount of underlying connective tissue to be removed (Figure 16.1 C2) in order to produce the required thin flap and partly due to the relatively flat alveolar contour. Together, these mean that for the flap margin to be coapted to the bone it must be rotated about the arc of a circle passing through the crest of the bone (Figure 16.1 C3).

A close examination of the geometrical differences between thin and thick tissues shown in Figure 16.1 (A–D) reveals that for the same depth of pocketing the position of the outline incision is progressively more coronal the steeper is the slope of the gingival surface, namely the 'thicker' is the tissue. This is because some of the flap length is utilized in transposing the arc towards the bone. The most extreme application is where the surface of the gingiva, as at the front of some palatal vaults, forms a ledge against the tooth (Figure 16.1 D). In this situation the outline incision is located almost at the level of the gingival margin, the pocket depth being represented by the thickness of the palatal mucosa itself. This will be found to be even more evident at pockets related to edentulous zones, at which the gingival surface is at right angles to the tooth as shown in Figure 16.17 (A and B).

There are also a number of other difficulties experienced. Firstly, the precise contour of the outline incision in relation to individual adjacent root shapes is not easily ascertained, especially those located posteriorly in the arch, as shown in Figure 16.5. Secondly, even when the appropriate position of the outline incision has been established, it is very difficult to thin the bulky palatal gingiva because the palatal tooth surfaces obstruct the filletting action of the scalpel (Figure 16.1 C1). Thirdly, having prepared the flap, the tenacious attachment of the broad based cervical wedge to palatal bone makes removal of this tissue difficult. Finally, the poor visibility and access to the palate, compounded by copious bleeding and the tendency for the surgical flap to spring back into place about the teeth, complicates instrumentation of root surface and bone.

Applications of the surgical options

The numerous technical problems cited above are most readily overcome by altering the sequence of the direct inverse bevel resection technique for thin tissue. This technique is therefore described first, followed by that of the modified indirect technique, and its applications elsewhere. These relate to pocket correction at tooth surfaces adjacent to edentulous areas such as saddle areas, maxillary tuberosity and mandibular retromolar areas. It is also possible to apply this technique to the management of isolated interdental pockets. As the choice of resection technique in each situation cited depends primarily upon the tissue morphology, the surgical methodology is best considered under morphological headings.

Thin tissue (the direct resection technique)

Crest of bone identification

This is located by a process of pocket depth probing, supplemented by horizontal sharp probing through the pocket wall to identify the position of the bone as shown in Figure 16.1 (E). The surface of the gingiva forming the pocket is then punctured with the probe to denote the level of the crest of the bone about each tooth in the field. The importance of the level of the bony crest as opposed to that of the pocket base, as the critical landmark in pocket resection must be re-emphasized here, for the latter is often located within intrabony defects (see Figure 14.6).

Flap preparation

Outline incision

This shallow scalloped incision is located about 2 mm coronal to the puncture marks (Figure 16.1 A1) and is carried out as described in the previous chapter. This ensures that the margin of the surgical flap lies coronal to and just covers the crest of the bone at completion of operation.

Filletting (thinning) incision

This produces a gingival flap of physiological thickness and isolates the cervical wedge which incorporates all of the pocket wall tissue (Figure 16.1 A1). The incision is carried out as described before, and the same practical hints and precautions are applicable. Although there is little chance of entering the pocket space itself there is still a risk of external perforation, so should be guarded against. The appropriate angled filletting incision always makes contact with bone apical to its crest. Dissection extends only as far apically as necessary to create a surgical flap of physiological thickness for the area and to completely isolate the surgical wedge tissue.

Flap reflection

The flap is reflected only sufficiently to allow for the removal of the cervical wedge (Figure 16.1 A2) and for root surface and bony instrumentation. There is a greater tendency for the more fibrous palatal mucosal flap to spring back into position, so it must be constantly retracted from the field of operation.

Cervical wedge removal and management of root and bone

This too is carried out as described previously. The only difficulty likely to be encountered is when curetting the tough fibrous attachment of this tissue to palatal bone. Only that part of the root surface contributing to the healed dento-epithelial junction need be instrumented (see Figure 15.9).

Flap adaptation

The flap is adapted over the crest of the bone (Figure 16.1 A3) which it will just cover when the outline incision has been correctly sited as shown in Figure 16.1 A2 and C. When on the other hand the incision has been placed too far apically, the bone will be denuded (Figure 16.2 B), or if too far coronally, incomplete pocket reduction results (Figure 16.2 D). Any subsequent surgical reduction

of bone height will also contribute to flap tissue excess. (See also Chapter 19.)

The problem of mucosal deficiency and bony denudation at sites other than in the palate may be dealt with by an initial further flap reflection beyond the level of the vestibular fold, followed by coronal repositioning (Figure 16.2 B1). Whereas in the palate, such deficiencies at thin mucosal tissue sites are not easily overcome and healing by granulation must usually be accepted. (See also Chapter 19.) Attempts to pull the flap more coronally by tighter suturing alone cannot be recommended for it is liable to cause mucosal ischacmic nccrosis and even greater bony denudation. Where however the mucosal deficiency has arisen because the resection incision has been related erroneously to the base of an intrabony pocket, the denuded non-supporting bone could be removed to facilitate mucosal coverage as shown in Figure 16.2 (B2).

In contrast, any excess flap tissue is less of a problem. This is either accepted and surgical reattachment attempted (Figure 16.2 D) or the tissue excess trimmed away (Figure 16.2 D1). The

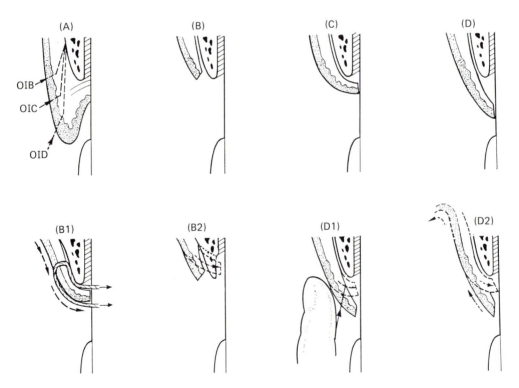

Figure 16.2 Management of surgical flap deficiency or excess in direct resection. (A) Outline incisions located too far apically (OIB), correctly (OIC) and too far coronally (OID) with their respective outcomes at (B–D). Mucosal deficiency at (B) corrected by (B1) coronal repositioning although at (B2) any associated non-supporting bone might also be removed to facilitate flap adaptation. Tissue excess at (D) accepted for surgical reattachment, (D1) resected or (D2) apically repositioned

latter can however sometimes be difficult to do on thin movable tissue, even when supported with a finger as shown in Figure 16.2 (D1). There is a further option at non-palatal sites of a selective apical repositioning (Figure 16.2 D2).

Flap stabilization

When the surgical flap margin contour conforms to the crest of the bone flap adaptation and stabilization can be achieved without difficulty. Indeed, as the base of the flap remains attached to alveolar bone it is inherently well supported and will be fixed into position over the bone by the blood coagulum. In practice, however, sutures are best inserted if only as a precaution against inadvertent postoperative displacement. Either continuous or interrupted sutures may be used, depending on the requirements at the opposing flap and individual operator preference. No periodontal dressing is necessary.

Thick tissue (the indirect resection technique)

The direct surgical sequence described above is modified in terms of first reflecting a full thickness mucoperiosteal flap, so that the pocket depths and the position of the bone can be assessed *in situ* to establish the appropriate resection incision. This means that unlike in the direct technique there is no need for detailed presurgical assessment. The indirect technique is most commonly utilized in the palate but is equally applicable to other sites presenting with gingival hyperplasia. The management of these other situations is described following that for palatal pockets.

Mucoperiosteal flap reflection

The palatal mucoperiosteal flap can usually be elevated and reflected by blunt dissesion and without any incision, although where difficulties arise (see below), sharp dissection should be used. Thus, the attachment at the pocket bases can be severed quite readily with a heavy curette (e.g. Goldman–Fox GF2 or Prichard PR1/2) or scaler (e.g. Hawe–Neos No.6) within the palatal and interdental pocket spaces (Figure 16.3 A and A1). The palatal pocket mucosa with the contiguous interdental papillary pocket tissues and mucoperiosteum related to the pocket bases, can then be reflected with a fine pointed periosteal elevator

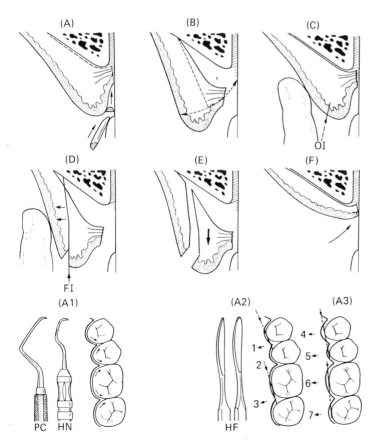

Figure 16.3 Indirect resection technique. (A) Pocket wall and papillary tissue detachment with (A1) Prichard surgical curette (PC) or Hawe–Neos No. 6 scaler (HW) and then (A2) Hu-Friedy No. 10 elevator (HF). (A2) Initial insertion of elevator with flat side against tooth, under detached papillae (arrowed sites 1–3). (A3) Further elevation at mid-palatal aspects of teeth via adjacent mesial papillary aspects (4–7). (B) Mucoperiosteal flap reflection. Appropriate position of outline incision assessed *in situ*. (C) Tissue replaced. Outline incision (OI) facilitated by digital support. (D) Tissue reflected into vertical posture, supported digitally and filletting incision (FI) carried out. (E) Surgical flap completed. Cervical wedge tissue comes away readily. (F) Flap adaptation

(Hu-Friedy No. 10) from within the loosened pocket spaces (Figure 16.3 A2 and A3). The palatal tissue is gently but firmly reflected with the curved surface of the instrument held against the mucosa to minimize trauma, by elevating against tooth and bone. The flap is reflected only sufficiently to provide adequate access and visibility to the palatal root surfaces and related bone (Figure 16.3 B).

The interdental pocket tissue usually lifts away quite readily from the interproximal spaces as part of the reflected palatal mucoperiosteal flap when the cervical wedge tissue at the facial aspects has already been curetted away as shown in Figure 16.4 (A and A1). In the absence of facial pocketing however, the interdental pocket tissue should be separated from the intact facial gingiva by a facial crevicular incision (Figure 16.4 B). Whereas, with palatal pocketing alone (and in cases of palatal gingival hyperplasia)

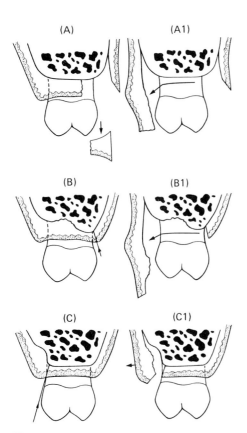

Figure 16.4 Palatal flap reflection and the interdental tissues. Interdental pocket tissue incorporated into palatal surgical field following (A and A1) removal of buccal cervical wedge tissue or (B and B1) its isolation from the buccal tissue by a crevicular incision. Intact interdental tissue (C and C1) isolated by palatal crevicular incision. Note tissue from within intrabony defects at (B1 and C1) lifting away as part of surgical flap

the intact interdental tissues are similarly isolated by a palatal crevicular incision (Figure 16.4 C). The palatal papillary and interdental pocket tissues are therefore incorporated routinely into any palatal surgical field. Intact palatal and interproximal dentogingival junctions within the surgical field must, as elsewhere, be freed by crevicular incisions or oblique relieving incisions used instead (see Chapter 17).

In summary, for the indirect technique a mucoperiosteal flap is reflected primarily by blunt dissection and sharp dissection used only when difficulties arise and at intact dentogingival junctions within the surgical field. The palatal flap consists of the entire pocket wall tissue and, where appropriate, the contiguous interdental tissues, the surgically disrupted supracrestal attachment and the bulk of any intrabony inflammatory tissue and lastly the contiguous palatal mucoperiosteum, as shown in Figure 16.3 (B) and Figure 16.4 (A1 and B1). This technique not only greatly reduces operating time but, as will be shown, also simplifies the subsequent surgical stages.

Practical hints and precautions

(1) Flap elevation is commenced at the most accessible part of the surgical field and within the thickest interdental papillary tissue. This usually proves to be at the distopalatal aspects of each tooth posteriorly, and anteriorly, at either the mesial or distal line angles of the teeth. In the former situations the elevator is thus inserted and the interdental papilla elevated coronopalatally from the interproximal spaces (Figure 16.3 A2). This is repeated at each tooth in the surgical field. Elevation is then extended distally about the palatal aspects of each successive tooth from within the deflected interdental papillary spaces (Figure 16.3 A3) to complete palatal flap reflection. Sites at which the mucoperiosteum is more tightly bound down to bone and does not come away easily are freed by sharp dissection rather than exerting greater force upon the flap with the elevator. Excessive force causes unnecessary mucosal trauma and possibly even mucosal tearing, as well as giving rise to greater postoperative pain. (See also Chapter 17.)

(2) The mucoperiosteal flap reflection technique advocated, obviates the tedious and difficult task of having to curette away the comparatively inaccessible interdental gingival tissues that would remain following the alternative use of palatal crevicular incisions. Similarly, the removal of inflammatory connective tissue from within any bony defects is greatly simplified, as this tissue usually comes away with the palatal flap instead as depicted in Figure 16.4 (B1 and

C1). In the same way, palatal pocket incision would tend to section such tissue from the inner aspect of the flap, leaving it within any palatal bony defects following flap reflection.

Management of root and bone

The flap is deflected from the teeth and any residual soft tissue tags attached to tooth or bone curetted away. The appropriate root surface debridement and osseous therapy is then carried out.

Surgical flap preparation

Assessment of flap form

This most critical and difficult stage of the operation aims to create a surgical flap that just covers the palatal bony crests and is of physiological thickness for the area. This necessitates trimming the edge of the mucoperiosteal flap and reducing its thickness. The operator must first establish what point on the flap keratinized surface will correspond to the crest of the bone and root contour at each site in the surgical field. This is judged by direct observation, having lifted the flap away (Figure 16.3 B), and making a mental note of the crestal bone position and individual root contours. The flap is then replaced *in situ* (Figure 16.3 C) and the appropriate level of the outline incision visualized. This incision line might instead be marked with an indelible pencil, or the tissue surface punctured at intervals with a probe.

Outline incision

The flap will at this stage, adapt closely to bone aided by the interdental papillary projections extending into the interproximal spaces. Supplementary digital support for the flap is, however, necessary as shown in Figure 16.3 (C) whilst making the appropriate apically directed shallow outline incision. Where any doubt exists about the appropriate position and contour of this incision, the mucoperiosteal flap is reflected once again and the situation reassessed before progressing further.

Practical hints and precautions

(1) A Swann–Morton No. 12 blade is best used at the back of the mouth, whilst anteriorly either a No. 12 or No. 15 blade may be preferred (Figure 16.5 A). Sharp blades are especially critical at this stage for effective incision of the movable tissue. The incision is best commenced at the distopalatal line angle of the last tooth in the surgical field, following root and bone contour as far mesially as possible. Posteriorly, the tooth crowns impede this cutting action of the blade resulting in an initially incomplete scalloping. This is disregarded at this stage. Elsewhere, access permitting, the individual incisions extend up to the flap margin.

(2) A series of semilunar shaped incisions is produced (Figure 16.5 A) crossing each other within the interdental papillae where access has allowed. The incomplete incisions elsewhere are extended and joined using a Swann–Morton

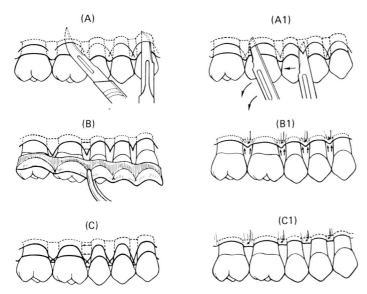

Figure 16.5 Indirect palatal flap preparation and adaptation. (A) Individual semilunar outline incisions, using Nos. 12 or 15 blade depending on access, follow flap margin contour and overlap where possible. (A1) Outline incisions completed by cutting coronally with No. 15 blade and subsequent filletting carried out in a similar manner. (B) Delivery of cervical wedge plus pocket inner wall tissue using curved forceps. Note papillary contour (arrowed) in relation to mesiodistal widths of interdental spaces. (B1) Flap papillary peaks adapted into interdental spaces but some bony denudation inevitable (arrowed). (C) Exaggerated scalloped outline incision to match (arrowed) greater mesiodistal interdental dimensions at level of crestal bone. (C1) Optimal mucosal coverage of interdental bone

No. 15 with a coronally directed cutting action (Figure 16.5 B). This dissection starts at the mid-axial points of each outlining incision and proceeds distally and mesially as necessary, towards the interdental papillae.

The contour of the mucoperiosteal flap is dictated by the crowns of the teeth to which it approximated, whilst that of the surgical flap must be related to greater curvatures of the roots at the level of the crest of the bone. Consequently where the outline incision follows the gingival margin, as advocated elsewhere, a discrepancy between the surgical flap margin and root contours is inevitable (Figure 16.5 B). In addition, the inherently wider interdental spaces related to the tapering palatal root forms of the molar teeth, in particular, demand both wider and longer interdental papillary peaks to the surgical flap to ensure optimal interdental bone coverage. This can be achieved by an exaggerated scalloped outline incision contour (Figure 16.5 C). This technique has also been referred to in Chapter 15 (see Figure 15.13). The ability to examine the root contours *in situ* following the initial flap reflection, greatly facilitates the preparation of appropriately shaped outline incisions. The effect of outline incisions that follow the initial mucoperiosteal margin are shown in Figure 16.5 (B1) and those with an exaggerated scalloped contour, which minimize interdental bone exposure, are shown in Figure 16.5 (C1). (See also Chapter 29 – Modified Widman flap.)

Filletting incision and removal of tissue

This aims to create a suitably thinned surgical flap by excising the underlying connective tissue from the mucoperiosteal flap (Figure 16.3 D). When carried out successfully tissue coaptation about the crest of the bone and necks of teeth is possible. Tissue reduction need only be limited to the 8–10 mm of mucoperiosteal tissue located immediately apical to the outline incision, although more extensive filletting is often necessary to facilitate subsequent flap coaptation. The mucoperiosteal flap is reduced by sharp dissection, using a No. 15 blade commencing within the shallow outline incision and passing with a filletting action progressively more deeply towards bone. The plane of dissection runs parallel to the keratinized surface and at a depth of about 2–3 mm and should ideally meet palatal bone just coronal to the level of flap reflection.

The interference by the palatal tooth surfaces to the filletting action is readily overcome by deflecting the already detached palatal mucosa into a more favourable vertical position away from the teeth. Where the initial mucoperiosteal flap reflection is inadequate for this it is simply reflected further as necessary. The flap deflection is achieved and maintained during filletting dissection by the simultaneous use of the blade as an elevator and a scalpel. Thus the blade is inserted into the outline incision and using its flat side as a retractor, dissection commences whilst at the same time supporting the keratinized aspect of the flap with the first finger of the other hand, as shown in Figure 16.3 (D). This digital support also helps the operator to assess the thickness of the flap being prepared.

The connective tissue dissected from the mucoperiosteal flap represents part of the cervical wedge. This tissue is gripped firmly with curved mosquito-type forceps as shown in Figure 16.5 (B) and delivered from the surgical field. As its attachment to bone will have already been severed by the initial flap reflection (Figure 16.3 B) the tissue is usually removed quite readily. Where, however, still attached to the surgical flap, because of incomplete dissection, or to the underlying bone, because of inadequate flap reflection, this is simply freed by the necessary further sharp dissection. The surgical flap can now be adapted over bone and about the teeth (Figure 16.3 F), prior to suturing.

Practical hints and precautions

(1) Where the position of the outline incision has been misjudged, the surgical flap may either be too long (Figure 16.6 A) or too short (Figure 16.6 B) in relation to the crest of the bone. In the former, the excess of tissue coronal to bone may be accepted for surgical reattachment or be trimmed away (Figure 16.6 A) at the appropriate level as described previously. Where the flap is too short at thick palatal mucosal sites, the bone denudation can sometimes be minimized by reflecting the palatal mucoperiosteum further to provide greater mucosal mobility. This, together with the inherent elasticity of the relatively thick tissue, may then allow the flap to be stretched over the bone when pulling up the sutures more tightly. This effect can be enhanced as depicted in Figure 16.6 (B) by making serial transverse incisions of the connective tissue surface, as when advancing a palatal mucoperiosteal flap to repair an oro-antral fistula. The hazard of mucosal ischaemic necrosis, with its sequelae of greater bony necrosis alluded to earlier, remains with each of these compensatory methods. Accordingly, as a forced choice, the existing inadvertent and ultimately smaller area of bony denudation would be the lesser of two evils, allowing healing to occur by granulation. (See Chapters 17 and 19.)

(2) The flap is reduced to a fairly even 2 mm thickness. Over-thinning should be avoided, for this and, worse still, any associated frank perforation, as shown in Figure 16.6 (C),

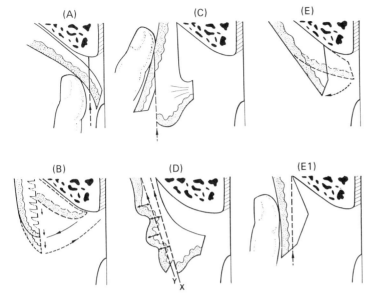

Figure 16.6 Palatal surgical flap defects. (A) 'Long' flap reduced by inverse bevel incision facilitated by digital support. (B) 'Short' flap elongated by connective tissue sectioning (arrowed) and mucosal stretching over denuded bone. (C) Flap perforation. (D) Filletting at prominent mucosal rugae based on tissue thickness between ridges (X); that on the crest of ridges (Y) predisposes to perforation. (E) Thick flap precludes close adaptation to tooth so (E1) reduced by further filletting

compromises the blood supply to the already comparatively poorly vascularized coronally related tissues of the palate, and frequently results in painful mucosal necrosis. Inadvertent or over-zealous tissue reduction is most likely to occur at the front of the palate where the prominent mucosal rugae will inevitably complicate the attempted even reduction of the flap thickness and may be associated with mucosal perforation. The degree of tissue reduction required at these sites should be based on the tissue between the mucosal ridges and not the thicker crests of the ridges (Figure 16.6 D). The rugae also complicate filletting itself, because the different tissue thicknesses lead to uneven mucosal flexing during dissection, whilst the ridge tissue tends to be tougher than the intervening tissues.

(3) Whilst preferable to err by leaving the flap too thick, this creates difficulty with flap adaptation. The resulting greater tissue rigidity means that a thick flap tends to spring back from its intended position (Figure 16.6 E). Further reduction of the bulk of the flap with a sharp No. 15 scalpel blade is then necessary using, once again, digital support as shown in Figure 16.6 (E1).

(4) The palatal flap at some second molars sometimes resists close adaptation to the teeth because of an apparently inadequate mucosal filletting. However this is sometimes due instead to a thin but prominent bony ridge extending anteriorly from the lateral wall of the greater palatine foramen, which interferes with flap

adaptation. This ridge is best reduced with a bur or bone chisel.

(5) Copious bleeding, often experienced during palatal thinning, is checked readily by the application of firm digital pressure over the flap for a short time. (See also Chapter 17.)

Flap adaptation and stabilization

The correctly contoured and thinned flap is closely adapted about the necks of the teeth and just covers the crest of the bone. The intervening blood coagulum holds the flap in place initially, but suturing is advisable to avoid the tendency for the margins to lift away or for the flap to sag as shown in Figure 16.7 (A). This occurs particularly in the presence of a relatively flat palatal contour. The application of a periodontal dressing (Figure 16.7 A1) is therefore necessary to help the flap in this situation but elsewhere sutures will suffice.

Practical hints and precautions

(1) Flap adaptation is more difficult when the flap has been inadequately thinned (be this inadvertently or because of the mucosal rugae) and is therefore more rigid and where the palate is flat. Adaptation can however be improved by increasing the tension of the sutures to pull the flap into position. This should be anticipated and the sutures inserted further away than usual from the flap margin. This not only minimizes the chances of the sutures tearing out but also

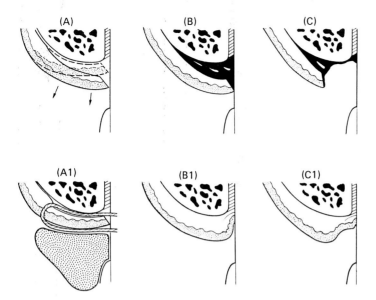

Figure 16.7 Palatal flap adaptation. (A) In shallow vaulted palates tendency for coronal displacement and sagging of flap tissue. Obviated by (A1) use of hammock-like suture and periodontal dressing. (B) Poor vertical adaptation with large blood clot predisposes to (B1) recurrent pocket. (C) Poor horizontal adaptation resulting in (C1) gingival deformity but no pocket

produces a hammock-like effect as depicted in Figure 16.7 (A1).

(2) Poor flap adaptation (in a vertical plane) over the bone in flat palates could result in recurrent pocketing (Figure 16.7 B and B1). The space between flap and bone becomes filled with blood clot, which organizes and is replaced by gingival connective tissue of similar thickness, which represents the depth of a potential pocket. Poor horizontal adaptation of a thick flap to the necks of the teeth, is comparable to bony denudation following overtrimming (Figure 16.7 C). A pouch-like gingival deformity without any associated pocketing is the most likely outcome, as shown in Figure 16.7 (C1).

Clinical case presentations

The direct and indirect resection techniques in a series of different clinical cases are shown in Figures 16.8, 16.9 and 16.10. The last of these incorporates the distal wedge technique which is described below.

Other situations

Having considered the technical features of the direct and indirect resection techniques in relation to thin and thick tissues respectively, the management of the remaining more specific situations can be dealt with. These are marked gingival hyperplasia, pockets related to edentulous sites and isolated interdental pockets and are described in that order.

Marked gingival hyperplasia

Gingival hyperplasia of developmental origin depicted in Figure 16.11 (A), that associated with, classically, the use of the anticonvulsant drug (Epanutin) therapy (Figure 16.11 B) and long-term maxillary prostheses (Figure 16.11 C), is regarded as thick tissue for surgical purposes and so qualifies for the indirect resection technique. There are however several peculiar difficulties.

Problems of tissue structure

The cauliflower-like structure of the tissues in many of these situations (Figure 16.11 B and C), compared with that of the more uniformly thickened dense fibrous hyperplasia elsewhere (Figure 16.11 A) complicates surgery. Indeed, the technical difficulties are very similar to those encountered at prominent palatal mucosal rugae, but on a very much larger scale. Accordingly, the uneven tissue thickness greatly increases the risk of inadvertent flap perforation and surgical flap margin laceration (Figure 16.11 B, C and C1). In addition, the comparatively thin tissue at the base of the reflected flap provides little support during filletting dissection of its bulky marginal parts. The sum total of these difficulties is that the preparation of the required surgical flap is often impossible.

Note: Even greater difficulties arise when these individuals also present with repaired developmental palatal clefts. These relate to flap reflection being impeded by the scarring and the potential risk of compromising the surgical repair and the post-surgical positioning of the prosthesis.

197

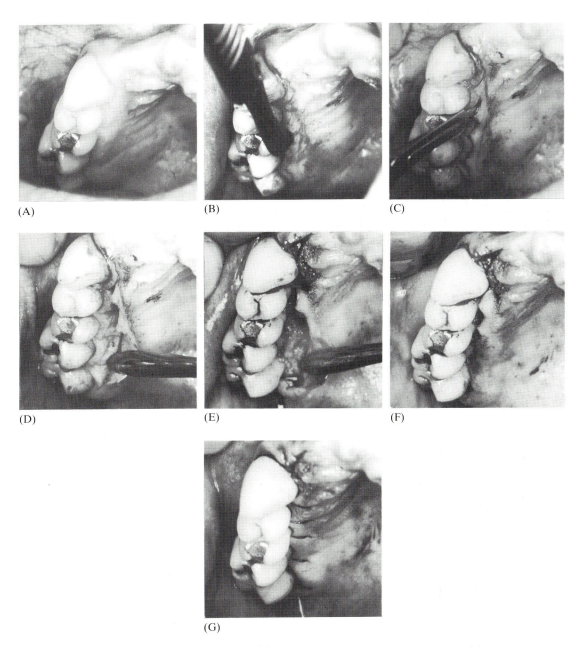

(A) (B) (C)

(D) (E) (F)

(G)

Figure 16.8 Direct resection. (A) Thin palatal tissue. (B) Outline incision using No. 12 scalpel blade. (C) Filletting incision with No. 15 blade not impeded by palatal cusps. (D) Cervical wedge tissue exposed by surgical flap reflection and then (E) removed. Note mesial relieving incision to enhance access for instrumentation. (F) Surgical flap prior to (G) coaption and stabilization by continuous suture. Note optimal tissue adaptation

198

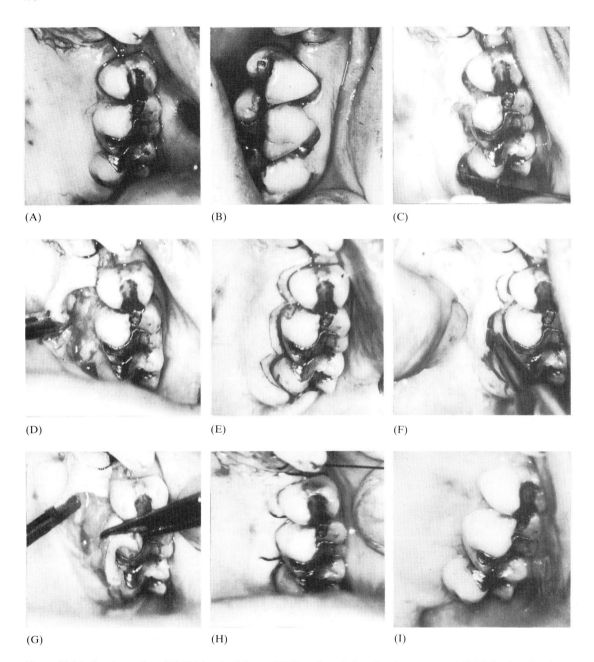

(A)   (B)   (C)

(D)   (E)   (F)

(G)   (H)   (I)

Figure 16.9 Indirect resection. (A) Thick palatal tissue. (B) Buccal cervical wedge tissue removed. (C) Palatal pocket tissue reflection with elevator incorporates contiguous interdental papillary tissue. (D) Exposure of root surfaces and bone for *in situ* assessment of location outline incision. Note mucosal thickness (E) Outline incision. (F) Digitally supported flap filletted with No. 15 blade. (G) Removal cervical wedge tissue. (H) Flap suturing. (I) 1 week postoperative

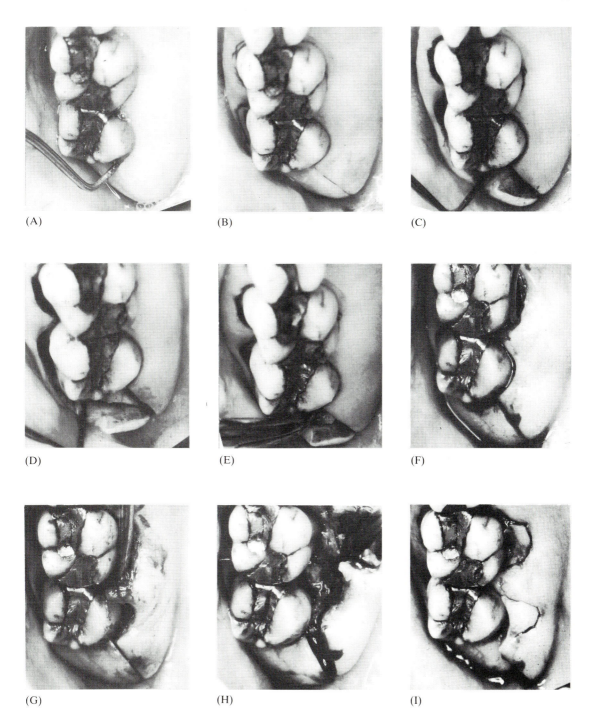

(A)　　　　　　(B)　　　　　　(C)

(D)　　　　　　(E)　　　　　　(F)

(G)　　　　　　(H)　　　　　　(I)

Figure 16.10 Indirect resection palatal and distal pocketing. (A) Initial presentation in 44-year-old woman. (B) Buccal outline and distal crestal ridge linear incisions. (C) Buccal and distobuccal tissue reflection reveals tissue thickness distal to 17. Neos 580-6 scaler was used to detach distobuccal tissue. (D) Distobuccal tissue filletted – resected tissue wedge *in situ*. (E) Wedge gripped with curved haemostat prior to incision of residual attachment with No. 12 blade. (F) Filletted distobuccal tissue in 'resting' position. Neos scaler disrupting palatal supracrestal attachments followed by (G) further mucosal detachment and elevation. Note rounded elevator surface towards tissue and interdental papillary tissue incorporated in mucosal flap. (H) Exposure of crestal bone and root forms for assessing appropriate (I) outline incision.

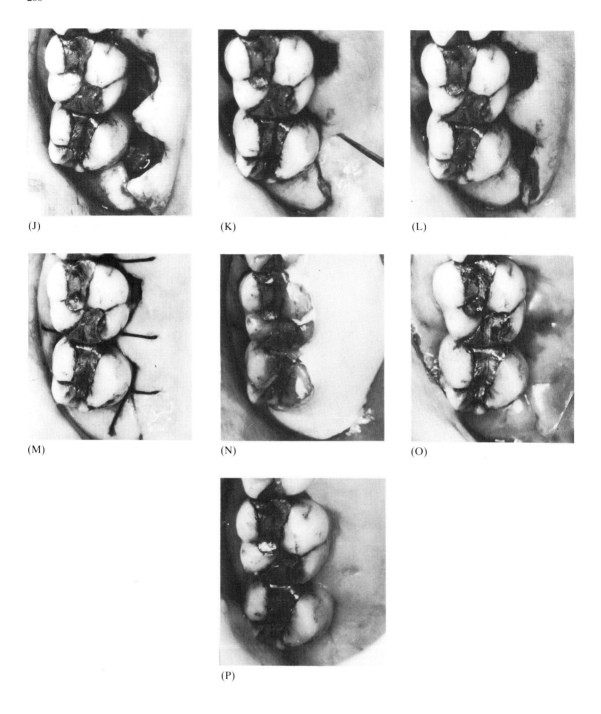

(J)　　　　　　　　　(K)　　　　　　　　　(L)

(M)　　　　　　　　　(N)　　　　　　　　　(O)

(P)

Figure 16.10 (*cont.*) (J) Palatal and distopalatal tissue filletting completed. (K) Surgical flaps coapted (palatal flap 'pegged' with probe for photography) following excision of distal overlapping tissue excess from distopalatal flap which results in close flap approximation. (L) Line of excision of excess tissue – small residual tissue tag to be removed. (M) Flap stabilization with continuous suture. Note positions of distal suture insertion points for optimal coaptation; also mucosal deficiency at 16 following imprecise initial outline incision. (N) Dressing to check tissue displacement coronally. (O) 1 week and (P) 2 weeks postoperatively. Mucosal deficiency granulating over with no deformity.

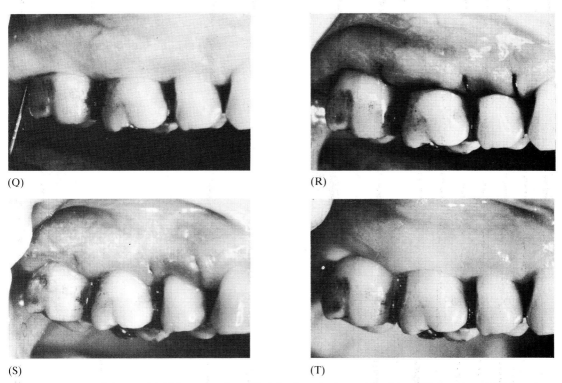

Figure 16.10 (*cont.*) (Q) Buccal initial presentation, (R) following suturing and healing at (S) 1 week and (T) 2 weeks

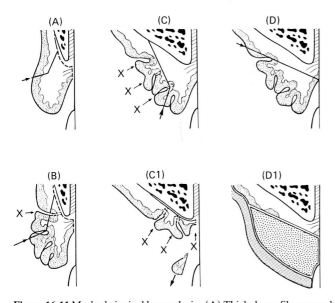

Figure 16.11 Marked gingival hyperplasia. (A) Thick dense fibrous pocket wall amenable to indirect resection but the (B) papillomatous structure characterized by epanutin hyperplasia and that (C) associated with prostheses is technically more difficult to dissect. This tissue is also prone to perforation (B, C and C1) at arrowed sites 'X' and loss of surgical flap margin. Access permitting, direct resection is easier but is subject to similar problems. (D) External bevel resection preferable. (D1) Wound protected by periodontal dressing located under prosthesis

Post-surgical prosthesis placement

It is often difficult to reseat any prosthesis at completion of operation because of altered palatal mucosal form. This appears to be due to mucosal oedema from tissue manipulation, local anaesthetic injections and possibly also submucosal bleeding. Acrylic partial dentures and orthodontic appliances are especially problematic for they tend to rock on the distorted palatal mucosa. The more rigid tooth supported cast metal dentures can however often be 'bitten into place' by the opposing teeth, but the risk of an ischaemic necrosis of the thus physically compressed mucosa does always exist. The appliance might therefore best be left out, but aesthetic and functional requirements or the maintenance of tooth position stability rarely permits this.

Other surgical options

As the indirect resection technique for marked gingival hyperplasia is fraught with both technical difficulties and postoperative complications, the aware operator must either take a chance on coping with these problems or utilize other surgical methods.

The first option is, access permitting, the direct inverse bevel resection shown at Figure 16.11 (C and C1), and the difficulties of establishing the appropriate outline incision regarded as a lesser evil and overcome by more careful judgement. It is preferable to err by resecting too little tissue at the outset. Any residual palatal tissue excess is then trimmed, while that occurring elsewhere in the mouth can be corrected by apical repositioning.

The external bevel (conventional) gingivectomy (Figure 16.11 D) is the second option. In the absence of bony defects this is the simplest technique and pockets are predictably eliminated. The disadvantage of the raw connective tissue wound surface is partly offset in these cases, by the protection of the overlying prosthesis and the interposed periodontal dressing (Figure 16.11 D1). A soft mix of Coe-pak is applied directly to the fit surface of the prosthesis which is then inserted promptly as if relining a denture. With skeleton type dentures it is easier to apply the dressing conventionally and inserting the appliance whilst the material is still soft. (See also Chapter 24.)

The final option is electrosurgery as shown in Figure 16.12. This is however not recommended as a routine technique so will not be considered further here.

Clinical case presentations

The applications of the indirect technique to a thick uneven tissue are shown in Figures 16.12 and 16.13 (developmental gingival hyperplasia), Figure 16.14 (denture hyperplasia) and Figure 16.15 (drug induced hyperplasia).

Edentulous sites – the surgical wedge technique

The applicability of indirect resection

Pockets at tooth surfaces adjacent to edentulous zones, the maxillary tuberosity and mandibular retromolar areas are most readily corrected by the indirect resection technique. This is because the tissue forming these pockets is comparable to an exaggerated thickened palatal pocket, with the keratinized tissue surface lying perpendicular to the long axis of the tooth. The pocket depth is in effect represented by the thickness of the tissue (Figure 16.16 C1) and is therefore amenable to the indirect resection technique. As wedges of connective tissue are removed to create thin surgical flaps, the procedure is described as the mesial or distal (depending on the site) or saddle area surgical wedge technique as shown in Figures 16.16 A and B respectively.

Difficulties may be encountered with flap preparation due to the tissue surface contour, interference from the adjacent teeth to instrumentation and the inherently poor access. These can be overcome by appropriate relieving incisions plus reflection of the facial and oral aspects of the edentulous pocket tissue into a more accessible vertical position (Figure 16.16 B). As the surgical wedge technique is essentially the same for each site, these will be dealt with together.

Mucoperiosteal flap reflection

The appropriate inverse bevel incisions are first completed at the facial and oral aspects of the related tooth. These extend only as far as the tooth line angles at which they are converted into crevicular incisions (Figure 16.16 A and B1). Where there is no facial or oral aspect pocketing present or where thick palatal tissue exists, crevicular type incisions are made at the outset. The respective crevicular incisions continue towards each other meeting over the crest of the edentulous ridge and should pass down to bone. No further flap preparation is carried out at this stage. This then ensures that the still attached facial and oral tissue provide optimal support for the contiguous edentulous site tissues during the subsequent wedge preparations.

A straight incision, commencing at the tooth and passing down to bone, is then made along the crest (Figure 16.16 A1, B1 and C1) of the edentulous ridge. Facial and oral mucoperiosteal flaps can now be reflected from the underlying bone (Figure 16.16 A2, B2 and C2). The respective flaps incorporate the pocket wall lining and connective tissue, which

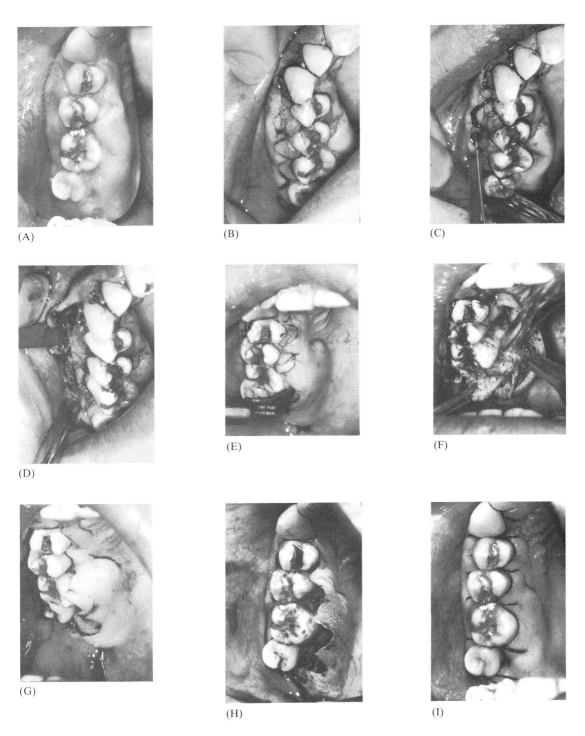

Figure 16.12 Developmental gingival hyperplasia. (A and O) Initial presentation 23-year-old woman with aesthetically displeasing gingival overgrowth mandibular anterior and right maxillary posterior quadrants. (B) Buccal outline resection incision. (C) Filletting with No. 15 blade. (D) Exposure of normal osseous form. (E) Palatal outline and (F) filletting incisions with Nos. 12 and 15 blades. Palatal crevicular incision preceded removal of cervical wedge tissue with haemostat. (G) Findings *in situ* necessitate additional resection at 17, 16. Note further outline incision. (H) Surgical flap prior to (I) coaptation and stabilization with continuous suture.

204

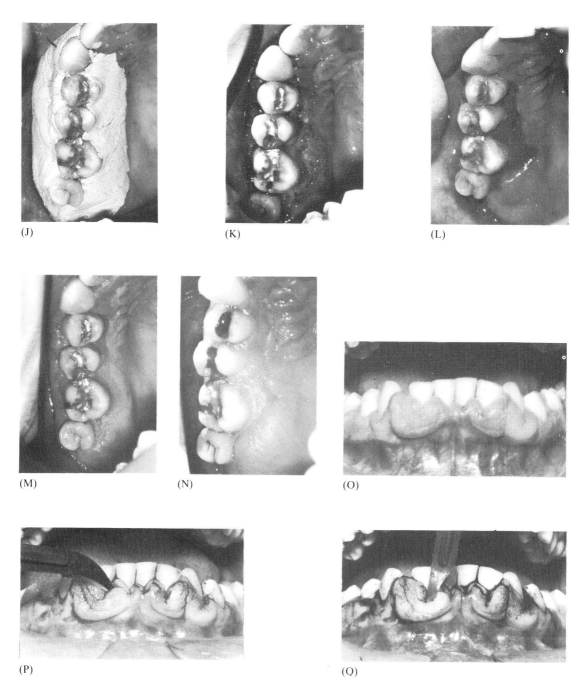

(J)

(K)

(L)

(M)

(N)

(O)

(P)

(Q)

Figure 16.12 (*cont.*) (J) Dressing critical for flap support. (K) Postoperative complication of mucosal ulceration finding at 1 week. (L) Ulcerated area healing at 2 weeks [note shape of area closely mirrors uneven mucosal surface contour at (I)], and (M) 4 weeks. (N) Presentation 10 years later with minimal recurrence hyperplasia. (O) Initial presentation mandible. (P) Outline incision No. 12 blade. (Q) Filletting incision – note complication of clefts at 43/42 and 32/33.

205

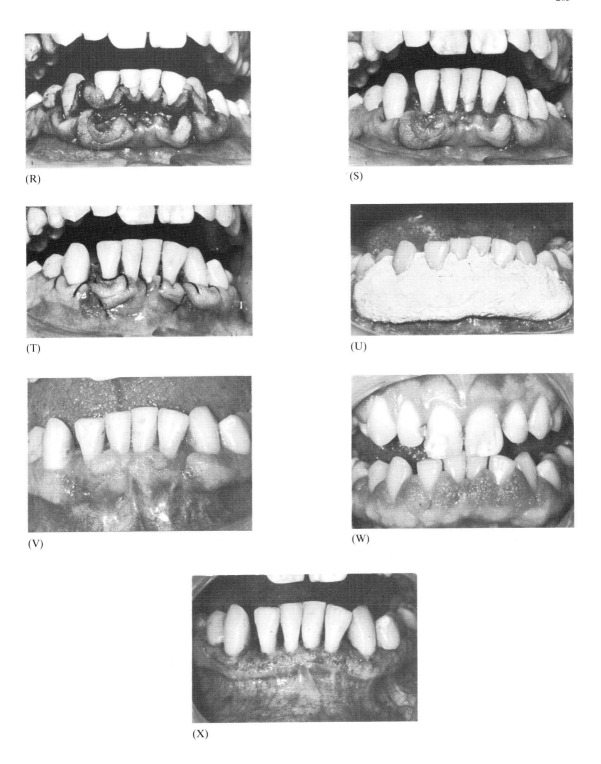

(R)

(S)

(T)

(U)

(V)

(W)

(X)

Figure 16.12 (*cont.*) (R) Surgical flap reflected – vertical mucosal breaches at 43/42, 32/33. (S) Cervical wedge removed. (T) Flap apically repositioned and sutured – note difficulty at 43/42, 32/33. (U) Periodontal dressing. (V) 1 month postoperative – effects of ulceration at 43/42, 32/33. (W) Recurrence hyperplasia after 2 years. Aesthetics unacceptable to patient. Option existed of external bevel excision or (X) electrosurgical embellishment of gingival form.

206

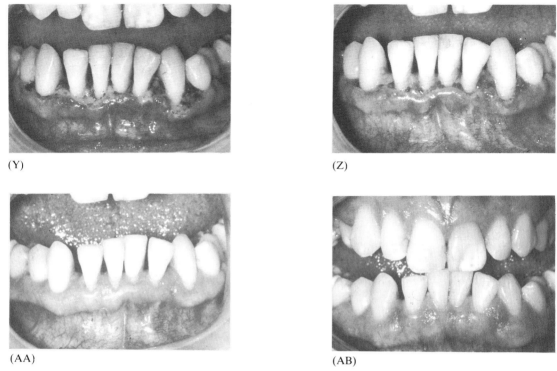

(Y)

(Z)

(AA)

(AB)

Figure 16.12 (*cont.*) Healing at (Y) 1 week (Z) 2 weeks and (AA) 4 weeks. (AB) Presentation at 10 years but with little tendency for further hyperplasia

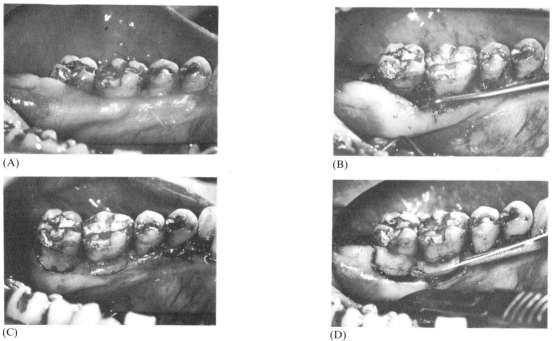

(A)

(B)

(C)

(D)

Figure 16.13 Indirect resection of developmental lingual and retromolar gingival hyperplasia. (A) Initial presentation in 28-year-old woman. (B) Mucosal reflection following lingual crevicular incision. (C) Outline incision. (D) Filletting with No. 12 blade.

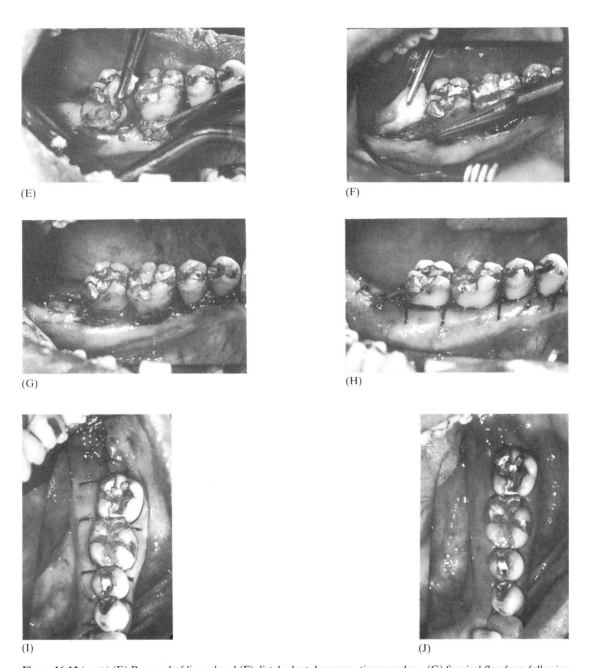

Figure 16.13 (*cont.*) (E) Removal of lingual and (F) distal edentulous zone tissue wedges. (G) Surgical flap form following resection of distal overlapping tissue excess. (H) Flap stabilization with continuous suture. (I) Occlusal views of sutured flap and (J) 1 week postoperatively.

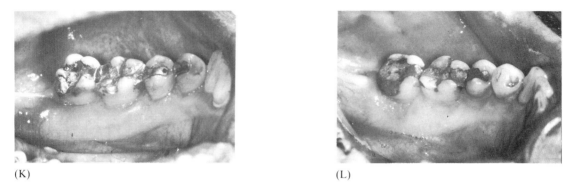

(K)   (L)

Figure 16.13 (*cont.*) (K) Healing at 4 weeks. (L) Presentation at 12 years – slight tissue proliferation lingually

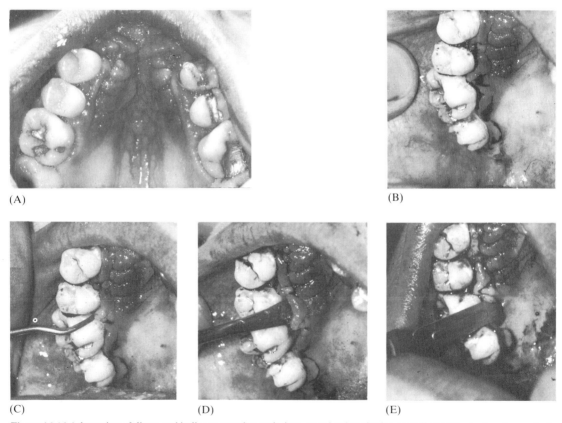

(A)   (B)

(C)   (D)   (E)

Figure 16.14 Adaptation of direct and indirect resection technique to palatal pocketing complicated by denture hyperplasia. (A) Initial presentation in 34-year-old woman – partial denture worn for 16 years. (B) Direct outline incision. (C) Use of Neos scaler to disrupt supracrestal attachment followed by (D) mucosal elevation to facilitate (E) indirect filletting technique with No. 15 blade. Note complicating effects of mucosal papillary hyperplasia and mucosal ridges.

209

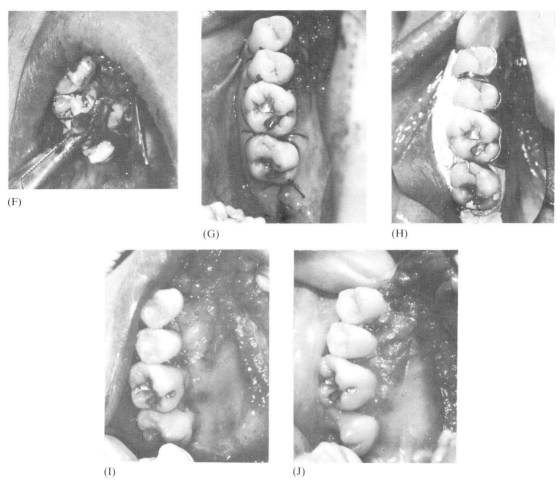

Figure 16.14 (*cont.*) (F) Removal of cervical wedge with haemostat. (G) Continuous suture for flap stabilization. Note uneven mucosal form at 15, 14. (H) Denture has been inserted whilst dressing material still soft. (I) Healing at 1 and (J) 4 weeks. Note interdental tissue proliferation and palatal mucosal hyperplasia

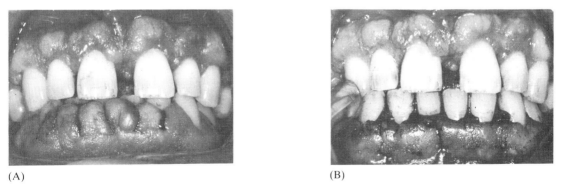

Figure 16.15 Surgical correction epanutin hyperplasia. (A) 22-year-old man 1 month following resection in maxilla and presurgical presentation in mandible. Note overgrowth represented primarily by interdental papillary hyperplasia. (B) External bevel resection of papillary component.

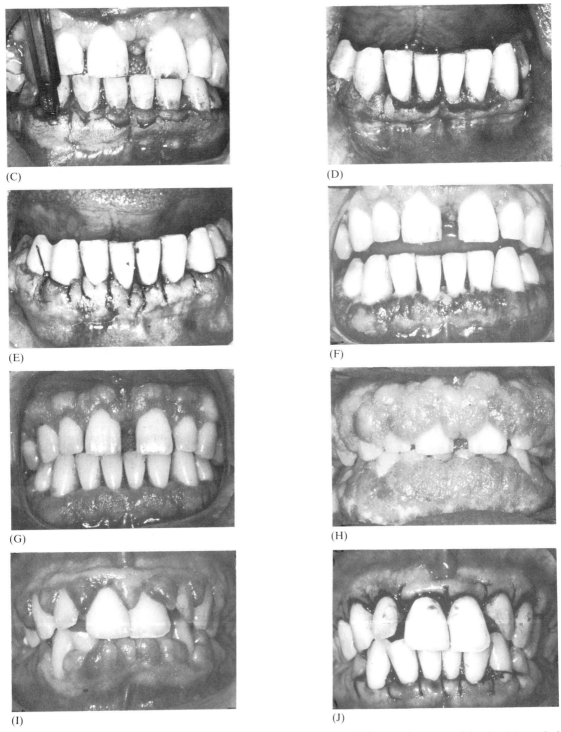

(C)

(D)

(E)

(F)

(G)

(H)

(I)

(J)

Figure 16.15 (*cont.*) (C) Inverse bevel filletting of labial tissue thickening. (D) Tissue wedge removed showing thin surgical flap and crestal bone. (E) Continuous suturing. (F) Healing at 1 week – some marginal tissue ulceration – and (G) 2 weeks. (H) Marked recurrence hyperplasia at 15 months. (I) Initial presentation 18-year-old woman. Greatly distressed by gingival overgrowth despite previous surgery. Oral hygiene indifferent. (J) Direct inverse bevel resection and flap coaption with continuous suturing in maxilla and at mandibular anteriors.

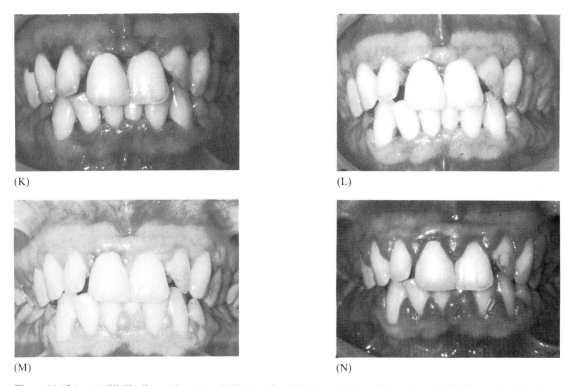

(K)   (L)

(M)   (N)

Figure 16.15 (*cont.*) (K) Healing at 1 week and (L) 4 weeks. (M) Presentation at 2 months and (N) 18 months with almost total relapse posteriorly and slightly, but acceptably so to the patient, anteriorly

are then excised (Figure 16.16 A3, B3, and C3) to reduce the flap tissue thickness, as in indirect pocket resection. This dissection is once again facilitated by the flap deflection into a more accessible vertical plane which is in line with that of the related facial or oral tooth surfaces.

Practical hints and precautions

(1) The linear incision is made along the crest rather than the centre (Figure 16.16 E) of the ridge to avoid complicating the subsequent filletting as depicted in (Figure 16.16 E1). However, in those instances where poor access for filletting is anticipated, such as when the distobuccal aspect of a maxillary molar is associated with a prominent coronoid process, the linear incision is best located at the buccal aspect instead, as shown in Figure 16.16 (D). This then allows filletting to be carried out upon the resulting larger, but more accessible, palatal flap and also minimizes the need for buccal flap filletting.

(2) The linear incision should be at least 1 cm long but extended only sufficiently to allow the flaps to be deflected into a vertical position. The incision may be limited by the presence of another tooth bounding the edentulous area as shown in Figure 16.16 (B1) and elsewhere by anatomical considerations. Thus, in the maxilla the distal incision should preferably not pass beyond the mucogingival junction and certainly not enter the soft palate. The unsupported mucosa in the mandibular retromolar area is also best avoided, although that related to and supported by the ascending ramus can be encroached upon more safely. (See also Anatomical considerations in surgery – Chapter 17.)

(3) Short oblique relieving incisions, extending laterally from the linear incision (Figure 16.16 A1) are used when any flap cannot be reflected into the required vertical position without stretching the tissue. Where, however, pocket surgery is necessary at the other tooth bounding a short saddle area, the crevicular incisions within the respective pocket spaces function as relieving incisions for the two flaps (Figure 16.16 B1). On the other hand, an intact periodontal attachment at any closely related bounding tooth is preferably not violated and oblique relieving incisions used instead. An

exception to this option is where the blood supply of the resulting very short flaps might be compromised, and when involvement of the intact attachment constitutes a lesser hazard.

Surgical flap preparation

Each mucoperiosteal flap is in turn carefully deflected into a vertical position with the flat side of a Swann–Morton No. 15 scalpel blade and the amount of tissue to be cut away estimated. Then, with the flap supported on its outer surface (Figure 16.16 C2) by the first finger of the other hand, where access permits and elsewhere with an elevator, the blade is withdrawn slightly and a shallow outline cut made. This runs parallel to the edge of the linear incision starting at its most accessible part. This outline incision serves subsequently to guide the blade and permit its simultaneous use as a retractor during the filletting dissection as described previously in the palate.

The dissection aims to create an evenly reduced surgical flap about 2 mm thick, extending to the level of mucoperiosteal flap reflection (Figure 16.16 A2, B2 and C2). The wedge of tissue thus separated from the flap represents the cervical wedge elsewhere. This then incorporates the pocket wall lining and connective tissue and the associated severed supracrestal attachment, plus the connective tissue from the inside of the edentulous ridge mucoperiosteal flaps (Figure 16.16 A3, B3 and C3). The tissue wedge may be found to be still attached in places to the underlying bone or the base of the surgical flap. This should be freed by further sharp dissection and the wedge then removed and discarded.

The deferred flap preparation at the facial and oral surfaces can now be completed. The then combined surgical flaps are reflected from underlying bone as necessary for root surface and any osseous instrumentation.

Practical hints and precautions

(1) The minimal initial mucoperiosteal flap reflection from the facial and oral plates of the bone, as depicted at Figure 16.16 (A, B and C2), is critical to the successful thinning of the edentulous site flaps by providing support to the tissues. Where reflected further, the resulting mucoperiosteal flap would be quite mobile, making the already difficult filletting dissection even more awkward.
(2) Filletting is always completed at the edentulous site flaps before proceeding at the facial and oral aspects of the related tooth.
(3) Dissection is usually best directed apically towards the base of the reflected mucoperiosteal flap. However, in Figure 16.16 (A2), the option

also exists of filletting in a coronal direction as well, should this be found to be easier.

Flap adaptation

The individual flaps are gently pressed back into place about the tooth, tending to overlap each other on the bony ridge (Figure 16.16 A, B and C4). The extent of this overlapping will vary according to the features of the case (see below). Similarly, close flap mucosal adaptation about the approximal tooth surface may not always be achieved at this stage. The reason for this mucosal deficiency is that the marginal contour of the flaps is predetermined by the formerly related tooth crown, which has a greater mesiodistal dimension than that of the root about which the flaps are adapted (Figure 16.17 A–C), making bony denudation inevitable. This deficiency will be even worse at approximal root surface concavities and furcations (*cf.* Chapter 18) and at tilted teeth (Figure 16.17 E–G). This bony denudation can fortunately usually be minimized by flap displacement towards the tooth, facilitated by oblique relieving incisions (Figure 16.17 D and H).

Practical hints and precautions

(1) The mucosal deficiency anticipated at a markedly tilted molars, as shown in Figure 16.17 (E), is most readily counteracted by using only a single flap over the edentulous ridge. The linear incision is therefore made along either the facial or oral aspect of the ridge (Figure 16.17 G), the decision depending upon the ease with which the reflected mucoperiosteal prepared flap can be filletted. Thus, at the mandible, dissection is generally simpler at the more accessible buccal aspects following a lingually placed linear incision; whereas, in most instances in the maxilla, the inherently thicker and more firmly supported palatal mucosa favours palatal filletting following a buccal linear incision.
(2) Oblique relieving incisions made at an acute rather than an obtuse angle to the linear incision, as shown in Figure 16.17 (C and G), will enhance flap displacement and adaptation about the tilted tooth (Figure 16.17 D and H).
(3) Bony denudation at relieving incisions to facilitate flap displacement can be minimized by bevelling the incision towards the tooth (Figure 16.17 B and F). Part of the inevitably resulting mucosal deficiency will then at least be occupied by connective tissue as shown in Figure 16.17 (D and H).

Management of flap excess

The operator first establishes which flap gives more complete mucosal adaptation about the tooth and,

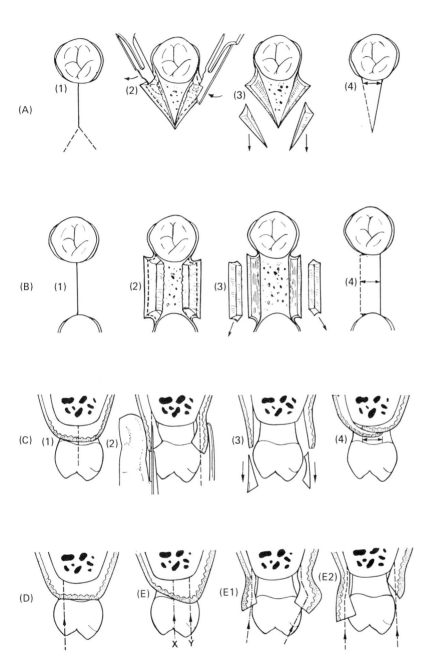

Figure 16.16 The wedge technique. Surgical sequence at (A1–4) mesial/distal pockets adjacent to edentulous sites is also applicable to (B1–4) saddle areas bounded by two teeth. (C1–4) Shows sagittal view and (D and E) effects of alternative locations of linear incision along edentulous ridge. Note: buccal aspects represented by left hand side of diagrams. (A and B1) Buccal and palatal inverse bevel incisions converted to crevicular incisions at tooth line angles. Linear incision on (C1) crest of ridge passes down to bone and may be associated with (A1) oblique relieving incision(s) or be (B1) bounded by tooth. (A, B and C2) Edentulous zone mucoperiosteal flap reflection to expose bone but note mucosa related to buccal and palatal aspects of teeth not reflected at this stage. Flaps supported (C2) digitally or with elevator during filletting. Dissection planes shown by broken lines in each situation and optional direction of dissection with No. 15 blade shown at (A2). (A, B and C3) Completed surgical flaps and discarded surgical wedges. (A, B and C4) Flap adaptation with extent of overlapping arrowed. (D) Buccal location linear incision where poor access necessitates filletting from palatal aspect. (E) Location of incision along crest (Y) rather than middle (X) of ridge ensures optimal facility for subsequent dissection shown at (E2) compared with difficulties depicted at (E1)

as shown in Figure 16.18 (A and E), the less well adapted one earmarked for subsequent management of any overlapping flap tissue. This tissue excess may be resected (Figure 16.18 E–G) provided no apical repositioning is intended at the contiguous flaps. This is because, with apical repositioning, an associated displacement also occurs at the overlapping tissues which simultaneously reduces or even eliminates (Figure 16.18 B and C) the tissue excess. In the former, any residual tissue overlapping is trimmed away (see below). In the event of flap separation occurring over the edentulous ridge, as a result of the apical repositioning required, a relieving incision is made at the tooth line angle and selective flap repositioning carried out as necessary (Figure 16.18 D).

The excess tissue is excised where surgical reattachment or resection has been carried out and, as necessary, upon completion of apical repositioning at the tooth related flaps. The less well fitting flap is first adapted into place and the other flap then placed over it (Figure 16.18 B and F). A mesiodistal incision of the deeper flap is made using the edge of the overlying flap as a cutting guide. A Swann–Morton No. 12 or No. 15 blade is used, depending on access. Upon removal of the resected tissue segment (Figure 16.18 C and G) the two flap margins will lie flush against each other (Figure 16.18 H).

The overlapping tissue at edentulous saddle areas, shown in Figure 16.16, is handled the same way so need not be considered further here. The facial and oral edentulous flaps will optimally butt close over the bone and be coapted to the approximal tooth surface(s). As this surgical flap tissue is of physiological thickness the pocket will have been eliminated and a normal healed dentogingival junction ensured.

Practical hints and precautions

(1) It is helpful to peg the flaps down to the bone with a probe when making the resection incision as depicted in Figure 16.18 (F1).
(2) In those instances where poor access impedes the use of the optimal tissue resection site elected, a surgical compromise and resection at the other flap should be accepted.
(3) The resection incision should preferably avoid intrinsically mobile tissue as in the soft palate and retromolar distolingual aspects. Such incisions tend to cause greater postoperative pain. Another complication at these sites is that flap coaptation is frequently counteracted by functional movements (see below).

Flap stabilization

Suturing is necessary to hold the flaps in position. When a continuous suture is required elsewhere, it is simply extended to include the edentulous site flaps as the terminal flap margin peak of the surgical

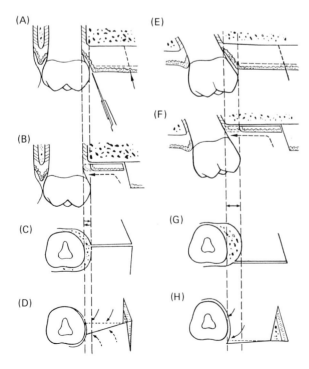

(A)   (E)   (F)   (B)   (C)   (G)   (D)   (H)

Figure 16.17 Problems with flap adaptation to approximal surfaces. (A) Greater mesiodistal dimensions of tooth crown compared to root results in (B and C) inevitable surgical flap mucosal deficiency with bony denudation. (E–G) Even greater discrepancy at tilted tooth. (C and G) Oblique relieving incisions facilitate (D and H) optimal flap coaptation. (G) Linear incision to create single flap for simpler flap management. Note bony denudation at relieving incision sites (G and H) minimized by (B and F) bevel of incision

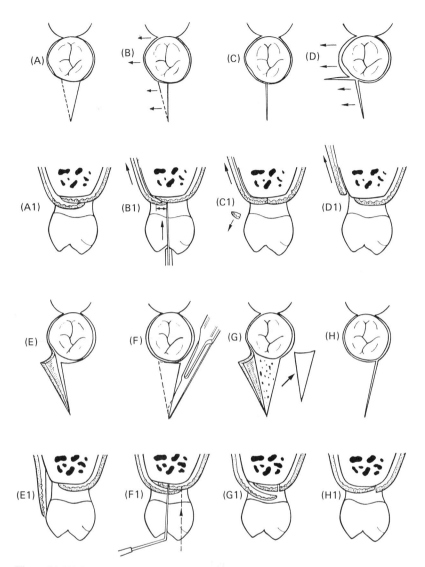

Figure 16.18 Management of flap tissue excess. Correction of overlapping tissue (A and A1) by (B–D) apical repositioning or (E–H) resection. Note buccal aspects represented by left-hand side of diagrams. (B and B1) Buccal flap apical repositioning only partially corrects overlapping necessitating (C and C1) trimming of palatal flap, but (D and D1) over-correction and exposure of bone compensated for selective degrees of apical repositioning. (E and E1) Placement of less well-adapted flap followed by (F and F1) other flap. Flaps pinned down with probe (F1) and overlapping tissue excess resected at edge of overlying flap. (G and G1) Removal of excised mucosa leaving (H and H1) butt joint to flaps

field (Figure 16.19 A). These flaps are best sutured independently of each other and of the contiguous facial and oral flap tissues. Thus, the suture having passed through the one terminal tissue peak passes right around the tooth before being inserted into the opposing peak as shown in Figure 16.19 (A1). The suturing is then continued as before (Figure 16.19

A2). This suturing method not only pulls the two flaps individually and closely about the tooth rather than towards each other, as when using interrupted sutures (Figure 16.19 B), but also ensures that there is no interference from any displacement of these contiguous flaps. The continuous suture may also be used for independent flap suturing about a single

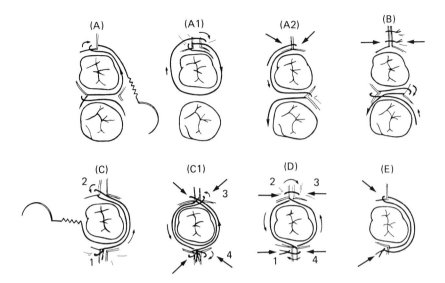

Figure 16.19 Wedge technique suturing. (A) Continuous suture from adjacent surgical field taken through one peak of wedge flap. (A1) Suture then passes around the tooth and then through the other peak of wedge flap. (A2) Suture now proceeds as conventional continuous suture. Note wedge flap peak optimal coaptation (arrowed) with continuous suture not achieved by (B) alternative use of interrupted suturing when continuous suture from adjacent surgical field has not been involved. (C and C1) Continuous suture at isolated single tooth (stages 1–4) with optimal flap coaptation (arrowed). (D) Simplified version of continuous suture precludes optimal coaptation and variable tensioning of opposing flaps. (E) Sling type suture

isolated tooth (Figure 16.19 C and C1). The alternative use of a sling-type suture is shown in Figure 16.19 (E).

Where the flaps can be sutured under similar tension, as in surgical reattachment or resection at both facial and oral aspects, the use of either the simplified continuous suture (Figure 16.19 D) or the interrupted suture as shown in Figure 16.19 (B) is optional. The latter does, however, offer no advantage when continuous suturing is already being used at adjacent units, although is well suited for the linear crestal incisions as shown at Figure 16.19 (B).

A periodontal dressing is necessary only where the tissues fail to remain adapted in position, as with sagging horizontally aligned flaps at the maxillary tuberosity, when mandibular retromolar tissue functional movements cause the flaps to lift or lastly, when the crestal bone level lies apical to that of the anatomical form of the related palatal and retromolar tissues. The tuberosity site can be dressed fairly easily, but in the mandible, retention of the dressing can be difficult because of jaw movements. Indeed, a dressing in the latter often leads to greater postsurgical pain, so is best avoided and a surgical compromise of pocket reduction accepted instead. Nevertheless, the removal of the tough retromolar fibrous tissues in the latter mandibular distal wedge

procedure does greatly improve access for post-surgical plaque control or tooth restoration.

Clinical case presentations

The applications of the wedge technique are shown in Figures 16.20, 16.21, 16.22 and 16.23.

Inverse bevel papillectomy

Interdental pockets

Interdental soft tissue pockets, as part of generalized pocketing, are corrected almost incidentally during the surgical therapy carried out at the facial and oral aspects of the related teeth. This is because the interdental septal tissues are removed together with the facial and oral cervical wedges and the respective thinned interdental papillary flaps then adapted over the exposed interdental bone during surgical pocket elimination surgery (i.e. apical repositioning or resection). However, in surgical reattachment some interdental soft tissue crater is inevitable (see Figure 15.11). Optimal management of any intrabony component to the pocket encountered is also facilitated by this technique (see Chapter 19).

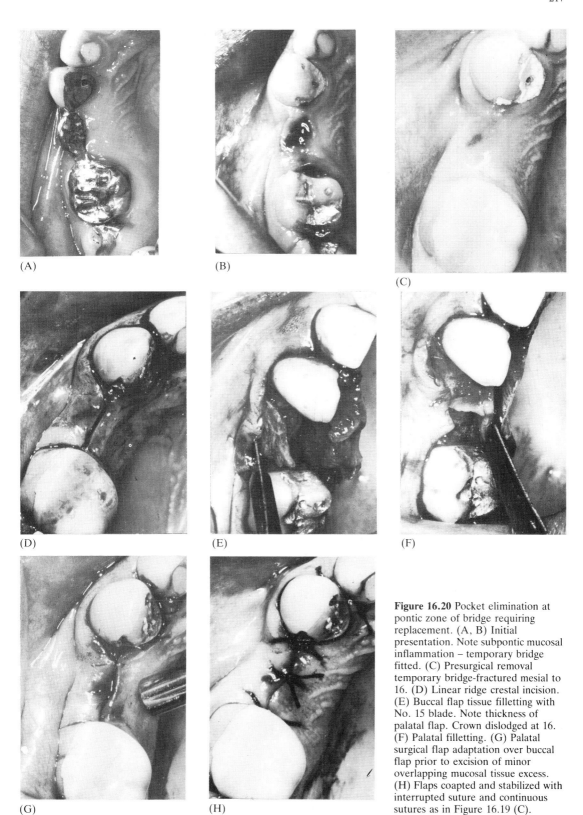

Figure 16.20 Pocket elimination at pontic zone of bridge requiring replacement. (A, B) Initial presentation. Note subpontic mucosal inflammation – temporary bridge fitted. (C) Presurgical removal temporary bridge-fractured mesial to 16. (D) Linear ridge crestal incision. (E) Buccal flap tissue filletting with No. 15 blade. Note thickness of palatal flap. Crown dislodged at 16. (F) Palatal filletting. (G) Palatal surgical flap adaptation over buccal flap prior to excision of minor overlapping mucosal tissue excess. (H) Flaps coapted and stabilized with interrupted suture and continuous sutures as in Figure 16.19 (C).

(A)

(B)

(C)

(D)

(E)

(F)

(G)

(H)

218

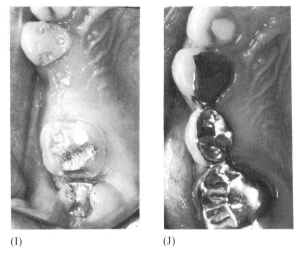

(I)   (J)

Figure 16.20 (*cont.*) (I) 4 weeks postoperative. (J) Replacement bridge fitted at 3 months

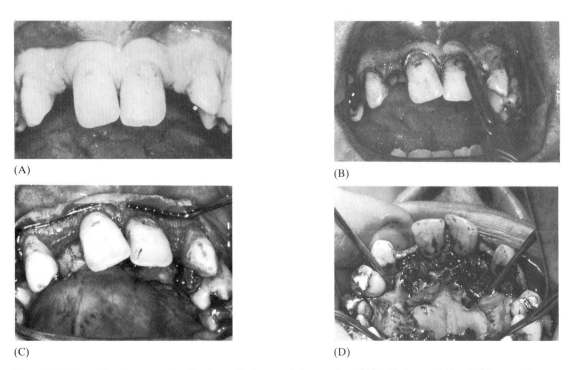

(A)   (B)

(C)   (D)

Figure 16.21 Prerestorative crown lengthening and minor pocket correction. (A) Initial presentation in 24-year-old man – partial denture removed. (B) Labial outline and crestal ridge linear incisions. (C) Flap reflection – note thickened labial and (D) palatal ridge tissue components.

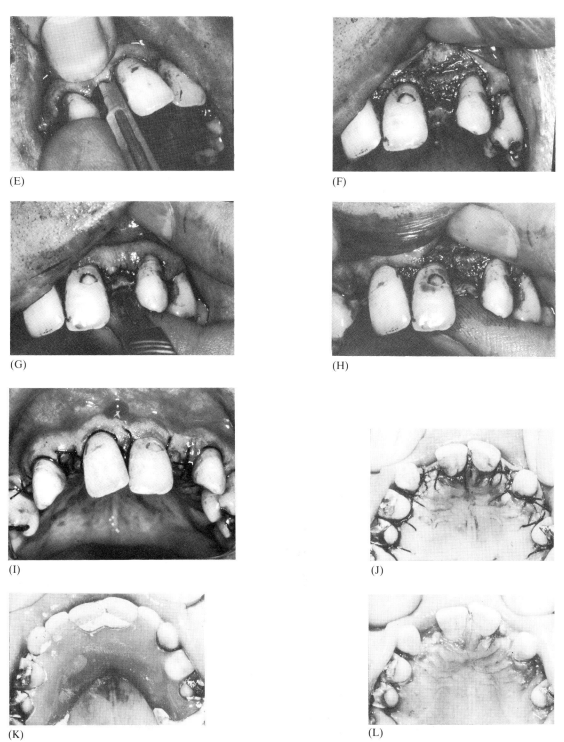

Figure 16.21 (*cont.*) (E) Filletting 12 labial tissue facilitated by digital support. (F) Filletted labial tissue at 22 ridge reflected and revealing thickened palatal tissue. (G) Filletting with digital support. (H) Filletted palatal mucosa adapted over bony ridge. (I) Labial and (J) occlusal views of sutured flaps and palatal mucosal rugae which complicated slightly the mucosal filletting. (K) Denture replaced over periodontal dressing. (L) 1 week postoperative healing. Note some mucosal ulceration.

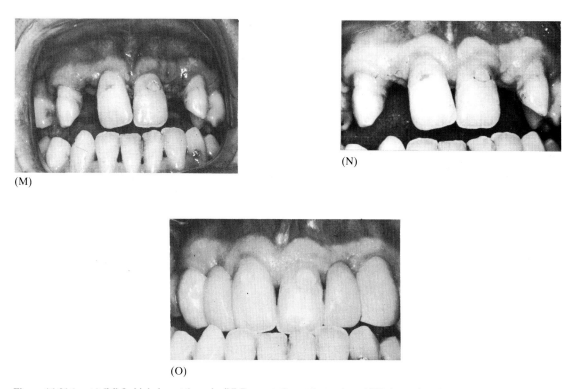

Figure 16.21 (*cont.*) (M) Labial view at 1 week. (N) Presentation at 1 month and (O) 6 months when cantilever bridges were fitted. Note inadequate embrasure spaces mesial to 13 and 23 abutments

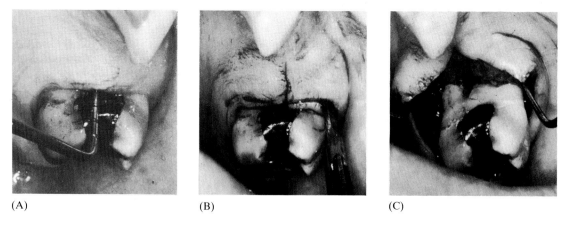

Figure 16.22 Mesial (and distal) wedge technique. (A) Isolated maxillary molar on presentation – proposed bridge abutment in 36-year-old woman. (B) Buccal, palatal and mesial outline incisions and mesial ridge linear incision. Note mesial aspect crevicular incision would have minimized extent of subsequent mucosal deficiency (as at G). (C) Removal of cervical wedges and reflection of thickened ridge mucosal flaps.

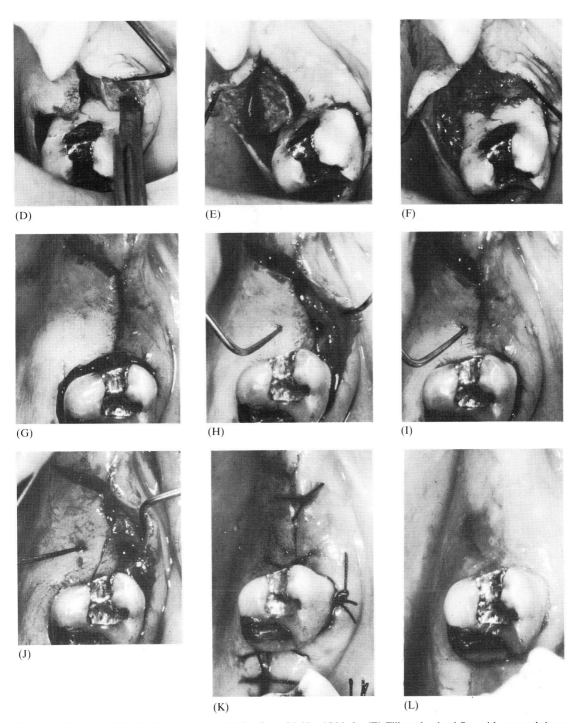

(D)

(E)

(F)

(G)

(H)

(I)

(J)

(K)

(L)

Figure 16.22 (cont.) (D) Filletting mesiobuccal ridge flap with No. 15 blade. (E) Filletted palatal flap with resected tissue wedge still *in situ*. (F) Surgical flap preparation completed. (G) Occlusal view of filletted flaps and mesiopalatal relieving incision. (H) Palatal flap displacement for optimal coaptation to mesial tooth surface. Flap 'pegged' down in place with probe to facilitate subsequent assessment of overlapping tissue excess. Note 'V' shaped zone of palatal mucosal connective tissue exposed at relieving incision site. (I) Buccal flap positioned over palatal flap which is sectioned along margin of buccal flap. (J) Incision line to eliminate mucosal tissue excess. (K) Flaps sutured as per Figure 16.19 (C). Note interrupted sutures across mesial and distal wedge linear incisions. (L) Healing at 1 week

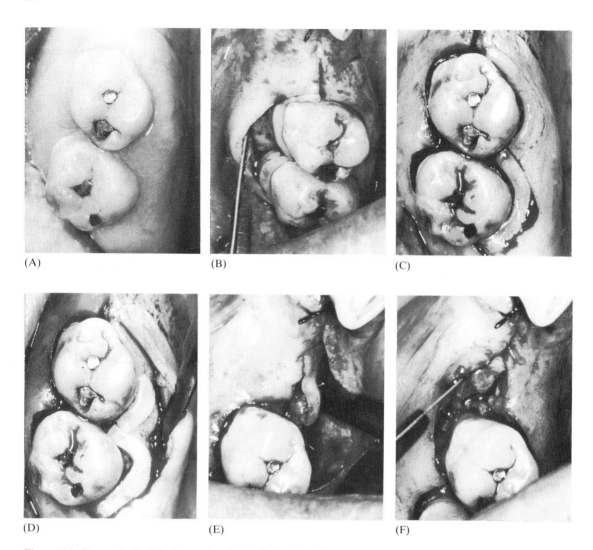

(A) (B) (C)

(D) (E) (F)

Figure 16.23 Preprosthetic clinical crown lengthening isolated maxillary molars. (A) Initial presentation 40-year-old man. (B) Buccal outline and filletting incision plus mesial linear incision. (C) Buccal cervical wedge has been removed and palatal mucosa reflected for assessment of outline incision shown completed. (D) Palatal flap filletting. (E) Mesiopalatal and (F) mesiobuccal ridge mucosal filletting.

223

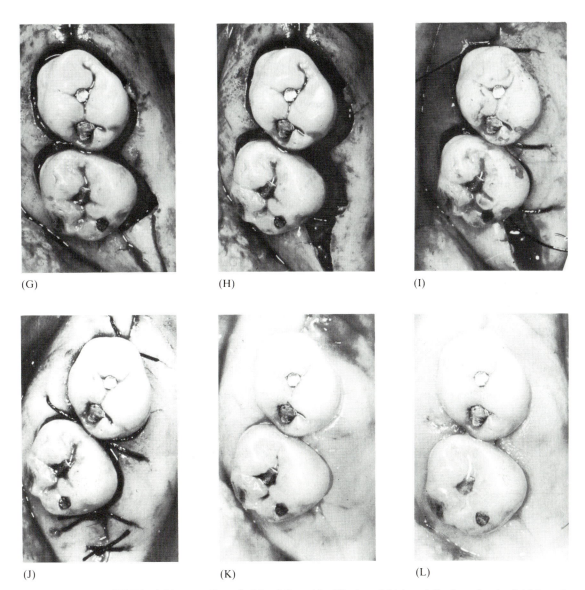

(G) (H) (I)

(J) (K) (L)

Figure 16.23 (cont.) (G) Distal ridge crest linear incision followed by filletting of thickened distobuccal and palatal tissue is completed, prior to palatal outline incision to resect overlapping ridge flap tissue. (H) Excess tissue has been removed and (I) palatal flap sutured into position with continuous sutures. (J) Suturing completed and knotted distal to 17. Note interrupted suture across distal linear incision. (K) Optimal healing at 1 week but for slight ulceration at mesiopalatal aspect. (L) Presentation at 2 weeks

Isolated interdental pockets are dealt with by a combination of the inverse bevel flap preparation for conserving facial and oral tissues and the technique of flap management utilized in wedge techniques. This technique is termed the inverse bevel papillectomy and is described below. No clinical case presentations are shown as the features have already been illustrated as parts of other cases (e.g. Figures 16.8 and 16.9).

Flap preparation

Crevicular incisions are commenced at the mid-axial points of the related teeth. These pass through the marginal gingival tissues at the tooth line angles and proceed towards each other as shallow inverse bevel outline incisions (Figure 16.24 A) which meet at the papillary crest. The papilla is then filletted with No. 15 blade cutting coronally from the more accessible of the outline incisions into a thin surgical papillary flap layer and the cervical wedge layer which is contiguous with the interdental pocket tissue (Figure 16.24 B and E). Dissection then extends apically to bone so that it isolates the cervical wedge tissue from the base of the papillary flap. The appropriate papillary flap preparation is carried out at the opposite aspect of the interdental space to completely isolate the cervical wedge/interdental gingival septal tissue complex (Figure 16.24 E).

Where the limited access at the posterior teeth (Figure 16.24 A) and especially at the palatal aspects (Figure 16.24 E) impedes papillary tissue thinning *in*

situ, the crevicular incisions are best continued to the tip of the papilla instead. The papilla is then deflected *in toto* into a more accessible vertical position and filletted as in the indirect resection technique.

Cervical wedge removal

The depth of the interdental pocket is comparable to that at edentulous sites and is represented by the vertical dimensions of the septal tissue shown as 'X' in Figure 16.24 (E). Consequently, when this tissue is removed (Figure 16.24 F) it will in effect eliminate the pocket.

Papillary adaptation inevitably alters the overall marginal gingival form. Furthermore, in many instances, the attachment of the contiguous facial and oral dentogingival junction limits the extent of the papillary tissue displacement resulting in interdental soft tissue cratering. This, together with the reparative granulation of the denuded interdental bone may lead to reformation of the interdental pocket. (See also Chapter 17.)

Flap adaptation and stabilization

Following the necessary root surface debridement, the exposed interdental bone is covered by the two thin scalloped papillary peaks being displaced apically into the interproximal space. While the opposing flaps adapt closely into the interdental spaces they will often not meet each other. This

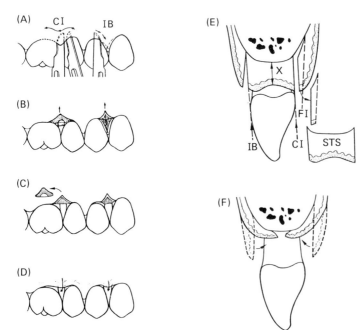

Figure 16.24 Inverse bevel papillectomy. (A) Crevicular incisions (CI) at 16, 15 and 14, 13 with conversion to inverse bevel incision (IB) at papillary peak between 14 and 13. (B) Papillary flap tissue reflection exposes interdental septal tissues plus residual papillary tissue at 14, 13. Papillary tissue filletting still required at 16, 15. (C) Removal of papillary tissue wedge at 16, 15 and interdental septal tissues at 16, 15 and 14, 13. (D) Papillary peak adaptation interproximally with loss of scalloped gingival form. (E and F) Sagittal section at 13 distal aspect. (E) Initial buccal (IB) and palatal (CI) to isolate septal tissue. Secondary palatal filletting incision (FI) following flap reflection in indirect resection technique. Note interdental pocket depth 'X' and total removal of soft tissue septum (STS). (F) Flap adaptation into interdental space effects pocket elimination. Some bony denudation inevitable

interproximal mucosal tissue deficiency is inevitable because the initial papillary incisions are separated by a distance equal to the facio-oral dimension of the interdental space. The resulting postoperative interdental bone denudation, as shown in Figure 16.24 (F), is greatest at the molar teeth as described earlier and illustrated in Figure 15.11.

The insertion of sutures is advisable lest any subsequent inadvertent displacement interferes with healing. The papillae may be supported equally well by a periodontal dressing alone, but this tends to be less comfortable postoperatively, despite the apparent advantage of the protection offered to the denuded bone.

Conclusion

The flexibility of the surgical approach advocated in dealing with interdental pockets, which represent the last possible type of soft tissue pocket encountered in therapy, substantiates the assertion of the existence of a periodontal pocket surgical panacea revolving about the inverse bevel incision. It remains only to deal with numerous miscellaneous aspects of this surgical regime in the next chapter. They are considered separately rather than in conjunction with the surgical techniques, in the interests of greater clarity.

17

Miscellaneous surgical considerations

This chapter considers important matters not covered in the preceding chapters on the basic periodontal surgical techniques. These are anaesthesia, the management of uninvolved sites, surgical bleeding, basic surgical precautions, anatomical considerations, postoperative care and complications, wound healing and the outcome of the different surgical options as an introduction to complex pocket surgery.

Anaesthesia

Periodontal pocket surgery requires anaesthesia and only local anaesthesia is advocated here. Any individually preferred proprietary anaesthetic solution containing a vasoconstrictor (e.g. 2% lignocaine with 1:80 000 adrenaline) may be used. Certain 'at risk' category subjects may, however, require non-adrenaline containing solutions (e.g. 3% prilocaine with felypressin).

The distribution and extent of anaesthesia is, for practical purposes, the same as that normally required for tooth extraction. In the maxilla, posterior superior dental infiltrations and infra-orbital blocks are required for the buccal aspects whilst palatally greater palatine and long sphenopalatine (incisal canal) blocks are needed. Additional infiltrations are sometimes necessary, as a result of individual subject requirements, at the labial aspects of the incisors and palatal to the premolars and

lateral incisors despite complete anaesthesia of adjacent sites.

In the mandible, inferior dental, lingual and long buccal anaesthesia is necessary for posterior sites. Mandibular blocks are also frequently required for anterior surgical fields, for which mental blocks even with the possible addition of labial and lingual infiltrations may be inadequate. Accordingly, bilateral mandibular blocks are advocated for mandibular incisor surgery, coupled with, where necessary, supplementary facial and lingual aspect infiltrations, to cater for upper cervical (C2,C3) aberrant branches.

Additional intrapapillary injections are sometimes needed in isolated instances but their routine use, although advocated by others, is not recommended. The claimed additional benefit of localized haemostasis is really applicable only to wound surfaces created by the external bevel gingivectomy, a resection technique which is rarely prescribed by the author. Marked bleeding at surgery is also an indication of undue inflammation which, in turn, suggests premature surgical intervention. This situation is one which will hopefully not often confront the readers of this text. Intrapapillary injections can be very painful, especially when given at the outset, so are best avoided. In addition, the possibility of an ischaemic necrosis of the injected surgical flap peaks cannot be discounted.

In those few instances when local anaesthesia alone is unacceptable to the patient its use in conjunction with pre-medication agents, relative analgesia or, alternatively, general anaesthesia should be considered. Any discussion of these specialized alternative methods of anaesthesia is beyond the intended remit of this text.

The management of uninvolved sites

The principles

Intact dentogingival junctions bordering the surgical field and any sites within the field at which pocket surgery is not required, are either excluded by oblique relieving incisions or incorporated into the field of operation via crevicular incisions. Whilst it is preferable to isolate peripheral units by relieving incisions, elsewhere this can result in multiple small flaps. This complicates overall flap management and may compromise the blood supply to the individual flaps. The alternative of crevicular incisions does, however, carry the potential risk of damaging the supracrestal attachment at these periodontally uninvolved sites. In addition, bony denudation will result from flap apical repositioning, although this bony complication can be minimized by utilizing appropriate vertical relieving incisions and selective flap repositioning, as shown in Figure 15.14 (D).

Relieving incisions are not advocated as a matter of course. Instead, the decision to use them and the type chosen should be deferred until filletting has been commenced so that the surgical requirements can then be judged more easily, and the postoperative integrity of the surgical flap and its underlying tissues be considered *in situ*.

Sites within the surgical field

Where several intact sites are present, it is expedient to incorporate them by crevicular incisions. The pocket site inverse bevel outline incisions thus pass through the gingival margin at each intact site and continue as crevicular incisions. These then function as horizontal relieving incisions which permit the reflection and elevation of a single, envelope-type, surgical flap spanning the whole surgical field (Figure 17.1 A). This is very much simpler to handle than several smaller flaps which would be created by the alternative of oblique relieving incisions. In addition, this ease of flap preparation and management outweighs the clinically insignificant attachment losses sustained by involving intact sites (see Chapter 31 – Effects of bone resection).

Isolated pockets

The initial inverse bevel pocket incision is converted to crevicular relieving incisions at adjacent sites (Figure 17.1 B). This usually provides an adequate envelope-type flap especially at interdental pockets and when the scalloped papillary form functions as oblique relieving incisions (Figure 17.1 B and C). Pocketing restricted to mid-axial tooth surfaces, or where greater flap reflection is necessary, usually demands oblique relieving incisions (Figure 17.1 C and E). The effect of a single relieving incision is first assessed. This is made at the surgical extremity that gives the best access whilst not stretching the flap tissue and which will not jeopardize the underlying periodontal tissues. The resulting surgical flap is triangular in shape as opposed to the trapezoidal flap form when the use of relieving incisions at both extremities proves to be necessary.

Edentulous zones

Relieving incisions at pocket sites adjacent to edentulous zones are dealt with in Chapter 16. They are represented by the linear incision along the crest of the ridge, supplementary oblique relieving incision(s) where necessary and crevicular incisions, when a short edentulous zone is bounded by an intact tooth.

Quadrant surgery

When full arch surgery is carried out by quadrants, the inverse bevel outline incision at the edge of the first surgical field simply passes, as though it were a crevicular incision, into the pocket spaces of the adjacent and, as yet, untreated field(s). When this subsequent quadrant is in turn treated, crevicular or oblique relieving incisions are made, depending on access. The inevitably uneven marginal tissue form at the initially treated/untreated sectors is corrected at the second operation.

Practical hints and precautions

(1) The oblique relieving incision is made on the far side of the intact interdental papilla bounding the surgical field (Figure 17.1 C–E). The incision commences at the tooth line angle, passes obliquely away from the surgical field and extends as far apically as necessary to permit adequate flap reflection which is, in practice, to the apical level of flap reflection. The surgical flap is therefore always bounded by an interdental papilla which facilitates subsequent flap adaptation and suturing.

The lateral edge of the flap produced by the relieving incision, is located ideally over interdental bone rather than mid-axial bone, which tends to be thin and might even be associated with dehiscences or fenestrations (see Figure 19.3). Thus, in the event of poor surgical wound margin approximation or post-surgical mucosal ulceration of the edge of the flap, the

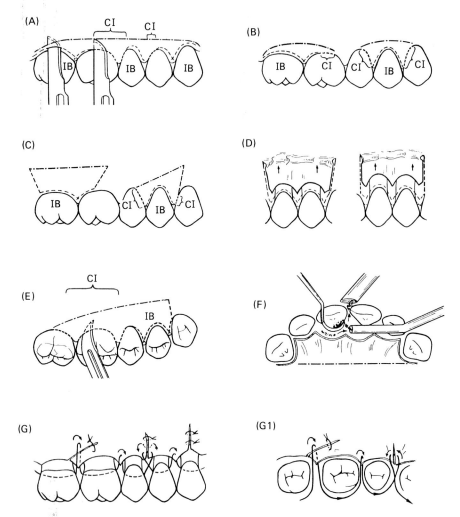

Figure 17.1 Miscellaneous surgical details. (A) Inverse bevel incisions converted to crevicular (CI) incisions at intact sites within surgical field. (B) Similar conversion of incisions about isolated pocket sites. Lines of reflection of (A and B) envelope-type flaps and of (C) trapezoidal and triangular flaps formed by the use of bilateral and unilateral oblique relieving incisions respectively. Note location of relieving incisions on far side of bounding papillae in (C–E). (D) Slight bony denudation adjacent to apically repositioned flap following use of oblique but not vertical relieving incisions. (E) Use of CI incision as in indirect resection and IB incision in direct resection technique coupled with mesial relieving incision for adequate flap reflection. (F) Curvature of maxillary arch permits flap reflection without use of relieving incisions. Note use of surgical tips for aspiration of blood and debris whilst ensuring unimpeded operator access and visibility. (G and G1) Suturing techniques at relieving incisions and unintended lacerations

resulting denudation of the underlying tissues will not then involve the potentially more vulnerable bony deficiencies and the related periodontal ligament. Similarly any post-surgical ischaemic necrosis and impaired healing at such sites, is bound to lead to localized gingival recession as shown in Figure 21.5 (B). As a rule, should any doubt exist about optimal healing at any proposed relieving incision line,

crevicular relieving incisions should be used instead.

(2) The relieving incisions are preferably bevelled towards the flap as shown in Figure 16.14 so as to minimize bone exposure, in favour of periosteum, should the incision line gape at completion of operation. Bevelled incisions are, however, of limited use in the presence of thin mucosa.

(3) A mucosal defect with bony denudation is inevitable following apical repositioning in relation to oblique relieving incisions (Figure 17.1 D). This complication should be anticipated and vertical relieving incisions used instead. The, then, narrower flap base means that the latter option is best restricted to surgical fields at least 2 cm wide to ensure an adequate blood supply to the flap.

(4) Relieving incisions are contra-indicated where underlying neurovascular bundles might be damaged. The mental and lingual nerves and, to a lesser extent, the greater palatine nerve are most vulnerable. Little risk of damaging the long sphenopalatine nerve exists for the curvature at the front of the maxilla affords adequate access following crevicular incisions (Figure 17.1 F). The palatal neurovascular bundle is liable to be sectioned when posterior palatal incisions are required (Figure 17.1 E), but no adverse neural effects are sustained. The initial copious bleeding caused is also readily controlled (see below).

(5) Relieving incisions are generally not sutured, as the flap suturing usually suffices. However, when the incision line gapes, interrupted sutures are best used. Similarly, flap surgical lacerations (euphemistically and most politically called in the teaching clinic, relieving incisions) are sutured as shown in Figure 17.1 (G and H). The continuous suture may also be modified to cope with such lacerations.

(6) The denuded bone at poorly approximated relieving incisions and at lacerations is preferably covered with a protective periodontal dressing, for patient comfort. However, it is not known whether this is beneficial or otherwise to healing, although when a firm dressing, fixed to the teeth, impinges on the movable alveolar mucosa it might cause greater postoperative discomfort.

Surgical bleeding

Bleeding at operation should represent little more than an interference to clear vision. Thus, provided pocket surgery is not undertaken prematurely, sharp dissection without tearing of the tissues ensured, and a local anaesthetic with a vasoconstrictor used, no difficulties should arise. Any marked localized gingival bleeding can be controlled easily by either giving a further local anaesthetic injection directly into the bleeding site and/or pushing the flap back into place and applying firm pressure with a damp gauze swab for about 1 min. Osseous bleeding can be checked by flap adaptation at accessible sites and elsewhere with a small swab pressed directly onto the bone. Sometimes, the bony trabeculation permits intra-osseous injections of a vasoconstrictor

within a local anaesthetic solution. The free bleeding during palatal filletting and palatal relieving incisions should not cause alarm for if the blood vessels have been incised cleanly they will constrict readily.

Good chairside assistance is absolutely essential. A high volume/low vacuum suction apparatus and the simultaneous use of two separate sucker tips is advocated. The finer (3-mm bore) tip is used at the site of instrumentation as shown in Figure 17.1 (F) whilst the other, the wider bore (6-mm) sucker, functions as a scavenger of blood, debrided debris and curetted soft tissue from the field of operation. It is also used for sucking away pooled blood, salivary and irrigation fluids from the mouth. This sucker performs its scavenging role most effectively by being placed on the opposite aspect of the teeth being instrumented. The suction effect operates from in between the teeth, whilst neither blocking the operator's field of vision nor impeding access. When clearing away fluids elsewhere, the sucker should not be placed end on to the mucosa lest the tissue is damaged by being drawn into its wide opening. The suction tip is always held obliquely against mucosa or preferably positioned carefully against a tooth instead, when it can be most usefully employed and easily controlled. Note: It is helpful to bevel the commercially produced straight ends of the wide bore surgical tips to that shown in Figure 17.1 (F).

Basic surgical precautions

The technical demands of periodontal flap surgery as advocated are comparable to any complex restorative technique or, say, the removal of impacted third molars, so the inexperienced operator need not feel unduly apprehensive. However, the comparatively long operating time (depending on the number of units involved), the repetitive nature of the exercise at each tooth, the difficulties of access and clear vision imposed by bleeding and the flap tissue itself and, not least, of limited surgical team-work experience makes flap surgery very taxing for patient and operator alike. Accordingly, only small surgical fields located at the front of the mouth in ultra-cooperative patients are attempted by neophytes to gain the necessary confidence and surgical expertise. Only then should larger and more complex exercises at inaccessible sites be undertaken. On the other hand, there should be no adverse reflection upon any clinician referring difficult problems to others more experienced.

Certain basic and common-sense precautions are mandatory in periodontal surgery. Precise and well-controlled handling of instruments is paramount, demanding a firm finger rest upon the adjacent teeth. Ultra-sharp scalpel blades and well-maintained, keen-edged hand instruments are equally critical. These ensure more delicate tissue manipulation and obviate the need for more vigorous and forceful instrumentation that characterizes the use of dull instruments. Such greater force is not readily controlled and could result in inadvertent slipping and laceration of the related tissues.

The mucosa should be handled gently and preferably not stretched lest it tears, whilst the bone should not be allowed to become dry (*cf.* Chapter 19). Together these precautions will do much to minimize post-surgical swelling and pain. The integrity of the related tissues must be safeguarded and not unnecessarily involved in the surgical procedure. The flap is, therefore, not reflected any further than is required and wherever possible vulnerable anatomical structures avoided.

Note: Surgical gloves were not used by the author at the time that some of the surgical sequences shown in this text were photographed. Gloves should now always be worn.

Anatomical considerations in surgery

Vulnerable structures

The greater palatine neurovascular bundle can be avoided as it emerges from the greater palatine foramen for it is rarely necessary to reflect the flap to that extent. However, its distal part is almost inevitably incised during palatal filletting and results in profuse bleeding already referred to. The sectioned nerve appears to present no adverse after-effects.

The integrity of the long sphenopalatine (incisive canal) neurovascular bundle is, in contrast, at risk as it emerges from its foramen. It should be carefully dissected away from the undersurface of the mucoperiosteal flap, and laid back upon the bone prior to pocket wall filletting. On the other hand, where mucosal perforation is likely, because of grooves between prominent palatal rugae, flap integrity is paramount and the bundle is best sectioned instead. This should be carried out as far away as possible from the foramen. Any resulting postoperative paraesthesia behind the incisors is of little consequence. This usually passes off within a matter of a few months suggesting that the nerve ends soon become reunited.

The mental nerve should always be avoided. Where any risk of damage arises, the procedure is best abandoned at that site, the flap replaced *in situ* and healing allowed. Following healing specialist advice and treatment can be sought if necessary. The lingual nerve is unlikely to become involved in routine periodontal pocket surgery because of its location. The delicate mucosa of the floor of the mouth and the associated sublingual vasculature and salivary glands in particular, are also rarely implicated, but are vulnerable to inadvertent trauma and so demand careful handling during lingual flap management. The soft palate is equally vulnerable but is even less likely to be involved in any periodontal surgical field.

Limited access

Limited mouth opening and restricted access to certain parts of the oral cavity may hamper surgery. Lingual aspects can be difficult if not impossible in the presence of a shallow lingual vestibule, a prominent and poorly controlled tongue or linguoverted teeth. Powerful lower lip activity can also be very troublesome. Palatal access can be impeded greatly by retroclined upper incisors in Class II Division 2 occlusions, whilst the associated deep overbite limits the interincisal opening. The mandibular coronoid process often impedes instrumentation at the buccal aspects of the maxillary molars but can be minimized by mandibular deviation to that side.

Barriers to flap adaptation

The external oblique ridge and its overlying vestibular mucosal form precludes apical repositioning of the mandibular buccal flap. Similarly, the root of the zygomatic arch impedes that of any related maxillary flap. The mandibular retromolar mucosal form and attachment of the pterygomandibular raphe complicate flap coaption over the bone in distal wedge procedures and thwarts pocket reduction. The vestibular mucosa at the distobuccal aspect of maxillary second and third molars also complicates flap positioning. On the distal and palatal aspects of these teeth effective distal pocket reduction is frequently prevented by the tuberosity mucosal surface and that of the soft palate being located at the same level as the distal gingival margin. Palatal flap adaptation at the molars is sometimes complicated by the presence of a bony ridge between the greater palatine foramen and the alveolus. Similarly, developmental bony exostoses (tori) in any situation will not only hamper flap preparation but also adaptation in pocket elimination surgery. The reduction of these bony prominences with chisels or burs is then frequently indicated. (See also Chapter 31 – Effects of bone resection.)

Reduced gingival dimensions

Sites with little or no gingival tissue (because of gingival recession) may be encountered in many surgical fields. The contiguous alveolar mucosa then forms the major part of the pocket wall and the management of the resulting technical difficulties is dealt with in Chapter 20. These difficulties are however summarized here. Firstly, surgical flap preparation is very much more demanding because the thinner alveolar mucosa is more difficult to dissect and handle and tears more readily. Secondly, the intrinsic tissue thinness means that filletting *per se* is not required, so that surgical flap reflection becomes the primary objective and associated retention of epithelialized pocket lining on the flap is disregarded. An initial crevicular type incision is therefore made at these sites. Thirdly, the thin alveolar mucosa will be found to be tightly bound to the crest of the bone at the pocket base and also surprisingly so to alveolar bone, from which it must be reflected by a combination of sharp and blunt dissection as required. This is complicated by the bone often being very thin at these sites and following an undulating path over the roots. Fourthly, reflection of any thin mucosa is always more difficult and the hazard of mucosal perforation constantly guarded against, lest painful postoperative ulceration and more importantly sloughing of the marginal mucosa ensues. Finally, care must be taken when suturing, as the thread tends to tear through the thin alveolar tissue quite readily.

Frenal insertions

Mucosal frena are simply regarded as variations of mucosal form which can be ignored during flap preparation. However, frenal insertions might complicate surgical flap margin adaptation by causing it to retract from the teeth and so possibly interfere with healing. This retracting effect can be overcome by a minor modification to the suturing advocated for inadvertent papillary tears shown in Figure 17.1 (G and G1). The suture, thus, both enters and makes its exit from the undersurfaces of the mucosa

on either side of the frenum (Figure 17.2 A), so that the short horizontal section of the suture lies over the frenum and pulls it interproximally.

An alternative method of coping with frenal tension is by simply making a shallow horizontal incision across the frenal base just apical to the point of insertion of the continuous suture (Figure 17.2 B and C). The importance of the minimal depth of this incision is to preserve the deeper connective tissue component of the frenum, which represents the flap tissue subsurface at that site as shown in Figure 17.2 (C). A deeper incision would be tantamount to flap perforation, which would compromise the blood supply and possibly lead to ischaemic necrosis of the flap marginal tissue. The technique of combining frenal resection with pocket surgery is dealt with in Chapter 22. On the other hand, where interference from bulky frenal insertions associated with wide diastemas is comparable to that prominent retromolar tissues described above, this is preferably corrected as a separate surgical exercise prior to any pocket correction. (See Chapter 22.)

Postoperative effects and care
Pain or discomfort

Some pain should be expected when the local anaesthetic wears off. However, as pain experience is subjective and variations in pain threshold levels exist it is difficult to predict any individual patient's response. Moreover, pain cannot be measured in any reproducible manner, which precludes any reliable investigation of either its causes and prevention in pocket surgery. In the majority of cases, post-surgical pain is controlled adequately by proprietary analgesics normally taken for a

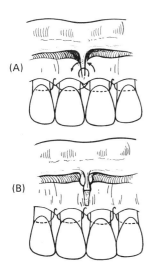

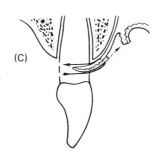

Figure 17.2 Frenal complications. (A) Modification of continuous suture to overcome flap papillary retraction by frenum. (B and C) Frenum sectioned just apical to insertion point of continuous suture. Note frenal body displacement (arrowed)

headache, but occasionally stronger analgesics are indicated. The pattern of postoperative pain varies greatly varying from a few hours to several days. It is important to reassure patients of these normal variations and that uncomplicated healing takes place in most cases. Furthermore, they should be informed that the teeth will be tender to touch and can become loose, lest undue concern be aroused. Chewing in the area is therefore to be avoided in the interests of patient comfort alone.

Oral hygiene

Only the occlusal surfaces of the teeth operated upon are brushed. Gentle brushing of the facial and oral tooth surfaces to relieve the dirty coated feeling that tends to develop is, however, permissible. A 0.2% chlorhexidine (e.g. Corsodyl, ICI plc, Macclesfield, Cheshire, UK) mouthwash is prescribed to compensate for the withdrawal of mechanical cleaning. Instructions are given to rinse with 10 ml of the solution for about 1 min, twice daily after routinely cleaning the other teeth.

A single 300 ml bottle lasting for about 2 weeks, is usually sufficient for most cases when routine cleaning can be resumed. When periodontal dressings are in place the solution is of limited benefit, for it appears unable to penetrate and to exert its bacteriocidal effects beneath a dressing. A comfortably hot saline mouthwash used four to five times a day, commencing the day following surgery has also been advocated. Although it appears to be quite soothing and mildly antiseptic there is little evidence to support its traditionally assumed benefits in healing.

Bleeding

Blood staining of the saliva is to be expected during the first day or so, and intermittent slight bleeding might also occur. These should not be cause for alarm and the products should either be swallowed or rinsed out with cold tap water. Assuming that no inherent tendency to bleed exists, freer and more persistent bleeding is unusual. This is most readily controlled by the patient first rinsing with cold water and then applying and holding firmly in place a cold moist paper tissue pad over the bleeding site itself (or any dressing present) for at least 10 min. The patient should rest in an upright sitting position while doing so, and continue to do so, for at least another 1 h after bleeding has been arrested and further mouth rinsing avoided. Hot drinks should not be taken lest the resulting vasodilation stimulates further bleeding. Similarly, it is prudent to refrain from alcohol, although its sedative effect might allay fear in some individuals and possibly help to check bleeding.

The patient should seek professional advice if bleeding persists. Essentially the same steps advocated above are then carried out in the dental chair. Further measures include the insertion of tight sutures plus the application of local haemostatic materials or the administration of systemic antifibrinolytic drugs (e.g. Cyklokapron 500 mg – KabiVitrum, Uxbridge, Middlesex UB8 2YF, UK) be considered on the merits of the case.

Limitation of jaw movement

Jaw stiffness and limited opening is not unusual particularly following mandibular surgery and the patient must be reassured accordingly. The symptoms can be attributed to muscle and joint strain from prolonged mouth opening at operation, detachment of vestibular muscle tissue and intramuscular bleeding during apical repositioning and, finally, post-local anaesthetic injection site pain leading to guarded jaw movements.

Swelling

Some facial tissue swelling is sometimes evident the day following operation. This is invariably due to tissue oedema following surgical trauma rather than the post-surgical infection, often suspected by the patient, who should be forewarned to avert unnecessary concern. Swelling may sometimes also be caused by postoperative bleeding into the tissues which produces a haematoma. This may be associated with bruising of the related skin and/or mucosa.

The application of an ice pack intermittently to the face covering the surgical area, for about 15-min intervals during the first 4–6 h following surgery is helpful. The ice is conveniently wrapped in a face flannel and placed in a polythene bag to stop water dripping down the patient's neck. Although ice packs have for long been advocated to check the development of swelling, but this has yet to be substantiated by controlled investigations. This deficiency is, in part, attributable to the practical difficulties of recording the extent of facial swelling in any such investigation.

Dressing displacement

A dressing that loosens within the first few days is either pushed back into place by the patient or, if too unstable, simply removed. Replacement is, however, rarely necessary at this stage, especially as any flap displacement will have already taken place. Consequently, application of a further dressing not only serves little purpose but also often causes greater discomfort.

Cervical sensitivity

Root surface sensitivity to thermal changes, especially cold, and also to touch, is not uncommon following surgery. This gradually subsides with effective oral hygiene but will be hastened by using fluoride toothpaste and mouth rinses – see Chapter 25. Where this sensitivity prevents cleaning, the chlorhexidine rinsing should be used for a longer period.

Interproximal tissue proliferation

In some instances there is a tendency for the reparative granulation tissue to proliferate excessively over the denuded interdental bone (and elsewhere at sites of inadvertent bony denudation). This tissue is tender to touch, bleeds freely and so may discourage effective plaque control which apparently aggravates the situation and leads to further proliferation. This might then occlude the interproximal spaces and thwart the surgical objective. However, provided careful cleaning is persevered with tissue shrinkage gradually ensues with no lasting adverse effects. Elsewhere the tissue might require resection.

The reason for this overgrowth is not clear, but clinical experience in the student clinic suggests that it might be related in part to residual tags of inflamed tissue at operation due to clinical inexperience or an endeavour to avoid prolonging operating time. Other possible reasons are poor plaque control alluded to above (but seemingly discounted by its development even in the presence of routine chlorohexidine rinsing) and trauma from oral hygiene devices. (See also Chapter 18 – Degree III furcations.)

Dressing and suture removal

It is a convention to remove dressings and sutures after 1 week, although this is based mainly upon when it is convenient for the patient to attend and orderly appointment systems. A difference of a few days either way appears to have little influence on healing, but patient comfort tends to be enhanced by early removal.

Coe-pak sets to a firm but flexible consistency, and is readily displaced by prising it away from the teeth with a sickle scaler. Occasionally, the suture thread will have become trapped in the material making its removal more difficult and more painful for the patient. Any dressing on the opposite aspect of the teeth is then best removed first to expose the sutures, which are cut where they pass through interdentally. This allows the offending dressing and its incorporated sutures to be lifted away together. The entrapped knot of the continuous suture may

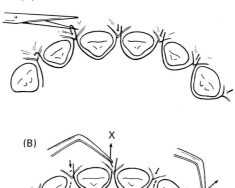

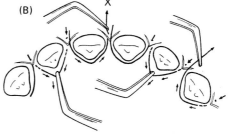

Figure 17.3 Suture removal. (A) Suture cut at each successive papilla. (B) Removal shown but avoiding drawing length of suture segment through tissue 'X'

similarly impede removal of the dressing. The common-sense solution to this problem is to nibble away, with fine suture scissors, the dressing material adjacent to the knot and once exposed, to cut the suture where it enters the tissue.

The continuous suture is removed by first cutting each part of the thread with fine scissors as it enters each tissue papilla (Figure 17.3 A). Each resultant U-shaped suture segments is then grasped with fine tweezers where it was cut or passes about the tooth and pulled away (Figure 17.3 B). The suture ends emerging from the tissue should not be used, because the debris accumulated on the suture is wiped off as the thread is drawn through and deposited on the tissue undersurface. The sequence is shown clinically in Figure 15.18 (G–J).

Undue postoperative pain

Early onset

Severe postoperative pain is shown, by retrospective clinical experience, to be due almost invariably to the patient's exaggerated subjective responses. The patient need only be reassured therefore and stronger analgesics prescribed. The possibility of secondary infection or of slow bleeding causing a haematoma cannot, however, be dismissed.

Infection is, fortunately and perhaps unexpectedly, an uncommon complication considering the extent of periodontal surgery undertaken sometimes. Where infection has supervened a firm and

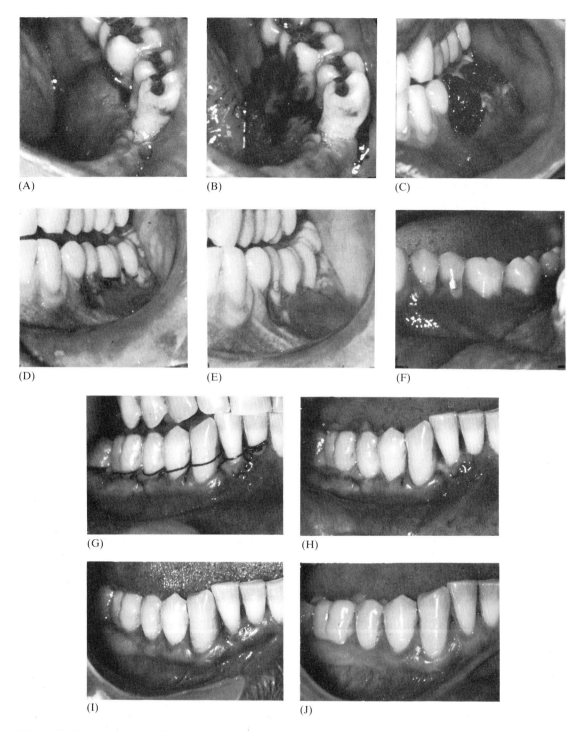

Figure 17.4 Post-surgical complications. (A) Unusual finding of abscess under surgical flap at fifth day. Dressing and sutures removed and (B) pus drained. (C) Development of submucosal haematoma on first day causing buccal displacement of flap. Blood clot removed, flap readapted and Coe-pak applied. (D) Dressing removed at 3 days. (E) Uneventful healing progressing at 1 week and (F) 4 weeks. (G) Suspected ANG coupled with marginal ulceration at 1 week – note suture isolation. (H) Presentation on suture removal. (I) Healing at 2 weeks and (J) 4 months with minimal residual effects.

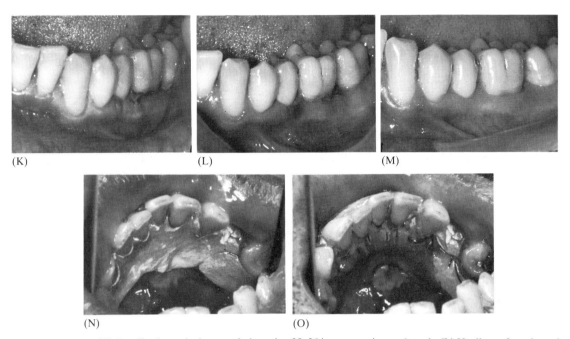

Figure 17.4 (*cont.*) (K) Localized marginal mucosal ulceration 35, 36 in same patient at 1 week. (L) Healing at 2 weeks and (M) 4 months with no deformity. (N) Over-extended lingual dressing resulting in (O) painful mucosal ulceration

very tender swelling develops, the regional nodes are enlarged and the patient's temperature will be raised. Dressings and sutures are removed to facilitate inflammatory drainage with the possible discharge of pus (Figure 17.4 A and B). An appropriate antibiotic is given and frequent hot saline rinses advocated.

The patient might also present with a strong foetor oris suggestive of acute necrotizing gingivitis (ANG). (See also Chapter 25.) This, coupled with the minor interdental mucosal cratering normally associated with interdental denudation and the occasional finding of a painful marginal ulceration of the papillary peaks, might appear consistent with such a diagnosis. In addition, the regional lymph nodes might be enlarged and a raised temperature exist, although neither are specific to ANG. On the other hand, this diagnosis is not wholly justified for spontaneous bleeding seldom occurs and the condition tends not to progress. Nevertheless a subacute form of the condition might occur (Figure 17.4 G and H) as a post-surgical complication and is best treated by the administration of metronidazole (May & Baker Ltd, Dagenham, UK) 200 mg thrice daily for 3 days.

Postoperative oedema and the development of a haematoma might also cause unexpected postoperative pain. This is presumably aggravated by the constricting effect of the dressing and/or sutures on the swollen tissues which often bulge up about these materials (Figure 17.4 C and D). A considerable relief occurs within minutes of such a dressing being removed, and/or when sutures that have become well bedded into the swollen tissues have been cut. These suture ends are best left *in situ* together with the remaining uninvolved continuous suture, to minimize operator interference although, at this stage, flap displacement is unlikely. More frequent hot saline rinses are indicated and the administration of an antibiotic considered prudent when haematoma formation is suspected.

Delayed onset of or gradually increasing pain

More marked pain in the absence of any other symptoms sometimes develops after 3–4 days, following an initially tolerable postoperative period. The patient should then be re-examined and the possible causes investigated.

(1) Bone denudation may occur following initially inadequate mucosal coverage as in Figure 24.7 (G) or a subsequent flap necrosis and ulceration as shown in Figure 17.5 (C and E). In the former it may be assumed that a localized osteitis, that is probably comparable to that of a 'dry'

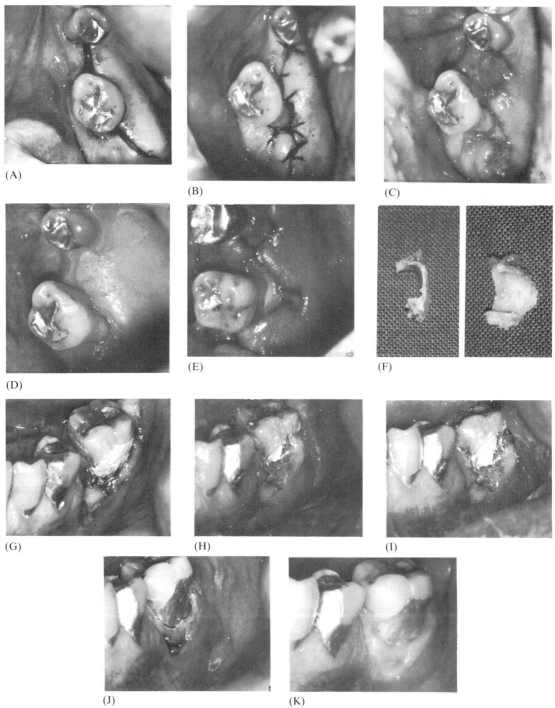

Figure 17.5 Sequelae of bony denudation following inadvertent flap displacement or mucosal ulceration. (A) Surgical stage prior to resection of palatal and wedge excess tissue. (B) Flap coaptation and suturing – note inter-radicular suturing. (C) 1 week – extensive flap ulceration and bony denudation at 17 palatal aspect. (D) Gingival regeneration with no residual deformity at 4 weeks. (E) Similar bony denudation in this case resulted in (F) bone sequestration. (G) Mucosal necrosis and bony denudation at 1 week following pre-restorative flap surgery (by student!). Probably related to inappropriately sited relieving incision and surgical trauma to bone. (H) Presentation at 2, (I) 4 and then (J) 6 weeks at which thin necrotic bone had been resorbed (undermining resorption) and resulted in (K) marginal gingival deformity at 10 weeks

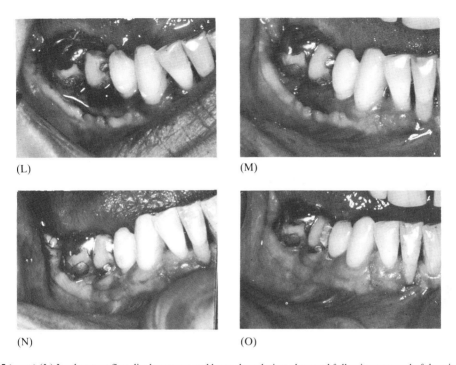

(L)

(M)

(N)

(O)

Figure 17.5 (*cont.*) (L) Inadvertent flap displacement and bony denudation observed following removal of dressing. Healing shown at 2 weeks with gingival regeneration from periodontal ligament. (M) Further regeneration stemming from undermining resorption with progressive mucosal coverage of thick buccal bone observed at 4 weeks and (N) 6 months. (O) 2-year findings

extraction socket, has developed. This may also occur following or indeed even be the cause of mucosal necrosis, but cause and effect cannot be readily established. Whatever the association, mucosal ischaemic necrosis may be the result of an inadequate collateral blood supply following over-thinning (as in Figure 17.5 C) or even frank perforation of the flap (as in Figures 15.21 E, 15.22 E), poor flap adaptation to bone (as is Figure 17.5 G and L), excessively tight sutures (as in Figure 16.23 K) or undue physical trauma to the tissues at operation as suggested at Figure 17.5 (G).

The patient will in most cases have accurately located the precise position of any flap necrosis and its associated mucosal ulceration (as at Figure 17.4 K), by the greater degree of pain experienced. Removal of any dressing and the sutures bring about an almost immediate pain relief, because the ulcerated mucosal margins are exquisitely painful to the touch and so might be expected to be irritated by the physical presence of these materials. The braided silk suture material may also function as a wick which facilitates the passage of both bacterial and endogenous pain-producing substances to within the tissues. The localized osteitis associated with flap ulceration presumably contributes to symptoms, although the surface of the necrosing bone itself is, as might be expected, not sensitive to touch.

The denuded bony sites are gently irrigated with warm saline and such rinsing carried out by the patient at frequent intervals. The bone gradually granulates over and heals fairly uneventfully although bone sequestration may follow in some cases (Figure 17.5 E and F) (see also Chapter 19). Where however the site is irritated by the tongue or not easily avoided during eating, a further dressing should be applied to protect it. This is retained for only a few days until symptoms subside and may then be removed by the patient using, for example, the sharp points of fine scissors.

(2) A loose dressing will remain in position where it is locked mechanically around teeth or held in place by sutures embedded within it. The normal functional movements of the lips, cheeks and tongue will then tend to displace slightly this mobile dressing causing it to rub against the underlying soft tissues or for the embedded sutures to tug on the mucosa. The frequency with which undue postoperative pain appears to be associated with a dressing and in turn relieved by its removal, suggests that dressings should be limited to only those sites that definitely demand flap support. An overextended dressing is liable to cause mucosal ulceration as shown in Figure 17.4 (N and O).

(3) Increased tooth mobility is normally experienced after surgery. Consequently during chewing, swallowing and clenching, any adherent dressing would tend to rub against the mucosa and cause pain. The loops of the continuous suture about mobile teeth will similarly pull on the soft tissues. The removal of the dressing and sutures effects an almost immediate relief. Hypermobile teeth also become slightly extruded so make premature contact with opposing units, causing a periodontic type pain during normal function and more especially parafunctional clenching. This pain is often not restricted to the offending teeth and may radiate along the surgical field, complicating diagnosis. Patient reassurance and, where necessary, occlusal adjustment to 'relieve the bite' is indicated.

(4) The development of pulpitis or an apical endodontic lesion may develop coincidently or as a result of surgical instrumentation and manifest at any stage following operation. Fortunately, such pulpal involvement is most unusual as it can make differential diagnosis at this stage extremely difficult. Careful attention to the restorative needs prior to undertaking periodontal surgery greatly minimizes the risk of pulpal problems. The likelihood of accessory root canals being exposed by root surface debridement and so leading to pulpitis is remote. (See Chapter 18.)

(5) Finally, in some instances healing is apparently quite normal and the cause for pain is not apparent. The possibility of tissue shrinkage with resolution of post-surgical inflammatory oedema causing the sutures to pull on the tissues cannot be ruled out, for relief of symptoms often ensues upon suture removal at this stage.

Post-surgical plaque control

Following removal of the dressing and sutures, the area is thoroughly irrigated with a warm dental spray and the teeth carefully cleaned with a soft rubber rotary cup and polishing paste. The difficulties of cleaning the interproximal areas at this early stage, because of tissue tenderness and dentinal sensitivity, means that it can rarely be accomplished. The former cleaning is nevertheless undoubtedly of some psychological benefit to the patient, especially as the staining from the chlorhexidine rinse at the front teeth can be polished away. That occurring elsewhere can be disregarded for it cannot be seen readily and is likely to recur anyway with continued use of the mouthwash.

The need for post-surgical professional cleaning is not altogether clear, for most patients will have been using a chlorhexidine mouthwash and this has been shown to be as effective as mechanical plaque control measures, even over a 6-month post-surgical period. However, the often unacceptable local side effects of chlorhexidine rinsing (see Chapter 35) means that the effective supragingival plaque control measures, established prior to surgery, must be reinstituted as soon as possible after surgery. This will be inhibited initially by the normal post-surgical findings of tissue tenderness, gingival bleeding, dentinal sensitivity and tooth mobility and tenderness. The patient should be advised accordingly lest he be deterred from cleaning and a softer toothbrush or the usual one, softened in hot water, used with a gentler action advocated. Similarly, dental floss and wood points are used more carefully lest they damage the healing junctional epithelium or traumatize the tissues and inhibit subsequent cleaning efforts.

The patient's plaque control is closely monitored over the first 6 months and supportive professional cleaning carried out as necessary. The respective benefits of such professional cleaning as opposed to that of patient supervision and motivation remains unclear. Initially, visits might be at 2-weekly intervals and then the time interval increased as dictated by the tissue response and the features of the case (see Chapter 27). Marginal gingival inflammation usually signifies inadequate cleaning but must be differentiated from that associated with the delayed healing at sites with poor flap adaptation.

Sites at which elective surgical reattachment was intended and those at which it has been imposed unintentionally, by apically repositioned flaps sliding back coronally or incomplete pocket wall resection, are especially carefully observed and maintained. This also emphasizes the need for careful documentation of the surgical technique carried out at each site. Care must, however, be taken during this professional cleaning to ensure that there is no interference with the possible development of the long junctional epithelium. A chart indicating the precise distribution of these sites is given to the patient for more careful home care. Such pocket closure sites, unlike those having minimal sulcus depths following predictable pocket elimination, are probably more vulnerable to recurrent disease although there is no documentary support for this. (See also Chapter 29 – Tissue curettage.)

Wound healing following surgery

In each of the surgical options of surgical reattachment, apically repositioning and resection, the flap is coapted to the dento-alveolar junctions, although this is frequently not possible interdentally. This optimal relationship results in comparable healing whatever the option used. The fact that the flap in surgical reattachment is, in addition, adapted to the exposed roots of the teeth, merely means that the potential exists for a correspondingly longer junctional epithelium. Interdental soft tissue cratering is inevitable in such instances, but the significance of this is considered later.

The common healing pathway

The closely adapted flap is fixed into place initially by the thin intervening blood clot. Within 24 h a band of polymorphonuclear cells develops on its connective tissue surface and over the denuded interdental bone. Epithelium proliferates over this minimally inflamed tissue surface by about the third day, progressing apically under the clot until the root surface is reached, establishing a new junctional epithelium within 7–10 days. There is a concurrent proliferation of richly vascularized granulation tissue from the periodontal ligament, the marrow spaces and the flap connective tissue, with flap attachment to bone occurring by about 21 days. In all instances, a minimal new connective tissue attachment associated with cementum regeneration (namely new attachment) occurs over the surgically exposed root located immediately coronal to the crestal bone. It seems that demineralization of root surface apatite crystals occurs first, followed by collagen fibrils deposition to establish the initial tissue continuity between connective tissues and tooth and, finally, cemental mineralization.

Bony denudation

The response of bone to flap surgery and its subsequent healing is dealt with in Chapter 19. Suffice it to say here, any denuded interdental bone undergoes necrosis. The initial intense inflammatory response to this insult is followed by granulation tissue proliferation from the adjacent periodontal ligaments, the interproximal bone marrow spaces and the scalloped flap margins (see Figure 17.5 L and M). This tissue gradually covers the bone allowing epithelial migration, the formation of a new supracrestal attachment and mucosal regeneration. Where close flap adaptation to tooth is not achieved, healing over the interposed denuded bone occurs in a comparable fashion. Healing can extend over several months depending on the extent of bony exposure and the structure of the bone involved. Bony sequestration may also occur in some instances (see Figure 17.5 E and F).

Interdental cratering

Where surgical reattachment is attempted, the marginal epithelial cells must migrate a greater distance and so will take longer to re-establish a new junctional epithelium. Healing is enhanced by close flap adaptation and minimal blood clot formation, but the influence of any residual pocket epithelium remains clear. The inevitable initial interdental mucosal cratering (see Figure 15.11) gradually becomes shallower by a combination of flap papillary tissue shrinkage and gingival septal tissue regeneration. The extent to which the latter is due an inflammatory tissue proliferation in response to inadequate plaque control at these comparatively inaccessible sites is also not clear. However where extensive interproximal bony defects are also present a tissue crater is more likely to persist. The resulting reverse gingival architecture does, nevertheless, appear to be consistent with periodontal tissue health in individuals capable of maintaining a high standard of cleaning.

Outcome of different surgical options

Investigations on different surgical techniques reveal broadly comparable results in respect of attachment levels and residual probing depths. It must, however, be appreciated that the former finding might not represent the result of surgical therapy, only that disease was not progressing at the time of surgery or, alternatively, that progressive destruction is still occurring at clinically undetectable rates. The other perhaps more unexpected finding concerning probing depth may be explained in part by the uneven patterns of periodontal destruction encountered precluding pocket elimination at every site and partly by the presentation of mean data for surgical fields (see Part III). The technical reasons for the former apparent surgical failure are summarized here as an introduction to complex pocket surgery.

(1) In apical repositioning the tissue displacement required for pocket elimination at the deepest sites, would result in an unacceptable exposure of bone at adjacent sites with lesser breakdown. Similarly it is very difficult to ensure that any resection incision follows closely the variable pocket depths at adjacent sites so that each pocket is actually eliminated and that bony denudation is avoided. Consequently, while suprabony pockets at the initially shallowest pocket sites can be predictably eliminated, those elsewhere can only be reduced by amounts equivalent to that achieved at the shallower neighbouring sites. Residual probing depths are therefore inevitable in many surgical fields.

(2) There is a problem in ensuring the stability of the flap margin positions during the immediate post-surgical period. That is the apically repositioned flap may become displaced coronally so assuming a surgical reattachment relationship to the tooth, while with intended surgical reattachment, the flap might become displaced apically. Consequently, at sites with the most commonly encountered initial suprabony pocket of about 5–7 mm there may be very similar dimensional outcomes.

(3) This equalizing effect would be increased during subsequent healing by progressive reparative tissue shrinkage (gingival recession) following surgical reattachment on the one hand, and on the other, coronal tissue proliferation at apically repositioned flap and indeed also flap resection sites.

(4) The intrabony component of any pocket cannot be eliminated by soft tissue surgery alone, and in many instances, correction by the removal of the supporting bone at adjacent tooth surfaces is not acceptable. Intrabony pockets can therefore at best be predictably reduced only by the extent of their suprabony component.

(5) The overall effect of the uneven pattern of breakdown in the surgical field is that in many situations pocket reduction must be accepted as a compromise solution to the initial surgical aim of pocket elimination, resulting in similar residual probing depths regardless of surgical technique.

Complex pocket surgery

The variable morphology of the roots, the uneven pattern of attachment loss and its effects on bony contour encountered at operation and, lastly, the extension of pocket bases to within vestibular mucosa will each be found to complicate simple pocket surgery. In essence, this means that the normal anatomical features of the periodontium rather than the actual extent of destruction are mainly responsible for thwarting the fundamental surgical objective advocated of pocket elimination. Fortunately, however, and despite the frustrating influence of these features, the basic surgical exercise described under 'Simple pocket surgery' is still applicable to every situation, for the additional surgical measures required can simply be incorporated as and when necessary. For this reason, these morphologically derived and essentially technical complications of pocket surgery are dealt with as separate entities under 'Complex pocket surgery', following the description of the simple pocket surgical techniques earlier and the miscellaneous surgical considerations in this chapter. Root morphology is considered first, followed by the problems associated with bony defects and lastly, those of vestibular morphology. The latter will then be expanded to cover the influence of variations of vestibular tissue on plaque control, the relationship between gingival recession and deep overbites and finally, the surgical correction of persistent vestibular tissue problems.

18

Complex pocket surgery:
I Root morphology

The variations of root form complicate simple pocket therapy more than any other single periodontal morphological feature so will be considered first.

The nature of the problem

Attachment losses involving root surface concavities, grooves and furcations complicate root surface management. This is because these situations are not easily debrided, not amenable to the required surgical flap adaptation at completion of operation, and optimal post-surgical oral hygiene cannot be ensured.

The complexity of mandibular and, more especially, maxillary root forms is clearly demonstrated by the cross-sectional contours shown in Figure 18.1. The various U-shaped and V-shaped configurations at concavities and grooves are depicted diagrammatically at Figure 18.2. The shapes of furcations themselves are dictated by not only the relationship of the roots to each other which range from fissures to patent spaces, but also the individual root contours. Similar variations are frequently also encountered at maxillary bicuspids, whilst in addition to the well recognized palatal grooves at maxillary incisors, other anterior teeth may also present with root surface grooves and concavities. The management of concavities, grooves and fissures will be considered apart from that of furcation involvement proper.

Concavities and grooves

Technical difficulties

Accessibility

Root surface concavities are readily accessible to oral hygiene measures at the facial and lingual aspects, and at approximal surfaces adjacent to edentulous areas. Elsewhere access is impeded by the neighbouring teeth (Figure 18.1 C and F). The operator can, however, invariably negotiate any such concavities.

Grooves, on the other hand, present difficulties to both patient and operator. They can be cleaned reasonably well with an interspace-type brush at accessible locations but not elsewhere. Similarly, debridement is feasible at only accessible locations and when using sickle type scalers or pointed ultrasonic inserts (e.g. Cavitron TF-10) as shown in Figure 18.3 (A and B); only the latter are likely to be really effective. Hoes are not suitable, and even the smallest Gracy type currettes cannot gain access to any groove, as their cross-sectional dimensions are too great (Figure 18.3 C–E) and indeed, are usually greater than those of even the entrances of most furcations. (See also Chapter 30 – Susceptibility to breakdown.)

Flap adaptation

The scalloped contour of the facial and oral surgical flaps permits reasonably close adaptation within any

242

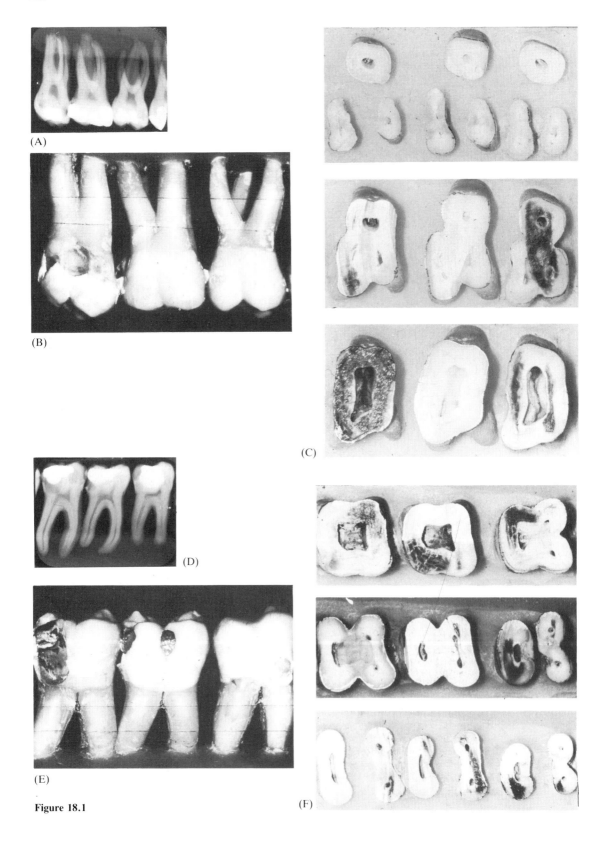

(A)

(B)

(C)

(D)

(E)

(F)

Figure 18.1

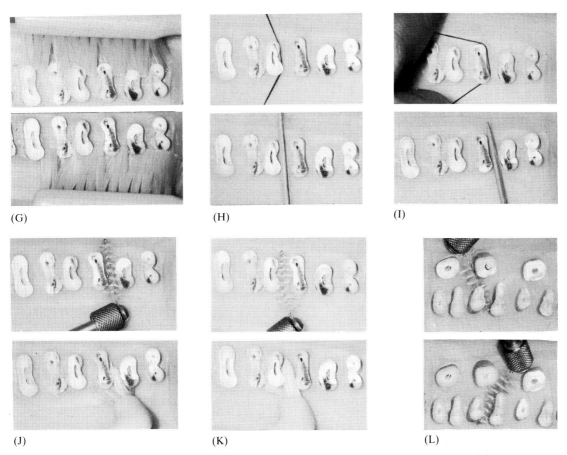

Figure 18.1 Molar root morphology and plaque control. (A and D) Radiographs and (B and E) buccal views of maxillary and mandibular molars with (C, C1 and C2 and F, F1 and F2) section planes at the cemento-enamel junctions, furcation entrances and at approximately mid-root levels. (G) Limitations of ordinary toothbrush for interdental cleaning shown at mandibular molars. (H and I) Limitations of dental floss and wood points at mandibular interdental and inter-radicular concavities respectively. (J and K) Feasibility of interproximal and interspace brushes at corresponding sites and of (L) interproximal brush within maxillary furcation spaces

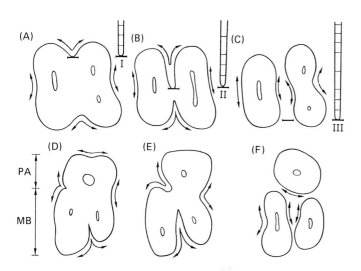

Figure 18.2 Diagrammatic representation of root morphology (adapted from Figure 18.1) of (A, B and C) mandibular and (D, E and F) maxillary molars. (A, B and C) On horizontal probing furcation involvement classified as degree I, II and III. Demonstration of root surface concavities and wide and narrow 'U' and 'V' shaped furcation grooves and fissures by correspondingly shaped arrows. Note: (C and F) inter-radicular root surface contours and (D) wider buccopalatal dimensions of maxillary mesiobuccal (MB) than the palatal (PA) roots resulting in palatally located furcation entrance

244

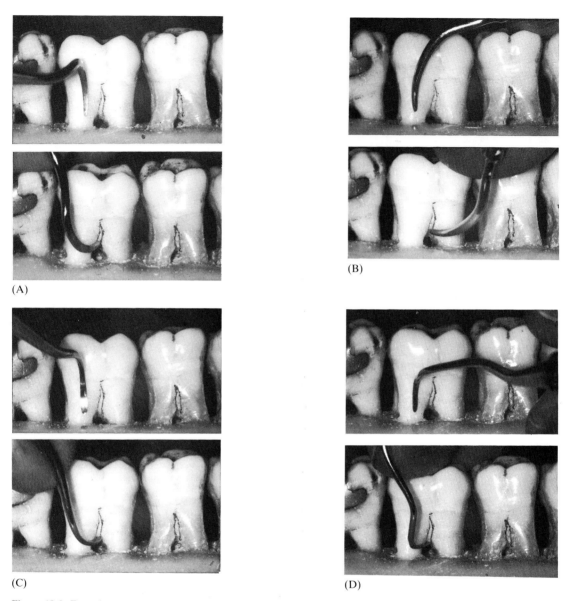

(A)

(B)

(C)

(D)

Figure 18.3 Furcation entrances and instrumentation. Use of (A) sickle scaler, (B) Cavitron TFI-10 insert, (C) Goldman–Fox and (D) Gracey curettes.

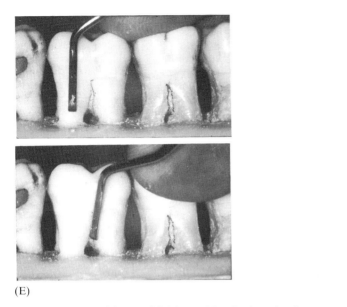

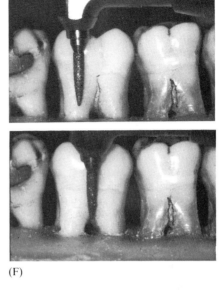

(E)

(F)

Figure 18.3 (*cont.*) (E) Hoe. (F) Diamond bur for furcationplasty

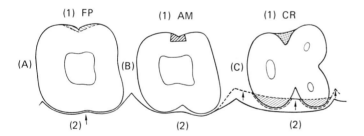

Figure 18.4 Operative options. Flap adaptation possible at (A2) surface depression (arrow) but not (B2) within shallow concavity. (C2) Flap contoured by trimming hatched segments to enhance adaptation (arrows). Groove (A1) eliminated by furcationplasty (FP) or occluded with (B1) amalgam (AM) or (C1) composite resin (CR)

related shallow concavities as shown in Figure 18.4 (A). Flap adaptation is, of course, not possible at interproximal root surface concavities as discussed previously. Deeper concavities (and grooves) would, in turn, be spanned by the flap tissue (Figure 18.4 B and C). This is of little practical significance during apical repositioning and resection, for the mucosal deficiency and the resulting denuded bone would granulate over and heal as at any denuded interproximal bone, but it would, as might be expected, preclude surgical reattachment. Adaptation can however be enhanced by reshaping (with difficulty!) the flap margin as shown in Figures 18.4 (C) and Figure 18.6 (C).

Operative options

There are several methods of dealing with root surface concavities and grooves encountered at

operation. Firstly, these could be flattened out or V-shaped contours converted to a less unfavourable U-shape by grinding away adjacent tooth material. Secondly, the recess could be filled with a restorative material. Thirdly, the offending root surface could be completely covered by coronally repositioning the surgical flap. Finally, a compromise could be accepted and the flap margin be reshaped where possible and then merely adapted in the most favourable fashion. The technical details of each option are now considered.

Reshaping of surfaces (Figure 18.4 A1)

This technique of odontoplasty is used mainly at furcation concavities and grooves, so is more precisely termed furcationplasty, but is also applicable to maxillary incisor palatal fissures. Tapered diamond or composite-type finishing burs are used (see Figure 18.3 F), to create about a 5-mm vertical span of flattened tooth surface, in relation to the intended level of the healed dentogingival junction, to ensure flap coaption and optimal postoperative plaque control.

The role of furcationplasty in contemporary periodontics has yet to be established and its simplicity belies its potential risks and limitations. Thus, the technique is possible only at accessible sites and so largely precludes interproximal surfaces. Only fairly shallow deformities can be dealt with because of the undue dentinal sensitivity and the risk of pulpal involvement. Similarly, the possibility of accessory pulpal canal exposure cannot be discounted, although neither the incidence nor the locations of these canals has been clearly established, if only because of the difficulties of doing so (see also Chapter 30 – Accessory canals). Nevertheless clinical experience suggests that the chances of exposure are remote and are further reduced by the cementum being thicker within furcations than elsewhere. Finally, it is not known whether furcationplasty sites are any more susceptible to caries, although the presence of root caries elsewhere should be taken as a contraindication to the technique. In any event, dietary sugar control to limit caries must be emphasized following furcationplasty.

Occlusion of deformities (Figure 18.4 B1 and C1)

Grooves and fissures can be filled in with amalgam, in situations where the necessary cavity preparation is possible. This then frequently precludes management of maxillary incisal grooves, although little difficulty arises when already endodontically treated. Once again, about a 5-mm section of groove, related to the proposed healed gingival margin, is restored to a smooth polished finish. Polishing is carried out at the 1-week post-surgical review with a fine tapered finishing bur under the healing flap. Alternatively, the restoration is inserted having reflected a flap specifically for this purpose, and then polished at the time of pocket surgery. The recently developed bonding-type resins represent a promising and potentially simpler alternative, but difficulties of isolating the field to gain dry conditions for placement may compromise the successful outcome. The efficacy of this particular method has yet to be established.

Coronal repositioning and surgical reattachment

This is possible only at accessible facial and lingual aspects and where the necessary flat tooth surface already exists or can be achieved by furcationplasty.

The surgical flap is reflected as for apical repositioning but then repositioned coronally instead to cover over the root deformity. (For technique see Chapter 22.) The success of the technique here has yet to be established, but appears to be primarily dependent on the flap being retained in position against the displacement effect of the contiguous vestibular mucosa. Coronal repositioning is only feasible when surgical reattachment is contemplated at adjacent units, so cannot be undertaken during pocket elimination surgery.

Compromise therapy

The adverse root morphology and tooth to soft tissue relationship is accepted and will, as such, represent one of the many enforced surgical compromises in complex pocket surgery. The offending root surface is therefore instrumented as well as possible and the flap positioned according to the intended surgical objectives. Surgical reattachment is, however, frequently imposed at such sites, because inconsistencies between the flap margin and the crest of bone are so commonly encountered at furcations. This, in turn, means that difficulties in post-surgical plaque control will remain on two counts, that of adverse root form and of residual probing depths. The outcome of compromise therapy at such sites is nevertheless more favourable than might be expected (see also Chapter 29 – Influence of root morphology), so is usually best attempted in the first instance and the need for alternative measures only considered later.

Optimal plaque control in these situations is best ensured by using interspace-type brushes. The apically directed bristles are first splayed out against the coronal tooth surface to produce a flattened chisel-like edge, and then pushed gently but firmly into the subgingival root surface concavity or groove (Figure 18.5 A). Interproximal surfaces are approached obliquely from both the facial and oral aspects (Figure 18.5 B, C, F and G). The angulation of the tuft can be altered by heating the neck of the brush over a flame and then bending it to suit individual requirements as is shown in Figure 8.6. Mesial interproximal surfaces and mesially tilted teeth are most readily negotiated with the obtusely angled tuft, whilst the acutely angled one is most suitable for the corresponding distal surfaces (Figure 18.5 B and C).

Although the interproximal-type brush is effective for supragingival cleaning at interproximal root surface concavities, it is not advocated here. This is because its subgingival cleaning action is impaired by the tendency for the relatively soft bristles to be deflected and easily distorted by the interdental gingival septum during use as depicted in Figure 18.5 (H). (See also Figure 11.11.)

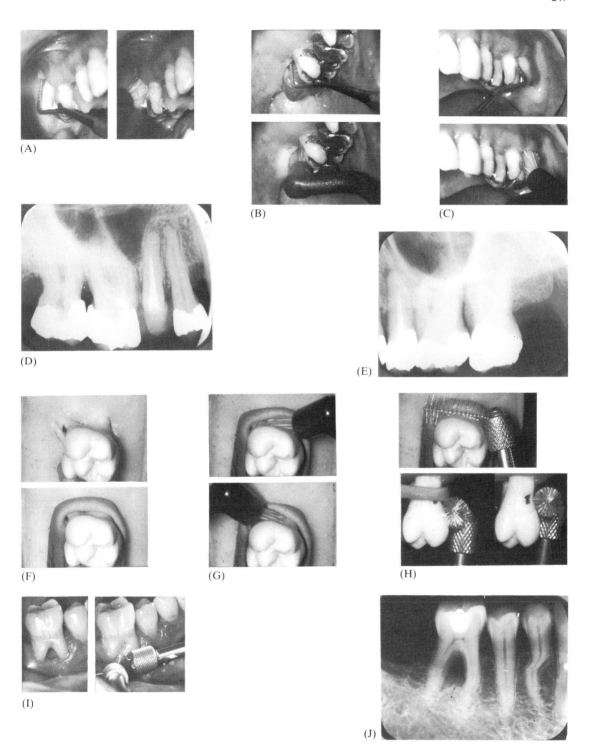

Figure 18.5 Furcation plaque control with (A–C) interspace brush. (A) Maxillary molar buccal furcation probed and negotiated. (B and C) Second molar mesial furcation approached bilaterally. (D and E) Radiographs of molar furcation involvement in (A–C). (F) Maxillary approximal root surface concavity and simulated soft tissue pocket below. (G) Subgingival concavity negotiated bilaterally by splayed out filaments of interspace brush. (H) Limitations of interproximal brush within such subgingival concavities. (I) Interproximal brush within furcation tunnel. (J) Radiograph of tunnel space

Furcations

Classification

Root furcation involvement represents the most complex morphological problem, for in addition to the usual vertical a horizontal component exists extending into the inter-radicular spaces. Although this section is devoted to molar furcations, it is equally applicable to bi-rooted maxillary bicuspids.

The findings at operation depend on a combination of the variable morphology of individual roots and their relationships to each other. The resulting inevitably complex clinical presentation demands some form of classification, if only for descriptive purposes. The following is commonly used as depicted in Figure 18.2

Degree I = Horizontal loss less than 1/3 width of tooth
Degree II = Horizontal loss greater than 1/3 width of tooth but not encompassing the total width of the furcation area.
Degree III = Horizontal 'through-and-through' destruction of the periodontal tissue in the furcation.

The extent and pattern of horizontal loss between the root surfaces is established by probing. Degree I and II involvements present respectively as shallow and deep cave-like spaces, whereas Degree III presents as a tunnel. Differentiation between these groups can be difficult when the roots are closely related and appear only as clefts as shown in Figure 18.2 (D and E). Furthermore, only shallow clefts between fused roots (Degree I) can be classified with any confidence. Thus, an apparent Degree I cleft involvement might, in reality, be Degree II, or in some instances even Degree III, when the roots are either too close together for probing or its passage checked by the third root of maxillary molars.

Practical implications

In practice the inter-radicular cleft is comparable to a developmental groove in that it cannot be adequately instrumented nor corrected by furcationplasty. However, it is also not amenable to either restorative correction or flap coronal repositioning and the operator is invariably obliged to accept a compromise solution.

With separated roots, differentiation between degrees of involvement is very much easier and the treatment options are widened. The relationship between the roots, their individual surface contours and the inter-radicular bone height will determine the accessibility of the furcation space for surgical instrumentation, surgical flap adaptation and most importantly, post-surgical plaque control. Access is most favourable, as might be expected, at the buccal and lingual furcations and very much less so interproximally.

Caves and tunnels can both be negotiated fairly easily, although tunnels tend to be more accessible because the passage of any mechanical device is not impeded and can be introduced from both directions. The root surface concavities of the individual roots within the furcation space, represent an added hurdle. These concavities are very common at maxillary molars and invariably present at mandibular molar roots (Figure 18.2 C and F). The resulting problems are comparable to those experienced at interproximal root surface concavities described previously, but occur within a very much more confined space.

The technical problems and management of Degree I furcation involvements are essentially the same as those at deep root surface concavities and grooves so need not be considered further here. The Degree II and Degree III involvements will now be dealt with.

Degree II furcations

Technical difficulties

Oral hygiene

Effective cleaning is feasible only at wide and deep (vertical) openings to the furcation cave and then usually only at the buccal and lingual aspects. Thus, the maxillary molar approximal surface furcation caves are, with the possible exception of the mesial aspect of the first molar and those associated with edentulous zones, seldom accessible. In the case of the first molar the combination of the palatal location of the mesial furcation as shown in Figure 18.2 and the smaller buccopalatal dimensions of the second bicuspid facilitates access from a mesiopalatal direction.

Access is generally better the greater the attachment loss, because of the divergent root forms and so, is enhanced by bone removal at operation (see below). Elsewhere at more closely related roots, a limited improvement in access could be gained by grinding the furcation root surfaces to widen the entrance, but this carries the risk of compromising the pulp, so is not recommended. Nevertheless, the signs of gingival inflammation in these relatively inaccessible cave-like furcation spaces appear to be surprisingly well-controlled by conscientious cleaning efforts alone, using interspace- and interproximal-type brushes and despite the periodic tendency inadvertently to traumatize the mucosa in the process. Thus, it seems that these efforts disturb the plaque sufficiently to keep its pathogenic potential in check, although the supplementary use of local chemotherapeutic measures should not be discounted in these situations (see Chapter 35 – Local antimicrobial therapy).

Professional cleaning

Provided the roots forming the furcation are adequately spaced, hand instrumentation is feasible, but few problems arise with the recommended use of ultrasonic devices. For practical purposes, the entire furcation space is carefully debrided, regardless of the intended flap positioning, although the roof of the furcation could be avoided where optimal pocket elimination is attempted.

The surgical options

Although the possible options are considered separately here, it is frequently necessary to use them in various combinations, as dictated by the features of the case.

Surgical reattachment

Success cannot be ensured because flap adaptation is not possible within the furcation itself. Complete coverage of the furcation by coronally repositioning the surgical flap could be attempted, but despite promising animal model findings, persistent pocketing is likely (see Chapter 31 – Intrabony defect healing). Recent clinical investigations on coronal positioning and, even more so, guided tissue regeneration are most encouraging (see Chapter 30 – The efficacy of therapy and Chapter 31 – Preferential repopulation investigations).

Surgical exposure of the furcation

Flap apical repositioning or resection will enhance access for subsequent plaque control measures. Adaptation of the flap margin into the furcation space may necessitate both mucosal shaping as shown in Figure 18.6 (C–E) and some bone removal. Even so, a surgical compromise is often imposed, because of the difficulties of achieving totally cleansible dentogingival relationships. These difficulties are in turn associated primarily with the need to remove extensive amounts of supporting bone (namely with an intact periodontal attachment) from about the adjacent root surfaces as depicted in Figure 18.6 (A and B). This is considered further below and in Chapter 19.

Conversion to Degree III

This should be considered when two molar furcation involvements present at the same tooth almost communicate with each other and if converted into a single tunnel would be readily accessible to an interproximal brush. This technique is, therefore, only feasible at reasonably spaced roots of mandibular molars and the maxilla where good access to the furcation entrances exists. The small amount of inter-radicular bone and periodontal attachment located between the two furcation cave lesions is removed to create the tunnel. This tunnel is, for the purposes of plaque control, then comparable to any interproximal space between two adjacent teeth. This bone removal is, however, technically difficult because of the confined nature of the furcation space and the obvious risk of inadvertent notching of the roots. The techniques of bone removal are considered in Chapter 19. Of these, only small dental burs and ultrasonic tips are able to negotiate the furcation spaces and extreme care is necessary to avoid damaging the roots.

Root resection

This is indicated when the inter-radicular dimensions will preclude cleaning, or where extensive loss of attachment or a questionable endotonic status exists at one of the roots. It should also be considered when complex coronal restorative treatment contemplated, demands a more predictable long-term periodontal prognosis for the tooth. This surgical option and its implications are considered in conjunction with Degree III involvement below.

Degree III furcations
Furcation accessibility

The Degree III involvement is merely the result of a horizontal merger of two lesser degree furcation involvements, so does not necessarily represent a more advanced disease, only a different pattern of periodontal breakdown. The essential feature is a horizontal buccolingual communication between two mandibular roots, or one, two or three interconnecting passages between maxillary molar roots. Access for plaque control and surgical instrumentation is, as elsewhere, again primarily dependent upon root morphology. Where totally accessible to a Williams-type periodontal probe, interproximal type brushes will also pass through readily and so are referred to as 'through and through' involvements (see Figure 18.5 I and J). On the other hand, where these tunnels are not accessible to the probe, because the roots are either too close together or the root positions, as at maxillary molars, impede the through passage of such mechanical devices, other measures are indicated. The management of these inaccessible situations are dealt with after that of accessible 'through and through' furcations.

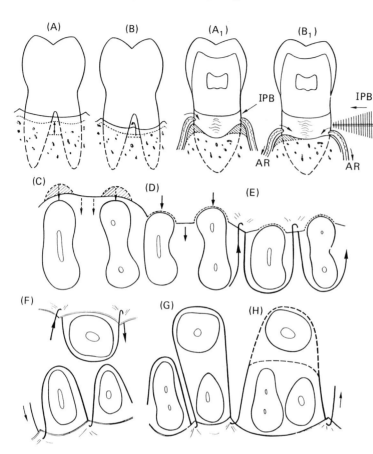

Figure 18.6 Furcation tunnels. (A and A1) Inter-radicular crater (arrowed in A) between buccal and lingual plates (cross-hatched in A1) complicates mucosal flap adaptation. Removal of (B) buccal and lingual supporting bone and (B1) hatched bone required to reduce depth of bony and mucosal crater. Note oblique (A1) and horizontal (B1) paths of insertion of interproximal brush (IPB) before and after bone removal. Crater eliminated by ramping effect following further bone removal (broken line) with flap apical repositioning (AR) for improved access for cleaning. The mucosal and bony management shown is equally applicable to degree II furcation involvements. (C) Improved mandibular flap adaptation by trimming hatched areas. (D) Trimmed flap in place. (E) Inter-radicular continuous suture for flap stabilization. (F, G and H) Variations of inter-radicular continuous suturing about maxillary buccal and palatal roots

Management of accessible furcations

Plaque control

The accessibility of any furcation passage for future cleaning is best assessed following the removal of the inter-radicular soft tissue, which corresponds to cervical wedge tissue elsewhere, and the exposure of inter-radicular bone. It should, of course, be borne in mind that the ultimate size of the space following healing will always be somewhat smaller due to soft tissue regeneration.

Interproximal brushes are best suited to molar furcation passages (Figure 18.5 I), especially as so many are associated with root surface concavities as shown in Figure 18.1. Any subgingival concavities present are, however, unlikely to be negotiated by the interproximal brush or any other device. The interspace brush is invariably too big to fit into tunnel spaces, and dental floss is effective only in the absence of concavities, thereby virtually precluding its use at lower molars. The expanding characteristic of Superfloss (Oral B Laboratories Ltd, Aylesbury, Bucks HP19 3ED, UK) would seem to be of limited

benefit here, but where floss is applicable, its stiffened end is most convenient for threading floss through the passage. Commercially available floss threaders (Butler Eez–Thru [John O. Butler Company, Chicago, IL, USA] and Janar Nupons [Janar Company, Grand Rapids, MI, USA]) are also available, although the latter could be readily constructed from 5-amp fuse wire instead. The comparative effectiveness of these different inter-radicular cleaning devices has not been adequately evaluated. This is due presumably to a combination of the infrequency with which furcation tunnels occur and the difficulties of reproducibly assessing the form of furcation spaces and measuring the presence or absence of any associated bacterial plaque.

Tissue curettage

The complete removal of inter-radicular tissue is critical for residual tissue tends to proliferate rapidly during healing and occlude the tunnel spaces and in turn impede oral hygiene measures (see also

Chapter 17 – Interproximal tissue proliferation). Removal is complicated by the limited access and poor visibility and not least by the difficulties of detecting any residual tissue. Upper molars are especially troublesome in this respect. Residual tissue can often only be identified by blood not passing freely through the tunnel with high volume aspiration, at one or other furcation opening, or the absence of a clear whistling sound produced by such suction. The Cavitron TF-10 tip is most effective for dislodging any stubbornly attached tissue, bone and for root surface debridement (see also Chapter 28 – Instruments for debridement and Chapter 31 – Surgical elimination of intrabony defects). Gracy curettes may be preferred by some, but they tend to become snagged against root and bone within the furcation and, although readily disengaged, leave the soft tissue behind.

Bone removal and flap adaptation

It is sometimes necessary to remove inter-radicular bone to create an unobstructed throughway for subsequent plaque control. The difficulties and risks involved have already been mentioned. The crest of the bone at the furcation entrances may also have to be reduced to allow the surgically recontoured flap margins shown in Figure 18.6 (C–E), to fit more closely into the furcations (Figure 18.6 A and B). This reduces the extent of post-surgical inter-radicular bony denudation and, in turn, possibly also tissue proliferation within the tunnel during healing. In addition, bony reduction also means that cleaning with an interproximal brush can be carried out in a horizontal rather than oblique plane (Figure 18.6 A1 and B1), which would tend to traumatize the inter-radicular mucosa and so inhibit the patient's efforts. Supporting bone must be sacrificed as shown in Figure 18.6 (A and B) to achieve the required bony contour, but as this may compromise adjacent teeth (*cf.* Chapter 19) will limit the clinical applications of the technique.

Suturing

The continuous suturing technique is readily adapted to furcation tunnels. The individual roots of a mandibular molar are simply regarded as two adjacent teeth (Figure 18.6 E). In the maxilla, several variations are possible (Figure 18.6 F–H), depending on the available access, what ensures optimal flap adaptation as determined *in situ* at the time of operation and finally, operator preferences. Thus the flaps may be sutured about the individual roots, singly or together. Suturing is, however, preferably commenced at the buccal aspect, because this is technically more difficult, and the palatal flap can at this stage still be deflected out of the way for improved visibility and access.

Healing within the furcation

The denuded inter-radicular bone heals as that at any interdental area (*cf.* Chapters 16 and 17), the regenerating tissue proliferating from the related periodontal ligaments, the alveolar bone marrow spaces, any soft tissue remnants and the surgical flap margins. Rolled collars of tissue develop initially about each root, partially occluding the passage and impeding cleaning. In addition, this tissue is tender to touch, readily traumatized and, being very vascular, bleeds easily. Each of these factors, together with plaque retention, may in turn perpetuate tissue proliferation, complicate cleaning and thwart the surgical objective. Further investigation is required.

Management of inaccessible furcations

The problem of inaccessibility

Furcations may be inaccessible to oral hygiene devices because the roots are too closely related, or in the case of maxillary molars, access is prevented by the neighbouring teeth or a direct passage precluded by root orientation. The removal of a root by root resection or amputation to provide access to the remaining root(s) should then be considered.

Clinical implications

The technique of root resection (sometimes called root amputation) has important endodontic and restorative implications. The practicality, predictability and, not least, the financial aspects of each component of treatment must therefore be carefully considered whenever root resection is contemplated. Furthermore the possibility that further periodontal breakdown may still occur cannot be discounted. Each will now be considered further.

In the first place, the likelihood of disease control at the remaining root(s) must be established. This will depend on the extent of breakdown sustained, the predicted efficacy of pocket elimination surgery contemplated and, where this is not possible, the resulting accessibility of the root(s) following surgical reattachment.

Secondly, the comparative cost in terms of professional time and patient discomfort, the technical expertise of the operators involved and the predictability of the necessary endodontic, periodontic and restorative measures must be weighed against other possible treatment options. For example, the possibly greater cost of prosthetic replacement following elective extraction might be offset by its greater predictability. The restorative status of neighbouring teeth and, indeed, the mouth as a whole, will also have an important bearing on this difficult decision. As these factors can be so variable each situation must be considered individually, the options discussed fully with the patient and a balanced decision then taken.

Finally, the existing inaccessible situations might be accepted in many instances, in the knowledge that, while further breakdown is likely, the rate of deterioration might have been retarded significantly by simple pocket surgery alone and the tooth retained for many years. This then once again represents compromise therapy and, while frequently the most appropriate approach, it may create other problems associated with tooth loss in later years (*cf.* Chapter 27). On the other hand, total tooth extraction instead is sometimes prudent where this would significantly enhance access for plaque control at an adjacent relatively inaccessible tooth deemed to have a better overall prognosis. This is especially applicable to maxillary molars.

The rationale for resection

Resection is warranted, first and foremost, when the removal of a root will resolve the localized problem of plaque control and of progressive breakdown at the tooth and where, furthermore, the presence of the existing condition is having a detrimental effect on the periodontal support of related roots. Unfortunately, these decisions are rarely so clear-cut and sometimes the more conservative alternative

of simple pocket surgery alone, followed by continuous reassessment, is preferable.

The identification of root to be resected

Where there is an obviously extensive periodontal destruction affecting one root forming the furcation and this is not amenable to pocket elimination surgery, root resection is clearly indicated. The relevant criteria at these clinical situations are, in essence, simply those applied when deciding whether a tooth is to be extracted; these are considered in Chapter 26. In short, the root to be resected should be, first and foremost, the one that is most severely involved periodontally and secondly, that which would provide the best access for plaque control at the remaining root(s). The predictability of the endodontic treatment at the remaining root(s) must also be assessed. It is not possible to lay down hard and fast rules here, but where, for example at a lower molar, the presurgical charting and radiographic findings show widely spaced roots with an almost totally intact support about one root and an extensive pocket at the other, as depicted in Figure 18.7 (A and B), the latter would be an obvious candidate for removal (see also Figures 18.9 A and 18.11 A). While at an upper molar, there might be a similarly extensive

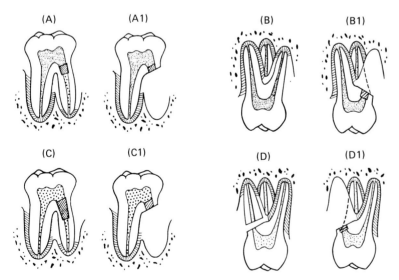

Figure 18.7. Endodontic implications. (A) Resection clearly indicated and preceded by endodontics and orthograde amalgam. (A1) Resection cut passes through amalgam. (B) Pre-existing root filling and obvious indication for root resection. (B1) Resection cut and retrograde amalgam insertion following root removal. (C) Uncertain periodontal prognosis of remaining root. Pulp extirpation and dressing followed by orthograde amalgam seal at proposed resection site. (C1) Root removed and healing assessed prior to completion of endodontics. (D) Vital pulp root resection. This may be left exposed postoperatively or sealed as at (D1)

periodontal defect restricted to a single buccal root (Figure 18.7 B). (See also Figure 18.10 A and G.)

The timing of root resection decisions

When to make the decision to resect a root, before, during or after pocket surgery, revolves very much about diagnostic difficulties encountered and endodontic implications of each situation. These are most expediently and clearly dealt with in conjunction with the following description of the root resection technique.

Root resection technique

Endodontic implications

Presurgical measures

Once it has been decided on periodontal grounds which root is to be resected, it must be established whether endodontics can be successfully undertaken and, if not, this should dictate against root resection in favour of acceptance of a compromise surgical reattachment or even tooth extraction instead. Thus, little merit exists in carrying out root resection on an endodontically compromised tooth. Where, however, successful endodontic treatment has already been achieved in the past as shown in Figure 18.7 (B), treatment planning is greatly simplified (see also Figures 18.10 G and 18.11 F).

Elective presurgical endodontics need only involve the root(s) to be retained, being both biologically and economically unnecessary at a root to be sacrificed. The pulp is extirpated from this root, a calcium hydroxide dressing inserted into the root canal, the coronal 4–5 mm of which is then enlarged and sealed with amalgam as shown in Figure 18.7 (A) (see also Figures 18.9 B and 18.11 L). The resection cut will then pass through this amalgam (Figure 18.7 A1), so eliminating the need for a retrograde apical restoration at the resected site. This technique is especially useful for mandibular molars at which access for retrograde restoration is usually inadequate, but is advocated for convenience elsewhere.

Where the choice between the resection of one or other root is not clear, root filling both would also be wasteful. Instead each canal is dressed with calcium hydroxide and sealed with zinc oxide cement. The decision on which root to resect is then made at the time of pocket surgery, and the resection carried out. Endodontics is completed at the remaining canal(s) following optimal surgical healing. Similarly, where the periodontal outlook of the potential remaining root is also uncertain, a calcium hydroxide dressing is again utilized in conjunction with an orthograde amalgam at the root to be resected (Figure 18.7 C and C1). The effects of pocket surgery and root resection can then be assessed after healing and where favourable, the root filling completed as shown in Figure 18.11 (N). Finally, any questionable decisions about root resections are, in principle, best deferred until the situation can be assessed more clearly at operation or preferably even following simple pocket surgical healing. These two options are considered next.

Surgical measures

When it is decided at operation that root resection is indicated at a previously root treated tooth (for example Figures 18.7 B, 18.10 G and M) there are no endodontic implications. Elsewhere at teeth with vital pulps, the resulting pulpal involvement can be handled in several ways. Firstly, endodontic therapy and root resection is deferred to a later date following surgical healing (see below). Secondly, pulp extirpation is performed at operation, the preserved canal(s) dressed and then sealed, and an orthograde amalgam inserted in the root to be resected. The endodontics is then completed at a later date.

In the last option, resection is carried out at operation (Figure 18.7 D) and the resulting small pulp exposure either left as it is (see also Chapter 30 – Vital root resection) or a minimal retentive cavity prepared and a quick setting calcium hydroxide dressing (e.g. Dycal [The L. D. Caulk Company, Milford, DE 19963, USA]), followed by amalgam, inserted (Figure 18.7 D1). In the former, endodontic treatment is best instituted within about 10 days, but in the latter could be deferred until (and if) symptoms or signs of dystrophic pulpal changes necessitate. This technique is not routinely recommended and is best restricted to only a single buccal root of upper molars as shown in Figure 18.11 (P). Elsewhere the comparatively larger pulpal exposure produced and/or difficulty in inserting a dressing predisposes to unacceptable pulpal symptoms. Differential diagnosis can often be difficult during the early post-surgical period. Furthermore emergency endodontic treatment at this stage would be more unpleasant for the patient.

Post-surgical measures

Whenever doubt exists at operation, the decision to resect should be delayed for some months after surgical healing and the situation then reviewed. Once the decision has been reached endodontic therapy is completed as described previously as in presurgical measures.

Operative technique

Provision of access

Flap reflection as for isolation of the cervical wedge in simple pocket surgery is usually sufficient, but

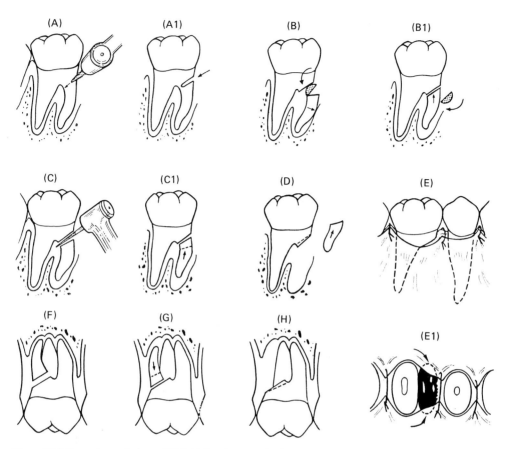

Figure 18.8 Resection technique. (A) Initial surface cut. (A1) Cut stops short of furcation. (B) Remaining segment fractured with elevator. (B1) Root elevated coronally for further trimming at (C) and again as necessary at (C1). (D) Root removed and coronal root face smoothed. (F, G and H) Similar sequence depicted at maxillary molar. (E and E1) Flap adaptation and suturing. Note mucosal deficiency equivalent to size of bony socket

should be extended where necessary. Where the need to resect has been established presurgically, this is carried out with the cervical wedge tissue *in situ*. This minimizes accummulation of the resection debris in the surgical wound, whilst any associated laceration of this tissue by the bur is of no consequence. Elsewhere, the cervical wedge tissue is removed as usual, but any residual granulation tissue retained about the root likely to be resected pending assessment at operation. This is because this tissue does not impede assessment, it limits contamination of the bony defect by debris and is very much easier to curette away following root resection and so simplifies technique. Alveolar bone is always carefully preserved, for it represents the bony component of what is, in effect, simply an extraction socket.

Resection cut

A high speed fine tapered fissure tungsten carbide or diamond bur is used, commencing at the most accessible coronal aspect of the root (Figure 18.8 A). The cut passes obliquely and apically towards the furcation, stopping just short of completely sectioning the root (Figure 18.8 A1), to ensure that the adjacent root surface and its periodontal attachment are not inadvertently damaged (see also Figures 18.9 G and 18.10 C). The dentinal and endodontic sealing material debris is then thoroughly flushed away.

Root delivery

A fine Coupland or straight Warwick James elevator is inserted into the resection cut and gently rotated to fracture the small remaining segment of intact root material (Figure 18.8 B). The thus completely sectioned root can then be carefully elevated from its residual periodontal attachment with the appropriate right- or left-sided Warwick James elevator (Figure 18.8 B1) and access permitting, removed from its socket. The cervical wedge plus granulation tissue together with any remaining adherent debris is then curetted away.

The alveolar bony crater and the length and contour of the resected root may sometimes interfere with root delivery, for its coronal cut edge becomes wedged against the under surface of the tooth as depicted in Figures 18.8 (B1) and 18.9 (H). Bone removal to free the root could compromise the remaining support for the tooth, whilst further trimming of coronal tooth material might weaken the crown, so both are best avoided. The coronal edge of the resected root is instead sectioned further (Figure 18.8 C), whilst in its coronally wedged position. The remaining shorter root is then elevated further coronally and removed (Figures 18.8 D and 18.9 I). In some cases, this sectioning sequence needs to be repeated especially when the root is curved (Figure 18.8 C1). On the other hand, although bone preservation is advocated, common sense must prevail and bone removed, where technical difficulties arise as shown in Figure 18.10 (D). These difficulties include the risk of damage to adjacent root surfaces and of the surgical flap being caught up and lacerated by the bur. In addition, the buccopalatal dimensions of the mesiobuccal root of maxillary molars often prevents its removal from in between the crown and the buccal alveolar crest and when bone removal becomes necessary.

Crown surface management

The under-surface of the crown is only smoothed down sufficiently at this stage to not irritate the cheek and tongue or impede post-surgical cleaning. The final coronal recontouring with respect to long-term plaque control is always delayed until after the socket has healed fully. There are several reasons for this. In the first place, it is easier for visibility is not impeded by bleeding and the risk of surgical flap damage by the bur is removed. Furthermore, the added risk of surgical emphysema and further possible contamination of the socket are avoided. Finally, and most importantly, the requirements of access for plaque control can only be judged properly once the healed soft tissue contour has been established. Otherwise the crown might be weakened unnecessarily by removing coronal tooth material at the outset, in an effort to improve access for cleaning, when a comparable outcome might be forthcoming by post-surgical tissue shrinkage alone as shown in Figure 18.11 (B–F).

Surgical socket management and flap adaptation

The extraction socket is finally irrigated again and any residual granulation tissue curetted away in conjunction with debridement of the adjacent root surface(s), as in any other surgical field.

Optimal mucosal coverage of the bone about any remaining root surfaces must be attempted. There will invariably be insufficient flap tissue available at the outset, this deficiency being equivalent to that of the dimensions of the extraction socket as shown in Figure 18.8 (E1). Mucosal adaptation may be enhanced by either coronally repositioning the flaps or making relieving incisions and rotating the flap tissue about the root(s), although complete crestal bone coverage is rarely achieved. The resulting heaping of the tissues about the tooth and its adjacent units is an insignificant penalty in the interests of optimal mucosal coverage over the resection site. However, care must be taken to avoid mucosal blanching where the flap overlies bony margins of the socket, lest ischaemic necrosis ensues. This bone is then best reduced when it may also enhance flap adaptation as shown in Figure 18.10 (D and E). The flap suturing method is optional. Interrupted sutures are shown in Figure 18.8 (E and E1).

Note: Preservation of the periodontal support of the remaining root surface(s) is critical and is best ensured by minimizing its operative involvement. Thus, in some instances, the surgical damage sustained by the combination of root extraction and pocket surgery might ultimately prove to be comparable to the not uncommon sequelae of the loss of distal periodontal support of the second molar following the surgical removal of an impacted lower third molar (*cf.* Chapter 25 and Chapter 31 – Third molar post-extraction healing). For this reason pocket surgery and root resection might best be carried out as separate surgical exercises. This does however demand further investigation.

Coronal restoration

Contrary to popular expectation fracturing of the crowns of root resected teeth is not inevitable as demonstrated by the clinical cases, shown in Figures 18.9–18.11. Thus, the size of any pre-existing restoration as an indication of coronal tissue destruction and of the endodontic access cavity itself, appear to be more important factors to the risk of subsequent fracture than the effects of the root resection itself. Tooth selection may therefore be critical in this respect. Furthermore, in the resection technique advocated minimal coronal tooth material will have been removed. Similarly reduction of the width of the occlusal surface overlying the resection site is contra-indicated lest

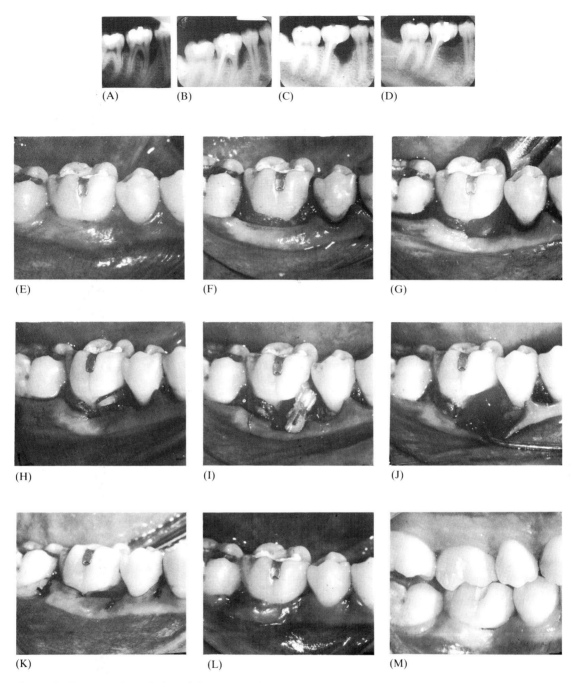

Figure 18.9 Root resection technique. (A) Isolated rapidly advancing periodontitis in 23-year-old woman – initial radiographic presentation. (B) Post-endodontics with amalgam seal in mesial canal opening. (C) 1 week and (D) 2 years post-resection mesial root. (E) Presurgical presentation. (F) Buccal (and lingual) surgical flap reflection via crevicular incisions leaving periradicular inflammatory tissue and 46, 45 interdental septal tissue *in situ*. (G) Oblique resection cut from mesial cemento-enamel junction to furcation. (H) Root elevated coronally, impacted against undersurface of crown and exposed coronal root segment sectioned almost completely (as shown) then cracked free with chisel. (I) Delivery of remaining root segment – note buccolingual dimensions compared to size of surgical aperture between crown and buccal bony plate. (J) Edges of crown smoothed off, residual inflammatory tissue curetted and related root surfaces debrided. (K) Interrupted sutures. (L) Healing at 1 week. (M) Presentation at 2 years. Marginal tissue health maintained by use of dental floss. Note occlusion and slight coronal tilting mesially but absence of mobility

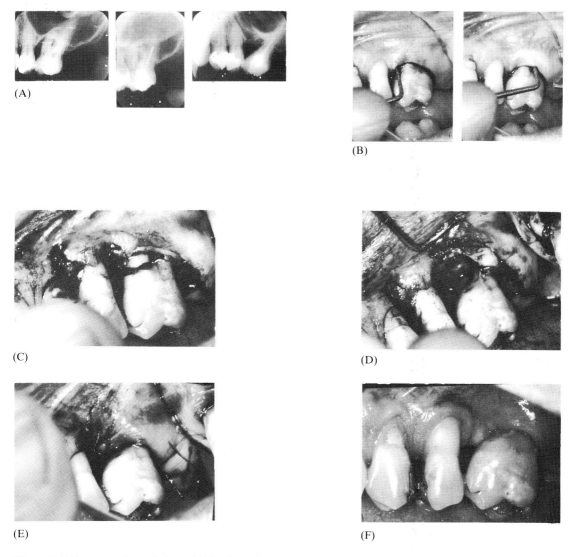

Figure 18.10 Root resection technique. (A) Radiographs on presentation, post-endodontic and 6 months post-resection. (B) Presurgical probing of mesial and buccal furcations maxillary molar in 37-year-old woman. (C) Initial root resection cut mesiobuccal root. (D) Despite coronal reshaping (as shown) and attempted trimming of resected root, operative difficulties necessitated buccal bone reduction for delivery of large (buccopalatally) curved root. (E) Bone removal did however facilitate optimal flap adaptation. (F) 6-month presentation. Note slight gingival recession.

coronal integrity be compromised. Finally, the increased tooth mobility sometimes noted following root resection, might serve as a possible buffer against potential fracturing forces. As this mobility appears to be due primarily to persistent plaque induced marginal inflammation as in Figure 18.11

(H and O), rather than the traditionally suspected occlusal overloading, extracoronal support (splinting) is rarely indicated. The restorative requirements are therefore dictated simply by the intrinsic intracoronal restorative needs. (See also Chapter 24 and Chapter 30 – Post-resection implications.)

258

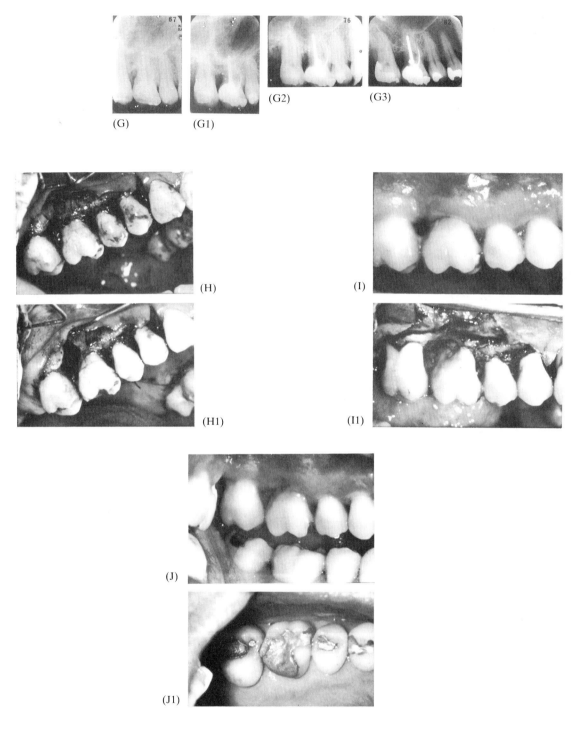

Figure 18.10 (*cont.*) (G–G3) Radiograph of existing endodontics at 16 associated with large restoration. Distal furcation involvement in 30-year-old man. (G1) 3 months post-resection distobuccal root. (G2) 9-year and (G3) 15-year presentation. (II) Surgical exposure bony defect. (III) Bone reduced for removal of root. Retrograde amalgam inserted. (I) Persistent subgingival inflammation resection site noted at 9 years. (I1) Surgical re-entry – note bony regeneration at resection site but loss at 17 buccal aspect. (J and J1) Presentation at 15 years. Note occlusion (in precentric position) and intact existing restoration.

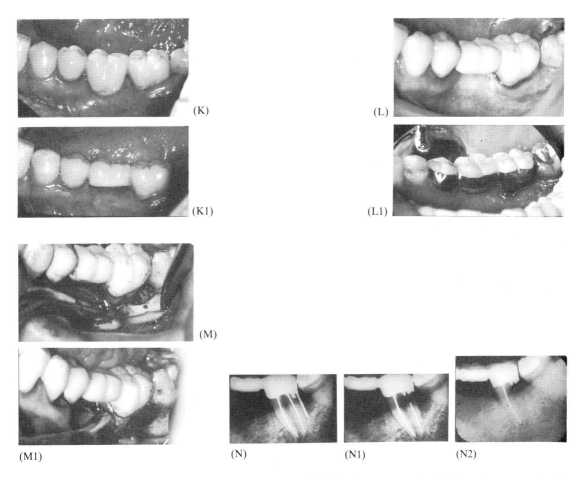

(K)

(K1)

(L)

(L1)

(M)

(M1)

(N) (N1) (N2)

Figure 18.10 (*cont.*) (K) Mandibular bridge 43-year-old woman. (K1) Pontic recontoured to facilitate plaque control at 35 and 37. (L and L1) Clinical improvement at 2 months but extensive distal pocket [confirmed by probing–radiograph at (N)] coupled with secondary caries at root filled tooth warranted resection of distal root. (M) Flap reflection and exposure of extensive bony defect. (M1) Root removed and sharp crestal bony margin rounded off for optimal flap adaptation. (N1) Resection cut and reduction of root height prior to elevation. (N2) 6-month presentation

260

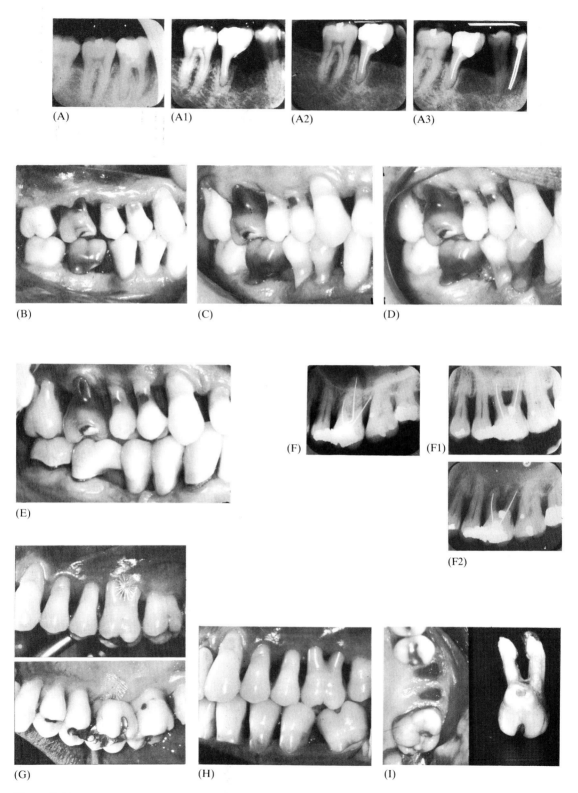

Figure 18.11

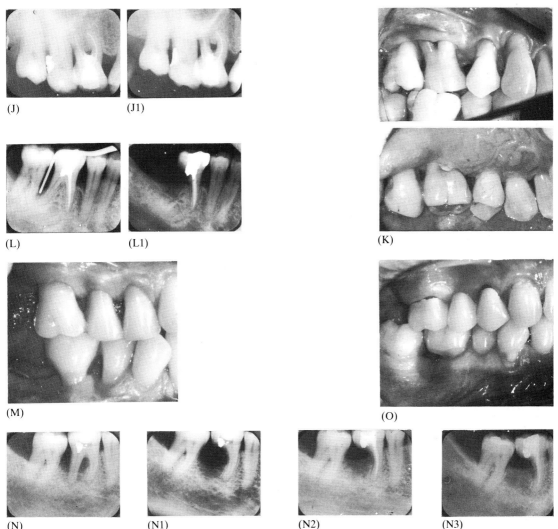

Figure 18.11 Post-resection findings. (A) Radiographs combined periodontal–endodontal lesion 46 mesial root in 28-year-old man in 1966. (A1) Endodontics at distal root and mesial root resected plus retrograde amalgam – 2-month post-resection presentation (1967). (A2) 3-year and (A3) 14-year radiographic findings – minimal further attachment loss at 46 but note deterioration at 45, 44. Clinical findings at (B) 3 years, (C) 9 years and (D) 14 years during which 46 displayed no mobility. (E) Bridge fitted 1 year later. Note 16 distobuccal root resection carried out in 1976. (F) Radiograph combined lesion of possibly endodontic origin at palatal root of long-standing asymptomatic root-treated 26 in 43-year-old man. (F1) 6-month post-resection – note apical radiolucencies buccal roots. Further endodontics not feasible. (F2) Development, after nearly 4 years, of combined lesion of probable endodontic origins. (G) Clinical presentation at 6 months. Inter-radicular cleaning with interproximal brush. (H) Tooth maintained Grade I mobility until acute episode and (I) extraction. Note good gingival status at sockets and combined lesion inflammatory tissue on both roots. (J) Radiograph 3 months post-resection palatal root of 16 in 65-year-old woman. Tooth had sustained extensive external root resorption within furcation. (J1) 10 years later. (K) Tooth remained in good function and firmly supported despite further attachment loss over assessment period. (L) Radiograph progessive attachment loss between 47 and 46 in 47-year-old woman with development of retrograde pulpitis. Endodontic treatment (by courtesy of Mr L.M. Fick) mesial root and distal root opening occluded with amalgam and root then resected. Note 47 deteriorated so extracted 15 months later. Presentation (L1) radiographically and (M) clinically after 6 years. Tooth in good function with no mobility and tight mesial contact. (N) Radiograph uncertain periodontal prognosis of furcation involved 46 mesial root in 63-year-old woman. Pulp extirpated, canal dressed and distal canal opening occluded with amalgam prior to resection of distal root. (N1) 1 month post-resection. (N2) Optimal healing at 6 months when endodontics completed (by courtesy of Mr C.J.R. Stock). Presentation (N3) radiographically and (O) clinically after 5 years. Good function but periodic slight mobility as some difficulty experienced in disease control within concavity on distal surface of root. Note some occlusion adjustment carried out by dental practitioners in this and the above case

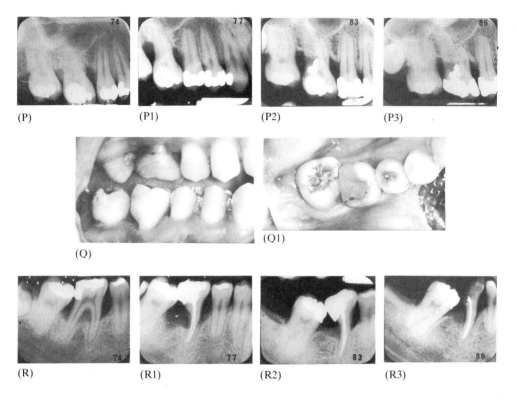

Figure 18.11 (*cont.*) (P) Radiograph 16 on presentation and (P1) 3 months after vital pulp root resection of distobuccal root with extensive furcation involvement in 21-year-old woman with localized sites of rapidly advancing periodontitis. Dycal dressing later sealed with amalgam. (P2) Pulp maintained vitality radiographically and (Q) clinically over 12-year assessment period. 46 distal root resection was performed at same time following elective endodontic therapy. (Q1) Large amalgam replaced after 4 years because of secondary caries. Tooth remains firmly supported despite difficulties in plaque control adjacent to tilted 47. (R) Radiographs 46 on presentation, (R1) 3 months post-resection and (R2 and R3) at 9 and 12 years when amalgam fractured once more

Summary

The technical problems resulting from the complex root morphology of molar teeth in particular, but also bi-rooted maxillary bicuspids and other root aberrations have been shown to complicate pocket surgery and in many instances thwart the overall surgical objective. Complex technical solutions with respect to root resections, and even extraction in conjunction with prosthodontic therapy are, nevertheless, feasible in some cases. In the majority, however, compromise solutions are imposed and at best a slowing down of the rates of periodontal destruction hoped for. The morphology of periodontally involved roots thus constitutes a major hurdle in surgical therapy. The influence of osseous morphology can now be considered.

19

Complex pocket surgery:
II Bone morphology

Pattern of bone resorption
Pathogenesis of bony defects
Operative implications
Management of intrabony defects

Bone behaviour in surgical therapy
Post-surgical management of bony defects
Summary

The crest of the bone is an important landmark in simple pocket surgery representing, for the purposes of surgical flap positioning, the base of the pocket. The management of any complications due to inconsistencies encountered between the contours of the flap margin and crest of bone, following different degrees of periodontal destruction, has been described in Chapters 14 and 15. Additional and often insurmountable complications arise however when bony resorption is found to extend apically from the crest of the bone. The resulting intrabony defects not only complicate root surface instrumentation, but more critically prevent surgical flap margin coaptation. The management of these defects constitutes part of complex surgery, but will be better understood if the nature and pathogenesis of bony defects is considered first. This chapter is concluded by examining the response of bone to operative treatment and to post-surgical denudation.

Pattern of bone resorption

When bone resorption has occurred in an uniform manner, its overall contour remains unchanged and its crest merely becomes located more apically to the cemento-enamel junctions (Figure 19.1 A). Where overall resorption has been uneven (Figure 19.1 B) the overall bone form becomes irregular resulting in marginal bony inconsistencies (Figure 19.1 B1 and B2). Bony defects are deemed to be present where bony craters are encountered about the periodontally involved roots (Figure 19.1 C). The above description is however an over-simplification for various combinations are usually encountered in any surgical field and even around single teeth. The individual components of the bony defects will now be considered. (See also Chapter 31 – The nature of bony defects.)

The bone adjacent to the necks of the teeth is called the crestal bone and together with the supporting bone is associated with the periodontal ligament fibre insertions (Figure 19.1 B1). Where a bony crater develops about a tooth the crestal bone is located within the crater, so described as the intrabony crest, whilst the term crest of the bone is reserved for the coronal edge of the crater (Figure 19.1 C1). Bone forming the crater no longer invests intact periodontal ligament fibres and so is regarded as non-supporting bone (Figure 19.1 C1). A periodontal pocket associated with a bony crater is logically described as an intrabony pocket (Figure 19.1 C2) with its base located at the intrabony crest, which in this case is synonymous with crestal bone. Similarly, at suprabony pockets no bony defect exists so the crestal bone and the crest of the bone are then synonymous (Figure 19.1 B1).

Bony defects present as four basic types depicted in Figures 19.2 and 19.3.

(1) The simple crater (SC) is situated at the facial or oral aspects of the teeth or adjacent to an edentulous zone. It has three bony walls facing the periodontally diseased root surface. Where a simple crater extends around more than one surface of a tooth it is more aptly described as a gutter (G).

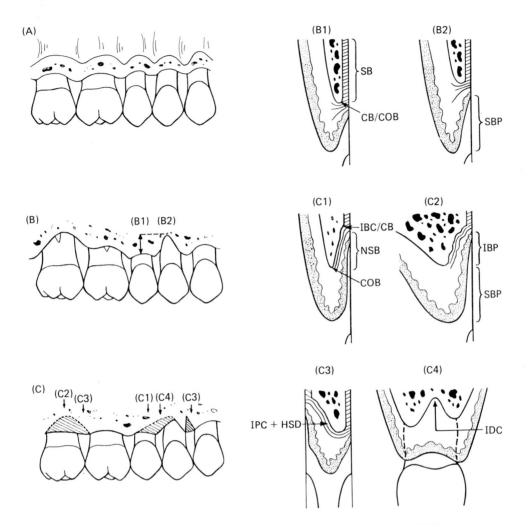

Figure 19.1 Pattern of bone resorption. (A) Surgical flap form with even bone pattern. (B) Uneven resorption with bone inconsistencies, those at 15 and 14 depicted at (B1 and B2). Note furcation involvement 17 and 16. (C) Intrabony defects, with thin bony wall at 15 but thick wall at 17 depicted at (C1 and C2). Interproximal crater at 14 mesial aspect forming a hemiseptal defect and the more extensive interdental crater between 15 and 14 depicted at (C3) mesiodistal view and (C4) buccopalatal view respectively. Key: CB, crestal bone; COB, crest of bone; IBC, intrabony crest; SB, supporting bone; NSB, non-supporting bone; SBP, suprabony pocket; IBP, intrabony pocket; HSD, hemiseptal defect; IPC, interproximal crater; IDC, interdental crater

(2) The interproximal crater (IPC) has a similar configuration but is located about a single interproximal root surface.

(3) The interdental crater (IDC) in turn involves both interproximal surfaces so has only two (facial and oral) bony walls.

(4) The angular septal or hemiseptal defect (HSD) results when the interproximal crater is associated with the loss of the facial and/or oral bony plates as well (the term hemiserum (HS) describes the remaining interproximal bony plate).

Each of these bony defects may be accompanied by various marginal bony inconsistencies which merge with each other or become associated with root furcation involvement creating complex clinical presentations (see Figure 19.3).

The commonly encountered use of the terms 'loss of attachment', 'loss of bone' and 'bone loss', as applied to radiographic findings needs to be clarified. A widened funnel-like periodontal ligament space that occurs during orthodontic movement (Figure 19.4 A), may appear radiographically as a loss of bone and so be misinterpreted as an

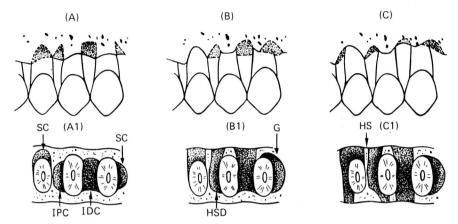

Figure 19.2 Bony defects. Destruction at (A, B and C) showing progressive changes in bony defects. (A1, B1 and C1) show occlusal views of defects. Key: SC, simple crater; IPC, interproximal crater; IDC, interdental crater; HSD, hemiseptal defect; G, gutter; HS, hemiseptum

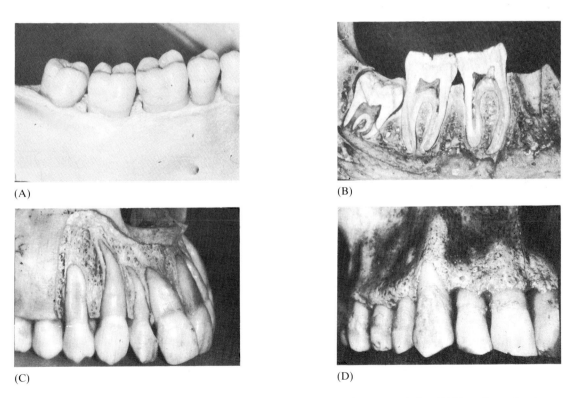

Figure 19.3 Bony defect form shown here on dry skull rather than clinically for greater clarity. (A) Normal crestal and interdental cortical bone. (B and C) Sections showing medullary structure and impending impaction of 48. (D) Uneven thickness buccal bone with prominent root bulges at 16 and at 13 associated with bony dehiscence.

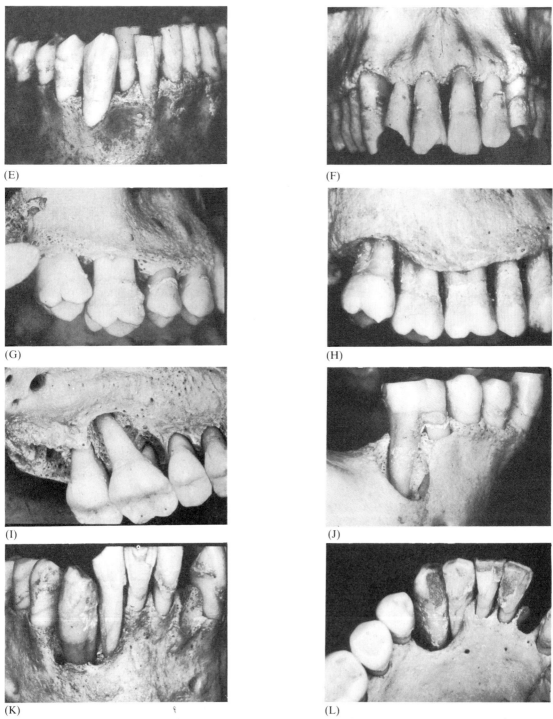

Figure 19.3 (*cont.*) (E) Uneven crestal heights associated with different tooth positions. (D and E) Slight IDC at 13/12 and 44/43 and 43/42. (F and G) Even bone loss, some IDCs and IPC at 13/12 and mesial 17/16. Note 16 mesiobuccal fenestration. (H) Uneven loss with marginal bony inconsistencies and development ledge-like crestal form and extensive IDC and IPC. (I and J) Extensive craters involving molar furcations and possibly also root apices. (K and L) Extensive gutter about 43 with hemiseptal defects at 44 and 42 but little loss elsewhere highlighting localized nature of disease. 43 mesial groove possible contributory factor

intrabony pocket. Whereas no loss of periodontal ligament attachment will have occurred, only a bony rarefaction associated with a degradation of the inorganic content of bone (bone loss), and which is reversible when the applied force is removed. The similar radiographic appearances of bone loss in a true intrabony pocket, which is often also associated with tooth hypermobility, represents a loss of attachment characterized by loss of both the inorganic and organic components of the bone (Figure 19.4 A, C, F and L). This change is in turn essentially irreversible, although treatment may achieve an increased radiographic density of bone. This may be indicative of bone remineralization, associated with reduced coronal mobility, or bony regeneration and remodelling (bone fill) of the former bony defects as shown in Figures 19.4 (L) and 23.2 (M and N), although it must be stressed that this is rarely associated with the development of new connective tissue attachment to the root surface. (See below and Chapter 31 – Intrabony defect healing.) As the radiographic findings are liable to misinterpretation, the relationship between plaque-induced bony defects and the potentially comparable findings with increased tooth mobility must be examined.

The radiographic finding of a funnel-like widening of the periodontal ligament space of hypermobile teeth in periodontal disease is commonly attributable to the mobility itself and, as such, is regarded as a cardinal sign of so-called occlusal trauma. There are however reasons to question the validity of this assumption. These are considered here, rather than in the chapter devoted to tooth mobility, for they relate to a combination of the site-specific nature of the disease and the influence of bony morphology on the resulting pattern of bony resorption.

In the first place, the characteristic radiolucencies occurring during active orthodontic therapy in the presence of normal bone support (Figure 19.4 B) are rarely encountered elsewhere, and then possibly only as a result of an unrealistically gross occlusal interference from coronal restorations or highly eccentric patient habits. In addition, the biomechanics of tooth mobility (see Figure 23.3) dictate that with normal bony support, such a periodontal ligament space widening could only be effected by a Grade III coronal mobility, which is not normally observed in clinical practice. Indeed, the fluctuating mobility levels between Grade I and II, recorded at the maxillary incisors, which have been attributed to inconsistent oral hygiene efforts coupled with a functional occlusal overloading and possibly also, but not readily measurable, parafunctional clenching habits in the case shown in Figure 19.4 (B), have not been accompanied by any obvious radiographic changes.

However, with reduced horizontal bony support following loss of periodontal attachment, the altered fulcrum of rotation (Figure 23.3 A1 and B1) during tooth mobility greatly decreases the effect of lateral tooth displacement upon the remaining bone. This, in turn, means that even with Grade III mobility, only slight widening or radiographic funnelling of the periodontal ligament space occurs. This is well illustrated by the barely perceptible widening associated with tooth hypermobility at the markedly reduced bony support in the case shown in Figure 23.2 (G–I).

In contrast, where intrabony pockets exist, as for example in Figure 19.4 (F and L), funnel-like radiolucencies about the affected roots are often encountered. However, these will reflect primarily the peculiar pattern of periodontal destruction and of bony resorption at the site. These situations are, moreover, invariably accompanied by supracrestal tissue inflammation and therefore increased tooth mobility which may influence the radiographic findings as shown in Figure 19.4 (C). The corollary to this is clearly supported by clinical observation of tooth mobility being almost invariably associated with periodontal attachment loss (*cf.* Chapter 23). Furthermore, with inflammatory resolution following root surface debridement and maintained oral hygiene, the accompanying reduction in tooth mobility is generally associated with little change in the radiographic findings (Figure 23.4 A and B). This would seem to endorse the limited influence that tooth mobility *per se* may have on radiographic presentation and that the changes observed should instead be attributed to the co-existing plaque-induced periodontal breakdown. Similarly, the reductions in the radiological width of intrabony defects occurring following treatment appear to more closely represent bony repair than the concomitant improved tooth stability (see Figure 19.4 L and M). Unfortunately, the ultimate clarification of this issue is dependent upon histological evaluation of human block sections, the procurement of which is extremely improbable.

Pathogenesis of bony defects

The pattern of bony defects observed in any surgical field reflects a combination of the varying degrees of attachment loss matched against the initial bony morphology. Thus, with progressive loss of attachment at, for example, the labial aspect of the mandibular left cuspid with a thin labial bony plate shown in Figure 19.5 (A), the associated osseous resorption leads to total loss of the related supporting bone, resulting in a suprabony pocket. Whereas, at the mandibular right canine a comparable loss of attachment and bony resorption in the presence of a thick labial plate, results in an intrabony pocket, although there is also a suprabony component to this pocket. The interproximal crater

268

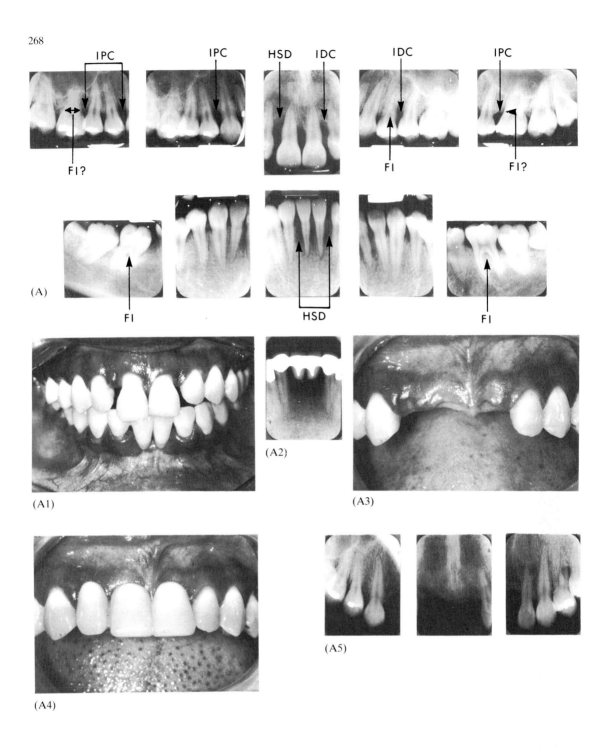

Figure 19.4 Radiographic signs of bony defects and tooth mobility. (A) Full mouth radiographs of 20-year-old woman with varying degrees of breakdown and of furcation involvement (FI) in rapidly progressive periodontitis associated with pathological drifting of incisors and fluctuating grades of mobility. (Key to defects as in Figure 19.2.) Grade II to III mobility at 41, 31 so early removal and provision bridge requested. (A1) Clinical and (A2) radiographic presentation 1 year later. Aesthetics and mobility (Grade I) at 11, 21 remained unacceptable so 12, 11, 21 removed and partial denture fitted pending outcome of therapy at 24. (A3 and A4) Clinical and (A5) radiographic 1 year post-extraction presentation.

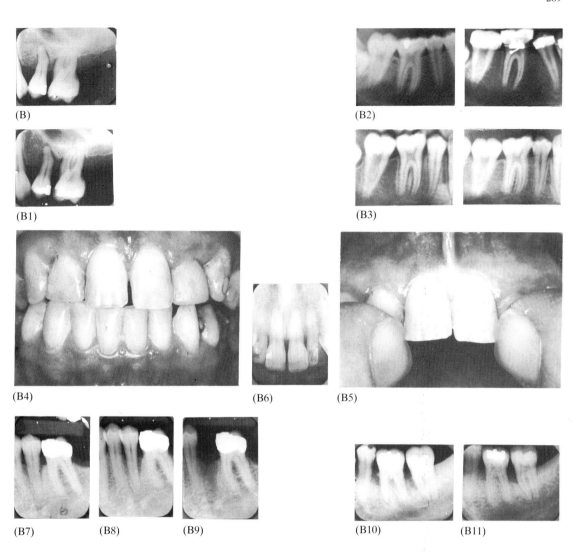

(B)

(B1)

(B2)

(B3)

(B4)

(B6)

(B5)

(B7)

(B8)

(B9)

(B10)

(B11)

Figure 19.4 (*cont.*) (B and B1) Radiographs middle-aged woman with progressive periodontal deterioration over 5-year period at infrabony pocket at 25, 26. Mobility at 25 gradually increased from Grade II to Grade III associated with mobility funnelling (MF), widened periodontal ligament space and apical radiolucency (AR) but with maintained pulpal vitality. (B2) Orthodontically induced funnelling of periodontal ligament space (B3) resolves on completion of therapy. (B4) Traumatic incisal relationship with fluctuating Grade I to II mobility at 11, 21 in 52-year-old woman with long-standing loss of posterior support, minimal attachment loss and marginal tissue health. (B5) Note mesial displacement of 11, 21 on digital pressure. (B6) Radiograph – slight apical radiolucency but no obvious widening of periodontal ligament space. (B7 and B8) Progressive periodontal breakdown at intrabony pocket at 35 with Grade II to III mobility culminating in (B9) extraction after 2 years in adult man with poor oral hygiene. Note funnelled mesial and distal periodontal ligament space represents pattern of periodontal destruction (namely infrabony pocket) rather than effect of mobility, which would be precluded by interproximal contacts. (B10) Grade II mobility at 36, 37 associated with marked gingival inflammation and infrabony pocketing. Note: periodontal widening and apical radiolucencies. (B11) Inflammatory resolution and pocket closure accompanied by tooth stability and disappearance of radiographic signs of mobility.

270

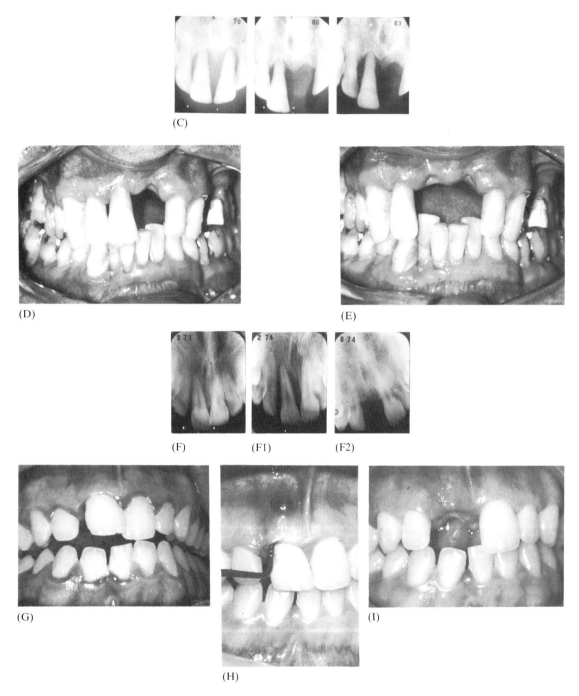

Figure 19.4 (*cont.*)(C) Radiographs of maxillary incisors of middle-aged male with progressive attachment loss plus intrabony pocketing and increasing mobility. Initial presentation (1970) 11 Grade II and 21 Grade III mobility. 21 Exfoliated (1975). 11 Mobility increased Grade III and exfoliated in 1985. Note 'funnelling' effect about mobile teeth. (D) Clinical presentation 1980 and (E) following loss of 11. (F and G) Initial presentation drifted 11 with Grade I mobility in 15-year-old girl with localized rapidly advancing periodontitis. Note 41 extracted due to 'looseness' 2 years previously. Extensive distal interproximal and labial crater at 11. (F1 and H) Orthodontic retraction following improved oral hygiene and incisal edge shortened for aesthetics. Further loss of attachment ensued despite careful debridement and after 6-month retention period acute abscess developed. Note labial sinus. Tooth then extracted lest extensive mesial bony defect compromised 21. Immediate partial denture fitted. (F2 and I) Presentation at 6 months.

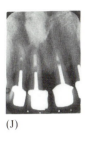
(J)

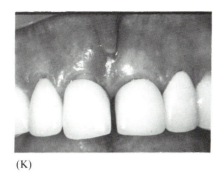
(K)

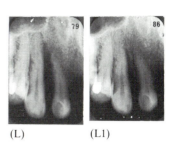
(L) (L1)

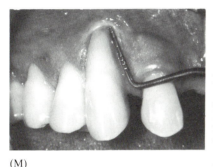
(M)

Figure 19.4 (*cont.*) (J and K) Extensive funnelled mesial intrabony defect at 11 associated with drifting and mobility Grade II. Inadequate root filling suggests primary endodontic lesion. Patient declined treatment. (L) Radiograph extensive mesial interproximal crater associated with marked inflammation and Grade I mobility in 52-year-old man. Surgical reattachment performed. (L1 and M) Pocket closure with some evidence of 'bony fill' and tooth again firmly supported. Maintained for over 6-year assessment period

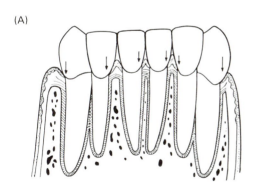
(A)

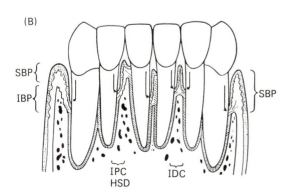
(B)

can be similarly explained by a single interproximal surface lesion at a wide interdental space, depicted between the right incisors in Figure 19.5. Here, an angular bony septal (hemiseptum) defect will develop following resorption of, or in the presence of, developmental labial and lingual bony deficiencies. Where, on the other hand, the teeth are more closely related, as at the central incisors, a total loss of the thin interdental bone septum is inevitable following periodontal destruction at one root surface without attachment loss necessarily occurring at the other. Finally, the interdental crater results from attachment loss at each bounding root

Figure 19.5 Pathogenesis of bony defects. (A) Alveolar bone depicted at 43 and 33 labial aspects is thick at 43 but thin at 33. Note arrows representing sites of advancing plaque fronts. (B) Periodontal destruction with development of an intrabony defect at 43 but suprabony pocket at 33. Note widths of interdental bony septa coupled with the location of advancing plaque fronts (arrowed) dictates form of bony defect. Key: SBP, suprabony pocket; IBP, intrabony pocket; IPC, interproximal crater; IDC, interdental crater; HSD, hemiseptal defect

surface, in the presence of thick facial and lingual bony plates.

The influence of developmental bony dehiscences and fenestrations as shown in Figure 19.3 (D, E and G) (see also Figure 2.3) on bony changes in disease must also be considered. The finding of a dehiscence at operation might be interpreted initially as a localized, but more extensive, loss of attachment; whereas, in reality, the existing supracrestal attachment will merely have been severed during flap preparation. Similarly, periodontal destruction of marginal bone will ultimately transform a fenestration into a dehiscence which may also be subject to clinical misinterpretation. There is no evidence that either of these developmental bony deficiencies increase susceptibility to plaque-induced loss of attachment. (See also Chapter 31 – The nature of bony defects.) However, where surgical exposure is necessary the related root surfaces should be avoided during debridement and optimal post-surgical mucosal coverage always ensured. (See also Figures 15.3 and 15.7 – Split thickness flaps.)

Operative implications

Access for root surface instrumentation

Gaining access and then ensuring adequate instrumentation can be difficult for several reasons as shown in Figure 19.6.

(1) Any residual cervical wedge tissue within bony craters (Figure 19.6 B and C) gets in the way and is difficult to remove.
(2) The bony walls of the defect create difficulties comparable to those encountered during any subgingival instrumentation. However, access and vision are complicated by the inability to, temporarily, displace the bony tissue and, moreover, the instrument tips tend to become wedged between tooth and bone impeding debridement.
(3) The uneven intrabony crestal levels and contours within defects require instrumentation to different depths about the circumferences of each tooth, whilst any complex root morphology involved compounds this difficulty.
(4) Clear vision within these confined sites cannot be readily maintained by surgical aspiration without also obstructing the operator's view with the sucker tip.

Flap adaptation

The existence of bony defects is irrelevant in surgical reattachment. Thus, the flap is simply adapted about the teeth as shown in Figure 19.6 (D), resulting in a relationship with both suprabony (as elsewhere) and intrabony surgical reattachment

components (see below). But in apical repositioning and resection, the intended adaptation of the surgical flap margin to crestal bone (in this case the intrabony crest within an intrabony defect) is impossible. At best the margin can be displaced only just apical to the crest of the bone, in conjunction with the creation of a residual intrabony surgical reattachment relationship (Figure 19.6 E and F).

The interdental morphology usually precludes total mucosal coverage of bone post-surgically even with the benefit of exaggerated scalloping, rendering the presence of any interdental bony defect of little practical importance at this stage (Figure 19.6 G). The postoperative implications of this bony denudation are considered later in this chapter.

Management of intrabony defects
Operative field accessibility
Cervical wedge tissue

Although it is prudent, as in simple pocket surgery, to preserve the supracrestal attachment at the base of the defect (Figure 19.6 C) this is frequently impractical. All soft tissue within bony defects including the supracrestal and transeptal fibre apparatus depicted in Figure 19.6 (C1), is therefore curetted away *in toto*. Any resulting damage sustained to the supracrestal attachment is, in turn, accepted in the interests of expediency, a reduced tendency for bleeding from the otherwise highly vascular inflammatory tissue present and of optimal direct vision for root surface debridement.

The transeptal fibre apparatus constantly remodels during loss of attachment, being maintained between the infiltrated gingival connective tissue and the resorbing bone. Its retention could potentially interfere with optimal bony regeneration within bony defects, by impeding the early passage of osteogenic cells from the bone marrow spaces. The presence of a sclerosed wall to the intrabony defect might similarly hinder healing. Perforation of this bone as shown in Figure 19.6 (C2) to expose the marrow spaces and facilitate the migration of osteogenic cells thus appears to be a reasonable albeit unsubstantiated measure. (See Chapter 31 – Intrabony defect healing.)

Bone form

In some instances the removal of bone may be required to gain access for intrabony root surface debridement. Only non-supporting bone should be sacrificed (Figure 19.6 C2) and the amount dictated by the individual situation and the operator concerned. Thus, a persevering and dexterous operator might succeed without removing any bone while others may need to do so. Recontouring of

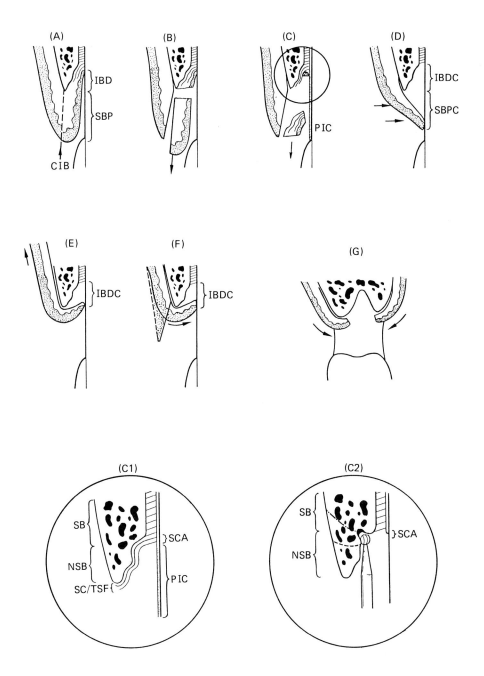

Figure 19.6 Operative implications of intrabony pockets. (A) Conserving (CIB) inverse bevel incision depicted here located within the suprabony (SBP) component of the pocket leaving intrabony defect (IBD) component intact. (B) Removal of suprabony cervical wedge tissue. (C) Removal of intrabony tissue and exposure of 'periodontally involved' cementum (PIC). (C1) Intact supracrestal attachment (SCA), supracrestal/transeptal fibre apparatus (SC/TSF) lining bony defect. Supporting (SB) and non-supporting (NSB) bone also shown. (C2) Curettage of intrabony tissue exposes bone and disrupts SCA. Note instrumented root surface, perforation of medullary spaces with bur and resection of NSB component of defect and recontouring of SB (osteoplasty). (D) Surgical reattachment with suprabony pocket component (SBPC). (E) Apical repositioning and where appropriate (F) resection flap margin adaptation. Flap margin may become slightly displaced into some defects. Residual intrabony defect component (IBDC) present in each instance. (G) Postsurgical interdental bony denudation not complicated significantly by presence of interdental bony crater

bone (osteoplasty) to enhance subsequent flap adaptation is also considered by some, but is not advocated here.

Practical hints and precautions

(1) The availability of appropriate instruments for intrabony root surface debridement is obviously critical. Fine 'Gracy' type curettes are preferable but the more recent wider acceptance of ultrasonic devices during surgical procedures has greatly simplified instrumentation. (See also Chapter 31 – Surgical elimination of intrabony defects.) Indeed, the Cavitron TF-10 insert is advocated for routine use and has the added advantage of greatly reducing operator fatigue.

(2) Periodontal surgery involving bony defects is undoubtedly more difficult and time consuming. Individual operator conscientiousness, endurance and experience and, not least, patient tolerance and cooperation must be acknowledged in treatment planning. Thus, too large a surgical field must not be undertaken at any one time, lest difficulties encountered compromise the intended successful completion of surgical objectives.

(3) Residual tissue tags within interproximal bony defects should ideally be avoided lest an exuberant tissue overgrowth results during healing and compromises the ultimate outcome of surgery. This is especially true of furcation associated bony defects. (See also Chapter 18.)

Flap and bone management

Intrabony crest/flap margin relationship

In practical terms an inconsistency exists between the crestal bone and surgical flap margin contour with respect to flap adaptation as shown in Figure 19.8 (E). During surgical reattachment this is irrelevant and may possibly even be more advantageous than a purely suprabony reattachment relationship (see below). Whereas in pocket elimination surgery the inconsistency has important practical implications. The removal of the non-supporting bone forming the defect will, in itself, not resolve the problem of flap adaptation to the crestal bone because the inconsistency still remains (Figure 19.8 F). As a component of surgical reattachment is thus enforced and is furthermore often mandatory at suprabony pocket sites elsewhere, because of bony inconsistencies, (see Figure 15.14), its feasibility as an elective surgical option at intrabony crestal inconsistencies cannot be dismissed.

Operative options

During apical repositioning and resection techniques, bony defects may, in the first place, be simply accepted and the flap adapted over the crest of the bone, as shown in Figure 19.6 (E and F) for intrabony surgical reattachment (see Figure 19.7). Secondly, the defect could be filled in with bone from other sources as in orthopaedic grafting procedures (Figure 19.8 B), or the non-supporting bone displaced (swaged) into the defect (Figure 19.8 A). Thirdly, this bone could be removed *in toto* (osteo-ectomy), so converting the defect into a suprabony pocket (Figure 19.8 C) which is then eliminated by a further inverse bevel resection or apical repositioning (Figure 19.7 D). This bone removal is prudent only when the adjacent supporting bone will not be compromised or additional problems of furcation involvement introduced. Furthermore it must be reiterated that removal of non-supporting bone is of limited benefit where problems of flap margin/crestal bone inconsistencies will persist as shown in Figure 19.8 (E and F). The likely nature of healing to be expected with each surgical option is now considered.

Reparative potential of bone

Surgical reattachment

As optimal healing in suprabony situations demands close adaptation of the surgical flap to root surface, the same might reasonably be expected to apply within intrabony pockets. Although flap coaptation is obviously not possible within the intrabony part of the pocket (Figure 19.7 A), bony regeneration (bone fill) is possible. The presence of any non-supporting bone thus appears to be advantageous during healing and should be conserved wherever possible. Defects bounded on all sides by bony walls (three-walled defects) apparently have the best chance of success, but the clinical findings are inconsistent. Some resorption of the crest of the bone does, however, always occur and bony regeneration is possible only to this level (Figure 19.7 C) and never coronal to it. (See Chapter 31 – Intrabony defect healing.)

It must be stressed that bony regeneration within an intrabony defect is not synonymous with the development of a new periodontal ligament (new attachment) depicted in its ideal form at Figure 19.7 (B). A very limited extent of new attachment is however possible immediately coronal to the existing periodontal ligament as in suprabony surgical reattachment (*cf.* Chapter 15). Similarly, a long junctional epithelium is the best that can be hoped for, with or without and bony fill (Figure 19.7 C), although pocket closure alone (Figure 19.7 C) is most commonly encountered.

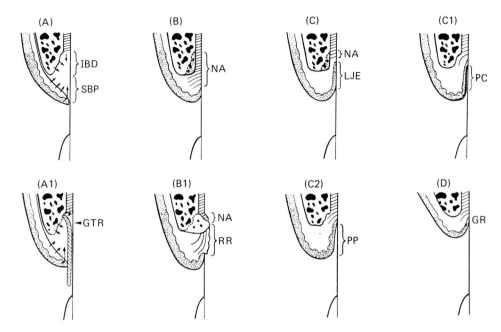

Figure 19.7 Osseous response to surgical options. (A) Flap margin/intrabony crest inconsistency accepted for surgical reattachment with intrabony defect (IBD) and suprabony pocket (SBP) components. Origins of reparative tissue cells arrowed. (A1) Potential for biological tissue filter placement (*cf.* Figure 14.3) to guide periodontal ligament tissue regeneration (GTR) and favour new attachment. (B) Theoretically ideal healing with bony regeneration and both intrabony and suprabony new attachment (NA). (B1) Root resorption (RR) from gingival connective tissue and from regenerating bone coupled with bony ankylosis observed following experimentally retarded epithelial downgrowth. (C) Optimal healing with minimal new attachment, crestal bone resorption and bony regeneration (bone fill), plus an interposed long junctional epithelium (LJE). (C1) Usual outcome of slight resorption of bony crest plus minimal bony fill associated with primarily suprabony soft tissue pocket closure (PC). (C2) Persistent pocket (PP). (D) Possible gradual crestal bony resorption plus gingival recession (GR) with progressive pocket reduction

Periodontal ligament cells alone have the capacity to establish a new attachment. The other three periodontal tissue components, the surgical flap epithelium and its connective tissue and the bone depicted in Figure 19.7 (A) each demonstrate peculiar healing patterns in relation to the root surface, as shown in experimental models. These are, in turn, a long junctional epithelium as described above (Figure 19.7 C); connective tissue apposition with fibre orientation parallel to but not attached to the root and possibly associated with what is described as cervical root resorption and, finally, bony ankylosis in conjunction with root resorption, referred to as resorption ankylosis (Figure 19.7 B). (See also Chapter 31 – The role of bone in new attachment.)

Of the possible outcomes of healing, the most frequent finding of an epithelium can be attributed to the differential rates of cell repopulation of the wound. Epithelial cells proliferate rapidly over wound surfaces such as the surgical flap, thereby thwarting ideal healing via a new connective tissue attachment. On the other hand, this epithelial

downgrowth does serve to prevent possible root resorption and ankylosis mediated by osteoclasts and gingival connective tissue cells (see Chapter 31 – Bone grafting). A technique for favouring the selective proliferation of periodontal ligament tissue cells coronally over the root surface during healing, for enhanced new attachment, referred to as guided tissue regeneration (see Figure 19.7 A1), appears most promising. (See also Chapter 31 – Preferential repopulation investigations.)

A few clinical investigations on single rooted teeth, have demonstrated the considerable potential for bony regeneration within intrabony defects although associated with a slight loss at the crest of the bone, following surgical attachment therapy that ensured optimal postoperative mucosal coverage of bone and a high standard of plaque control during healing. There have also been numerous other clinical reports and experimental model findings claiming successful bony regeneration and new attachment following intrabony surgical reattachment therapy alone, and when combined with root surface 'conditioning' with citric acid, although other investigators have consistently failed to achieve this. (See Chapter 31 – Intrabony defect healing and acid conditioning.)

In conclusion, current knowledge indicates that bone regeneration following intrabony surgical reattachment is a feasible if not predictable clinical objective. Where successful, this occurs in association with a long junctional epithelium, the long-term outcome of which has yet to be established. The technique is therefore advocated as routine clinical practice in anticipation of this type of healing and pending the outcome of controlled clinical investigations. On the other hand, it must be conceded that the outcome in most instances is, at best, likely to be one of pocket closure alone or with the development of a long junctional epithelium, but with little or no bone regeneration (Figure 19.7 C and C1). The pocket may also persist in some instances as shown in Figure 19.7 (C and C1). This is most likely at molar teeth, presumably as a result of poor access for plaque control and the influence of furcation morphology. Even so the suprabony component and, to a lesser extent, the crests of the bony defects at residual pockets do tend to remodel over a period of time, gradually reducing the pocket depths (Figure 19.7 D).

Bone grafting

Bony regeneration might be enhanced by packing the defect with bone (Figure 19.8 B) or by bone swaging (Figure 19.8 A). In the latter the bony wall of the defect is partially detached at its alveolar base with a bone chisel and then deflected against the root. Whereas in grafting, bone is used in a bone chip-blood mixture, derived from non-supporting bone in the surgical field, healing extraction sockets, the maxillary tuberosity or extra-oral haemopoietic sites like the iliac crest. Bone substitutes have also been used. The techniques merely represent adjuncts to the intrabony surgical reattachment and none have been shown, in controlled studies in humans, to be consistently advantageous and may even carry the risk of root resorption and ankylosis. (See Chapter 31 – Bone grafting.)

Bone resection

The removal of non-supporting bone with the view to merely reducing flap margin/crest of bone contour inconsistencies is not advocated. However, this bone might reasonably be removed when it is possible to not only eliminate the defect altogether, but if the resulting greater suprabony soft tissue component of the pocket can also be corrected, by the appropriate tissue resection or selective apical repositioning, as shown in Figure 19.8 (C and D).

Removal of prominent bone margin crests that cause mucosal blanching following flap adaptation is prudent, so as to further minimize the intrinsic risks of ischaemic necrosis of the unsupported suprabony parts of the flap at intrabony sites (see Figure 19.6 E and F). Similarly, reduction of non-supporting bone may be preferable to post-surgical bony denudation

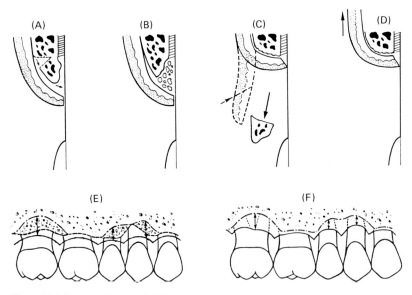

Figure 19.8 Osseous therapy. (A) Bone swaging. (B) Bone grafting for intrabony surgical reattachment. (C) Bone resection and optimal flap adaptation following further trimming and (D) apical repositioning. (E) Vertical discrepancy (arrowed) between the flap margin and intrabony crests. (F) This is improved but not corrected by removal of non-supporting bone

where flap margin deficiencies arise through surgical misjudgement although, when supporting bone is involved, denudation should be tolerated as a lesser evil.

The simple technique of removing non-supporting bone to correct intrabony defects must be kept in perspective. First and foremost, it should be reiterated that inconsistencies between flap margin and crestal bone contours may not be significantly reduced so that a surgical reattachment relationship is still imposed. Furthermore, there appears to be little advantage in eliminating the bony component of any such mandatory surgical reattachment procedure and indeed, surgical interference might possibly even be inimical to healing. Secondly, an unacceptable removal of adjacent supporting bone about the tooth itself and, more importantly, its neighbouring units, might also become necessary to create the overall bony contour that is commensurate with flap adaptation for pocket elimination at the initial intrabony defect site. Thirdly, this bone removal might introduce an additional problem with respect to furcation involvement. Finally, as will be discussed below, the mere surgical exposure of bone at operation and even more so its surgical reduction will result, in many instances, in a further net loss of crestal bone and possibly also periodontal attachment. (See also Chapter 31 – Effects of bone resection.)

Flap adaptation

The surgical flap is, as elsewhere in simple pocket surgery, adapted about the necks of the teeth and over the crest of the bone and an intrabony and, where necessary, a suprabony surgical reattachment relationship accepted as shown in Figure 19.7 (A). Interproximally, mucosal inadequacies, both laterally and mesiodistally should be expected, although where this has been anticipated and initially exaggerated scalloped flap margins created (see Chapters 14 and 16), greater interproximal coverage can be achieved as shown in Figure 19.9 (A and D1). Interproximal flap adaptation may also be enhanced by short oblique relieving incisions over supporting bone at the contralateral line angles of the related teeth (Figure 19.9 D1 and F1). This has a localized elongating effect on the interdental papillary peaks and also permits tissue adaptation into any defects. The latter results in an overall soft tissue contour

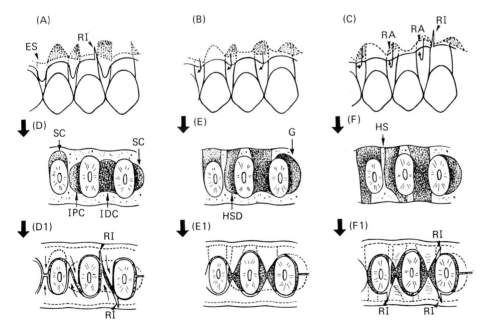

Figure 19.9 Flap adaptation at interproximal intrabony defects. (A) Surgical flap margin prior to adaptation showing exaggerated scalloped (ES) contour between 16 and 15 and relieving incision (RI) at 14. (B) Flap adaptation into interproximal spaces. (C) Papillary tissue adaptation into intrabony defects between 15 and 14 and 14 and 13 facilitated by RI but creates reverse gingival architecture (RA). (D, E and F) Sectional views of different degrees of bony defects as in Figure 19.2. (D1) Optimal interproximal mucosal coverage from exaggerated scalloping with papillary peaks butting end-on between 16 and 15 and papillary tissue overlapping between 15 and 14 and 14 and 13, the latter enhanced by relieving incisions. (E1) Mucosal deficiencies predispose to postsurgical cratering. (F1) Relieving incisions for papillary adaptation

with interdental craters rather than peaks – this is aptly described as a reverse gingival architecture (Figure 19.9 C).

Summary

As the resection of bone may create other, potentially more serious, problems each situation must be carefully assessed and, where necessary, a surgical compromise of intrabony surgical reattachment resorted to. The alternative option of only a partial bony reduction in situations where total removal is not feasible, raises the fundamental question of the rationale for the elective tolerance of a residual, but less extensive, bony defect. Thus, might the initial intrabony defect not have been equally acceptable? To find the answer to this question further controlled investigation will be required.

Some bony regeneration is possible within bone defects, particularly at single rooted teeth, following optimal postoperative mucosal coverage and high standards of plaque control during healing. Other methods to stimulate bone growth are insufficiently predictable and, coupled with the risk of side effects, are not recommended. In most instances, attempted intrabony surgical reattachment results in pocket closure with, at best, a long junctional epithelium with little or no bony regeneration. Elsewhere, reduced and hopefully more manageable pockets persist, although these together with pocket closure sites tend to become shallower by further tissue shrinkage and remodelling. Finally, the results of guided tissue regeneration are promising and warrant further investigation.

Bone behaviour in surgical therapy

Response to surgical intervention

In the surgical approach advocated, bone is routinely exposed. This, in itself, has been shown to cause some superficial bony necrosis followed by resorption coupled with the possibility of some attachment loss. The damage sustained from the trauma of surgical exposure alone, is furthermore increased by direct instrumentation of the bone and even more so by the failure to cover bone with mucosa postoperatively. (See also Chapter 31 – The treatment of intrabony defects.)

The bony necrosis can be attributed to a combination of factors: initially, the physical disturbance of its overlying periosteum by surgical flap elevation; the exposure of bone to an unphysiological external environment; and the associated temporary disruption of its superficial blood supply derived from the mucosa. In addition, there is the unavoidable physical instrumentation during operation and

aggravated by elective osseous surgery and, most importantly perhaps, postoperative ischaemia following post-surgical denudation. Finally the possible influence of post-surgical microbial damage cannot be excluded.

The necrotic bone is first resorbed during healing and is then followed by a compensatory bony regeneration, but a net bone loss and an associated attachment loss is almost always sustained. This is most marked, amounting to about 1 mm of crestal bone height under the most adverse surgical conditions cited, and more especially at situations with only intrinsically thin cortical type bone. Thick cancellous type bone on the other hand, does ultimately tolerate these assaults more favourably. Finally, it must be reiterated that bony regeneration occurs only within bony defects and never coronal to the presurgical crestal bone level.

Handling of bone during surgery

There are a number of basic common-sense precautions that should be observed, some of which have already been referred to in previous chapters.

(1) Bone should be exposed only sufficiently to satisfy the immediate surgical objectives; that is, flap reflection should routinely be as conservative as possible.

(2) Surgically exposed bone should be maintained in as physiological an environment as possible throughout the operation. Only the immediate area being instrumented needs to be clearly visible, elsewhere the surgical flap being put back in position over bone. Where this is not practical, a layer of blood is best retained over the bone. This, in turn, means that super-efficient aspiration efforts by the chairside assistant to establish bloodless surgical fields, coupled with extensive surgical flap retraction to enhance visibility during operation should be avoided. Where, however, technical considerations demand prolonged exposure and a totally clear vision of bone a saline drip is essential. The likelihood of bone desiccation is greatly reduced by the use of an ultrasonic scaling device for root surface debridement. This is because it not only speeds up operating time in difficult situations, but also constantly irrigates the surgical field by virtue of the coolant water spray. The use of mains water pressure precludes the desired optimal isotonic environment and also introduces the possible risk of extraneous contamination. However, in practice, neither appears to be of any clinical significance, but each is readily overcome by using saline in a chemically sterilized, pressurized garden-spray type apparatus that has been adapted for clinical use.

(3) Where bone removal is indicated, and especially for pre-restorative purposes (*cf.* Chapter 24), this must always be carried out under either bloody conditions, although visibility will be slightly impeded, or a saline drip. Burs are most commonly used for gross reduction but some dentists prefer bone chisels (e.g. Ochsenbein, Rhodes – see Figure 24.5). Enamel chisels and gingival margin trimmers and ultrasonic sealer tips (TF-3 and 10) are also suitable for any finer reductions required. Ultrasonic devices are especially helpful in confined interproximal and inter-radicular spaces (*cf.* Chapter 18) and do not have any apparent adverse effects – see also Chapter 31 – Bony resection techniques. Indeed, as yet, there is no substantial evidence to support the superiority of any one method of bone removal, so the choice remains a personal one.

When using burs, frictional heat is generated which, despite irrigant cooling, may cause further damage. The largest round bur that can be accommodated in the surgical field and used at the lowest possible speed, to minimize heat production, is advocated. The ever-present risk of catching the overlying flap and notching the related tooth surfaces must always be guarded against. The latter is most readily prevented by refraining from burring thin crestal bone and removing these small remaining parts with hand instruments instead as shown in Figure 24.5–24.7.

(4) A periosteal connective tissue 'protective' layer could be retained over bone by routinely preparing split thickness type surgical flaps. That means the filletting incision extends all the way to the base of the flap, (as shown in Figure 15.7) leaving the periosteum *in situ*. The simple pocket surgical approach permits this facility in all situations including, with appropriate modification, the indirect resection technique. However, the preparation of such flaps is technically more difficult and carries the risk of flap perforation, which might ultimately prove to be a greater hazard than surgical bone exposure. Furthermore, available evidence (see Chapter 31 – Surgical mucosal coverage) suggests that provided the mucosal flap is closely adapted about the teeth at completion of operation, healing is the same regardless of whether periosteum is retained or not. For these reasons split-thickness flaps are not recommended for routine use.

Bone healing following surgery

The reparative fronts

Healing of bone can occur on three separate fronts, the surgical flap connective tissue and any associated periosteum, the marrow space endosteum and the periodontal ligament as shown in Figure 19.10 (B). The influence of gingival epithelium need not be considered further here.

The pattern of healing depends on a combination of the bony morphology itself and the relationship of the reparative fronts to the bony wound site, of which the most critical appears to be that of the surgical flaps to crestal bone. Flap margin crestal bone approximation is precluded in many parts of the surgical field because of the uneven pattern of periodontal destruction commonly encountered and, as might be expected, also interproximally. Fortunately, the reparative potential of the interdental bone is, by virtue of its cancellous structure in common with that of thick facial and oral alveolar bone with substantial endosteal marrow spaces, better suited to withstanding the effects of surgical trauma than thin cortical type bone elsewhere. The periodontal ligament may contribute to healing at its coronal edge adjacent to the necrosing crestal bone and from within the ligament space itself. However, the potential at the former might initially be impeded by the trauma inevitably sustained during root debridement.

The reparative roles of each of the individual tissue fronts are first considered under conditions of optimal flap adaptation. Then the influence of post-surgical bony denudation and of the subsequent mucosal regeneration will be dealt with. Due to the lack of suitable human histological material, much of current knowledge stems from experimentally induced lesions in animal models.

Optimal mucosal coverage

The necrosed bone first undergoes osteoclastic resorption in an initial resorptive phase and is followed by a reparative phase in which new bone is formed by osteoblasts. The resorption of the superficial necrotic bone stemming from mucosal connective tissue, is called frontal resorption (Figure 19.10 B). This commences within 3–4 days and continues for approximately 2 weeks. An undermining resorption of necrotic bone also occurs from the related marrow spaces and when the bone is thin (Figure 19.10 E), from the periodontal ligament thereby enhancing the overall rate of resorption. In undermining resorption, the still vital bone located between the superficial necrotic layer and the resorbing osteoclastic cells is removed first.

When the rate of undermining resorption exceeds that of the frontal resorption and the residual necrotic bone becomes separated from the alveolus, a bony sequestrum results. Sequestration has however been encountered only infrequently in clinical practice. This may reflect the mandatory mucosal coverage of bone advocated, which both minimizes bony necrosis and facilitates a more complete frontal resorption. Furthermore, the few instances of sequestration witnessed have each been associated with inadequate flap preparation and post-surgical bony denudation or postoperative mucosal ulceration (see Figures 17.4 and 17.5).

The osteoblastic reparative phase commences within about 10 days with granulation tissue proliferation from the gingival connective tissue, periodontal ligament and marrow spaces. Repair progresses for 4–5 weeks although when complicated, as with bony denudation and sequestration (see below), total functional repair (Figure 19.10 C and F) may take up to several months.

Influence of osseous morphology

Thin compact supporting bone at suprabony pockets (Figure 19.10 D) is primarily sustained during healing by the overlying flap mucosa and periodontal ligament and so is more vulnerable to irreversible bone loss, although not necessarily to attachment loss. The limited crestal bone reformation results in a slightly increased supracrestal soft tissue attachment as depicted in Figure 19.10 (F). In contrast, thick cancellous supporting bone (Figure 19.10 A) is sustained additionally by its generous medullary component, so withstands surgical intervention with little crestal loss (Figure 19.10 C).

As non-supporting bone at intrabony craters (Figure 19.10 A1 and D1) is susceptible to superficial bony necrosis on both its outer (as elsewhere) and, as a result of the removal of intrabony connective tissue at operation – its inner aspects as well, a greater overall resorption is to be expected. The net loss of bone at the crest of the defect, following healing, has the effect of reducing the vertical dimensions of any residual bony deformity especially at thin bony sites (Figure 19.10 E1 and F1). The potential for bony regeneration is in turn greater at thick non-supporting bone as depicted in Figure 19.10 (B1 and C1), by virtue of the enhanced reparative potential of the adjacent medullary spaces. The potential for post-surgical gingival recession is also rather less initially, at thick than at thin bony sites (Figure 19.10 C1 and F1), although recession may occur with time (Figure 19.10 C2). On the other hand pocketing might recur instead as depicted at Figure 19.10 (C3).

Finally, the interdental bone withstands the effects of surgical intervention in the most favourable fashion. This is presumably because it is more adequately sustained by the combination of its inherent generous medullary blood supply and that stemming from the adjacent periodontal ligaments (Figure 19.10 G and H). The effects of the almost inevitable post-surgical denudation on healing is examined next.

Influence of interdental denudation

In simple pocket surgery the denuded interdental bone is covered initially with a blood clot (Figure 19.11 A and A1). This granulates over within a few days by tissue proliferation from the adjacent periodontal ligaments, the underlying exposed marrow spaces and the facial and oral flaps (Figure 19.11 B and B1). The small surface area of superficial necrotic interdental bone soon undergoes undermining resorption from the medullary spaces and regenerates with no bony deformity. Similarly, the regeneration of a new gingival septum is uneventful (Figure 19.11 C and C1).

Healing at interdental bony defects (Figure 19.11 D, E and F) is essentially comparable, but is slower because of the greater size of the lesion and the pattern of bony regeneration is unpredictable (Figure 19.11 F and F1). An interdental gingival deformity results, initially conforming to the shape of the residual bony crater and creating a reverse gingival architecture in which the interdental soft tissue lies apical to that of the facial and oral tissues. The mucosal crater tends gradually to become reduced by a combination of soft tissue proliferation, resorption of the crests of the defect and bony regeneration within the defect as shown in Figure 19.11 (F and F1). Residual probing depths are, however, frequently encountered. The clinical outcome at intrabony sites cannot be predicted with any degree of certainty and further carefully controlled investigation is required. (See also Chapter 31 – Preferential repopulation investigations.)

Inadvertent denudation

Facial or oral bone may become denuded through excessive tissue resection or apically repositioning or be the result of flap margin necrosis as depicted at Figure 19.12 (A and D). Healing is more complex and delayed compared with interdental denudation. This is because of the extensive bony necrosis that occurs and the need for mucosal regeneration and the re-establishment of a new dentogingival junction. (See also Chapter 20.)

Bony healing at thick bony sites (Figure 19.12 A–C) is very similar to that at denuded interdental bone. The bone thus granulates over a period of 2–3 weeks by tissue proliferation from the marginal periodontal ligament, the bony marrow spaces via existing channels to the surface or following undermining resorption of superficial necrotic bone and, lastly, from the surgical flap tissue (Figure 19.12 B). These proliferating tissues gradually merge as shown in Figure 19.12 (G) and form a new mucosa. Maturation of this regenerated mucosa occurs within about 6–8 weeks (Figure 19.12 C and

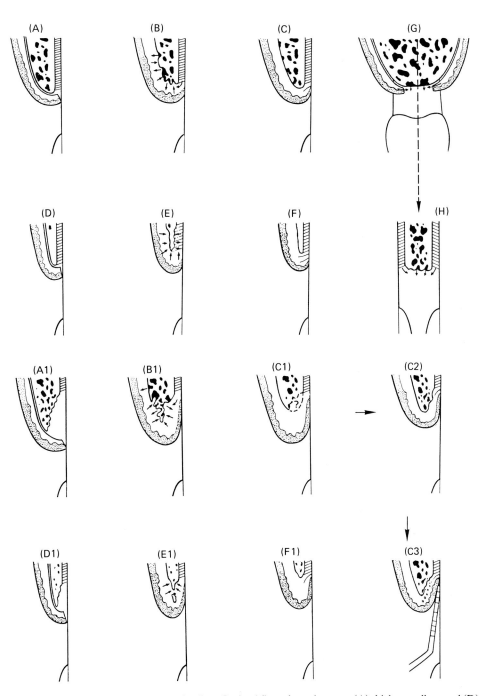

Figure 19.10 Suprabony pocket bony healing. Optimal flap adaptation over (A) thick cancellous and (D) thin cortical bone. (B) Origins of proliferating reparative connective tissue cells (arrows) in frontal and undermining (medullary) resorption. (C) Total repair. (E) Frontal plus undermining resorption from the periodontal ligament. (F) Net bone loss and slight attachment loss associated with increased length of supracrestal attachment. (G) Interdental mucosal deficiency and (H) mesiodistal view at plane of dotted arrow line showing origins of reparative tissue proliferation. (A1–F1) Show comparable intrabony healing but (B1 and E1) greater necrosis and resorption at non-supporting bone. Note loss of crest of bone with reduction of intrabony defect coupled with potential for subsequent bony regeneration (?) at (C1), but elimination of defect at (F1). (C2) Usual healing with residual intrabony defect associated with gradual gingival recession and reduction of suprabony component of pocket. (C3) Probing depth with recurrent inflammation

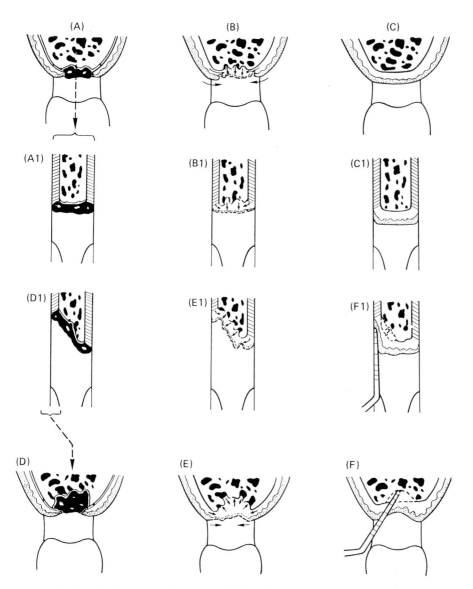

Figure 19.11 Interdental bony healing. (A and A1) Suprabony mucosal deficiency occluded by blood clot. (B and B1) Undermining resorption and granulation tissue proliferation from medullary spaces, periodontal ligament and flap margins followed by wound epithelialization. (C and C1) Healing with no deformity. (D–F) Similar healing sequence at intrabony defects. Note residual bony crater and probing depth but with possibility ? of bony fill (broken lines) at (F and F1)

H). Small bony sequestra might sometimes discharge via sinuses through the regenerating mucosa which then heal.

Where the denuded bone is thin and cortical in structure (Figure 19.12 D), healing is similar but the undermining resorption is mediated by the periodontal ligament cells instead (Figure 19.12 E). A total and irreversible loss of denuded bone usually results and while under favourable conditions will be associated with a long supracrestal attachment (Figure 19.12 F), attachment loss often occurs instead, leading to localized gingival recession as

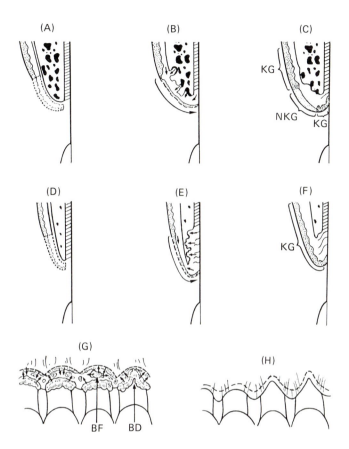

Figure 19.12 Bony denudation. Denudation of (A) thick and (D) thin bone following flap margins necrosis (ghosted) or mucosal deficiencies. (B) Reparative granulation tissue derived from remaining intact surgical flap, the medullary spaces and the marginal periodontal ligament, following undermining resorption of necrotic bone and epithelialization (E) Thin bone and lack of medullary spaces minimizes bony contribution, but that of periodontal ligament enhanced by undermining resorption which may be associated with bony sequestration. (C) Slight attachment loss and minimal residual bony deformity compared to (F) marked bone loss coupled with some loss of attachment and establishment of long supracrestal attachment. Note distribution of healed keratinized gingiva (KG) from surgical flap and periodontal ligament sources and non-keratinized tissue (NKG) from medullary spaces in (F and C). (G) Granulation stemming from surgical flap margin and marginal periodontal ligament as well as from bony fenestration (BF) and bony dehiscence (BD). (H) Healed gingival contour with recession at both dehiscence site and fenestration following loss of marginal bone and its related attachment

shown in Figure 19.12 (H). As thin bony sites tend to be associated with bony dehiscences and fenestrations, this greatly facilitates periodontal ligament involvement in healing and, in turn, influences the nature of the regenerated mucosa.

Mucosal regeneration over denuded bone

The characteristics of the regenerated mucosa are dictated by the origins of the proliferating granulation tissue. When derived from the surgical flap margin, the resulting mucosa is, as might be expected, of a similar structure. In most instances the surgical flap is comprised of gingiva which induces keratinized tissue. The periodontal ligament tissue also induces the development of keratinized tissue as shown in Figure 19.12 (C and F). Alveolar bone and its marrow spaces will in turn induce the development of a non-keratinized mucosa (Figure 19.12 C), although the ultimate nature of the mucosa developing over bone also depends in part upon the structure of the denuded bone. Thus, if the bone is thin, the undermining resorption exposes and involves periodontal ligament and keratinized

tissue is induced at that site instead (Figure 19.12 E and F). Consequently, a mixture of keratinized and non-keratinized mucosa tends to develop, depending on the features of each surgical field and the competitive rates of proliferation of each contributing component, although the final outcome at any single inadvertently denuded bony site cannot be predicted. This intriguing issue is considered further in Chapter 20. The sequence of healing following inadvertent bone denudation is shown clinically in Figure 17.5. (See also Chapter 32 – Gingival dimensions and gingival health.)

Post-surgical management of bony defects

The post-surgical management of any intrabony defect depends as elsewhere on a high standard of plaque control. The peculiar difficulties of negotiating these must therefore be pointed out and the appropriate methods of cleaning demonstrated to the patient. The interspace brush is advocated, its bristles first being splayed out against the coronal tooth surface and gently passed pressed apically into the defect as shown in Figure 18.5. Care must, however, be taken during the first few months not to damage the newly forming junctional epithelium.

Interdental craters are less easily negotiated and as they may be associated with an exuberant tissue overgrowth (e.g. see Figure 26.6), bleed freely when cleaning and may deter the patient. Nevertheless, diligent and careful cleaning efforts with a softer type interspace brush (e.g. Mentadent Inter) is often rewarded by gingival shrinkage and the maintenance of a stable reverse gingival architecture. It does, however, appear that the facial and oral bony margins of these defects gradually reduce with time for they do become shallower. Whether this remodelling is a physical effect of the brush used as advocated, or is simply a spontaneous tissue change is not clear.

Summary

The pattern of bone resorption in periodontal breakdown can be attributed to a combination of the variable behaviour of bacterial plaque and the bony morphology at different parts of the dental arches. The resulting bony defects impede root surface instrumentation and thwart the creation of the surgical flap margin crestal bone relationship necessary for pocket elimination. Although the outcome of bony regeneration procedures is not predictable, it is usually preferable to the attempted surgical contouring of these defects to satisfy the local requirements. This is because the penalties sustained by bone removal at adjacent sites and, more especially, root furcations rarely warrants it. Compromise solutions of surgical reattachment are therefore once again necessary. Even so, as with the technical difficulties imposed by root morphology, the prognosis at sites with bony defects appears to be very much better than traditionally thought. The influence of the last of the three morphological barriers to successful simple pocket surgery, that of vestibular tissues, can now be considered.

20

Complex pocket surgery:
III Vestibular morphology

Vestibular form
Variable clinical presentations in disease

Operative implications
Summary

Vestibular form

The vestibular tissue morphology constitutes the last
of the periodontal anatomical features liable to
complicate simple pocket surgery. Although the
gingiva is part of the vestibule both functionally and
anatomically, the vestibular tissues are deemed, for
descriptive purposes in this chapter, to commence at
the mucogingival junction. Thus, only the alveolar
mucosa, its contiguous vestibular mucosal fold and
the opposing facial and lingual oral mucosa, are
considered.

In health, the form of the facial vestibular tissue is
trough-like, its depth being dictated by the variable
levels of the lip and cheek mucosal reflections
(Figure 20.1 A). It is shallowest where it merges
with the mandibular retromolar tissues, the maxillary tuberosity and the soft palate and at muscle
(frenal) insertions. The lingual vestibule is, on the
other hand, rather shelf-like in relation to the floor
of the mouth and sublingual salivary glands and only
forms a trough at the base of the tongue and where
prominent lingual frena exist.

Variable clinical presentations in disease

Involvement of vestibular tissue in pocket surgery
depends on the extent of breakdown in relation to
the gingival dimensions (namely amount of keratinized tissue) and vestibular morphology. For
example, buccal pockets of moderate depth at
maxillary molars, where a wide gingival band and

deep vestibule usually exist, would be contained
within gingiva (Figure 20.1 B). Whereas, labial
pockets of similar depth at mandibular incisors,
associated with a narrower gingival band and
shallow vestibule, could extend to or even be apical
to the mucogingival junction (Figure 20.1 C3).
Deeper pockets will, in turn, involve alveolar
mucosa or even reach the vestibular reflection
(Figure 20.1 C1 and C2). Vestibular tissue involvement in periodontal pocketing thus depends primarily on the existence of reduced gingival dimensions,
as determined developmentally for the particular
site or following marginal gingival recession.

Despite the numerous permutations of the variables shown in Figure 20.1, only three basic
situations (which tend to occur most commonly in
the mandible and so are represented diagrammatically as such here) need be considered:

(1) The pocket base is adjacent to the mucogingival
    junction so that the pocket wall is comprised of
    gingival tissue alone (Figure 20.1 C).
(2) The pocket extends beyond the mucogingival
    junction and so incorporates an alveolar mucos-
    al component (Figure 20.1 C1).
(3) The pocket base is located apical to the level of
    the vestibular fold (Figure 20.1 C2) which then
    also forms part of the pocket wall.

In each situation an added possible complication of
a reduced or complete lack of gingival tissue may
exist, as depicted in Figure 20.1 (C3 and D). The
effects of this on surgical therapy itself and on the
maintenance of marginal tissue health must therefore also be considered.

285

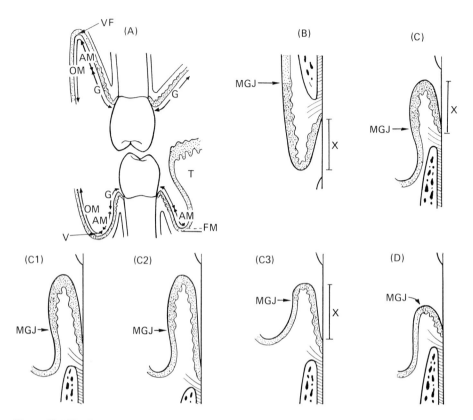

Figure 20.1 Vestibular morphology. (A) Composite representation of vestibular form. Key: G, gingiva; AM, alveolar mucosa; VF, vestibular fold; OM, oral mucosa; FM, floor of mouth (depicted as broken line); T, tongue. Varying relationship of mucogingival junction (MG) and vestibular fold is shown in B–E. Moderate pocket 'X' (B) contained within wide gingival band, (C) base is level with and (C3) apical to mucogingival junction (MG). With progressive attachment loss at (C), pocket extends (C1) into alveolar mucosa, and (C2) beyond vestibular fold. Note pocket at (C3) associated with a narrow gingival band. (D) Loss of gingival band following surgery or gingival recession resulting in location of MG at the gingival margin

Operative implications

The surgical management of pockets becomes progressively more difficult with each successive pocket relationship cited above. Thus, whilst surgical flap preparation and management technique described for simple pocket surgery is still applicable, certain refinements are demanded by the difficulties imposed by the different tissue characteristics and vestibular mucosal form. In addition, the intended flap positioning and stabilization is often impossible, thwarting the overall surgical objective. These technical difficulties and their management are examined next.

Flap preparation

Pocket base adjacent to mucogingival junction (Figure 20.2)

In simple pocket surgery the filletting incision is contained within gingival tissue and so meets bone coronal to the mucogingival junction (Figure 20.2 A). Any further flap preparation required is then carried out by blunt dissection, facilitated by the cleavage plane between mucosa and bone (Figure 20.2 A1). When, however, the mucogingival junctional mucosa forms the apical part of the pocket wall, as in Figure 20.2 (B), the sharp filletting dissection must extend beyond it. This dissection is

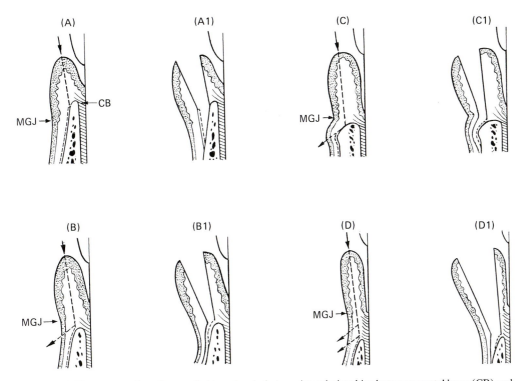

Figure 20.2 Flap preparation when pocket base located at varying relationships between crestal bone (CB) and mucogingival junction (MGJ). (A and A1) Simple pocket surgical filletting incision and blunt dissection over alveolar bone applicable when MGJ located apical to CB. (B and B1) Greater attachment loss and MGJ adjacent to CB. Filletting dissection must then extend beyond MGJ with risk of perforation (arrowed) because of uneven mucosal and bony crest contours. (C and C1) Underlying bony form further complicating surgery. (D and D1) Greater problems caused by existence of thin mucosa and bony dehiscences

complicated by the abrupt transition of the intrinsic tissue characteristics and surface contour of the mucosa at the mucogingival junction. Thus, the readily dissected comparatively thick, tough and immobile keratinized gingiva forming the pocket wall, gives way to the less manageable, thin, soft and loosely bound-down alveolar mucosa that will form the base of the surgical flap. Dissection is further complicated by variations in gingival thickness at adjacent units, any undulating contour of the underlying bone and roots (Figure 20.2 C), and differences in crestal bone heights at adjacent units, as a result of uneven attachment losses or bony dehiscences as shown in Figure 20.2 (D).

The dissection ideally traverses the tissues at an even depth, the blade angle being adjusted appropriately as the variable mucosal and bony morphology is encountered. Progress can fortunately be monitored fairly easily by the slight mucosal bulge produced by the blade. The risk of perforation is ever present at the mucogingival junction and even more so within the contiguous thin alveolar mucosa forming the apical part of the flap. The risk is increased in the presence of an uneven bony form. Sharp dissection is preferable in all such situations, but is converted to blunt dissection more apically over the alveolar bony plate (Figure 20.2 B1 and C1).

Pockets extending into alveolar mucosa (Figure 20.3)

The coronal gingival and mucogingival junctional components of the surgical flap are prepared as described above. A very careful, precise surgical technique is demanded for the alveolar mucosal component because of its thin structure and movable nature (Figures 20.2 D and D1 and 20.3 A). Ensuring the excision of the pocket lining

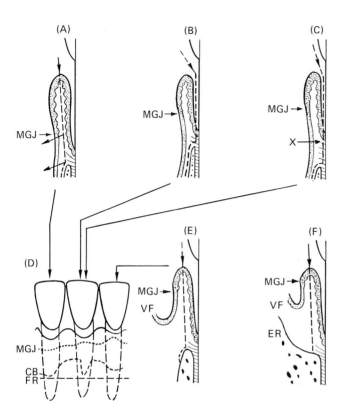

Figure 20.3 Problems caused by pocket base being apical to MGJ. (A) Abrupt reduction in tissue thickness at MGJ, mobility of the thin alveolar mucosal component to pocket wall, plus ledge created by crestal bone complicates filletting and carries risk of mucosal perforation. (B) Difficulties averted by use of crevicular-type incision instead of the inverse bevel. This extends as sharp split-thickness dissection over the crestal and alveolar bone as necessary to cater for (D) variable crestal bone (CB) levels at adjacent sites. Note level of dissection for flap reflection (FR). (C) Similar dissection required at long supracrestal associated with bony dehiscence. Note location of horizontal incision 'X' when necessary to isolate intact supracrestal tissue. Pocket base apical to (E) vestibular fold (VF) and associated with thicker labial mucosa and (F) external oblique ridge (ER)

epithelium is especially difficult (Figure 20.3 A), as is avoiding perforation of the alveolar mucosal pocket wall tissue. Fortunately, the elasticity and comparative translucency of the tissues allow the blade depth to be observed more closely than elsewhere, partly offsetting the greater risk of mucosal perforation. The blade inevitably contacts the root or bone in these cases, quickly dulling its cutting edge and impeding progress, necessitating early replacement. A keen edge to the blade is critical for the successful sharp dissection, but ironically is also most likely inadvertently to perforate the tissue. Avoiding perforation is paramount in all instances even at the expense of retaining pocket epithelium by making a crevicular type incision into the pocket space instead, as shown in Figure 20.3 (B).

Sharp dissection is extended, as elsewhere, to just beyond the pocket base to the crest of the bone. This can be difficult to judge where there are uneven pocket depths (Figure 20.3 A, B and D) and more especially bony dehiscences, as depicted in Figure 20.3 (C and D), when crestal bony landmarks are not available. In these instances, sharp dissection is extended well beyond the suspected level of the pocket base (Figure 20.3 C) before passing down to bone. Following reflection of this, then essentially split thickness flap, the pocket base is located by vertical pocket space probing within the cervical wedge tissue. The coronal pocket-related segment of cervical wedge tissue adjacent to the root is then sectioned from the intact supracrestal attachment component by a horizontal incision as depicted in Figure 20.3 (C) and then removed.

Pockets extending apical to the vestibular fold (Figure 20.3)

The gingival and alveolar mucosal components of the pocket wall are dissected as above. As the apical component is comprised of vestibular fold sub-mucosal tissue which is, in effect, quite thick (Figure 20.3 E and F) the pocket lining epithelium can be excised quite readily. On the other hand, however, it is not possible to create a surgical flap as elsewhere. This is because the oral surface of the mucosa related to the apical part of the flap lies at right angles to the root and creates, instead, a surgical pouch between the cervical wedge and the mucosa (see Figure 20.4 A and C). Where, as is often the case, there are also uneven pocket depths the dissection will initially not pass apical to the crestal bone at the deepest pocket sites. The further necessary dissection is then greatly complicated by the poor visibility within the surgical pouch and the frequently copious submucosal tissue bleeding encountered.

Influence of a lack of gingival tissue

Each situation cited above could potentially be associated with an absence of gingival tissue through marginal tissue recession or previous resective surgery. The surgical flap would then be comprised exclusively of alveolar mucosa as shown in Figure 20. 1 (D) and so be subject to the difficulties of dissection already described. Very careful handling is necessary to avoid tearing or incising the margin of, or perforating, the flap tissue. Difficulties also arise in subsequent management of this readily traumatized thin mucosa (see below).

Flap management

Flap retraction during cervical wedge removal, root debridement and any osseous administration is in all instances as for simple pocket surgery. However this can be awkward at 'surgical pouch' situations and more especially where there is little or no marginal gingival tissue. This is because surgical margin comprised of alveolar mucosa tends to curl inwards under itself, forming a rolled edge which impedes visibility, slips away readily during attempted flap retraction and is easily torn.

The surgical objectives of apical repositioning and surgical reattachment are with a single exception (see below) as readily achieved here in complex, as in simple, pocket surgery. This in turn means that the existence of surgical flap comprised predominantly of alveolar mucosa is of no clinical significance, although suturing can be more difficult where no gingival component at all exists. This is because the thinner non-keratinized tissue tears more easily during the insertion of sutures and often also

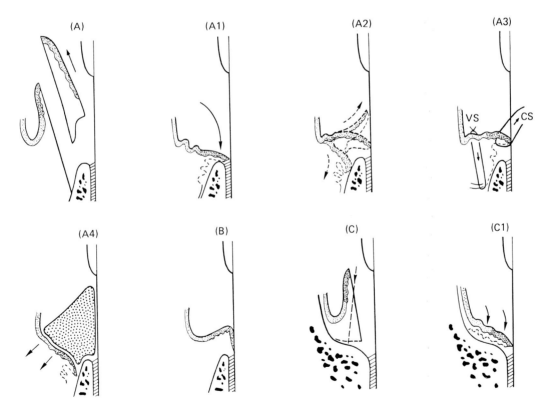

Figure 20.4 Flap management. (A) Cervical wedge removal at pocket extending beyond vestibular fold. (A1) Attempted apical repositioning limited by level of vestibular fold. (A2) Difficulties of flap positioning showing excessive displacement with bony denudation, and different degrees of coronal relapse resulting in a surgical reattachment relationship. (A3) Vestibular suturing (VS) for flap support and to counter coronal relapse from continuous suture (CS) used in surgical field. (A4) Inadvertent flap displacement by dressing resulting in bony denudation. (B) Optimal healing. (C) Secondary filletting of vestibular tissue and (C1) difficulties of apical repositioning caused by external oblique ridge

postoperatively. In the latter, the thread will appear to have pulled out in association with a painful mucosal ulceration, although it is not clear whether this has been the cause or effect. Taking a greater compensatory 'bite' of the mucosa during suturing, in an attempt to counter this, is helpful but may also increase postoperative pain, so it is not advocated.

When the pocket base has been located apical to the vestibular mucosal fold as shown in Figure 20.4 (A) major difficulties arise in apical repositioning and an attempted surgical reattachment is often imposed instead. This is because tissue displacement is limited by the level of the vestibular fold itself, whilst being precluded elsewhere by the presence of an underlying external oblique ridge, depicted in Figure 20.4 (C and C1) or the root of the zygomatic arch. Even where the surgical flap margin can be forcibly displaced apically (Figure 20.4 A1) it cannot be readily maintained in that position and, as illustrated in Figure 20.4 (A2), may become displaced either further apically or relapse coronally. Furthermore, the necessary use of any interdental type suturing for flap support, tends to pull the flap back coronally, although this can in turn sometimes be countered by suturing the vestibular fold to the deeply located intact facial muscle attachments (Figure 20.4 A3). This vestibular type suturing together with the other option of applying a bulky periodontal dressing to hold the tissue in place (Figure 20.4 A4), causes considerable postoperative pain. The dressing may, unknown to the operator, also inadvertently displace the flap margin apically away from crestal bone and tooth, resulting in an even more painful osseous denudation. In most instances however, the attempted apically repositioned flap tissue and its contiguous vestibular mucosa tend to slide back coronally assuming a surgical reattachment relationship to the teeth. This will heal, hopefully, with a long junctional epithelium (Figure 20.4 B), but may equally recreate the pocket at which surgery had been directed. This relapse appears to occur mainly in the immediate postoperative period but may also progress gradually over a period of 4–6 weeks.

Post-surgical healing

Gingival flaps

The pattern of healing of optimally positioned facial and oral gingival type flaps, is no different from that described following surgical reattachment and apical repositioning in simple pocket surgery. Similarly, the tissue regeneration over any denuded interdental bone stems from the gingival inductive capacity of the papillary flap margins and the adjacent marginal periodontal ligaments and from the bone itself, which, in turn, induces a non-keratinizing tissue (Figure 20.5 A and A1). The extent of the

latter reparative contribution is, however, limited by the effects of the inevitable superficial bony necrosis.

Alveolar mucosal flaps

Where, on the other hand, the flap margins are comprised of alveolar mucosa rather than gingiva (Figure 20.5 B) a predominantly non-keratinized interdental tissue septum develops instead (Figure 20.5 B2). Healing elsewhere depends on the relationship of these facial and oral flaps to the associated crestal bone. There are three possible relationships: the alveolar mucosal flap margin is adapted about the teeth, as in surgical reattachment; it just covers the crestal bone, as in apical repositioning; or it lies apical to the crestal bone. Each situation must be considered more carefully.

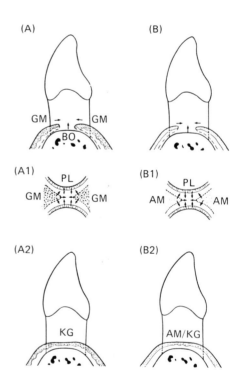

Figure 20.5 Interdental mucosal regeneration. (A, A1 and B) Tissue proliferation from gingival flap margins (GM) and periodontal ligaments (PL) induce gingival tissue and that from bone (BO) alveolar mucosa, resulting in (A2) a predominantly keratinized tissue (KG) regeneration. (B and B1) Alveolar mucosal (AM) flap margins resulting in (B2) a very much greater proportion of alveolar mucosa (AM) during healing

Reattachment relationship (Figure 20.6 A)

A loose alveolar mucosal type attachment is established over the alveolar bone itself (Figure 20.6 A1). This also occurs in the other two situations (Figure 20.6 B1, C1 and D1) described further below so this aspect need not be referred to again. The coronal part of the surgical flap, coapted to the root surface, becomes re-epithelialized as in simple pocket surgery and results in, at best, a long junctional epithelium as shown in Figure 20.6 (A1). It is not known whether this is any more susceptible to the effects of plaque accummulation than that of a long junctional epithelium associated with gingival tissue in simple pocket surgical reattachment. (See also Chapter 29 – Tissue curettage.)

Optimal relationship (Figure 20.6 B)

The proliferating connective tissues from the non-keratinized flap and the periodontal ligament merge to form the new supracrestal attachment. Although

this will initially appear to the naked eye to be comprised of alveolar mucosal tissue, the marginal attachment is via gingiva, to form a dentogingival junction (Figure 20.6 B1). (See also Chapter 32 – Gingival dimensions and gingival health.)

Denudation relationship (Figure 20.6 C and D)

Healing is as described over denuded bone in the previous chapter (see Figure 19.12). Although a greater proportion of alveolar mucosa develops, stemming from both the flap and the bone, a dentogingival junction always results (Figure 20.6 C1). Healing is, however, also influenced by the structure of the alveolar bone. Thus, where this is thin and cortical in nature (as depicted in Figure 20.6 D), the regenerative potential of the periodontal ligament is enhanced via undermining resorption and an increased amount of gingival mucosa develops, albeit usually at the expense of some loss of periodontal attachment (Figure 20.6 D1).

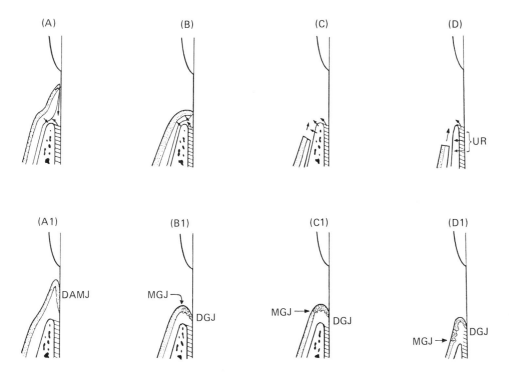

Figure 20.6 Healing of alveolar mucosal flaps. (A) Surgical reattachment relationship and origins of reparative cells (arrows) from alveolar mucosal epithelium and connective tissue and from periodontal ligament. (A1) Healing by long junctional epithelium to form dento-alveolar mucosal junction (DAMJ). (B) Optimal relationship with development of (B1) a clinical (DAMJ) but histological dentogingival junction (DGJ). (C) Denudation of thick bone and healing with (C1) predominantly alveolar mucosa but DGJ. (D) Thin denuded bone results in (D1) greater proportion of gingiva following undermining resorption (UR). Note location of mucogingival junction (MGJ) in each situation

Summary

The nature and morphology of the vestibular tissues have been shown not only to complicate but, in some instances, even to preclude optimal surgical pocket management. The additional technical problems encountered, by virtue of a coexisting lack of gingival tissue at the surgical flap margin and its influence on healing, have also been described. It remains only to examine the effects of these gingival deficiencies on the maintenance of health. Furthermore as recession is sometimes associated with deep incisal overbites, the nature of this relationship should also be examined.

21

Vestibular morphology and gingival health

Potential problems
Functional implications
Clinical implications
Patient concern

Site management and future assessment
Rationale for surgical intervention
Influence of deep overbites on disease

Potential problems

There are several features of vestibular morphology that might complicate routine oral hygiene measures and so predispose to marginal disease or might cause some patient concern. More specifically these relate to the vestibular depth and width on the one hand, and on the other, reduction in gingival dimensions and alteration of marginal coutour, manifesting as gingival recession. Each feature might occur in isolation or in different combinations in any one mouth. Variations of vestibular sulcus form are primarily of developmental origin, while those of the gingivae are predisposed to by the local tissue morphology and usually develop as a result of long-standing subclinical plaque-induced inflammation or traumatic oral hygiene practices. Where associated with deep incisal overbites, the opposing teeth might also be implicated (see below), thereby reinforcing the influence of tissue morphology in the development of recession.

This chapter will evaluate the clinical implications of these vestibular morphological variations. Firstly, the manner in which vestibular morphology might impede plaque control and the appropriate alternative cleaning methods are examined. Secondly, as surgical corrective measures are frequently recommended where marginal disease persists despite these cleaning efforts, the rationale for this intervention must be examined. Cosmetic requirements may, however, sometimes demand surgical treatment. Thirdly, as patient reassurance to allay fear of impending tooth loss and concern about poor appearances following gingival recession depends on an understanding of the nature of recession, this must be clarified here. Finally the relationship of deep incisal overbites to gingival recession must be considered.

Functional implications

Mucosal variations

The vestibular dimensions are determined primarily by the attachment of the buccinator and related muscles of facial expression buccally; and lingually by those of the floor of the mouth as depicted in Figure 21.1. Any developmental variations which reduce, in particular, the vestibular depth will impede access for plaque control (Figure 21.1 A).

Mucosal frenal insertions are merely very localized aberrations of vestibular form. The frenum is most commonly of an acute triangular shape, flaring out as it merges with the vestibular fold (Figure 21.1 B). Narrow sheet-like frena may extend between lip and gingiva and insert close to the tip of the interdental papilla (Figure 21.1 C–E). Where a diastema exists the frenum may be quite broad, passing between the teeth, and be inserted into the lingual or palatal gingival papilla (Figure 21.1 F). Frenal attachment to the lip, cheek or the tongue may also vary greatly as shown, for example, in Figure 21.1 (G and H). A frenum not only reduces vestibular depth at the site, but where especially prominent also makes the vestibule narrower by restricting displacement of the related lip as shown in Figure 21.2 (C), cheek or tongue.

294

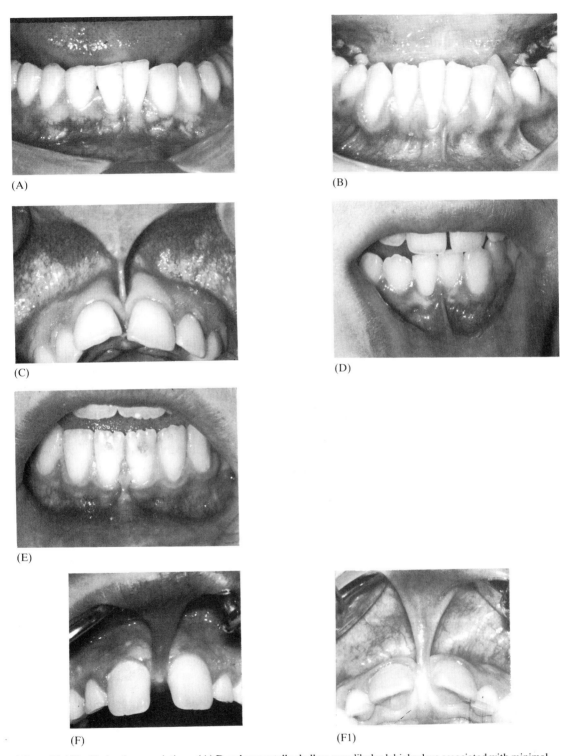

Figure 21.1 Vestibular tissue variations. (A) Developmentally shallow mandibular labial sulcus associated with minimal gingival dimensions. (B) Narrow labial frenal insertions at 43, 33 and between 41, 31. (C–E) Sheet-like frena extending between (C) upper and (D) lower lip and attached gingiva and (E) into tip of papilla. (F) Broad frenum associated with diastema (F1) inserted into incisal papilla.

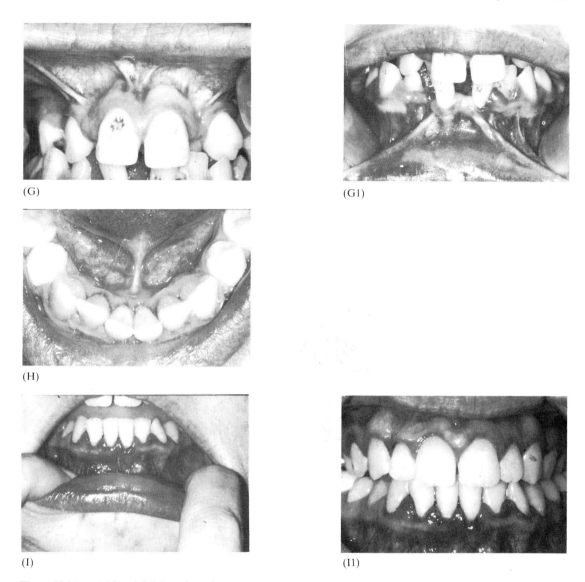

Figure 21.1 (*cont.*) (G and G1) Prominent frenal insertions into lips and (H) tongue. (I) Strong involuntary lower lip action impedes cleaning and is associated with (I1) more marked lower anterior gingival inflammation than elsewhere

A strong labial (especially lower) muscle tone may resist lip displacement. When combined with a powerful involuntary lip activity detected in Figure 21.1 (D and I) or a prominent, poorly controlled tongue, this can severely limit accessibility for patient and operator alike. Vestibular dimensions are also determined by the underlying bone. The depth is, in effect, reduced by the external oblique ridge and root of the zygomatic arch whilst the mandibular coronoid process reduces the functional width of vestibule in the maxillary molar area.

Gingival variations (Figure 21.2)

Gingival hyperplasia (overgrowth) of idiopathic or familial origins, or that induced by drugs or bacterial plaque-associated inflammation (see Figure 9.1) has no adverse influence on vestibular form and is of no relevance here. However, as the increased bulk of the tissue results in shorter clinical crowns, cleaning might become more difficult. In contrast, marginal gingival recession may impede plaque control by both reducing the vestibular depth and by the effects

296

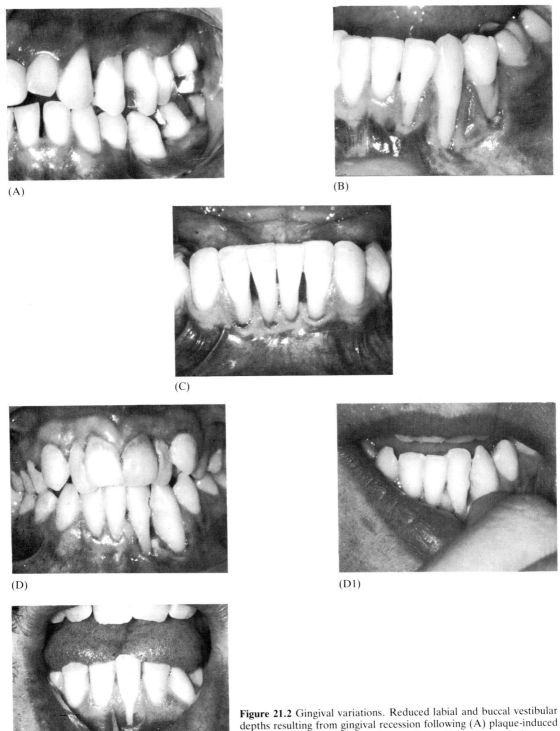

(A)

(B)

(C)

(D)

(D1)

(E)

Figure 21.2 Gingival variations. Reduced labial and buccal vestibular depths resulting from gingival recession following (A) plaque-induced attachment loss, (B) over-zealous tooth-brushing, (C) surgical resection or (D and D1) pernicious habits. (E) Uneven marginal gingival contour, reduced gingival dimension, localized shallow vestibular depth and prominent frenum restricting lip displacement, may each impede cleaning in this case

of the irregular marginal tissue contour. Gingival recession may occur in long-standing disease (Figure 21.2 A), over-zealous toothbrushing (Figure 21.2 B), other pernicious traumatic habits (Figure 21.2 D) or even surgical resection (Figure 21.2 C). The resulting altered gingival form may present at only localized sites or be more generalized, with adjacent units being similarly affected or displaying different degrees of recession.

The functional importance of gingival tissue is that it constitutes a band of immovable tissue about the teeth, to check any potential physical interference from the contiguous movable vestibular tissues, during routine oral hygiene practices. The corollary to this is that reduced gingival dimensions predispose to such interference. This means, in practical terms, that in the extreme situation of an apparent total lack of gingiva coupled with a shallow vestibule, the juxtapositioning of the dentogingival junctions and vestibular fold severely restricts access for cleaning. In addition, the intrinsic vulnerability of non-keratinized mucosa to incidental toothbrush trauma during routine cleaning, might provide a further disincentive to plaque control. Finally, in cases of uneven degrees of gingival recession the resulting inconsistent marginal contour makes cleaning even more difficult.

Clinical implications

Multifactorial influence

The extent to which there is actual interference with cleaning is extremely variable and depends very much on the individual patients and their willingness to overcome any difficulty. There can never be a simple assumption that vestibular tissue aberrations will automatically present cleaning problems, and each situation must be assessed on an individual basis. Difficulty arises when, as is often the case, more than one potential hurdle to plaque removal exists at the same site, as shown especially well in Figure 21.2 (E), and when the influence of each must be separated before corrective measures can be instituted. The manner in which each individual vestibular tissue feature might impede cleaning, and the appropriate modifications in technique advocated, must therefore be considered more closely.

Vestibular form

A shallow sulcus restricts the amount of space available for toothbrushing in particular. An analogous situation can be created in the normal mouth by attempting to brush the labial surfaces of the lower incisors whilst pressing horizontally with a finger against the lower lip just below the vermillion border (Figure 21.3 A and B); both the initial

positioning of the brush-head and its brushing action will be inhibited. Interference is greatest with the roll and least with the miniscrub technique; it will also be found that the bristles tend to scratch the tender lip mucosa, which will further inhibit cleaning.

Clinically, the difficulties can often be overcome, either by initially displacing the lip or cheek with the back of the brush-head, or by pulling the offending tissue outwards with the other hand. A strong reflex lip activity is also best controlled by digital displacement (Figure 21.3 D). Interference from the underlying bony external oblique ridge or the root of the zygomatic arch, or that of the retromolar tissues is, however, insurmountable. Interference by the proximity of the floor of the mouth is not readily overcome, but that from the tongue is best countered by positioning the tip of the tongue to the site being brushed as shown previously in Figure 8.1. This not only automatically displaces the bulk of the tongue to the opposite side but also means the tongue can direct the bristles into position. This technique is also very effective in controlling strong gagging reflexes, for this displaces the sensitive posterior part of the tongue from the area being cleaned.

The mucosal frenum has comparable effects to a shallow vestibular sulcus. Its sheet-like structure further complicates cleaning at the otherwise accessible adjacent sites by obstructing the toothbrush or by impeding lip or cheek displacement during cleaning (Figure 21.3 F). The frenum is prone to inadvertent trauma which will further discourage cleaning at related teeth (Figure 21.3 G). Careful manipulation of the interspace brush will, however, often overcome this problem (Figure 21.3 H–J).

Gingival form

Gingival recession has several consequences with respect to oral hygiene measures. Firstly, and most importantly, pocketing will have been reduced but this beneficial effect need not be considered further here. Secondly, the reduced gingival dimensions mean that the gingival margins approximate to the vestibular sulcus which become shallower and restricts access for cleaning. However, this recession is only of consequence when the existing non-keratinized component of the vestibular trough is already shallow, as shown at Figure 21.2 (C), for the proportional reduction in overall depth elsewhere is insignificant. Thirdly, where recession progresses unevenly, the influence of the resultant uneven marginal gingival contour on plaque control becomes increasingly important. It must also be appreciated that the superimposed effect of gingival sensitivity associated with plaque-induced marginal

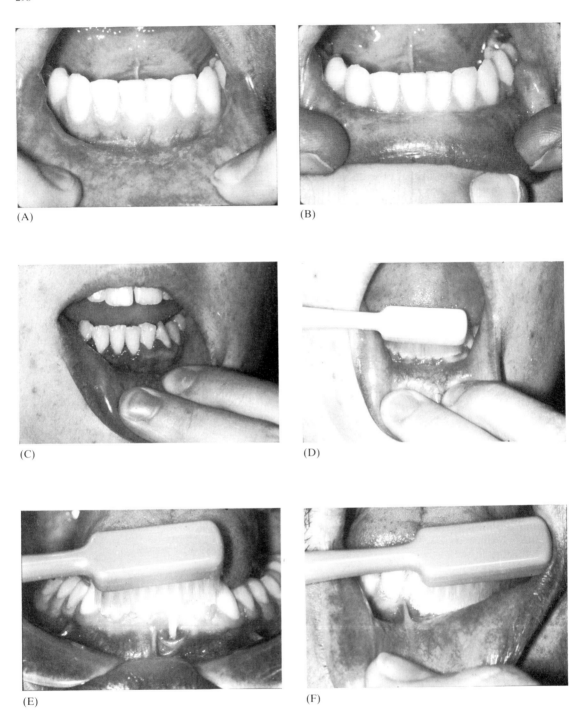

(A)

(B)

(C)

(D)

(E)

(F)

Figure 21.3 Influence of cleaning. (A) Normal vestibular space (B) elimination by digital pressure shown by everting lip. (C) Strong lower lip action of patient shown in Figure 21.1 (I) produces effect of shallow vestibule. Overcome by digital displacement of lip (D) during cleaning. (E) Case shown in Figure 21.2 (E). Toothbrush only effective at non-receded sites. Efforts to reach receded sites may traumatize (F) adjacent labial and alveolar mucosa and

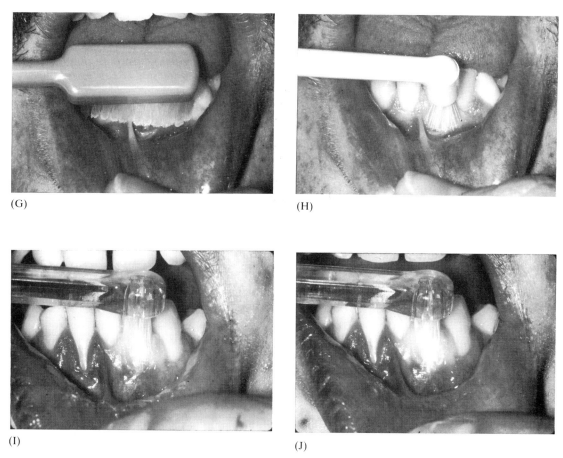

(G)   (H)

(I)   (J)

Figure 21.3 (*cont.*) (G) frenum. (H) Frenal interference overcome by labial retraction and careful use of interspace brush, but in this case, brush is too large for receded site. (I) Narrower more pointed brush appropriate at cleft-like recession sites; bristles first splayed out against tooth then (J) carefully pushed apically into crevice (I and J reproduced from *Restorative Dentistry,* by permission of A. E. Morgan Publications Ltd)

inflammation may also inhibit cleaning in all these situations, so setting up a vicious circle.

Reduction in gingival dimensions

Gingival deficiency has, in itself, not been shown to jeopardize marginal tissue health (see Chapter 32 – Gingival dimensions and gingival health) so need not be discussed further here with respect to plaque control. On the other hand, when the dentogingival junctions and the mucogingival junctions approximate, the risk of inadvertent trauma to the potentially more vulnerable adjacent alveolar mucosa does exist so could discourage brushing at the site. The presence of non-keratinized mucosal margin might be similarly significant, although clinical investigations have demonstrated that the total lack of keratinized tissue is consistent with the maintenance of marginal tissue health in subjects carrying out high standards of cleaning, as shown in Figure 21.7. Furthermore, animal model investigations have demonstrated neither an increased susceptibility to disease nor severity of the inflammatory response to plaque-induced disease (see Chapter 32 – Gingival dimensions and plaque-induced disease). Finally, although the intrinsic mobility of alveolar mucosa predisposes to marginal tissue retraction during function, especially in the presence of frenal insertions, this is not significant with respect to plaque retention. See also 'tension' and 'blanching' tests – Chapter 32 – Gingival dimensions and plaque-induced disease.

Changes of marginal gingival contour

Situations with an even pattern of gingival recession manifest primarily as a loss of interdental papillary form as shown in Figure 21.2 (C). The resulting patent interproximal spaces make cleaning even easier, for they allow the use of wood points or interproximal brushes, where previously only the passage of floss was possible. The exaggerated scalloped gingival contour, resulting from more localized gingival recession (as in Figure 21.2 E), does however complicate cleaning in several ways. Firstly, the filaments of the ordinary toothbrush cannot reach easily into the gingival sulcus at the more apically located receded margins. This is because the other filaments on the brush-head are checked by the adjacent non-receded gingival margins (Figure 21.3 E) and efforts to negotiate the receded site are likely to traumatize the adjacent non-keratinized mucosa (Figure 21.3 F) and so further inhibit cleaning.

Secondly, a V-shaped receded marginal gingival contour presents a specific problem, for even with the pointed interspace brush (Figure 21.3 H) the adjacent non-keratinized mucosa tends to become traumatized. The more careful use of a finer single-tufted brush is thus demanded as shown in Figure 21.3 (I and J). The greater expenditure of time with surfaces being cleaned individually might, in turn, possibly present a further disincentive to the maintenance of oral hygiene.

Thirdly, some individuals will be totally unaware of recession and so make no special effort to clean recessed areas, while others will deliberately refrain from cleaning such sites because of tissue tenderness or a fear of increasing the recession. In summary, the finding of marginal inflammation related to sites of isolated gingival recession is not only predictable, but can also be explained quite simply on grounds of difficulties or oral hygiene alone.

Patient concern

Gingival recession might be aesthetically displeasing in some instances or be interpreted as a sign of impending tooth loss.

Aesthetics

Poor appearance due to recession is a more common cause for patient concern than the redness and swelling with gingival inflammation. This concern may only appear during therapy when recession develops following inflammatory resolution. Moreover, the gradually increasing clinical crown lengths, following an even pattern of gingival recession, is traditionally accepted as an inevitable age change – 'getting long in the tooth'.

When recession is evenly distributed the loss of interdental papillary form and the resulting dark spaces between the teeth rather than the gingival shrinkage *per se* tend to cause most concern (Figure 21.4 A). When, in contrast, recession is restricted to single or several isolated units the resulting different crown lengths may be even more displeasing (Figure 21.4 B). This type of recession does, however, tend to occur in the mandibular teeth and at maxillary cuspids, so is often masked by the lips as shown in Figure 21.4 (C). Indeed the patient frequently needs to resort to aggressive animal-like grimaces accentuated by digital retraction of the lips to even demonstrate the offending units! Genuine aesthetic problems arise in individuals with broad smiles which might even be altered in an attempt to conceal the elongated teeth, and also where the margins of crowns become exposed, especially when associated with darkened roots (Figure 21.4 D). Acrylic gingival veneers should then be considered (Figure 21.4 E–J). (See also below – Cosmetic problems.)

Fear of tooth loss

The patient must be reassured that gingival recession in itself does not mean the tooth loss is imminent and that it essentially only represents one of the signs of a long-standing plaque-induced disease. This, and the mechanism of gingival recession in disease (described in Chapter 13), need not be considered further here.

Recession may also develop in the absence of periodontal disease as a result of the liability of thin marginal tissue to irreversible damage and tissue loss following minor trauma. This occurs most commonly, albeit inadvertently, during toothbrushing as shown for example in Figures 21.1 (B), 21.2 (B1) and 21.4 (B). Recession is also encountered following careless operative treatment adjacent to the gingival margins, or as a result of complications of routine endodontics (Figure 21.5 A), apical surgery (Figure 21.5 (B–D)) and orthodontic fixed appliance therapy (Figure 21.5 E). It is claimed that labial tooth displacement might also result in gingival recession, but the exciting factor is more likely to be direct physical trauma to the thin overlying mucosa. Similarly, poorly supported prostheses might potentially also cause recession as might the opposing incisors in the presence of deep incisal overbites especially when biting, for example, hard crusty rolls (see below). Localized recession resulting from trauma is very obvious to the patient and arouses great concern about possible tooth loss. However, apart from cases with unpredictable endodontic implications the prognosis is good. The pathogenesis of recession must therefore be explained to the patient (*cf.* Chapter 24).

301

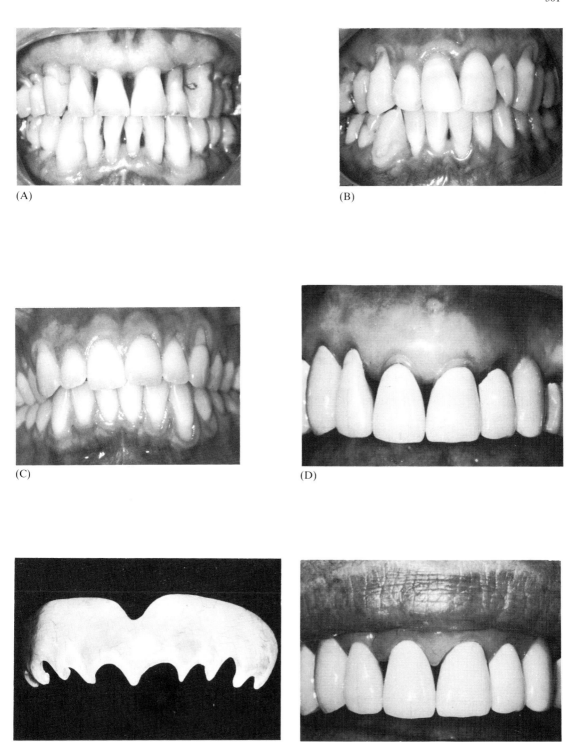

Figure 21.4 Aesthetic consequences of recession. (A) Dark interdental spaces. (B) Uneven marginal gingival form and thus crown heights – appearance may be aggravated by cervical abrasion cavities. (C) Recession mainly restricted to cuspids less apparent. (D) Exposure of restoration margins. (E) Acrylic gingival veneer to (F) mask effects of recession.

302

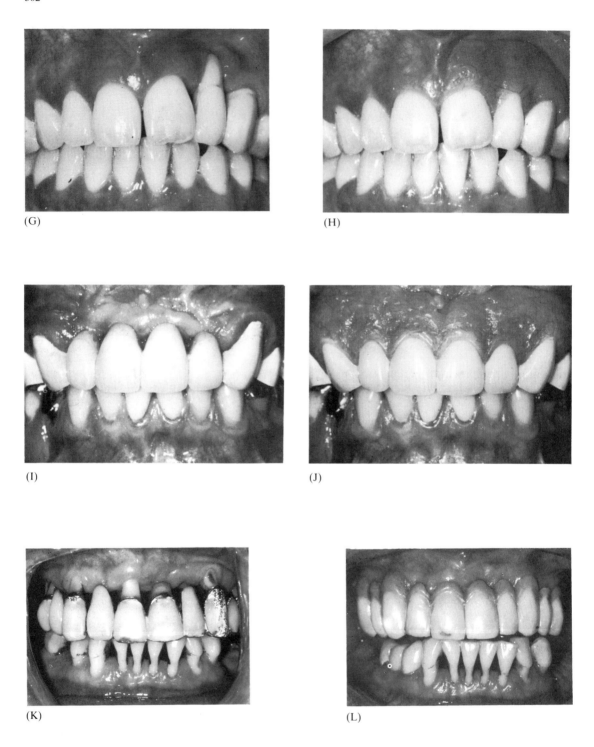

(G)

(H)

(I)

(J)

(K)

(L)

Figure 21.4 (*cont.*) (G) Localized tissue loss at 22 pontic site masked by (H) unilateral veneer. (I) Similarly aesthetics of pontics at 12, 11, 21, 22 enhanced by (J) veneer. (K) Attempt to mask major aesthetic problem of postsurgical recession by (L) incorporating false gingiva within fixed reconstruction. This precludes oral hygiene and is therefore contraindicated

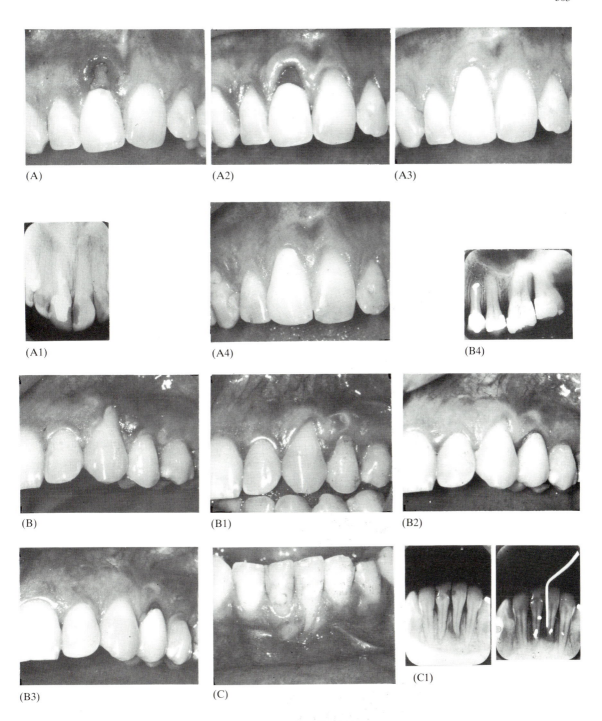

(A)   (A2)   (A3)

(A1)   (A4)   (B4)

(B)   (B1)   (B2)

(B3)   (C)   (C1)

Figure 21.5 Iatrogenic gingival recession. (A) Labial gingival necrosis from chemical leaching through endodontic accessory canal. (A1) Radiograph amalgam seal following surgical exposure. Presentation (A2) 2 years, (A3) 3 years following crown replacement and (A4) 7 years later – note further recession elsewhere. (B) Recession followed inappropriate location of relieving incision over 23 for apical surgery at 24 – presentation at 2 weeks postoperative, (B1) 1 year, (B2) 3 years and (B3) 9 years. (B4) Radiograph after crown fitted at 5 years. Note recession at 24 but gradual coronal creeping at 23. (C) Recession following attempted apical surgery 31. (C1) Radiographs pre- and postoperative (with probe in receded area).

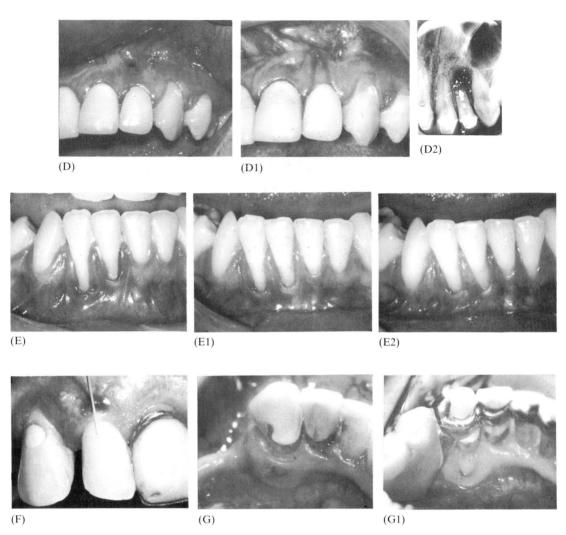

Figure 21.5 (*cont.*) (D) Gingival fenestration over failed apicectomy with further tissue breakdown and recession (D1) 1 year later. (D2) Radiograph. (E) Gingival recession 43, 42 following mucosal trauma apparently sustained during removal of orthodontic bands. Presentation at (E1) 5 years and (E2) 9 years. (F) Traumatic fenestration of gingiva at 12 at recession level of adjacent teeth – clefting imminent. (G) Gingival perforation from ill-fitting lingual connector (cut away) with subsequent breakdown of mucosal band and (G1) presentation of recession

Pathogenesis of recession

The depth of any physically induced minor gingival lesion in relation to overall tissue thickness at thin tissue sites (Figure 21.6 A), means both the junctional epithelium and its subjacent attachment fibres become involved. This leads to an almost inevitable loss of marginal attachment, as shown in Figure 21.6 (A2 and C). In contrast, a lesion of comparable depth within thick gingiva will be fairly superficial and only a slight reduction in overall thickness sustained following healing (Figure 21.6 B2). For this reason, the progressively thicker form of the investing tissues more apically, coupled with the presence of underlying crestal bone, means that recession tends to be self-limiting (Figure 21.6 C and C1). That is, recession cannot extend apical to the level of the vestibular mucosal reflection in response to physical trauma in marginal tissue health while in disease, only pocket formation can result. It should

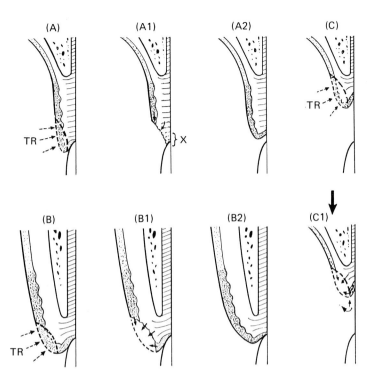

Figure 21.6 Trauma and gingival form. (A) Thin gingiva sustains substantial wound from trauma (TR) involving (A1) junctional epithelium and most coronal (X) attachment fibres. (A2) Healing results in recession. (B) A similar lesion at thick tissue results in (B1) proportionally less damage and a greater potential for repair with (B2) minimal marginal tissue deformity. (C) The thicker more apically located remaining tissue following repeated trauma at (A) responds as in (B) so that (C1) gingival recession tends to be self-limiting

be appreciated that the crestal bone has a limiting effect upon traumatically induced recession, while developmental bony dehiscences in gingival health, as depicted in Figure 21.6 (A), predispose to gingival recession from toothbrushing. On the other hand, it should be emphasized that while such situations are no more vulnerable to plaque-induced disease (see above), once attachment loss has been sustained, recession occurs readily as described in Chapter 13.

In summary, gingival recession is likely following both trauma and attachment loss at sites with inherently thin gingiva. It may also occur where subclinical levels of marginal inflammation exist and are accompanied by gradual attachment losses, manifested by increasing clinical crown heights but without any overt signs of disease being present. However, periodic phases of bleeding on gentle probing of normally healthy gingival crevices, may be observed in some cases. The difficulties of differentiating between recession resulting from marginal tissue trauma (which may either be subclinical or simply happen to occur between review appointments) and low grade gingival inflammation precludes any clearer analysis. Finally, where pocketing does exist, further recession is to be expected but, as in all instances elsewhere, will be arrested at the level at which the supracrestal

tissues assume the critical thickness. An effective but non-traumatic toothbrushing technique must therefore be achieved and be based upon a delicate balance between cleaning sufficiently well to control plaque and inflammation but not so vigorously as to damage the tissues. The use of a disclosing agent is invaluable in establishing this balance.

Site management and future assessment

Marginal tissue health

Where marginal gingival health is maintained by an atraumatic cleaning regime at sites with thin tissue form, further recession is unlikely, as shown by the cases presented in Figure 21.7. The patient must be reassured about this, and the fact that healthy dentogingival junctions are well able to withstand both normal functional stresses and mechanical irritation produced by a toothbrush used sensibly. In those few instances where the recession does progress, this occurs to only a minimal extent and is usually of little or no clinical or aesthetic importance. Furthermore, in some individuals similar degrees of recession will also gradually develop at other, previously unaffected, sites with thin gingival morphology, as a result of possible trauma or

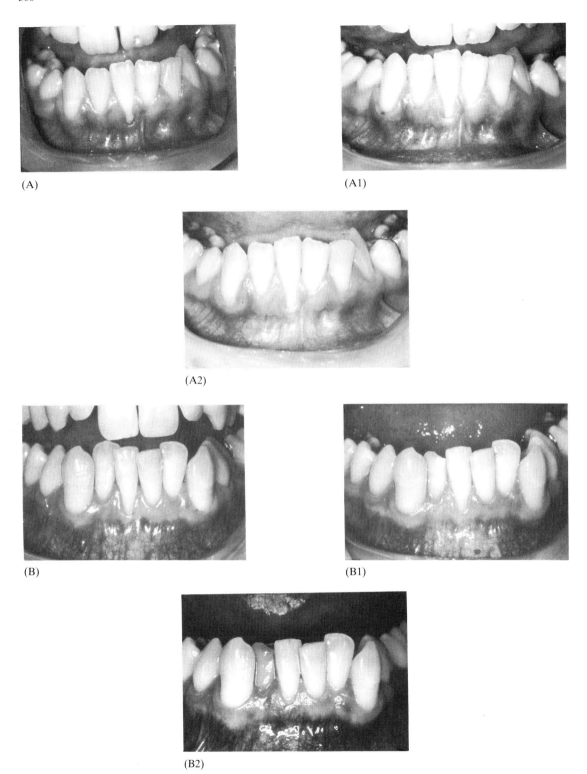

Figure 21.7 Long-term effects of recession. (A) Recession 41 plus frenum and shallow vestibule in 15-year-old girl. Findings at (A1) 26 and (A2) 29 years. Note slight coronal creeping but recession at 43, 32. (B) Localized recession 41 24-year-old man with coronal creeping at (B1) 26 and (B2) 38 years.

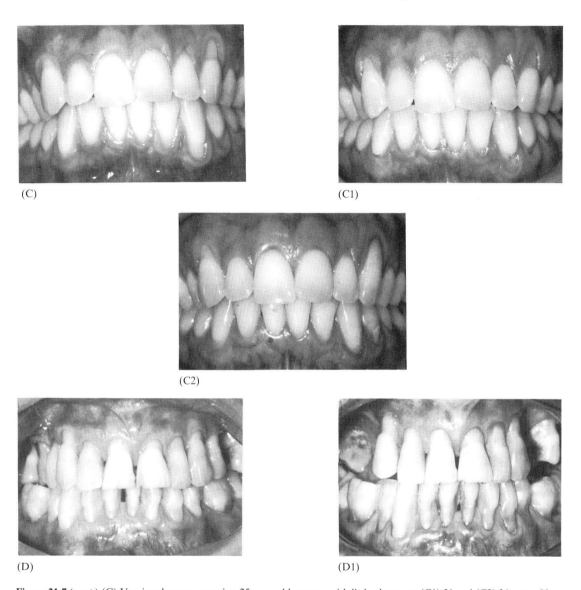

Figure 21.7 (*cont.*) (C) Varying degrees recession 25-year-old woman with little change at (C1) 31 and (C2) 36 years. Note marginal inflammation 23 and 33 associated with recently inserted adversely contoured cervical restorations. (D) Generalized recession in 68-year-old woman (D1) some progression by 80 years (A–A2, B–B2 and C–C2 reproduced from *Restorative Dentistry,* by permission of A. E. Morgan, Publications Ltd)

subclinical inflammation, as shown for example in Figure 21.7 (A–E). The overall effect then becomes one of a more generalized recession, but which is self-limiting by virtue of the thicker tissue that is ultimately involved. Thus, it is evident that sites with recession are no more vulnerable to further recession than other sites at which no recession has occurred. Additionally, the normal gingival dimensions at these uninvolved sites will not in itself preclude the subsequent development of recession (see also Chapter 32 – Gingival dimensions and gingival health).

Persistent disease

Where marginal inflammation and slight detachment exist, the patient must be warned that a further, albeit minimal recession frequently results

308

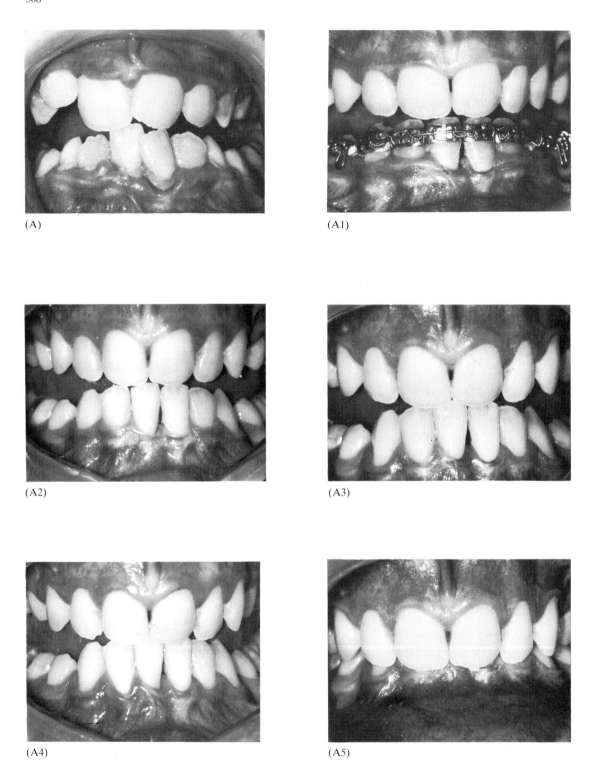

(A)

(A1)

(A2)

(A3)

(A4)

(A5)

Figure 21.8 Mucogingival deformities and influence of plaque control. (A) 9- year-old boy. Findings at (A1) 13 years during orthodontic treatment. (A2) 16 years, (A3) 19 years and (A4) 21 years of age and showing (A5) overbite; Note interdental inflammation in maxilla.

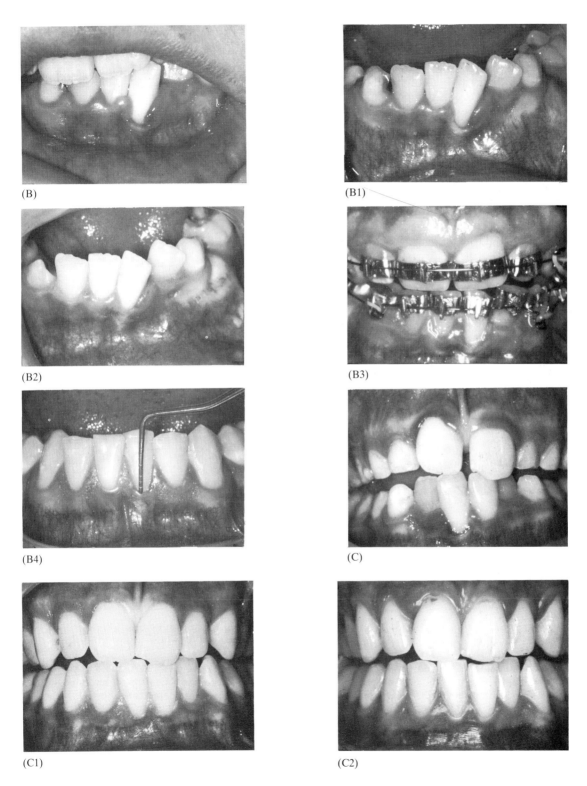

Figure 21.8 (*cont.*) (B) 8-year-old boy. Findings at (B1) 9 years, (B2) 11 years, (B3) 13 years and (B4) 21 years of age. (C) 7-year-old boy. Findings at (C1) 11 years and (C2) 19 years of age.

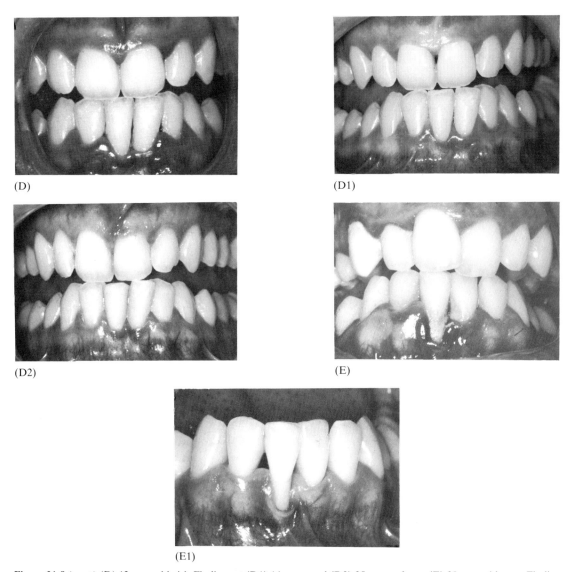

(D)

(D1)

(D2)

(E)

(E1)

Figure 21.8 (*cont.*) (D) 12-year-old girl. Findings at (D1) 14 years and (D2) 25 years of age. (E) 28-year-old man. Finding (E1) 2 years later. Note optimal plaque control possible in each case (cases in B and C reproduced from *Restorative Dentistry,* by permission of A. E. Morgan Publications Ltd)

from resolution of inflammation following improved plaque control. The patient might otherwise refrain from the cleaning measures advocated and more especially as the technique, which requires the brush filaments to be placed gently but firmly subgingivally, might be construed to be pushing the tissues more apically. In fact, any such gingival recession should be regarded as a bonus instead, because the associated pocketing will have become shallower and future cleaning made easier. In addition, the recession will at worst be limited to only the

detached component of the tissue and the patient advised accordingly. On the other hand, where there are persistent or fluctuating levels of marginal inflammation, because of inefficient and inconsistent plaque control further recession should be anticipated. The clinical case presentations in Figures 21.7 and 21.8 demonstrate that periodontal health can be achieved despite the presence of gingival deformities, reduced gingival dimensions, shallow vestibular depth and prominent mucosal frena. The recognition of this is fundamental to treatment planning. Furthermore, the possible relevance of any mucogingival aberrations cannot be adequately assessed until after the patient has had the opportunity of mastering the necessary cleaning techniques.

Site recording

Sites with gingival recession should be assessed periodically for any possible changes. Accurate records of the pattern and extent of recession are necessary for both reference purposes and patient reassurance. Study casts may be preferred when many surfaces are involved but localized areas at recession are best recorded *in situ,* using dividers to measure the clinical crown lengths (Figure 21.9 B and C). The divider points are then simply indented into the clinical charting grid and the puncture marks used for future reference. It can, however, often be difficult to locate reproducible occlusal surface reference points. The use of alternative reference points such as cemento-enamel junction, a suitable restoration margin or most accurately (and expensively) a soft PVC occlusal overlay (Figure 21.9 D) may be considered. Even these are subject

to change through tooth surface abrasion or erosion, occlusal wear or restoration replacement. Finally, clinical photographs might also be used, although standardized camera angulation is not easily assured. The exigencies of individual clinical practices will dictate which method is actually used.

Cosmetic problems

Where recession results in unacceptably long clinical crowns or restoration margins become exposed an acrylic gingival veneer can be considered as shown in Figure 21.4. The possible surgical options are dealt with in the next chapter.

Insurmountable difficulties of access

Persistent marginal inflammation at sites with gingival recession, a shallow vestibule or a prominent frenum despite carefully supervised and conscientious cleaning efforts would suggest that a genuine difficulty in negotiating the area exists. This would be confirmed by finding marginal tissue health at the adjacent units at which there is clearly no interference from the vestibular morphology to cleaning. It

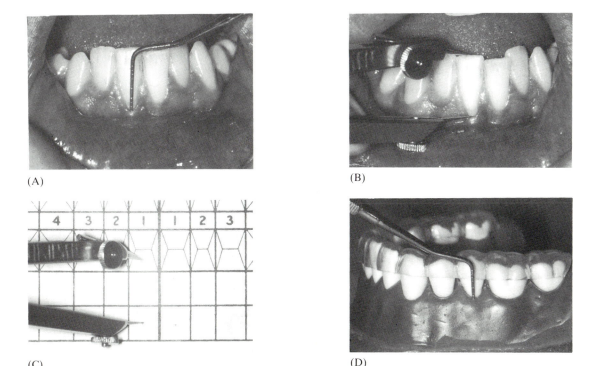

(A)

(B)

(C)

(D)

Figure 21.9 Recording recession. (A) Localized recession 41 and attempted reading of probe measurement from cemento-enamel junction. (B) Use of dividers for recording clinical crown height and (C) then puncturing clinical chart. Note reproducibility difficulties when measuring for example 32 or 33. (D) Use of soft acrylic stent on model

is, nevertheless, prudent to check the cleaning method once again and review the situation after a further period of time. In the vast majority of instances the technical difficulties will eventually be overcome and inflammation will resolve. In the few remaining instances, and provided the patient acknowledges that difficulty of access is actually responsible, surgical correction of the offending tissue morphology should be contemplated. However this does often, even at this late stage, stimulate some patients to reveal previously hidden talents for effective plaque removal, to avoid surgery.

Rationale for surgical intervention

Surgical intervention should not be based merely on persistent marginal inflammation or even bleeding on probing. Progressive gingival recession in the absence of detectable pocketing or a measurable progressive loss of attachment must be demonstrated to exclude the possible existence of a stable lesion. In most cases, repeated re-evaluation over a period of years rather than months is required to demonstrate any changes considered to be significant clinically. Consequently, the decision to intervene surgically, based on these parameters here, can be as difficult to make as that regarding pocket surgery elsewhere. There is, however, an added complication here. That is it is necessary to establish which of the commonly encountered co-existing features of a shallow vestibule, inconsistent gingival form or reduced gingival dimensions represents the problem, for upon this will the appropriate corrective surgical technique selected depend. Thus, for example, a situation with localized recession at a single unit might impede cleaning because of its V-shaped contour, the overall uneven marginal contour, the associated reduced vestibular depth or the predisposition of the related non-keratinized mucosa to inadvertent trauma.

This surgical dilemma is resolved by a logical process of elimination in close consultation with the patient. The difficulty most likely to be experienced is a lack of space available for cleaning because of shallow vestibular form. This is most readily and predictably corrected by surgically displacing the vestibular fold in an apical direction. Fortunately, in most instances, the improved access gained by this procedure proves sufficient also to overcome any remaining potential cleaning problems relating to gingival form and dimensions, so that no further surgical attention is required. Continuous reassessment is, therefore, fundamental in these cases. Where, on the other hand, the patient is concerned primarily about poor appearance at sites of gingival recession, the decision to intervene surgically is much simpler although the solution is rather less predictable. The improvement of aesthetics to

satisfy the patient's wishes then becomes the sole objective. The appropriate corrective surgical techniques are described in the following chapter.

Influence of deep overbites on disease
Nature of the problem

Subjects with deep incisal overbites may present with gingival recession suggestive of a direct causal relationship. The association could however be purely coincidental, as a high frequency of gingival recession can be found in other sites following loss of attachment and/or traumatic oral hygiene methods alone. This possibility is supported by the frequent finding, in individuals with deep incisal relationships, of a thin periodontal tissue morphology that is susceptible to recession. It is, however, evident that the incisal edges are potentially capable of traumatizing the opposing mucosa either directly, from sharp unevenly worn edges, or indirectly by the forced impaction of hard foods.

The observation of incisal edges in direct contact with opposing receded gingival margins and that of incisal indentations in the attached gingiva might initially appear to result from an increasing overbite. However, in the former, it could be that the position of the incisal edges is secondary to an independently occurring gingival recession. Alternatively, the incisal relationship could be stable and the recession have merely halted at the point of contact between incisal edges and the opposing gingiva. Similarly, the mucosal indentations might be due to either a plaque-induced gingival swelling being moulded by the presence of the opposing teeth in a stable position, or to tooth over-eruption as a result of an unstable incisal relationship.

The variable clinical presentation in these cases coupled with the lack of long-term controlled data on tooth to soft tissue relationships in gingival health and disease, complicates both differential diagnosis and treatment planning. The resulting clinical dilemma can, however, be clarified by first examining the possible influence of tissue morphology upon the development of gingival recession in deep overbites, before considering the potentially traumatic effect of the opposing teeth.

Periodontal morphology and recession
Predisposition to recession

The mandibular labial periodontium is comprised of thin gingiva and minimal bone incorporating developmental bony deficiencies. The palatal gingiva tends to be thick, other than in steeply vaulted palates, and the underlying bone support substantial, being part of the palatal bony vault (Figure 21.10 A and B). Gingival recession is therefore to be

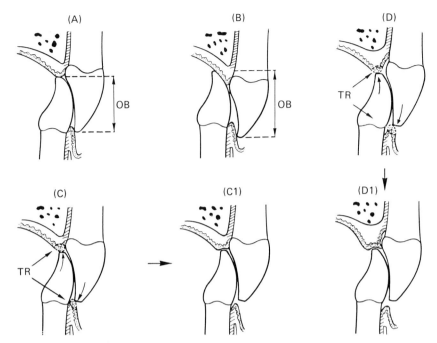

Figure 21.10 Periodontal tissue morphology. Increased overbite (OB) relationship of incisal edges to (A) gingival margin and (B) attached gingiva in situations with 'thin' mandibular labial tissue but 'thick' palatal tissue. (C) Trauma (TR) from food impaction or toothbrush results in (C1) recession in mandible with loss of tooth to soft tissue contact but overgrowth in maxilla. (D) Loss of attachment with development of maxillary pocketing but tendency for mandibular labial recession. (D1) Increased plaque induced inflammatory changes and/or any superimposed trauma establishes a vicious circle accentuating palatal hyperplasia and causing further labial recession. Note: uneven sharp incisal edges depicted

expected in the mandible following both plaque-induced attachment loss and marginal tissue trauma, whereas in the palate, pocketing and reparative hyperplasia of any traumatized tissue respectively, is more likely to occur (Figure 21.10).

Risk of periodontal disease

The marginal tissues in deep overbites are potentially more liable to plaque-induced disease than elsewhere, because of their comparative inaccessibility for routine oral hygiene measures. Thus in the mandible, access is impeded by strong lip muscle activity resisting displacement and the shallowness of the vestibular sulcus. Whereas in the maxilla, the depth of overbite effectively reduces inter-incisal opening and thereby access to the palatal aspects (Figure 21.11 A and B). Retroclination of the maxillary incisors and the associated, relatively ledge-like, palatal gingival form may further complicate access.

Vulnerability to trauma

The difficulties of access for plaque control does in turn predispose to inadvertent toothbrush trauma.

Similarly the clinician may experience greater operative difficulties at these sites and thereby increase the risk of inadvertent tissue damage from inadequate instrument control, as during scaling.

Occlusal implications

The potential for direct trauma to healthy gingiva from the opposing incisal edges is improbable during normal chewing and swallowing. However, with nocturnal clenching and grinding habits the tissues could become scratched, especially when opposed by uneven sharp incisal edges (Figure 21.10). Irregular incisor wear can be attributed to parafunctional habits (attrition) but is both accelerated and modified by acidic demineralization from dietary constituents or gastric regurgitation. Thus, when incisal edge enamel has been lost from the initial incisal wear, the subsequent differential rates of acidic erosion of the exposed dentine and surrounding enamel results in incisal edge 'cupping'. The unsupported peripheral enamel then fractures easily with further clenching which leaves jagged edges (Figure 21.11 B). Deep overbites are prone to mucosal trauma from the impaction of hard crusty foods. Although this in itself is highly unlikely to

314

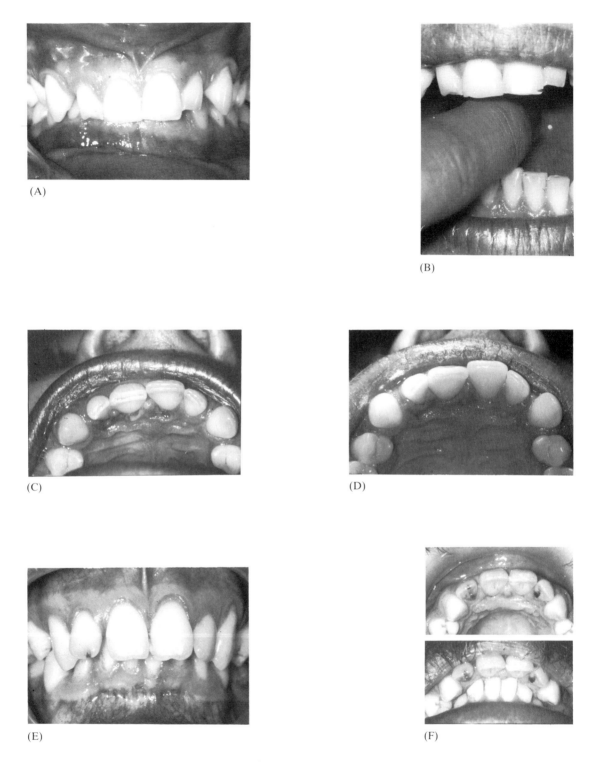

(A)

(B)

(C)

(D)

(E)

(F)

Figure 21.11 Clinical features. (A) Deep overbite in 26-year-old woman reduces (B) interincisal opening. Note unevenly warn sharp incisal edges liable to traumatize opposing mucosa. (C) Palatal mucosal hyperplastic tissue indentations and inflammation but no loss of attachment. (D) 1 year later following inflammatory resolution. (E and F) Palatal gingival hyperplasia but no inflammation associated with deep overbite and overjet. Note recession at 23 labial aspect.

315

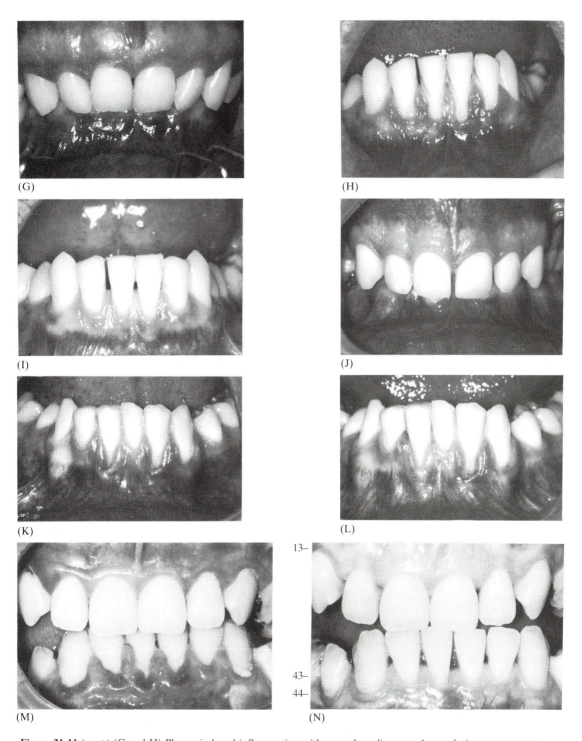

(G)

(H)

(I)

(J)

(K)

(L)

13–

(M)

43–

44–

(N)

Figure 21.11 (*cont.*) (G and H) Plaque-induced inflammation with secondary direct tooth to soft tissue trauma at mandibular labial gingivae associated with recession in 28-year-old man. (I) 1 year later following plaque control. Note slight coronal gingival creeping. (J and K) Gingival clefting 41, 32 associated with tooth to attached gingiva relationship in deep overbite 23-year-old man. (L) Improvement by plaque control measures over 2-year period. (M) 24-year-old woman with marked gingival inflammation and increased tooth mobility associated with deep overbite. (N) Symptoms resolved completely by plaque control alone over 2-year period but note residual inflammation at 13, 44, 43.

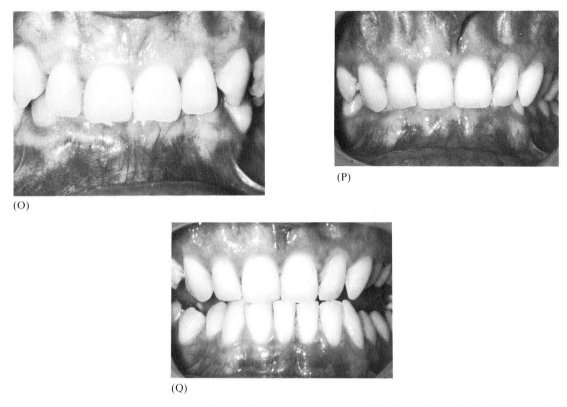

Figure 21.11 (*cont.*) (O) Extent of overbite. (P and Q) Elder sister of patient at (M) with similar occlusion, high standard of oral hygiene yet no gingival lesions

cause gingival detachment, the thin tissue morphology, predisposes to gingival recession (Figure 21.10 C and C1).

When, on the other hand, the marginal gingiva is inflamed in gingivitis or as a result of trauma from, for example, a hard crust or toothbrushing, the swollen tissue is liable to a secondary direct trauma from the opposing incisal edges (especially if worn) and a vicious circle is established (Figure 21.10 C). When inflammatory resolution is accompanied by marginal tissue recession this eliminates the potentially traumatic tooth to soft tissue relationship (Figure 21.10 C1). A similar sequence occurs following loss of attachment in chronic periodontal disease (Figure 21.10 D and D1), but the tissue responses tend to be exaggerated. Thus, recession predominates in the mandible, while pocketing with gingival hyperplasia is more likely to persist at the palate. As the patient frequently presents at the acute stage of secondary trauma, the long-held, but mistaken, clinical impression that the complaint is primarily of occlusal origin, tends to be perpetuated.

The possible pathogenesis of the associated periodontal breakdown and marginal recession in these individuals can now be examined.

Pathogenesis of recession in deep overbites

At the outset, the incisal edges may be related either to the intact gingival margins (located at the cemento-enamel junctions) or to attached gingiva as shown in Figure 21.10 (A and B). With the development of labial recession in the former situations, and assuming a stable incisal relationship exists, the incisal edges will become located coronal to the gingival margins (Figure 21.10 C1). Whereas, with a similar degree of recession in the latter deeper overbites, a tooth to soft tissue relationship would still remain in which the incisal edges would either approximate or lie apical to the opposing gingival margins. The possible pathogenesis of each clinical presentation is considered before the effect of a superimposed unstable incisal relationship is examined.

Tooth to gingival margin relationships

When, in health, traumatic breaches of marginal gingival epithelium from, for example, hard crusts or vigorous toothbrushing, is associated with gingival swelling (Figure 21.10 C) this results in further (direct) trauma from the opposing teeth. This may establish a vicious circle, but most individuals will carefully avoid the area until healing occurs. The outcome of healing and the ensuing gingival form depends on the depth of the lesion in relation to gingival morphology. Thus, relatively shallow wounds heal uneventfully, whilst deeper wounds as in the mandible result in irreversible tissue destruction (gingival recession) and loss of the relationship between incisal edge and gingiva (Figure 21.10 C). The thicker (usually palatal) tissue responds to repeated trauma by epithelial hyperkeratosis and possibly also fibrous hyperplasia, with minimal or no loss of attachment.

The greater gingival swelling occurring with increased inflammatory changes in plaque-induced disease (Figure 21.10 D) leads inevitably to direct trauma from the opposing incisal edges. This sets up a vicious circle, which may be aggravated by gingival tenderness which inhibits cleaning. Symptoms subside as the inflammation resolves, be it spontaneous or following improved oral hygiene, but periodic exacerbations are likely. Where gingival shrinkage occurs, as shown in the mandible in Figure 21.10 (D1), the vulnerability to direct trauma ceases. The thicker pocket wall tissue in the palate is less likely to recede, and a chronic inflammatory fibrous hyperplasia tends to occur instead. The resulting mucosal indentations then give the impression that the teeth have incised into the gingiva. While this may appear to be endorsed by blanching or tissue displacement when the teeth are clenched together, it should be appreciated that both blanching and displacement occur quite readily at inflamed tissue sites in response to only a small amount of pressure.

Tooth to attached gingiva relationship

Direct trauma to attached gingiva from an opposing incisor is improbable, but may occur secondarily, following indirect trauma from impacted hard foods causing mucosal inflammatory swelling (Figure 21.12 A and A1). Most injuries heal uneventfully, but with repeated trauma in the palate gingival hyperplasia develops (Figure 21.11), while in the mandible, where the attached gingiva is thin and associated with a bony deficiency, the inevitable involvement of the underlying periodontal ligament may lead to an irreversible loss of attachment and a tooth to gingival margin relationship (Figure 21.12 A2). (See also Figure 21.14.) The gingival fenestration that might be expected in these instances (Figure 21.12 A1.1 and A 1.2) is almost never seen

clinically. This is probably because the lesion also involves the gingival margin and recession results instead, or where occurring more apically, the intervening band of tissue shown in Figure 21.12 (A1.2), soon breaks down. In either event, this might provide an explanation for the cleft-like gingival recession sometimes encountered in subjects with deep overbites (Figure 21.11).

In the presence of pocketing (Figure 21.12 B) trauma to thin mandibular detached gingival tissue is likely to result in mucosal perforation and merger of the gingival and pocket lining epithelium (Figure 21.12 B1.2) (*cf.* Chapter 13). The detached gingiva coronal to such fenestrations is liable to break down even more rapidly than that described above, establishing a marginal gingival cleft. Once again this is rarely seen clinically, although comparable lesions, but which are unrelated to the opposing teeth, have been observed elsewhere as shown in Figure 21.5 (D, F and G). The thicker palatal detached gingiva is, in contrast, unlikely to be perforated and chronic inflammatory fibrous hyperplasia develops instead located both coronally and apically to the point of incisal contact (Figure 21.12 B2).

Unstable occlusal relationship

In each of the clinical situations cited above, a stable occlusal relationship has been assumed. This implies that, where on presentation, the incisal edges meet the receded gingival margins as shown in Figure 21.13 (A2), they must have initially been in contact with the attached gingiva as depicted in Figure 21.13 (B), and the gingival tissue has then receded until the two components coincided. It is, however, also possible that an increased incisal overbite has developed instead, in the presence of an unstable occlusion, as depicted in Figure 21.13 (B and B1). As the incisal changes in such instances might have followed, coincided with, or preceded the gingival recession, the occlusal implications must be considered.

The development of an increasing incisal overbite following marginal gingival recession in an otherwise stable occlusion, depicted in Figure 21.13 (A2), implies that the anterior occlusal stability has been dependent upon the position of the opposing gingiva. Any increase in overbite would therefore be regarded as a secondary adaptive change to gingival recession. On the other hand, were a primary increase in overbite to have developed instead, as a result of an unstable occlusion, the incisal edges would inevitably lead to the physical detachment of the opposing gingival margins. The gingival recession would then constitute the secondary adaptive response to the occlusal changes. Similarly, at incisal edge to attached gingiva relationships, any primary

318

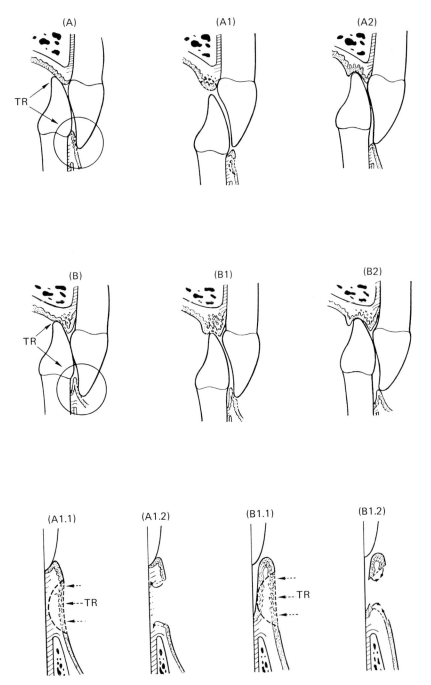

Figure 21.12 Tooth to attached gingiva relationship. (A) Deep overbite with attached gingiva vulnerable to trauma. (A1) Traumatic swelling of attached gingiva, with teeth in precentric position to avoid further trauma and creation of vicious circle. (A2) Teeth in intercuspal position following inflammatory resolution; palatal tissue hyperplasia with tooth indentation but labial recession resulting in the upper incisal edge meeting lower gingival margin. (B, B1 and B2) Comparable but exaggerated tissue responses in presence of pocketing. Note (A and B) balloon areas bottom row. Pathogenesis of recession (A1.1) gingival trauma results in underlying periodontal ligament necrosis and (A1.2) mucosal fenestration followed by loss of coronal marginal tissue band and creation of cleft-like gingival recession. (B1.1) Traumatic perforation of detached gingivae with creation of epithelialized mucosal fenestration and ultimately marginal tissue recession. See comparable situation Figure 21.5 (F and G)

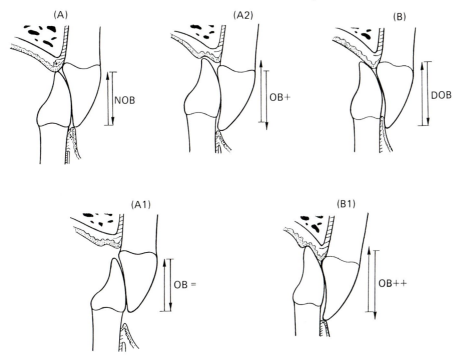

Figure 21.13 Stability of incisal relationships and disease. (A) Incisal edge to labial gingival margin relationship and normal overbite (NOB) with onset of early disease. (A1 and A2) Periodontal breakdown and development of gingival recession in both arches. With (A1) stable occlusion (OB=) loss of contact occurs between tooth and opposing gingival margins, but contact maintained in (A2) unstable occlusion associated with increasing incisal overbite (OB+). Possibility of progressive recession being caused by primary increasing overbite cannot be discounted. (B) Deep overbite (DOB) with tooth biting on attached gingiva. In presence of stable occlusion, attachment loss and gingival recession will result ultimately in relationship of incisal edge to palatal mucosa but to labial gingival margin. (B1) With increasing overbite (OB++) in an unstable occlusion, tooth to gingiva relationship established may result in further recession labially and greater palatal mucosal indentations

increase in overbite would inevitably cleave the thin labial gingiva leading to mucosal fenestration and then recession, but elsewhere would once again cause only mucosal indentations and fibrous hyperplasia (Figure 21.13 B1). Finally, recession and increasing overbite could occur simultaneously making it impossible to differentiate between cause and effect.

There has been very little documented information about any of the possibilities cited above, but it does appear from clinical observations that an increasing overbite in an otherwise stable occlusion does not often occur. The reader is referred to texts on occlusion for the possible influence of posterior occlusal instability which might have adverse effects on incisal relationships. Suffice to say that occlusal slides causing incisal edge impaction against the opposing gingivae and loss of posterior support with incisal over-eruption, might conceivably traumatize the gingivae and so lead to recession.

Management of the problem

The initial gingival lesion

Where a normal dentogingival relationship exists, any marginal gingival lesion related to the opposing incisal edges can be regarded simply as a traumatic ulcer and the patient advised accordingly. Effective cleaning is best maintained with the interspace brush. Uneventful healing ensues, but symptomatic relief may be gained from the topical application of chlorhexidine (Corsodyl Gel, ICI plc, Macclesfield, Cheshire SK10 4TG, UK) or other proprietary oral ulcer preparations (e.g. Bonjela, Reckitt & Colman, Hull HU8 7DS, UK; Medilave, Martindale Pharmaceuticals, Romford, Essex RM1 4JX, UK). The apparently offending incisal edges should not be trimmed as this may be followed by over-eruption, but irregularly worn sharp edges are best smoothed using a fine sandpaper disc. A reduction in acidic food intake is prudent, and fruit juice preferably taken instead and sucked through a straw to minimize contact with the teeth. Acid regurgitation, suspected by the loss of palatal enamel should also be counteracted, in consultation with the patient's physician (*cf.* Chapter 26).

Recurrent gingival lesions

When the above preventive measures are found to be ineffective, a full coverage occlusal bite guard may be considered. This can be fitted in either arch to disclude the teeth and so preclude gingival trauma and be worn as and when necessary.

Lesions in the presence of disease

The measures described above, in conjunction with the appropriate routine periodontal care dealt with in previous chapters, are indicated and need no further consideration here. Where gingival recession already exists, a similar treatment regime is directed at preventing further loss of attachment.

Lesions with anterior occlusal instability

Where instability is suspected, any obvious or predisposing occlusal relationships are first corrected. Only where a progressively increasing overbite and gingival recession does occur, or where aesthetic considerations demand it, should complex multi-disciplinary orthodontic or skeletal surgical restorative solutions be considered. These are beyond the scope of this text.

Prognosis

Standardized clinical photographs are helpful, but periodontal attachment measures, appropriate extra-oral radiographs and study casts are essential for future reference purposes. Clinical experience suggests that where marginal health is maintained and trauma from toothbrushing and hard foods avoided, neither the initial onset nor progression of recession will occur in subjects with deep overbites in stable occlusions as shown in Figures 21.11 and 21.14. In practice, these sites appear to be no more vulnerable to gingival recession than any other sites with a comparable dentogingival morphology and indeed respond in similar fashion to variations of plaque control.

Conclusion

It is, at present, not possible to forecast those situations where recession will actually develop and, where it has occurred, whether it will progress. This coupled with the lack of control documentation of the different forms of occlusal treatment carried out also precludes the evaluation of the role of occlusion in these cases. Consequently, until such time that clear indications for any such specific interceptive measures have been established, the operator is best advised to concentrate simply on containing the associated plaque-induced lesion, as in any other patient, without reference to the apparently peculiar intermaxillary relationship.

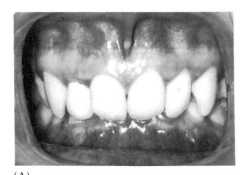

(A)

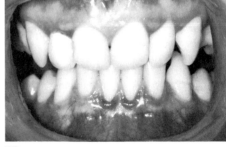

(B)

Figure 21.14 Longitudinal assessment. (A and B) Deep overbite and plaque induced gingival inflammation and minimal recession at 41, 31 in 20-year-old.

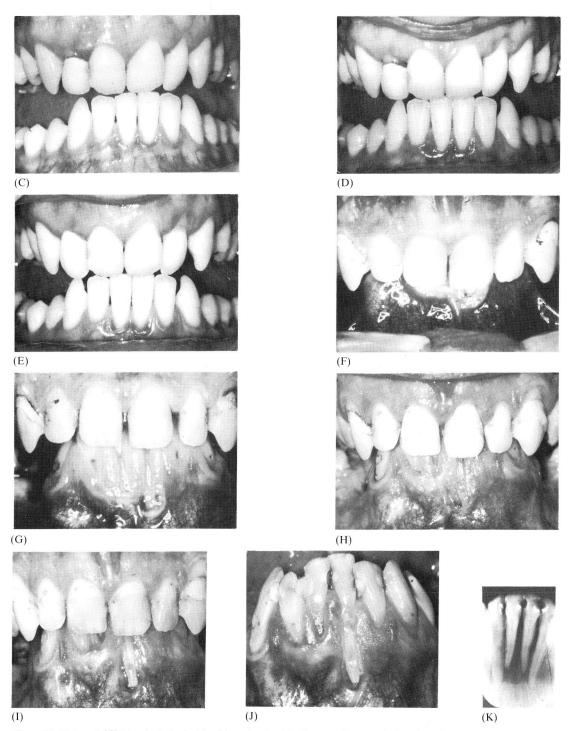

Figure 21.14 (*cont.*) (C) Marginal gingival health maintained for 2 years; fluctuated after that with development of further recession at 41, 31 but also at other sites unrelated to overbite. (D) 6 years, and (E) 9 years. Occlusion remained stable. (F) Deep overbite in 22-year-old man, (G) corrected by orthognathic surgery. Residual gingival recession to 31 root apex plus clefting at 42, 41, 32. Findings (H) 6 years later and (I) 12 years later – no change in 31 recession but some coronal creeping at 42, 41, 32. (J) At 15 years widening of cleft with greater exposure of root apex, but also further recession elsewhere; (K) radiographic presentation.

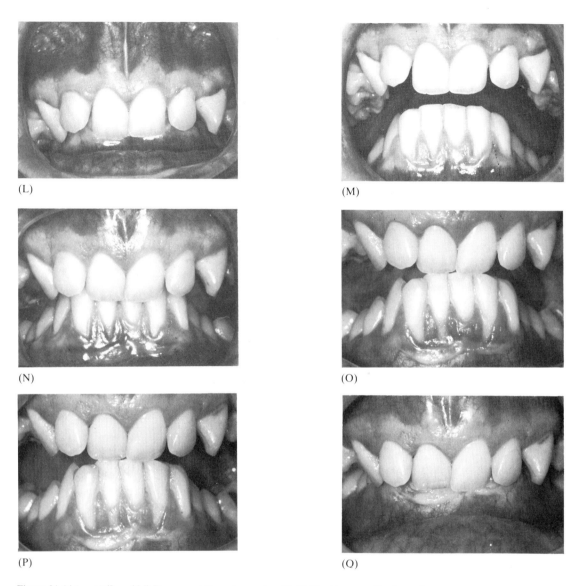

(L)

(M)

(N)

(O)

(P)

(Q)

Figure 21.14 (*cont.*) (L and M) Deep overbite and recession 42, 41 32 with generalized marginal inflammation in 24-year-old man. (N) Free gingival graft (6 week healing shown) at 2 years (1971!). Further slight recession noted 42, 32 and at other sites by (O) 10 years and (P) 14 years. Note (Q) overbite and apparently stable occlusion

22

The surgical correction of vestibular problems

Increasing vestibular depth
Mucosal frenal surgery

Marginal gingival inconsistencies

The correction of vestibular problems will be dealt with in the following order of shallow vestibules, prominent mucosal frena and, lastly, adverse gingival contour. This is in line with their relative clinical importance and because the respective surgical measures to be described follow a sequential technical pattern.

Increasing vestibular depth

Vestibular fold displacement technique

Mucosal fenestration

Apical displacement of the vestibular fold is achieved by first making a horizontal incision, preferably just coronal to the mucogingival junction (Figure 22.1 A and A1). This ensures that an intact band of marginal tissue, of at least 2 mm in width, is maintained about the teeth to avoid damaging the supracrestal attachment. For this reason, where the gingival dimensions are also minimal the incision would be located within non-keratinized mucosa (Figure 22.1 B1). This incision is then progressively opened up like a buttonhole, by an apically directed split-thickness sharp dissection. This technique is described in greater detail below (Figure 22.1 B and B1) under the free gingival graft recipient bed preparation, with which it has so much in common. The displacement of the apical margin of the mucosal fenestration has the effect of deepening the vestibule. Provided this displaced tissue is prevented from returning to its former position during healing, vestibular depth is maintained.

Fenestration healing

The reparative tissue cell proliferation stems from bone, periosteum, the surrounding gingival mucosa and the periodontal ligament where developmental bony fenestrations and dehiscences are present or where undermining resorption of thin necrotic bone occurs during healing (Figure 22.1 B1). In situations where the fenestration wound is bounded by alveolar mucosa, the potential for keratinized tissue regeneration is rather limited, being restricted to only those sites with periodontal ligament involvement. Consequently a variable combination of alveolar mucosa and gingiva develops during healing (Figure 22.2 B and G).

Post-surgical relapse

The characteristics of the healed mucosa are of clinical importance because only gingival tissue, by virtue of it being firmly bound down to the bone, is capable of maintaining vestibular fold displacement. Any such deficiency, coupled with the tendency for the physically displaced vestibular tissue to gradually move back to its original position, means that some coronal relapse is inevitable during healing, so thwarting the surgical objective. This relapse appears to occur mainly within the initial 6-week healing period. The presence of a physical barrier, like a periodontal dressing, is therefore necessary. When, as in apically repositioned flap surgery, this dressing is retained for only 1 week an almost complete relapse occurs; whereas when it is retained

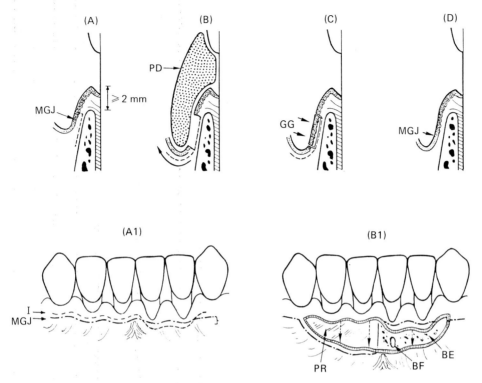

Figure 22.1 Mucosal fenestration and grafting. (A and A1) Initial incision (I) not less than 2 mm from gingival margin located just coronal to mucogingival junction (MGJ) at 42, 41, but located within alveolar mucosa at 31, 32. (B and B1) Mucosal fenestration created by vestibular tissue displacement apically. Fenestration bounded by gingival mucosa at 42, 41 and alveolar mucosa at 31, 32. Periodontal dressing maintains tissue displacement. Note periosteal retention (PR) at 43, 42, 41, bone exposure (BE) at 31, 32, 33 and bony fenestration (BF) with root surface exposure at 31. (C) Placement of gingival graft (GF) in fenestration. (D) Healed graft with more apically located MGJ. Note slight shrinkage of graft and coronal relapse of vestibular tissue

for up to 6 weeks, as much as half of the surgical fenestration opening intended may still be lost (Figure 22.2 C and H).

The clinical applications of the fenestration technique are *very limited*, because of the great technical difficulties of maintaining tissue displacement and the considerable postoperative discomfort experienced. Each can, however, be readily overcome by inserting keratinized mucosal tissue, represented by a free gingival graft, within the mucosal fenestration (Figure 22.1 C). (See also Chapter 32 – Vestibular morphology.)

Rationale for grafting

Free gingival grafting offers several advantages to the vestibular fold displacement technique. Firstly, the graft takes readily so that healing is rapid and postoperative discomfort is minimized, although this

is partly offset by the creation of a second (donor site) wound. Secondly, as the grafted gingival tissue retains its inherent tissue characteristics, an ideal tissue with which to inhibit coronal relapse is provided from the outset, although some shrinkage of the graft itself does occur. Finally, it is no longer necessary to separate the surgical fenestration wound edges with a bulky mechanical dressing.

Free gingival grafting

Graft bed

Preparation of the graft recipient bed is essentially that of the mucosal fenestration technique, but it is considered in more detail here. The lip or cheek is first gripped and pulled outwards to define the mucogingival junction more clearly and while maintaining this tension, the initial incision is made

325

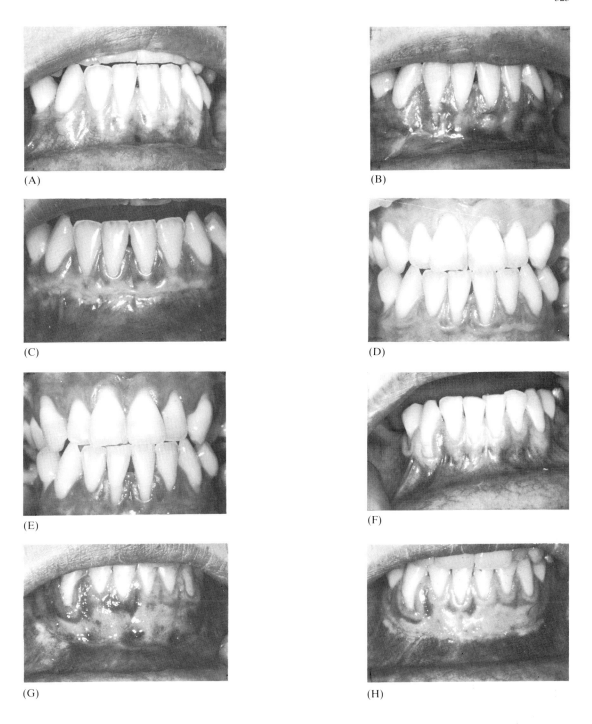

(A)

(B)

(C)

(D)

(E)

(F)

(G)

(H)

Figure 22.2 Mucosal fenestration healing. (A) Gingival 'inadequacy' deemed to exist despite gingival health (1967) in 24-year-old woman. (B) Fenestration wound healing at 4 weeks, when dressing removed (note root exposure at 42) and (C) 10 weeks. Some coronal relapse coupled with mucosal scarring, almost complete repair at 42 and slight coronal creeping of gingival margins elsewhere. Presentation at (D) 10 years and (E) 18 years. Further recession at 41, 31 and at several other sites but not at 42. (F) Fenestration surgery considered necessary (1967) for recession at 43 and 41, 31 and shallow vestibule in 20-year-old woman. (G) Fenestration healing at 6 weeks when dressing removed (associated with marginal tissue inflammatory proliferation and possibly displacement by presence of dressing) and (H) 10 weeks.

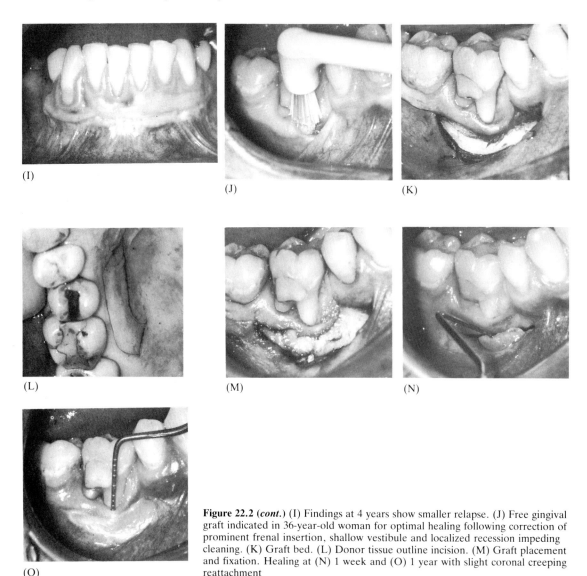

Figure 22.2 (*cont.*) (I) Findings at 4 years show smaller relapse. (J) Free gingival graft indicated in 36-year-old woman for optimal healing following correction of prominent frenal insertion, shallow vestibule and localized recession impeding cleaning. (K) Graft bed. (L) Donor tissue outline incision. (M) Graft placement and fixation. Healing at (N) 1 week and (O) 1 year with slight coronal creeping reattachment

with a Swann Morton No. 15 blade. This incision is at right angles to the gingival surface and ideally runs just coronal to the line of the mucogingival junction (Figure 22.1 A) producing a narrow buttonhole-like slit apical to the line of the incision. Where, however, bony dehiscences are suspected the blade is best directed apically from the outset, to minimize the risk of root surface exposure and of compromising the viability of the donor tissue subsequently. The apically directed split-thickness dissection of the mucosal fenestration next prepared separates the vestibular mucosa and any related muscle fibres from the periosteum which is retained

in situ to form the graft bed (Figures 22.1 B and B1 and 22.2 K). This dissection may however be complicated by the mucosal thinness and the often corrugated bone contour over the roots and results in inadvertent periosteal perforation. Fortunately the clinical outcomes at periosteal and osseous recipient beds are no different, although root surface exposure at bony dehiscences or fenestrations does carry the risk of periodental ligament necrosis and the graft not taking at the site. It should be obvious that the technique should not be attempted in the presence of pocketing, for not only is the periosteal bed lacking, but mucosal pocket wall tissue perforation to the underlying periodontally involved root surface is almost inevitable.

Dissection is extended as far laterally and apically as necessary for vestibular fold displacement, and is simply judged at the time by the amount of space required for subsequent toothbrush placement. Sometimes oblique relieving incisions are necessary at the lateral edges of the field to expedite displacement. The graft bed tends to be semilunar in outline with a gently scalloped coronal margin, associated with the undulating mucogingival junction, and a rounded apical edge (Figure 22.1 B1), and depending on the relationship of the initial incision to the mucogingival junction, is bounded by either keratinized or non-keratinized mucosa.

A warm saline gauze swab is pressed gently but firmly over the graft bed on completion and retained in position, between it and the displaced vestibular mucosa, during donor tissue preparation. Absolute haemostasis is critical to ensure the subsequent intimate apposition of the graft tissue to the recipient bed.

Donor tissue

The smooth surfaced keratinized mucosa of the postero-lateral walls of the palatal vault are the sites of choice (Figure 22.2 L), but the maxillary buccal aspects may also be used. Marginal gingiva is not involved to avoid damaging the supracrestal attachment. The anterior part of the palate is best avoided as the rugae make it difficult to obtain donor tissue in the required even thickness and could also make the healed grafted site look peculiar.

A shallow (1–2 mm) outline incision conforming to the required shape and size of the recipient site is made with a Swann Morton No. 12. blade. This is judged visually, using the scalloped palatal gingival margin contour as a guide to the required shape of the coronal edge of the graft. Alternatively, the shape can be traced about a tin-foil template cut to fit the recipient site. The filletting dissection, using a sharp Swann Morton No. 15 blade, is commenced at the most accessible mesial part of the outline incision and is then extended distally, preparing the thinnest possible layer of tissue (i.e. about 1 mm). The appropriate tissue thickness is readily confirmed by the dull grey colour and contour of the blade observed through the comparatively translucent mucosa.

Where free bleeding obscures vision this is best controlled by further injections of vasoconstricting (1:80000 adrenaline) local anaesthetic solution into the surrounding tissues. Low pressure aspiration is maintained immediately adjacent to the blade, using a 3-mm diameter aspirator tip, which is also used to deflect the progressively enlarging donor tissue from the palate during dissection. A second, wider bore nozzle is used as necessary for overall oral clearance.

Graft tissue transfer and placement

When dissection is nearing completion the tip is placed end on against the outer keratinized surface of the graft tissue and with suction pressure carefully controlled so that the tissue becomes gently attached to the tip end, the graft is finally separated from the palate. It is transferred in this fashion directly to the recipient site, from which the gauze swab has just been removed. Once positioned, the graft tissue is pressed gently into place using a moist gauze swab. The carefully prepared donor tissue fits closely against the coronal edge of the graft bed (Figure 22.1 C and 22.2 M) for optimal healing. The fit apically is less critical for any associated denuded periosteum or bone, heals as described previously.

Graft fixation

The fibrinous blood coagulum virtually glues the graft in position, but application of a few small drops of quick-setting cyanoacrylate contact adhesive (e.g. Powabond – Powabond 102, Double H International Ltd, Staines, Middlesex, UK) along its coronal edge is advocated. The vestibular mucosa is retracted until the adhesive sets. (The graft may if preferred be sutured in place instead.) A soft Coe-pak dressing is then applied to the dried necks of the teeth and gently moulded over the graft using the moistened lip with a prosthetic muscle-trimming manipulation to avoid over-extension apically. Failure to do so may cause subsequent graft displacement during functional movements and interfere with healing. The apical part of the dressing approximates to any denuded connective tissue surface at the base of the vestibule.

Donor site protection

A warm saline gauze pressure pack is used first to control bleeding. A soft Coe-pak is then applied to the adjacent dried tooth surfaces, to which it sticks readily, and as the material hardens it is patted apically, with a moist finger over the donor site wound. Alternatively, the wound could be protected with pre-processed acrylic palatal prosthesis lined with Coe-pak.

Postoperative care and healing

The graft site is merely carefully avoided and no special post-surgical instructions are necessary (*cf.* Chapter 17). Healing is generally uneventful and the dressings are removed at 1 week, although that in the palate will sometimes have dislodged earlier. The coronal margin of the carefully prepared graft blends imperceptively with the related tissue, whilst a greyish-pink tissue and blood slough presents apically at the base of the vestibule (see Figure 22.2 N). The epithelial surface of the graft usually desquamates as a thin friable surface layer that is readily flushed away, but may sometimes appear ulcerated in parts which soon re-epithelialize.

The grafted tissue is sustained initially by tissue fluid diffusion. Revascularization by endothelial outgrowths from the underlying recipient vascular bed, commences by about the fifth day with a peripheral vascular plexus being re-established by about 10 days. Healing at the donor tissue site is as described for the essentially comparable mucosal fenestrations, so need not be considered further here. (See also Chapter 32 – Gingival dimensions and plaque-induced disease.)

The clinical effects

As the grafted tissue retains its intrinsic characteristics, a new mucogingival junction is established at the apical edge of the graft and the vestibular sulcus displacement maintained (Figure 22.1 D and 22.2 O). Some shrinkage occurs during healing but its limited extent is of little clinical significance. In some instances the related receded gingival margin will undergo coronal creeping (Figures 22.2 O and 22.3 E) although this phenomenon may also occur spontaneously as shown in Figures 21.5 B; 21.7 A and B and 21.11 I.

The benefits of gingival grafting apparently accrue from the improved access for plaque control, provided by the wider band of immobile keratinized tissue established about the teeth displacing the

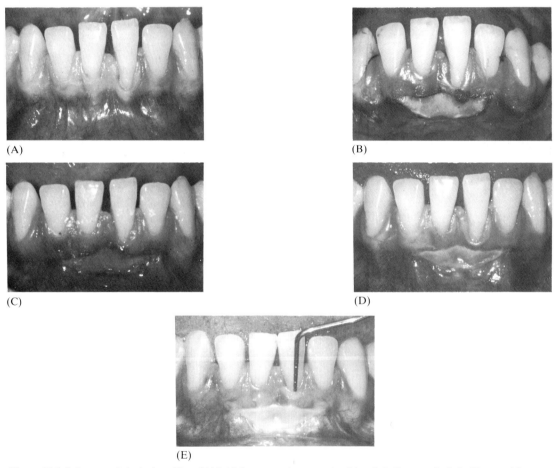

(A)

(B)

(C)

(D)

(E)

Figure 22.3 Influence of gingival grafting. (A) Initial presentation recession 31 and shallow vestibule in 22-year-old professional model with possibly unstable incisal relationships. Anticipated (in 1974) that risk of further recession associated with tooth displacement would be obviated by provision of gingival graft. (B) Graft fixation. Healing at (C) 1 week and (D) 3 months. Note graft shrinkage. Coronal creeping reattachment first observed at 4 years maintained to (E) 9 years. Note altered tooth alignment.

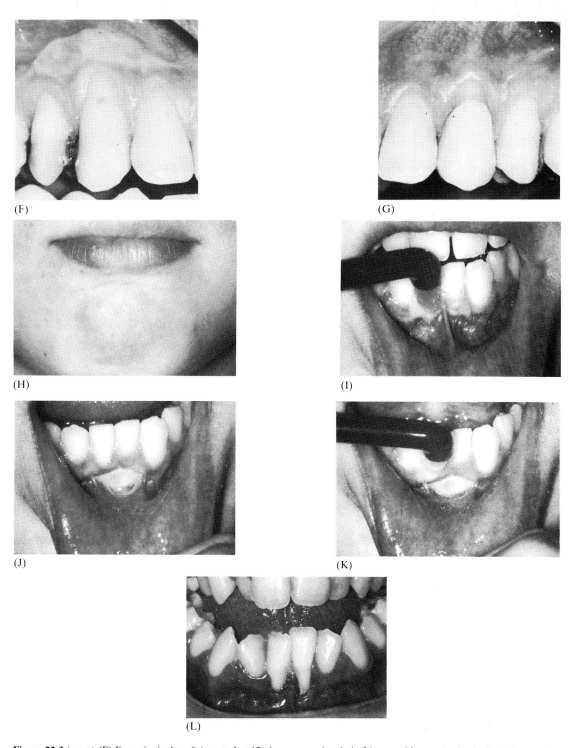

Figure 22.3 (*cont.*) (F) Free gingival graft inserted at 1⟨3⟩ 4 years previously in 36-year-old man, to check gingival recession with (G) ⟨2⟩3 serving as control. Clinical records showed no change at either site. (H) Powerful lower lip tone plus prominent labial frenum in 15-year-old girl (see also Figure 21.1 (D)) complicated oral hygiene. (I) Labial retraction and use of interspace brush inadequate so frenal resection requested. (J) Gingival graft inserted at resection site (K) facilitates cleaning. (L) Vestibular tissue impeding cleaning in 17-year-old girl – orthognathic surgery contemplated.

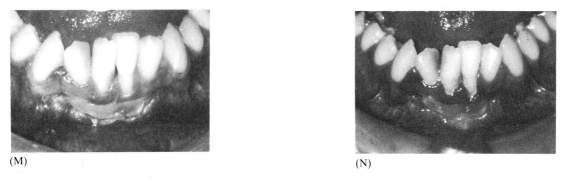

(M)   (N)

Figure 22.3 (*cont.*) (M) Vestibular displacement with graft – 6 month healing. (N) Recurrent inflammation 12 months later despite improved access

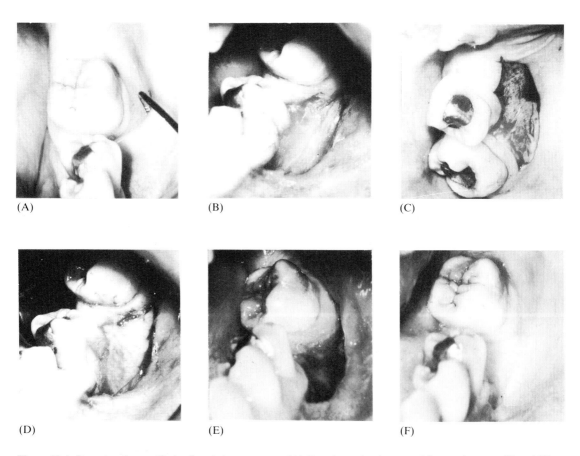

(A)   (B)   (C)

(D)   (E)   (F)

Figure 22.4 Prerestorative vestibular frenal tissue surgery. (A) Prominent developmental frenum between 35 and 37. Orthodontic uprighting 37 indicated in 38-year-old woman. (B) Displaced frenum and graft bed. (C) Palatal donor bed after delivery graft tissue. (D) Graft fixation. Healing at (E) 1 week and (F) 4 weeks.

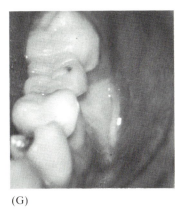

(G)

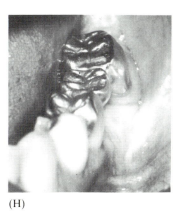

(H)

Figure 22.4 (*cont.*) (G) Post-orthodontic retention with provisional restoration. (H) Bridge in place (by courtesy Department of Conservation, Institute of Dental Surgery, London) – note effective tissue displacement

interfering influence of the movable vestibular tissues (Figure 22.3). When, on the other hand, improved plaque control does not accrue as shown in Figure 22.3 (L–N), the true cause of the problem will have been misjudged by the operator. In conclusion, it must be emphasized that the need for vestibular deepening and grafting arises very rarely in clinical practice. (See also Figure 22.4.)

Mucosal frenal surgery

The gingival insertion of the frenum is a handicap to plaque control, by representing a localized shallow vestibule. It is, therefore, amenable to surgical correction by the vestibular displacement technique in which the outline fenestration incision is dictated by the frenal form. The simplest application of the technique, that for the narrow steeply 'V' shaped labial frenum described here, is, with appropriate modifications, applicable to all other frenal forms.

Frenal displacement

Outline incision

The lip is retracted to clearly delineate the lateral borders of the frenum. Separate outline incisions, aligned at right angles to the gingival surface, are made down to bone with a Swann Morton No. 15 blade along each of the lateral borders of the frenal attachment. These incisions commence at the level of the adjacent vestibular folds and pass coronally to meet at the frenal apex (Figure 22.5 A). These outline incisions will not meet coronally at wider,

more 'U'-shaped frena (Figure 22.5 E) so need to be joined by a short horizontal incision. Where displacement of the adjacent vestibular tissues is also necessary, the appropriate additional incisions are made along the mucogingival junctions and the two procedures then carried out together.

Filletting incision

This sharp dissection frees the frenal body connective tissue from the underlying bone. It commences from within either one of the outline incisions, and extends towards the other with the blade held fairly flat against the adjacent gingival surface (Figure 22.5 A and A1), whilst simultaneously retracting the lip. The frenum comes away readily revealing a narrow tapering strip of denuded periosteum and/or alveolar bone. This bony surgical wound is contiguous apically with the mucosal wound on the frenal body suspended from the retracted lip (Figure 22.5 B and B1), at the point representing the level of the new vestibular fold.

The mucosal wound contracts almost immediately (see Figure 22.6 B and G), resulting in a marked reduction in the size of the frenal body. This tissue is retained intact on the inner surface of the lip, as its total resection would simply create a larger wound with more complicated healing and increased postoperative discomfort, but without any commensurate benefit. Furthermore, the frenal body tissue shrinks progressively over a period of time, leaving but a small and clinically insignificant fibrous nodule in most instances (Figure 22.5 D and 22.6 E and I).

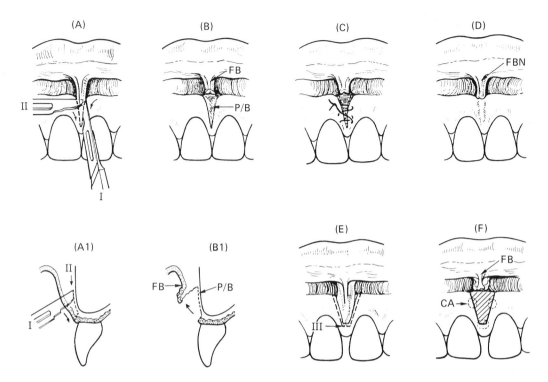

Figure 22.5 Frenal displacement. (A and A1) Initial (I) outline incision along lateral border of frenal body and passing down to bone followed by (II) filletting incision. (B and B1) Frenal body (FB) displacement apically. Note contiguous periosteal/bony (P/B) and frenal body (FB) wounds. (C) Mattress-type suturing of periosteal/bony wound. (D) Healed wound and residual frenal body mucosal nodule (FBN). (E) Wider frenum necessitates additional coronally located (III) horizontal incision, and (F) insertion of free gingival graft stabilized with cyanoacrylate adhesive (CA)

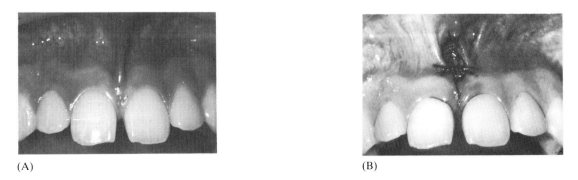

Figure 22.6 Labial frenal displacement. (A) Initial presentation in 15-year-old girl. (B) Frenal body displacement plus suturing.

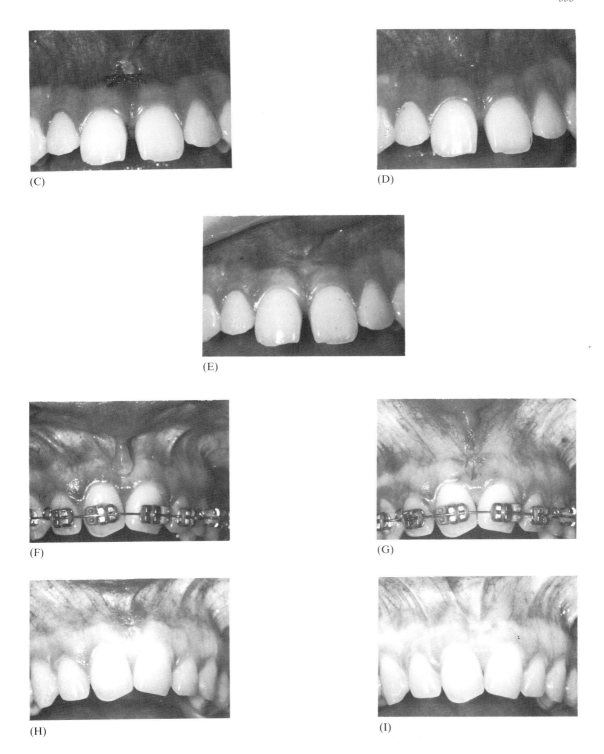

Figure 22.6 (*cont.*) Healing at (C) 1 week, (D) 6 weeks and (E) 8 months. Note scarring and shrinkage of former frenal body. (F) Prominent labial frenum limiting upper lip movement in 23-year-old woman. (G) Fenestration suturing – note frenal body displacement apically. (H) Healing at 4 weeks, when sutures and orthodontic appliance removed and at (I) 2 years. Note shrinkage of frenal body.

334

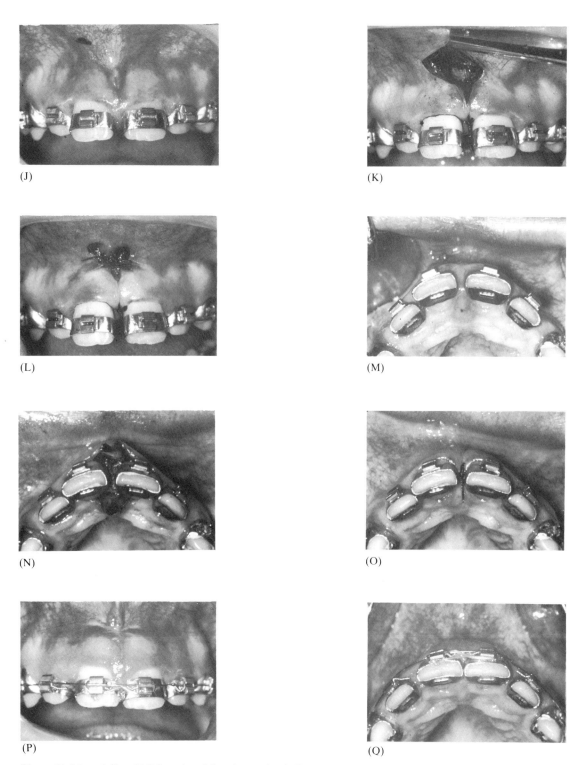

Figure 22.6 (*cont.*) (J and M) Interdental frenal resection indicated in 14-year-old girl in conjunction with orthodontic closure of maxillary spacing. (K) Labial component of frenum displaced and (L) sutured. (M) Frenal insertion into incisive papilla. (N) Labial and palatal papillary flap reflection for removal of interdental component of frenal tissue. (O and L) Papillae adapted interdentally and sutured. (P and Q) Healing at 4 months

Wound surface separation

The frenal body will revert to its approximate presurgical position when lip retraction is ceased. The approximating wound surfaces will then heal with reformation of the frenal attachment. It is therefore necessary, as in vestibular fold displacement surgery, to separate the wound surfaces during healing. This can be achieved in several ways. The first two options of frenal body tissue resection and of periodontal dressing placement as in fenestration surgery, to minimize the chances of reunion, carry disadvantages cited above. Next, the insertion of a gingival graft should be considered when a comparatively large wound area exists as depicted in Figure 22.5 (F), but requires a further surgical procedure. The last is the insertion of a mattress-type suture across the mucosal split (Figure 22.5 C) which proves to be the simplest and most practical method. The suturing is retained for 3–4 weeks, its physical presence impeding approximation of the opposing wound surfaces until each has epithelialized individually. The delayed healing at the points of entry of the suture is associated with some scarring but no adverse clinical effects have been observed. In addition there is negligible postoperative discomfort and most importantly, little tendency for frenal reformation, the former frenal body simply shrinking progressively to a small residual fibrous nodule (Figure 22.6 E and I). The clinical surgical sequence is shown in Figure 22.6.

Interdental frenal tissue resection

Labial frena that pass between the teeth and are attached to the lingual or palatal interdental papillae are handled as described above, but with minor modifications and coupled with an interdental papillectomy for the interdental tissue component. Thus, the labial outline incisions are extended coronally only to the level of the mid-labial gingival margins of the related teeth, at which they are joined by a horizontal incision passing through the frenal body (Figure 22.7 A). The frenum is then displaced and suturing inserted. The papillectomy crevicular incisions should commence at the respective mesial line angles of the bounding teeth and are joined interdentally as shown in Figure 22.7 (A and A1). The labial papillary flap is then reflected only

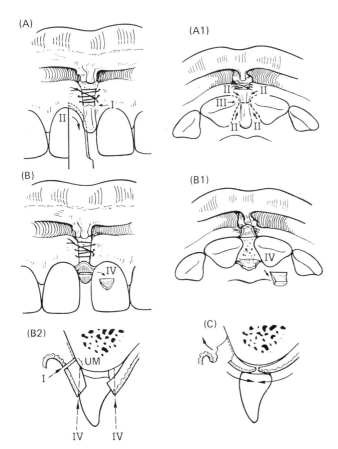

Figure 22.7 Frenal displacement and interdental frenal resection. (A1, B2 and C) Initial labial frenal body displacement and suturing as in Figure 22.5 (C). (A and A1) Interdental frenum resected by (arrowed) horizontal incision (I) followed by labial and palatal papillary crevicular incisions (II) which are joined (III) interdentally. (B2) Labial and palatal papillary tissue reflection and filletting followed by removal of (B and B1) the respective (IV) tissue wedges. Note band of undisturbed labial mucosa (UM) between surgical fields. (C) Frenal displacement and papillary adaptation interdentally

minimally for filletting, to ensure that a band of intact undisturbed mucosa separates the two surgical fields (Figure 22.7 A1 and B2). This in turn maintains the integrity of the papillary flap blood supply, which might otherwise lead to its ischaemic necrosis.

The palatal papillary flap is prepared quite routinely, any residual interdental septal tissue curetted away and the papillary flaps coapted,

meeting interdentally (Figure 22.7 C). The flaps are stabilized by the application of cyanoacrylate tissue adhesive or suturing. The clinical surgical sequence is shown in Figure 22.6 (J–Q).

Note: Frenal displacement is sometimes necessary in conjunction with pocket surgery, when the interdental frenal tissue resection is indicated. The technique is shown clinically in Figure 22.8 (A–H).

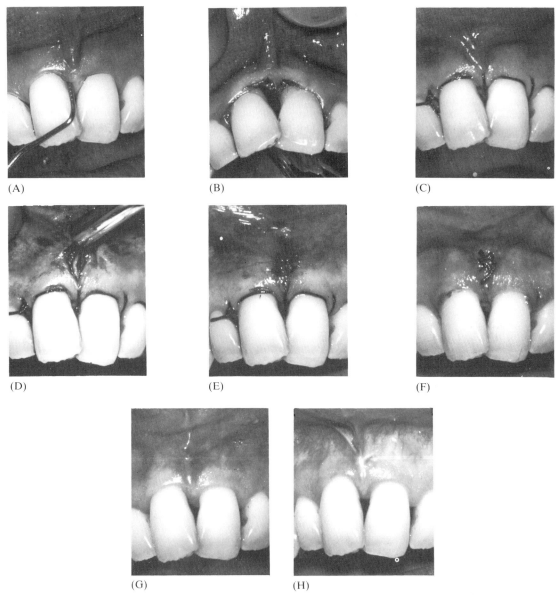

Figure 22.8 Frenal displacement in conjunction with pocket surgery. (A) Pre-operative probing. (B) Pocket surgery flap elevation and (C) suturing. (D) Frenal displacement and (E) suturing. Healing at (F) 1 week, (G) 4 weeks (when frenal sutures removed) and (H) 6 months.

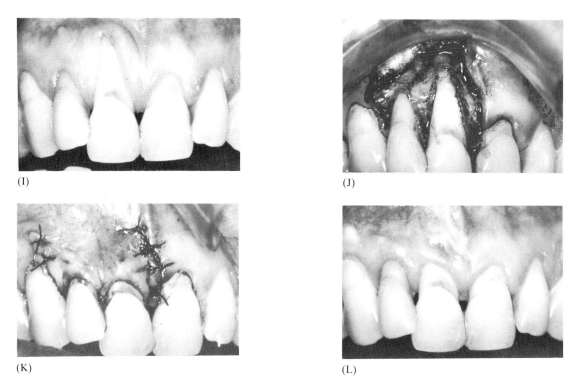

Figure 22.8 (*cont.*) (I) Coronally repositioned flap at aesthetically displeasing 11 – initial presentation. (J) Mucoperiosteal flap prepared and (K) positioned coronally. (L) Healing at 2 years. (By courtesy Dr J. J. Wennström)

Marginal gingival inconsistencies

The type of corrective surgery will depend on the nature of the problem, which may relate to poor aesthetics or difficulties in oral hygiene. A displeasing localized gingival tissue overgrowth is readily corrected by inverse bevel resection, as described in Chapter 16. At the other extreme, root surface exposure following localized recession could be masked by an acrylic gingival veneer, by surgically transposing the adjacent mucosa by pedicle grafting or the provision of a free gingival grafting. In pedicle grafting either neighbouring tissue (laterally repositioned flap) or that about the tooth itself (coronally repositioned flap) is utilized (Figure 22.9). It is fortunate that the difficulties in cleaning at sites of localized recession usually resolve following vestibular fold displacement surgery alone. This is because the alternative surgical options of grafting are not always predictable and are liable to relapse. This is due to the grafted tissue to root surface relationship being represented primarily by a long junctional epithelium, although the potential for some new attachment does exist. This stems from the bounding (apical and lateral) periodontal ligament tissues. In some instances, however, a pocket might even be created at the site, whilst at the donor site in lateral repositioning, the marginal attachment may be compromised with the development of gingival recession (see Figure 22.9 A2). Free gingival grafting is, as might be expected, the least predictable and is only feasible at very narrow (less than 2 mm) cleft-like sites of recession.

There are numerous variations to these techniques, each of which is designed to enhance healing, cater for inherent limitations of potential donor sites and safeguard the integrity of the donor site supracrestal attachment. These variations need not be considered here, because the principles involved are as described below and so are applicable to all situations, and the clinical and cosmetic indications for the techniques are so limited. (See also Chapter 32 – Gingival dimensions and plaque-induced disease.)

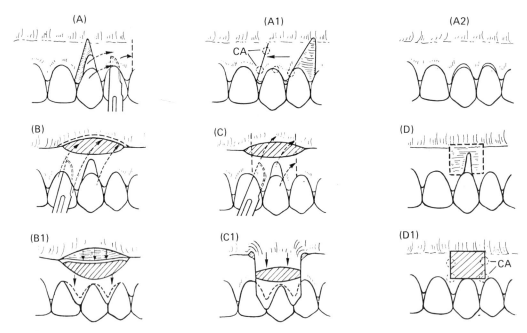

Figure 22.9 Localized gingival recession root coverage techniques. (A) 23 Laterally repositioned flap recipient bed and 24 donor tissue preparation. (A1) Flap positioned and stabilized with cyanoacrylate adhesive (CA). (A2) Healing with slight relapse (recession) and possible recession at donor site. (B and C) Healed free gingival graft and flap tissue preparation for coronal repositioning. Note respective horizontal fenestration incision apical to grafted tissue at (B) and bilateral linear relieving incisions at (C). (B1 and C1) Coronally positioned tissue excess over adjacent coronal surfaces resected along broken lines. (D) Free gingival graft bed preparation over narrow gingival cleft. (D1) Gingival graft stabilized

Laterally repositioned flap

The donor tissue constitutes a pedicle graft with its own blood supply, which sustains that part of the graft tissue located over the root surface. The graft is additionally sustained by the recipient connective tissue bed about the initially exposed root surface. On the side of the tooth remote to the donor tissue, the recipient bed is prepared by paring away, with an external bevel incision, a 2–3 mm wide band of surface mucosa as shown in Figure 22.9 (A), whilst on the near side, the bed is created by the split-thickness dissection of the donor tissue.

The width of donor tissue required is first established and appropriate oblique incisions made from the respective gingival margins to beyond the mucogingival junction, followed by a crevicular incision coronally. Care is taken to minimize damage to the supracrestal periodontal attachment at both the recipient and donor sites. The recipient root surface is carefully debrided to enhance compatibility with the donor tissue mucosal flap when rotated and positioned over the exposed root and its surrounding periosteal connective tissue bed (Figure 22.9 A1). This pedicle graft is closely

adapted with a moist gauze swab and following haemostasis, fixed by suturing or tissue adhesive at its margins. A soft mix of Coe-pak is applied to protect primarily the exposed donor site.

Coronally repositioned flap

A free gingival graft is best first inserted to displace any potential vestibular tissue interference, as depicted in Figure 22.9 (B and C). Following healing, a crevicular incision is made about the receded unit and its two adjacent teeth and the tissue to be repositioned coronally is dissected free in one of two ways. In the first, a linear incision is made apical to the graft and a mucoperiosteal mucosal tunnel created between this and the crevicular incision, by both sharp and blunt dissection commencing from the coronal aspect (Figure 22.9 B). The mucosa is then displaced coronally creating a mucosal fenestration apically (Figure 22.9 B1). In the other, vertical relieving incisions are made at the mesial line angles of the neighbouring teeth (Figure 22.9 C). A mucoperiosteal flap is then reflected beyond the vestibular fold and the, thus, totally mobilized flap displaced coronally over the receded root surface (Figure 22.9 C1). Where the adjacent tooth coronal surfaces become covered by the repositioned flap tissue, this is trimmed away as necessary prior to fixing the flap into position. The latter technique, but without previous incorporation of a gingival graft, is shown in Figure 22.8 (I–L).

Free gingival grafting

The graft bed and root surface preparation depicted in Figure 22.8 (D) are as for the laterally repositioned flap and the grafting technique is as described before. The narrow zone of graft tissue located over the root surface itself (Figure 22.8 D1) must be sustained initially by diffusion from the contiguous graft connective tissues. The tendency for breakdown at its coronal margin results in less complete root coverage than anticipated.

Section III

Allied problems

23

Mobility and drifting

The nature of the problem
The clinical significance of increased mobility

The management of unacceptable degrees of
    mobility and drifting
Conclusion

In this chapter the contentious question of increased mobility of the teeth will be considered under three separate headings. Firstly, the nature of the problem of increased mobility, then its significance in health and disease and, finally, the management of mobility that influences patient function and comfort.

The nature of the problem

A tooth will become displaced and then display mobility when forces are applied to it. Normally, these forces originate from the opposing teeth during functional (chewing and swallowing) and parafunctional (e.g. clenching and grinding) activities. Similar displacement forces also operate in orthodonic therapy and, in some instances, from prostheses.

In health a barely perceptible, physiological or functional, mobility of the teeth exists and every tooth with healthy periodontal support will have a physiologic range of mobility. The incisors are more mobile than posterior teeth and mobility is usually greatest on awaking, and gradually decreases through the day. When teeth are subjected to greater forces, as from bruxism or clenching, an increased degree of mobility develops as a physiological adaptation to these forces.

Increased tooth mobility also occurs in plaque-induced disease. Indeed this is so commonly encountered as an accompanying feature of gingival inflammation and pocketing that it is regarded as characteristic of chronic disease. The degree of mobility present in any situation is influenced by both the levels of inflammation of the supracrestal tissues, with which it is in turn liable to fluctuate, and by the extent of attachment loss sustained (see Figure 23.3). Mobility is sometimes associated with drifting of the teeth. The significance of mobility and drifting in therapy and more importantly, patient concern about the possible functional, cosmetic and prognostic implications must be examined.

Signs and symptoms

Patient awareness of mobility

Few patients are aware of mobility until it is pointed out to them, although periodic phases of looseness will have sometimes been experienced but disregarded, as a transient spontaneously resolving and so apparently insignificant phenomenon. Mobility may, however, be detected quite incidentally when the patient's attention is brought to the tooth by tenderness experienced on chewing. Food impaction between mobile units is often simply attributed to poor restorative contact points, and is tolerated as a lesser inconvenience than that of restoration replacement. Similarly, 'squeaking' experienced with clenching may be dismissed as a normal effect of restorations rubbing against each other. For these reasons, increased tooth mobility is frequently not complained of until the fairly advanced stages of disease (e.g. Figures 23.1 L and 23.2 O). Once conscious of this mobility, most patients become apprehensive and may equate this with impending tooth loss. Chewing on the involved tooth and, more importantly, normal cleaning in the area is then

344

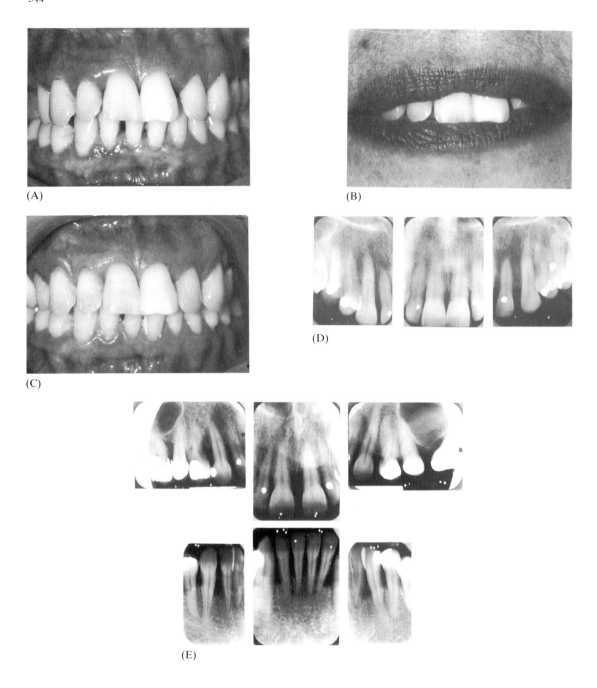

(A)

(B)

(C)

(D)

(E)

Figure 23.1 Features of increased and increasing mobility. (A) Maxillary incisor drifting and Grade I mobility developed over a 9-month period in 45-year-old woman. Associated with moderate palatal gingival inflammation and slight attachment loss. (B) Influence of lower lip. (C and D) Clinical and radiographic presentation 11 years later following plaque control measures alone. Note no change in tooth alignment. (E and F) Initial and 6-year radiographic findings of (G) extensive inflammation, Grade II mobility and drifting in 36-year-old woman. (H) Inflammatory resolution and marked reduction in mobility with improved plaque control over 2-year period. (I) Recommendation of maxillary pocket reduction surgery (as in mandible) rejected on aesthetic grounds. Progressive periodontal destruction followed with increasing mobility and further drifting by 6 years. (J and K) 58-year-old man shown in Figure 19.4 (C–E) with Grade III mobility at 11. Apparently adequate functional support provided by chrome cobalt denture replacing 21. (L) Degree of mobility shown by tooth being displaced labially by tongue pressure alone.

345

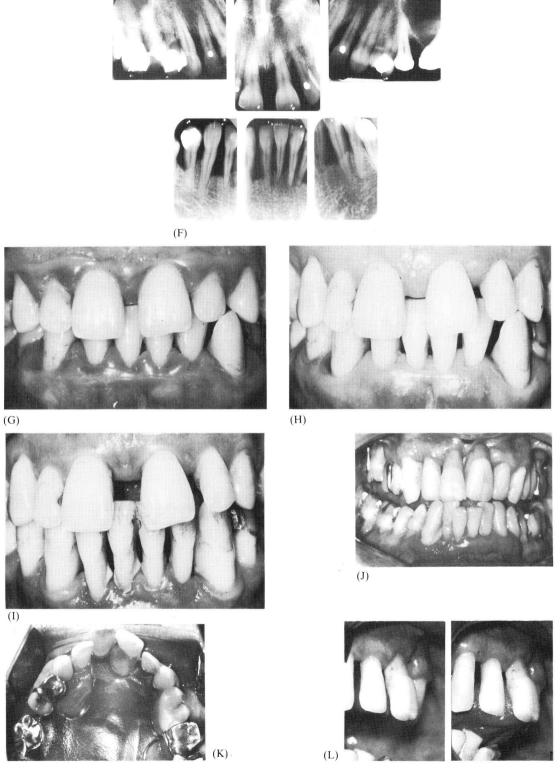

(F)

(G)

(H)

(I)

(J)

(K)

(L)

Figure 23.1 (*cont.*)

346

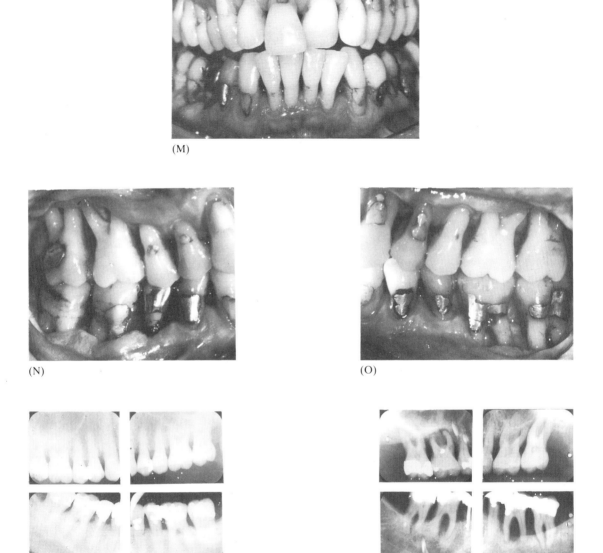

(M)

(N)

(O)

(P)

(Q)

Figure 23.1 (*cont.*) (M) Rapidly progressing molar periodontal destruction with gradually increasing mobility in 55-year-old over the previous 3 years, despite excellent oral hygiene and regular subgingival debridement. (N and O) Note extensive recession plus furcation involvement at molars. (P and Q) Initial and 3-year radiographic findings

frequently avoided, lest further loosening results, thereby aggravating matters. In this context, the fact that normal function will have prevailed without ill-effect prior to the recognition of the mobility or of clinical diagnosis ought to be, but rarely is, reassuring to the patient.

Functional discomfort

Pain is not a characteristic feature of hypermobile, periodontally involved teeth, although discomfort may periodically be experienced on chewing. Pain is, however, to be expected following sudden tooth displacement when biting on hard foods or with inadvertent trauma. Similarly, with any plaque-induced acute inflammatory episode the associated increase in mobility coupled with slight extrusion of the tooth results in pain on chewing. The effect is comparable to that experienced with an acute apical abscess and will subside once the acute phase passes. Finally, functional impairment, when chewing tough foods or biting things like cotton thread, may be experienced when there is increased mobility or drifting.

Aesthetics

Drifting (tooth migration) may occur with or without obvious signs of increased mobility. Anterior labial or lateral tooth displacement results in fanning and elongation of clinical crowns with consequent poor appearance. Where upper incisors become displaced labially outside the stabilizing influence of the lower lip, this may perpetuate drifting (Figure 23.1 A and B). In contrast, the posterior teeth which tend to tilt mesially, particularly with broken arch form, have little untoward aesthetic effects. However, such a deranged posterior occlusion often proves to be a major factor in drifting of anterior teeth with a reduced periodontal support.

Associated clinical findings

Variable degrees of gingival inflammation, loss of attachment with pocketing or gingival recession are encountered in keeping with the characteristic presentation of chronic disease. However, as a rule, mobility will increase in line with the level of inflammation even for the same depth of pocketing, whereas with resolution of inflammation, the mobility decreases gradually (e.g. Figure 23.1 G and H). Thus for example, a transient increase in mobility is to be expected with the development of an acute lateral periodontal abscess, which is characterized by a painful gingival swelling with or without the expression of pus from the pocket at a tooth with a vital pulp. Similarly with lesser

subclinical increases in inflammatory levels (subacute inflammation) at such sites, correspondingly smaller changes in the pattern of mobility occur. Indeed the patient may, under these circumstances, be rather more aware of the slight tooth mobility than the heightened underlying periodontal inflammation, something which unfortunately also appears quite frequently to escape the notice of the occlusion-conscious clinician. Teeth with furcation involvement are more prone to this phenomenon and, moreover, tend to be more mobile than others displaying comparable levels of destruction. This is because of the greater predisposition to both plaque-induced inflammation and, more importantly, periodic greater inflammatory cycles in association with the comparatively inaccessible furcations as shown in Figure 23.1 (N and O).

A correlation does exist, as might be expected, between mobility and residual attachment levels, but the findings can vary widely. Thus, in many instances, initially mobile teeth with markedly reduced support may become surprisingly firm following plaque control (Figures 19.4 M and 23.2 E and O), thereby endorsing the primary role of inflammation in the production of increased mobility (Figure 23.1 H and Figure 23.3 C and C1). Finally, although signs of occlusal surface wear consistent with parafunctional clenching and grinding habits, are often present at mobile and drifted teeth, this does not necessarily imply any correlation. That is, occlusal wear occurs at firmly supported teeth as well (e.g. Figures 24.6 and 24.7).

Radiographic changes

While the radiographic findings are reliable indicators of the extent of periodontal breakdown this does not hold true for the degree of mobility (*cf.* Chapter 19). Thus, a marked horizontal radiographic loss of bony support may be associated with minimal mobility as in Figure 23.2 (G), whereas a modest degree of breakdown may be accompanied by pronounced tooth mobility. Furthermore, an increased mobility associated with extensive plaque-induced supracrestal tissue inflammation, becomes markedly reduced upon inflammatory resolution following plaque control without any obvious attendant radiographic changes, as shown in Figure 23.4 (A). Periodontally involved mobile units may also display funnelled periodontal radiolucencies resulting from the co-existing angular bony defects (Figure 23.2 M and P) and sometimes, apical radiolucencies suggestive of an endodontic lesion may be encountered (see Figure 19.4 B), but which may be excluded by the demonstration of a vital pulp. Similar radiolucencies may be evident within furcations at furcation-involved mobile teeth. The possible significance of funnel-like widening of the

348

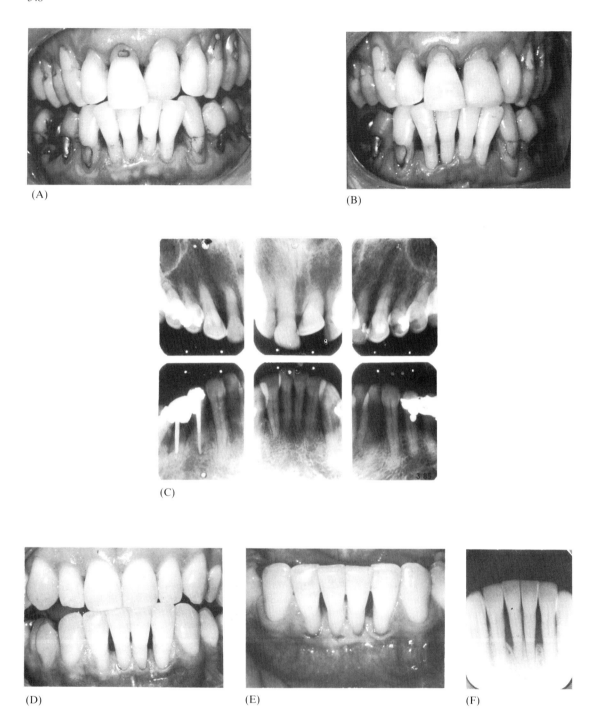

(A)

(B)

(C)

(D)

(E)

(F)

Figure 23.2 Management of hypermobility. (A and B) Mandibular incisor attachment loss over a 3-year period – same patient as in Figure 23.1 (M–Q). These teeth remained firmly supported despite loss of molars and is consistent with absence of clinical signs of inflammation. Note 21 has been built up with glass ionomer to satisfy aesthetics. (C) Radiographic findings. (D) Extensive periodontal destruction at 41, 31 associated initially with marked inflammation and Grade II mobility in 45-year-old woman. Presentation following plaque control and surgical pocket elimination. No residual mobility (see also Figure 21.2 C). (E and F) No change in clinical (but note toothbrush trauma) and radiographic findings at 5 years.

349

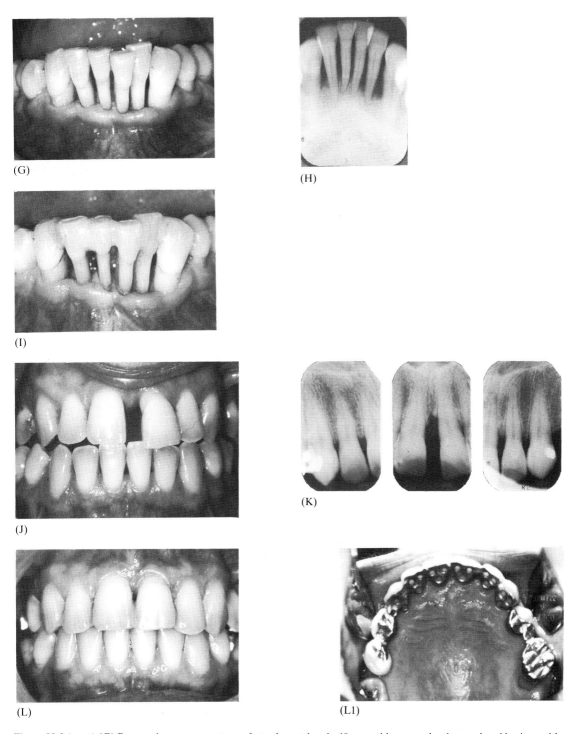

(G)

(H)

(I)

(J)

(K)

(L)

(L1)

Figure 23.2 (*cont.*) (G) Progressive uneven pattern of attachment loss in 48-year-old woman despite good oral hygiene with Grade I mobility at 41, 31 and Grade II at 32. (H) Corresponding radiographic presentation. (I) Mobility then increased with further attachment loss necessitating splinting for patient comfort. Note same patient as in Figure 26.5. (J) Pathological drifting maxillary incisors 37-year-old woman (same patient as in Figure 22.4). (K) Initial radiographic presentation. (L, L1) Orthodontically corrected and retained with rochette splint (by courtesy of Departments Orthodontics and Conservation, Institute of Dental Surgery).

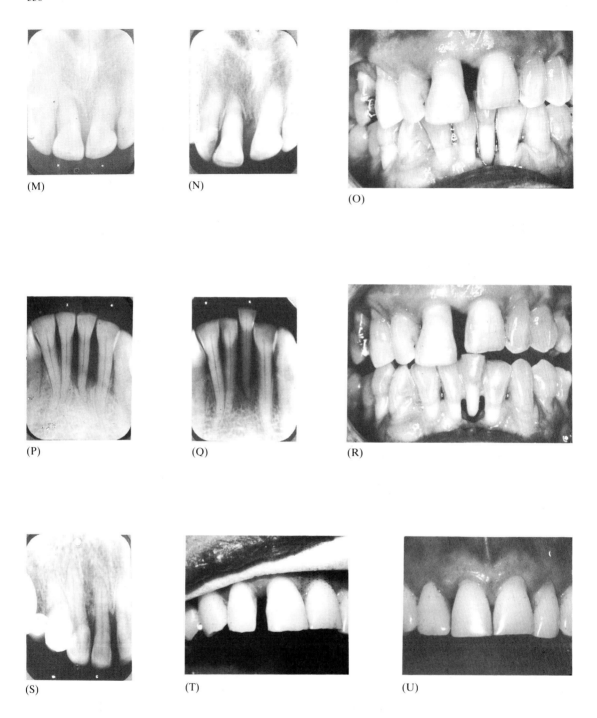

Figure 23.2 (cont.) (M and P) Presenting radiographic findings in 64-year-old woman. See also Figure 26.4. Sustained acute periodontal abscesses associated with extrusion and drifting plus increased mobility at 11 and 31. Surgical reattachment and cosmetic occlusal trimming carried out. (N and O) Radiographic and clinical findings 12 years later; 11 firmly supported despite residual widened periodontal ligament space associated with bony fill. (Q and R) Gradual attachment loss 31 associated with further extrusion and mobility increasing Grade I–III. Splinting with glass ionomer cement and incisal trimming at 31 to enhance comfort. Subsequent root resection converting natural tooth into a pontic (by courtesy Mr C. F. Invest). (S) Radiographic presentation of (T) spacing at 12, 11 in 45-year-old woman. (U) Corrected by building up the related tooth surfaces with glass ionomer cement (by courtesy Mr P. H. Rosenkranz)

periodontal ligament space has been considered in Chapter 19.

Other features

A mobile tooth might, in some cases, display a normal healthy periodontal support as shown in Figure 19.4 (B). The possible causes of this mobility include accidental trauma to the tooth, a periapical endodontic lesion, a recently inserted 'high' filling and ongoing orthodontic treatment, each of which presents little diagnostic difficulties. Less obvious causes are poorly designed and supported prostheses, parafunctional activities, unstable post-orthodontic occlusal relationships and idiopathic or post-traumatic root resorption. Finally, the possibility of underlying pathological osteolytic conditions should not be overlooked, but these need not be considered here.

Differential diagnosis

Chronic inflammatory periodontal disease is by far the commonest cause of increased tooth mobility, so must always be excluded first. The numerous other possible causes, cited above, should then be eliminated in a logical sequence. Unfortunately, in many instances, the pattern of periodontal destruction and more especially the furcation anatomy preclude optimal plaque control, so complicating differential diagnosis. Accurate diagnosis and formulation of the appropriate treatment then depends on careful examination of each situation. It is traditional practice to score on an index the degree of mobility encountered for initial record purposes and subsequent re-evaluation.

Measurement of mobility

Any tooth mobility present can be detected by simply displacing the crown of the tooth to and fro with the handle of a periodontal probe. The amount of movement noted can then be scored on ordinal scales such as:

Grade 0 = Physiological mobility
Grade I = Slight mobility
Grade II = Moderate mobility
Grade III = Marked mobility

Degree 1 = Movability of the crown of the tooth less than 1 mm in horizontal direction
Degree 2 = Movability of the crown of the tooth exceeding 1 mm in horizontal direction
Degree 3 = Movability of the crown of the tooth in a vertical direction as well

Clinical relevance of mobility scores

The disadvantages of any assessment of mobility are the subjectivity with respect to the imprecise gradings of the scales and their insensitivity; i.e. an inability to detect any minor fluctuations in mobility. However, these disadvantages ultimately prove to be of little significance in the overall management of disease. This is fortunate, for the more refined measuring devices used for clinical research are impractical for routine clinical practice. In addition, as mobility is only to be expected in disease it does, as a clinical sign, provide little more than confirmation of the already clinically obvious existence of disease. Similarly, longitudinal variations of mobility are primarily a reflection of the different degrees of inflammation present. Thus, it is worth reiterating here that, for comparable attachment levels, greater mobility should be anticipated at sites with more marked inflammation. Furthermore, mobility will always diminish with inflammatory resolution following plaque control. Consequently information about the initial levels of mobility and its subsequent predictable changes with plaque control is of little practical consequence, and is indeed superfluous to the associated already clinically obvious signs of the presence of disease and resolution of inflammation respectively. In summary, mobility recordings merely endorse the other clinical signs of disease and should be regarded as such. The motivational impact of reducing mobility upon the patient, may, however, be helpful in some cases.

Accordingly, at initial diagnosis of disease, only a fairly cursory assessment of the presence or absence of mobility is advocated and its extent is not considered critical while there is inflammation present. On the other hand, mobility may be significant if it persists following successful plaque-related periodontal treatment, or occurs in the absence of plaque-induced disease. Finally, the reader will no doubt encounter frequent references to the fact that tooth mobility associated with occlusal discrepancies in subjects with chronic inflammatory periodontal disease will lead to more rapid loss of attachment and, as such, will necessitate appropriate mobility measurements. This claimed modifying influence of the occlusion on disease has yet to be substantiated in humans, so is not to be considered here (see Chapter 33 – Occlusal trauma and the pattern of periodontal breakdown).

The clinical significance of increased mobility

As mobility is most frequently associated with plaque-induced disease, it is considered first.

Increased mobility in disease

Influence of gingival detachment

The supracrestal gingival and transeptal fibre attachment apparatus form a complex series of linked collagen bundles about adjacent teeth (see Chapter 2). This helps not only to maintain junctional epithelial adaptation but also to stabilize the teeth. Consequently degradation of this fibre apparatus and marginal tissue detachment in established disease reduces tooth support and results in increased mobility. With further loss of attachment the progressively flabbier inflamed detached tissues afford even less supracrestal support and so contribute to even greater mobility as depicted in Figure 23.3 (C and C1). Nevertheless, significant support is still provided by these detached tissues as demonstrated by the immediate increase in mobility observed upon removal of cervical wedge tissue during pocket surgery. There is also evidence that the supracrestal tissue inflammatory cell infiltrate, mediates significant volumetric (density) changes within the subjacent alveolar bone (see Chapter 33 – Occlusal trauma and the pattern of periodontal breakdown). Thus, in experimental plaque-induced disease, the marrow spaces enlarge and the alveolar bone related to the periodontal ligament, tapers coronally in conjunction with the development of increased tooth mobility. These histological changes were then reversed when oral hygiene measures were instituted.

To summarize, the finding of increased mobility of vital teeth in the presence of periodontal disease must be regarded simply as a feature of disease and the patient reassured accordingly.

Response to plaque control

As disease is controlled, mobility will gradually decrease. Any residual mobility following the attainment of periodontal health will then reflect a physiological adaptation to the loss of attachment sustained. However, when this mobility is greater than that at other comparable units secondary occlusal overloading should be suspected. The management of such occlusal problems is dealt with later.

Development of pain

A tooth with a vital pulp becoming progressively more mobile over a period of a few days in association with increasing gingival tenderness, pain on chewing and a feeling that it is proud suggests the development of a lateral periodontal abscess. Where, however, the tooth is non-vital the possibility of a coexisting apical abscess (that may or may not be communicating with the pocket) masquerading as a lateral periodontal abscess cannot easily be discounted. The management of such primary periodontal and of combined periodontal and endodontic lesions is described in Chapters 24 and 25.

Furcation involvements

The degree of mobility at such units tends to be somewhat greater and to fluctuate more than it does at anterior teeth with comparable attachment losses. This probably reflects greater inflammatory levels due to poor access for plaque control within furcations and the impaired drainage of inflammatory exudates. Any associated extrusion of the tooth results in premature occlusal contact with its antagonist and causes an even greater mobility. Such findings might then lead to the conclusion that mobility is primarily of traumatic rather than inflammatory origin. Occlusal adjustment is therefore inappropriate in these cases other than as a palliative measure to relieve discomfort. Treatment must instead be directed at the underlying plaque-induced disease. Where successful, a reduction in mobility will follow, but as plaque control is frequently precluded by furcation morphology, some residual mobility is inevitable.

Increased mobility might also be expected following molar root resection (Chapter 18), yet the available data suggest this need not be so (*cf.* Chapters 18 and 30). Clinical experience shows that the tooth will remain firmly supported, provided that effective cleaning is maintained (see Figures 18.9, 18.10 and 18.11). However, any assessment of potential mobility in these cases will be impossible when splinting of these mobile teeth to neighbouring teeth has been undertaken in a mistaken bid to compensate for loss of support.

Risk of tooth loss

A markedly mobile tooth seldom impedes normal chewing elsewhere and is rarely shed spontaneously. Indeed, it is salutory to fail in an attempt to remove such a tooth with the fingers in the belief that delivery would be easy, and more especially when no anaesthesia has been provided. The patient will also confirm how painfully resistant to removal such hypermobile teeth really are! The toughness of the few remaining attachment fibres is also demonstrated clearly by the comparable situation of attempting the quick removal of an apparently exfoliating primary tooth in an unwilling child.

The hypermobile tooth can be retained in acceptable function and comfort (Figure 23.1 J–L) provided that, in the first place, it is not inadvertently bumped during toothbrushing or hard things like apples, crusts or fruit stones are not bitten.

Fortunately, as each of the above encounters would be painful, any such force having extraction potential is carefully avoided by the patient, not unlike the chronic back pain sufferer avoiding bending and lifting heavy objects. Secondly, that intolerable pain from an acute exacerbation of the periodontal lesion, or pulpal involvement in a developing combined periodontal–endodontic lesion, does not arise. Thirdly, that an aesthetically displeasing progressive drifting does not occur. Drifting is however unlikely to progress when attachment loss has been checked. Patient reassurance of this encourages improved plaque control and enhances acceptance of the existing drifted appearances. Lastly, when the retention of the offending teeth is considered by the patient to be preferable to the alternatives of their complex and costly stabilization (to be described later), or their replacement by prostheses. The first option of stabilization has however been greatly simplified by the recent development of glass ionomer type bonding materials. In summary, factors which determine patient comfort and function will, in the majority of cases, dictate the ultimate fate of hypermobile teeth (see also Chapter 26).

Increased mobility with healthy intact periodontal support

Tooth mobility in the presence of a normal healthy support usually results from increased occlusal loading from inappropriate restorative or prosthetic treatment, or from parafunctional habits. Mobility encountered during orthodontic treatment and as a result unstable post-orthodontic tooth relationships or accidental physical trauma need not be considered here. Finally, teeth with shortened roots as a result of root resorption, may be less able to withstand occlusal loading and so might also account for tooth mobility in health.

'High' restorations

High spots on amalgam restorations may not be detected initially by the patient who avoids closure upon the newly inserted material. However, when the occlusal prematurity is encountered subsequently some pain is experienced. The site is therefore avoided by an adaptive path of closure or used more gently, until the prematurity is corrected professionally or disappears due to wear or fracture. Where, however, the interference persists, occlusal tenderness followed by an adaptive hypermobility ensues (see below).

High spots on cast metal and porcelain restorations are usually detected and corrected prior to cementation. Excessive occlusal contours may however only become apparent during subsequent parafunctional mandibular excursions. The resulting discomfort evokes the appropriate evasive mandibular deviation, but when this cannot be sustained and the occlusal interferences are contacted consistently an adaptive tooth mobility is to be expected. Whether the mobility is accompanied by discomfort or frank pain depends upon the extent of the interference and the frequency of the occlusal insult. A comparable situation is that of the initial tooth tenderness experienced with orthodontic appliance therapy, prior to increasing mobility.

The pain or discomfort experienced with occlusal interferences results from trauma to the periodontal ligament sustained from excessive occlusal forces. When these symptoms are tolerated by the patient, in the expectation of spontaneous resolution, the tooth is avoided whenever possible and during this time the periodontium gradually adapts to the occlusal overloading. This is achieved by osteoclastic resorption of supporting bone with a corresponding widening of the periodontal ligament space, which cushions the periodontal tissues from further trauma and the pain ceases. This compensatory mechanism manifests clinically as increased tooth mobility, representing a physiological adaptation to occlusal overloading. This implies that the changes are reversible following correction of occlusal form and that the periodontal ligament space is restored to normal functional width and tooth mobility to normal levels.

It is important to emphasize that the above adaptive changes need not involve the supracrestal attachment apparatus, for this is not traumatized. The inherent supracrestal tissue flexibility simply absorbs the effects of any increased occlusal loading or coronal displacement. Consequently, all the changes in primary occlusal trauma from the repeated application of excessive forces, are restricted to the periodontal ligament itself. Furthermore, any increased tooth mobility induced will not compromise the integrity of the supracrestal periodontal attachment; that is no loss of attachment will occur (see Chapter 33 – Occlusal trauma and the pattern of periodontal breakdown).

The insertion of anterior crowns that interfere with harmonious mandibular movements, result in not only increased mobility but also the possibility of labial drifting of the maxillary incisors. Similar displacement, such as tilting or drifting may also occur at posterior teeth subjected to iatrogenic occlusal prematurities, especially in incomplete dental arches. This sequence of occlusal changes in relation to primary occlusal trauma is somewhat simplistic and belies the existence of complex inter-relationships which are beyond the intended remit of this text. Suffice it to say that these relationships exist between poorly restored occlusal form, occlusal wear in parafunction, occlusal height loss due to erosion and occlusal disharmony following the non-replacement of missing teeth.

Prosthetic clasping

Teeth firmly clasped by poorly supported free-end saddle partial dentures will frequently display a gradually increasing mobility and perhaps also distal drifting. The resulting opening of interproximal contacts predisposes to food impaction and although possibly annoying for the patient, will be of no significance in periodontal health in the presence of effective plaque control. The potentially detrimental long-term effects of such removable prostheses on the occlusion as a whole and, more importantly, of progressive alveolar ridge resorption must not be overlooked. The reader is referred to the appropriate texts for further details.

Inadequate bridge abutments

A compensatory increase in mobility is also to be expected following the fitting of fixed bridge work upon inadequate abutments. However, the ability of abutment teeth to support pontics has been reviewed in recent years and the rigid application of Ante's Law is no longer considered essential (*cf.* Chapter 34 – The dilemma of tooth replacement).

Parafunctional habits

The habitual clenching or jiggling on a single tooth or other persistent habits, like pencil biting, could result in an adaptive tooth mobility. However this does not appear to be that common a phenomenon, for in most instances the teeth subjected to parafunctional stresses are firmly supported, provided always that marginal tissue health exists. The complex inter-relationships of parafunctional tooth mobility, tooth wear and tempero-mandibular joint dysfunction are also beyond the remit of this text.

Root resorption

This uncommon finding may be idiopathic or may follow orthodontic therapy resulting in significant root shortening. A comparable effect may also be produced by over enthusiastic apical surgery. The reduced root length alters the clinical crown/root ratio and so predisposes to tooth mobility in response to parafunctional clenching.

Increased mobility with healthy reduced periodontal support

Teeth with reduced bony support following successful periodontal therapy, might be expected to display some residual mobility because of the relative increase in occlusal loading yet, in many instances, are found to be remarkably firm. This suggests that interocclusal relationships may be more critical in producing mobility in these situations than the amount of remaining periodontal support. This mobility is often referred to as secondary occlusal trauma representing the effects of normal occlusal forces on teeth with reduced support. However, as the histological features of this periodontal lesion are no different from those occurring following an absolute increase in occlusal loading, as in primary occlusal trauma described above, trauma from occlusion or more simply occlusal trauma would be a more appropriate terminology. This may then be qualified according to the reasons for the resulting increased mobility in any particular situation (see also Chapter 33 – Occlusal trauma and reduced periodontal support).

The effects of occlusal trauma at sites with a healthy reduced periodontal support are the same as those occurring with normal support. That is, the changes do not involve the supracrestal tissues and no loss of attachment will be sustained. In addition, this clinical impression coupled with the patient's understandable apprehension that the persistent mobility itself at teeth with reduced support, would exert a greater physical distorting effect upon the marginal (crestal) bone than at sites with normal support and so possibly also a greater potential for damage to the periodontium, is not borne out by the pure mechanics of such situations. This is because of changes in the fulcrum of rotation of the tooth in response to displacement forces that occur with progressive loss of attachment. Thus, for the same degree of mobility measured at the crown, a tooth with reduced support is associated with less displacement. This phenomenon is considered below.

Mechanical implications

In the normal periodontium the fulcrum of tooth movement is located a little more than half way down the root length (Figure 23.3 A1) and the greatest amount of lateral displacement of the root, within bone, therefore occurs at the level of the crestal bone. With progressive loss of attachment however, the point of rotation shifts more apically (Figure 23.3 B1), so that when in those situations only the apical periodontal attachment fibres remain, the fulcrum is located at the root apex. The effect of this is that despite the marked increase in mobility developing coronally, there is not a corresponding increase in root surface displacement at the level of the crestal bone (Figure 23.3 A1 and B1).

Biological implications

The biomechanical implications are that as periodontal support is reduced, so does the potential for lateral displacement of the remaining intra-alveolar part of the root in response to occlusal

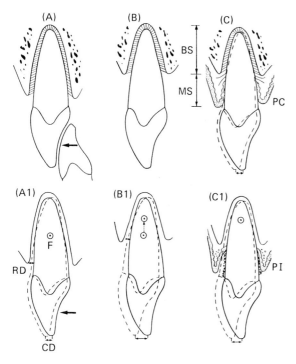

Figure 23.3 Biomechanics of tooth mobility. (A) Normal and (B) reduced alveolar bone support (BS). (A1 and B1) Fulcrum of rotation (F) to occlusal generated displacement forces located more apically with reduced support. Consequently similar amount of root surface displacement (RD) occurs at the crestal bone for different degrees of coronal displacement (CD). (C) Alveolar bony support supplemented by the supracrestal pocket mucosal support (MS) as represented by CD at (B1) being greater than at (C1). In addition greater resistance to displacement in presence of (C) pocket closure (PC) than (C1) pocket wall inflammation (PI)

generated forces (Figure 23.3 B1). The corollary to this is that the marginal periodontal tissues related to a tooth with a marked loss of attachment and extreme tooth mobility, as shown in Figure 23.3 (B1) experience stresses that are similar to those in situations with normal support and exhibiting only slight mobility (Figure 23.3 A1). Consequently, any concern that this marked mobility might in some way be detrimental to the remaining periodontal support is both mechanically and biologically unfounded. In addition, this reduced support can not only withstand any occlusal generated tooth displacement without risk to the marginal periodontal attachment, but in the unlikely event of this displacement reaching tooth extraction proportions, pain is experienced which reflexly triggers the appropriate mandibular deviation.

Clinical implications

First and foremost, increased mobility should not in itself be equated with imminent tooth loss. Secondly, the existence of increased mobility is not detrimental to the remaining reduced healthy periodontal support and there is no scientific basis for seeking to reduce this mobility (*cf.* Chapter 33). Thirdly, increased mobility and any associated drifting need be viewed with respect to the patient

comfort and function alone. That is, only where difficulty is experienced in eating or the patient feels insecure about loose teeth, or the appearances are unacceptable, is specific occlusal therapy indicated (see below). This treatment then reflects the wishes of the patient. Finally, whenever occlusal therapy is contemplated, the prior establishment of marginal tissue health is paramount, for it would otherwise be impossible to differentiate between the respective possible causative influences upon the offending increased mobility. Furthermore, when an expected reduction in mobility is not achieved following occlusal therapy the operator would be unable to judge whether this was due to incomplete occlusal equilibration or a co-existing marginal lesion.

Increasing mobility at units with reduced support

Small increases in mobility are not easily detected due to the limitations of measurement methods, making it difficult to assert that mobility is actually increasing between review appointments. Where obvious differences are apparent, this is due most commonly to a pocket related inflammation. The other reasons are a further loss of attachment with reduced support in a progressive periodontal disease, or a further adaptation to an absolute increase

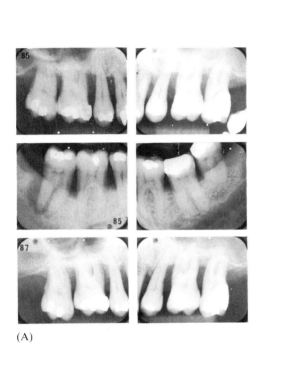

(A)

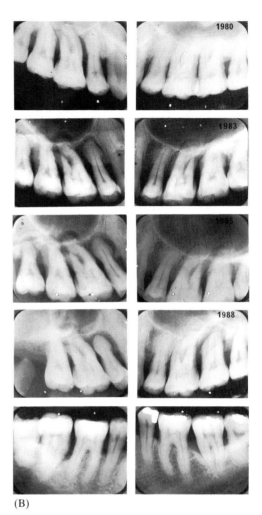

(B)

Figure 23.4 (A) Radiographic findings on initial presentation in 1985 of 42-year-old man with marked gingival inflammation. Tenderness on chewing and Grade II–III mobility in maxillary molar and premolars. Lesser destruction in mandible apart from at presenting complaint of combined lesion at 47 necessitating extraction. No obvious radiographic changes accompanied resolution of superficial clinical signs of inflammation and elimination of mobility patterns over a 2-year regime of plaque control and subgingival debridement. Note supereruption of unopposed 17 has reduced depth of intrabony component of pocket. (B) Radiographs of 36-year-old woman 1980. Extensive periodontal destruction, supracrestal inflammation and Grade II–III mobility. Improved oral hygiene instituted and regular subgingival debridement carried out. Marked reduction in mobility coupled with pocket closure resulted with functional comfort through to 1988. Very occasional minor inflammatory episodes at 16, 15 plus 26 (controlled by systemic tetracycline administration) associated with transient increased mobility. Note: despite several apical radiolucencies pulpal necrosis unequivocally demonstrated for the first time at 16, 15 (1985), and then at 27 (1988). Pulpal symptoms necessitated removal 18 (1987). Extraction 15 advocated in 1985 to safeguard distal support 13 but rejected as only minimal discomfort experienced. Opposing units at 1988 alone are shown below

in occlusal loading. Finally in the case of non-vital teeth, active periapical lesions might be developing, the implications of which are considered in Chapter 26.

Pocket related inflammation

A transient increase in the level of the plaque induced supracrestal inflammation is invariably accompanied by increased mobility (Figure 23.3 C and C1). When this subsides (spontaneously or following local treatment) the mobility decreases once again as shown in Figure 23.4 (A and B). The fluctuating pattern of mobility in such situations appears to be related primarily to variations of tissue tone. Thus, oedematous flabby inflamed detached gingiva provides less physical support about the

necks of the teeth than the firm relatively uninflamed tissue that characterizes pocket closure. This
need not be considered further here.

Progressive disease

An increasing mobility is to be expected with
reducing periodontal support in progressive
periodontal breakdown. This might represent either
recurrence of a successfully treated condition or
persistent existing disease, as at inaccessible molar
root furcations. Where the disease is then subsequently controlled, an initial slight reduction of
mobility (associated with inflammatory resolution)
followed by a maintained level of residual mobility
ensues. Elsewhere, when progression of disease
appears inevitable, a gradually increasing and
frequently fluctuating pattern of mobility associated
with periodic, more active, inflammatory episodes
occurs, with further loss of attachment. Indeed it
can in such cases be difficult to differentiate between
increasing mobility caused by greater inflammatory
changes and by loss of periodontal support *per se*.

In the latter situations the basic problem remains
one of progressive disease, with any net increase in
mobility or any drifting representing tangible signs
of disease. The patient should, however, be
reassured that the characteristic episodic fluctuations in plaque-induced inflammation means that
the levels of mobility will vary from time to time and
will not necessarily indicate further deterioration.
Furthermore, that the rate of deterioration is very
slow in the vast majority of instances and tooth loss
not imminent (*cf*. Chapter 26). Thus, teeth displaying even Grade III mobility may be retained in
tolerable function and comfort for many years by
plaque control measures alone (Figures 23.1, 23.2,
23.4 and 23.5). In some instances, however, occlusal
grinding to reduce the occlusal interferences and so
enhance patient comfort and confidence in chewing
may be necessary. Similarly, where aesthetically
unacceptable extrusion of the tooth (namely drifting) occurs periodic trimming of the incisal edges
might also be necessary (see below).

Further adaptation to increased occlusal overloading

Increased occlusal loading is most commonly
encountered in partially edentulous cases, where the
reduced periodontal support of the surviving teeth
cannot withstand the progressively greater occlusal
forces to which they are subjected. A further
compensatory widening of the periodontal ligament
with a corresponding increase in mobility and/or
drifting occurs. In the latter instance, the tooth may
then become somewhat firmer.

Pathological drifting

The facility for drifting is dictated by opposing and
neighbouring teeth and the related soft tissues. For
example, any intact arch will preclude both lingual
and distal drifting, whilst labial drifting in the
mandible is checked by the interincisal relationship.
The maxillary anterior units are only contained by
the lips, which makes them more liable to drifting.
They might then become displaced further labially
by the lower lip, when it falls behind the upper
incisal edges as shown in Figure 23.1 (B). Drifting of
mandibular and maxillary posterior teeth is limited
by interdental contacts in intact arches, but elsewhere mesial (and less often distal) tilting tends to
occur.

The 'over-eruption' or extrusion of isolated units
mentioned to above, represents a form of drifting.
That lower incisors are so frequently able to
over-erupt in spite of their former interincisal
relationships, presumably reflect altered mandibular
movements or deviations to avoid occlusal contacts
at these mobile teeth (see Figures 23.1 and 23.2).
This could also explain patient tolerance of extreme
degrees of mobility elsewhere in the mouth.

The management of unacceptable degrees of mobility and drifting

The nature of complaints about mobility and drifting
are likely to vary from patient to patient and should
be dealt with individually. Thus, looseness might
complicate chewing, inhibit cleaning of adjacent
units, lead to a feeling of insecurity or simply
become personally unacceptable to the patient.
Drifting might result in similar complaints, but poor
appearance is the main cause for concern. The
handling of these complaints will now be considered.

Mobility

The patient should be reminded that as mobility
may be due to both disease and on the force exerted
by opposing teeth, renewed plaque-control efforts,
despite past failures, are often rewarded by the teeth
becoming firmer. This should therefore remain the
primary line of therapy in all cases. Where
unsuccessful, the persistent mobility and elsewhere
the residual unacceptable mobility is best reduced
by selective occlusal adjustment of occlusal prematurities and interferences. The techniques are
well described elsewhere and need not be considered in detail here, save to say that effective
equilibration is technically difficult, especially in the
presence of marginal disease and when the objectives are often not attained. Where the symptoms
are related primarily to parafunctional activities a

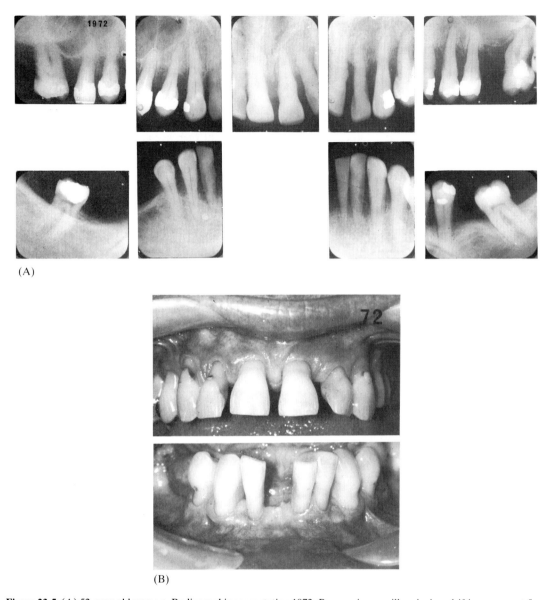

(A)

(B)

Figure 23.5 (A) 52-year-old woman. Radiographic presentation 1972. Progressive maxillary incisor drifting over past 5 years. (B) Post-gingival response 1975 – pockets self-correcting by gingival recession.

full arch bite guard is worth considering. This is worn as and when necessary, for in between periodic phases of occlusal hyperactivity the teeth become firmer again. These appliance might also be used prophylactically to prevent the onset of or to check further drifting.

Where occlusal adjustment has been ineffective or is not feasible and unacceptable mobility levels persist, splinting (mechanical linking) of mobile teeth to the neighbouring more stable teeth should

be considered (Figure 23.2 I – see also Figure 26.5). It must, however, be emphasized that splinting, whilst enhancing patient comfort and function, will not in itself, benefit the underlying plaque-induced condition. Indeed, it might even perpetuate the primary problem, because splinting inevitably complicates plaque control. Details of the numerous techniques available are well described elsewhere, so need not be repeated here. Suffice it to add that the recent development of restorative materials with

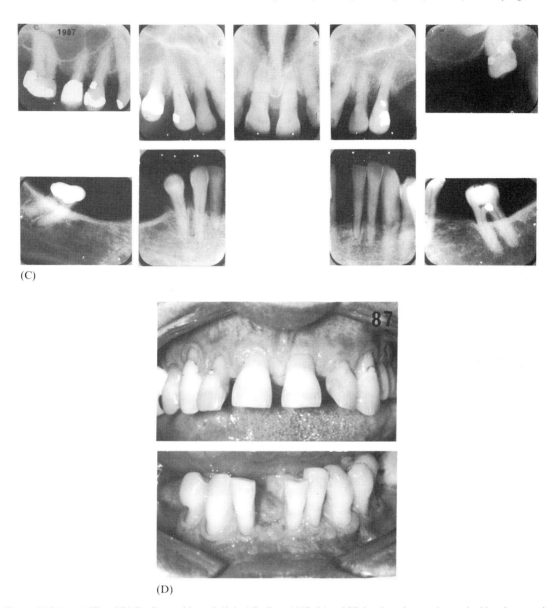

(C)

(D)

Figure 23.5 (*cont.*) (C and D) Radiographic and clinical findings 1987. 24 and 27 developed secondary pulpal involvement in 1974 so extracted and partial denture fitted. 25 lost as a result of endodontic complications. No further obvious drifting or significant attachment losses ensued. Grade II mobility 42, 31 associated with recurrent plaque induced inflammation. Note resulting slight widening of periodontal ligament spaces

a bonding capacity to enamel, have greatly simpli-fied splinting (Figure 23.2 I and R) especially when used in conjunction with Rochette/Maryland techni-ques (Figure 23.2 L). A certain proportion of bonding failures must however be anticipated over time with the present state of the art.

The possible option of extraction with fixed prosthetic replacement, especially when a cosmetic-ally unacceptable drifting has also occurred, should not be discounted as shown in Figure 19.4 (A), especially as the overall costs and efforts are often comparable to splinting. Furthermore, where re-movable prostheses are acceptable, the involvement of supporting units in otherwise needlessly complex restorative measures can be avoided. In most instances, the difficulties associated with satisfactorily stabilizing teeth has led to patient acceptance of mobility instead and the author has instituted splinting in very few instances over the past two decades.

Drifting

The technical and financial implications of the orthodontic realignment, followed by the necessary retention in the form of splinting (Figure 23.2 L) is a major barrier to the correction of drifted units. Consequently many patients simply accept drifting provided it does not get significantly worse. This is difficult to predict, although it does appear that following disease control drifting is self-limiting (Figure 23.1 A–C) or increases by only an insignificant and aesthetically acceptable degree (Figure 23.5). Indeed, in the latter instances, it seems that following the initial major concern about drifting, further minor deterioration is tolerated as might a gradually receding hairline or balding in middle-aged men! It would, nevertheless, be prudent to take study casts for the purposes of future reference purposes and patient reassurance. Furthermore, occlusal discrepancies deemed to predispose to drifting are corrected by the appropriate occlusal adjustment. In a few instances, reconstruction of the posterior occlusion will also be necessary but is often precluded by the costs involved. In addition, such complex therapy is often difficult to justify when the underlying periodontal prognosis is uncertain. In any event, whatever occlusal therapy is undertaken this must not de-emphasize the all-important issue of plaque control.

The aesthetically displeasing effects of drifting can frequently be masked by fairly simple means, especially where the drifted units appear to have adopted a stable position. Thus, the teeth may be built up with glass ionomer type materials (Figure 23.2 U) or where crowns are already in place, slightly wider ones fitted (Figure 11.7 G and H). The justification for the latter is strengthened by gingival recession which necessitates the provision of longer clinical crowns as well.

The role of orthodontics

Where it has been decided to realign drifted teeth by orthodontic therapy, it is always necessary to resolve the following considerations: the sequence of the orthodontic and periodontic phases of treatment; the possible influence of orthodontic therapy on the underlying periodontal pockets; the stability of the post-orthodontic occlusion; the appearances of longer clinical crowns following periodontal therapy and, finally, the implications of disease not being arrested.

Sequence of therapy

While orthodontics may be carried out before or after periodontal therapy, it is preferable to first establish periodontal health. There are several reasons for this. First, as loss of attachment has been primarily responsible for drifting, it is reasonable that this should be halted before dealing with its consequences. Secondly, there is a risk, suggested by animal experimental models (*cf.* Chapter 33), although not substantiated in humans, that orthodontic treatment might aggravate the pre-existing periodontal condition. Thirdly, the post-periodontal treatment aesthetics might prove to be unacceptable, so that a solution involving extraction followed by prosthetic replacement might be preferred. Finally, post-orthodontic retention might be enhanced by periodontal health although this has yet to be substantiated.

Orthodontics in the presence of pockets

Where the earliest possible tooth realignment is necessary to satisfy patient demands (Figure 23.2 J and K and as in the case shown in Figure 26.6), this should be commenced as soon as is practical, following the establishment of, at least, improved levels of oral hygiene and thorough subgingival root surface debridement. A carefully supervised plaque-control regime in conjunction with periodic debridement is also critical during active orthodontic therapy. No difficulties should be experienced when removable appliance therapy is used, although the plaque retentive hazard of the appliance upon the marginal gingival lesion must be guarded against.

Fixed appliance therapy even with the widespread use of bonded brackets complicates plaque control and root surface instrumentation. Pre-orthodontic surgical elimination of the pocketing to simplify future periodontal care might therefore be prudent in such instances and would, as such, represent another reason for the treatment sequence advocated above. On the other hand, orthodontic realignment can apparently be carried out with an equal, if not greater, facility in the presence of pocketing than elsewhere. Furthermore, the morphology of any bone defects might be altered favourably (with respect to subsequent pocket surgery) by becoming physically smaller when the teeth are moved into them. Controlled research investigation is called for (*cf.* Chapter 33 – Other orthodontal objectives).

Post-orthodontic retention

A stable occlusal relationship is unlikely to be achieved following orthodontic realignment so that some form of retention will be required. Sometimes only a bite guard for periodic nocturnal wear suffices. Where, however, permanent retention is necessary, the onerous responsibility of carrying this out to the requisite standard and without creating any other problems with respect to future plaque control, pulpal damage or recurrent caries rests with the operator. This burden is lessened when the teeth are already heavily restored, necessitating complex restorations anyway as in the case shown in Figures 24.3 and 26.6. Where none of the possible retention techniques, including even the more conservative Rochette/Maryland type splints (Figure 23.2 J–L) are feasible, orthodontic treatment would seem to be contra-indicated.

Post-periodontal treatment aesthetics

It is important that the patient, electing to undergo orthodontic therapy, is able to visualize at the outset the likely appearances of the teeth following the periodontal phase of therapy. Fortunately, the loss of gingival tissue can often be acceptably masked with an acrylic gingival veneer. Where prosthetic replacement of posterior teeth is required the veneer might be incorporated into a 'swing lock' type denture design. The obvious alternative to combined orthodontic–periodontal therapy with questionable aesthetics is simply extraction and prosthetic replacement of the drifted teeth as shown in Figure 19.4 (A) or where the posterior teeth are adequately supported, fixed bridgework considered instead.

Persistent periodontal disease

In some instances, disease might not be arrested because the optimal choice of pocket elimination will be precluded by the irregular pattern of breakdown or the need to carry out compromise surgical reattachment therapy in the interests of aesthetics. The justification for complex orthodontic and restorative treatment efforts then becomes highly questionable.

In conclusion, each case must be given careful individual consideration. Fortunately, the majority of patients when confronted with the combination of a likely persistent marginal periodontitis, major orthodontic and restorative treatment, opt to accept the pathologically drifted units (see Figure 23.1 (E–I)). Consequently, it is only the small minority of patients that do ultimately demand such complex treatment.

Conclusion

Provided the patient with increased or increasing mobility of teeth tolerates the inconvenience of loose teeth, any periodic phases of discomfort or acute painful episodes, and can function adequately by modifying chewing habits and, finally, is not concerned about the aesthetics of any associated drifting, the clinical situation can be accepted. Indeed, clinical experience shows that most individuals will accept the presence of often surprisingly mobile units over periods of many years even when they are deteriorating gradually. Similarly, drifted units are also tolerated. This is usually because the problems related to any attempted stabilization of the mobile teeth and orthodontically realigned teeth, or their extraction with the creation of an edentulous space with or without a prosthodontic replacement are greater than the existing ones. The patient may on the other hand decide upon extraction, at which stage the problems of the co-existing restorative and prosthetic treatment needs at adjacent teeth and of the arch as a whole, have to be solved. This is considered further in Chapter 26.

24

Periodontal restorative relationships

The presence of both caries and periodontal disease in the same individual means that several different problems often have to be coped with at once and so involve a number of inter-relationships. The placement of restorations in a periodontally healthy mouth and the difficulties in restorative exercises created by the presence of chronic inflammatory periodontal disease are considered first. Then the indications for periodontal surgery to expedite restorative treatment, the periodontal implications of combined periodontal–endodontal lesions, endodontic apical surgery and the effect of prostheses on the periodontium will be discussed.

Restorations in periodontal health

Operator difficulties

Restorative dentistry is concerned with the restoration of broken down teeth to their normal contour and function. The marginal gingivae are frequently involved in relation to the cervical or approximal margins of restorations. The tissues may be traumatized during cavity preparation, impression techniques or the insertion and finishing of restorations. Complex restorations may involve subgingival extension especially in the quest to obtain ideal appearance. In these situations, even where optimal restorative principles are observed, the restoration margins may retain plaque and so possibly compromise marginal tissue health.

Less than ideal restorations are often encountered which is not unexpected, bearing in mind the exacting and technically difficult nature of restorative dentistry. Limited access within the oral cavity,

the greatly differing levels of individual operator dexterity and care and, not least, of patient cooperation during treatment all combine to thwart the ideal restoration. These restorations impede plaque removal and as such constitute iatrogenic factors in chronic inflammatory periodontal disease.

Nature of adverse restorations

For the purposes of plaque control, adverse restorations are constituted by deficient or over-extended (overhanging) margins which trap plaque and, to a lesser extent, approximal surface over-contouring which reduces interproximal space dimensions for interdental cleaning (Figure 24.1). Over-contouring at facial and oral aspects is also a problem but presents rather less of a handicap in plaque removal. Defective contact points predispose to food packing, but this will not in itself compromise gingival health, the related plaque retention being the main problem at these sites.

Deficiencies will result from incomplete packing and condensation of amalgam, while overhangs result from poor matrix band adaptation, lack of wedging at approximal restorations or inadequate trimming of excess material at over-filled cervical cavity restorations. This excess material may be difficult to detect at the time of insertion, when occurring at buccal and lingual furcation grooves and more especially approximal tooth surface concavities at molars and maxillary first premolars. These defects are therefore frequently only recognized subsequently upon radiographic examination or by the finding of a localized marginal gingival inflammation adjacent to a restoration. The patient

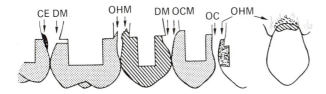

Figure 24.1 Restoration and plaque retention depicted diagrammatically at 17–13. Cast metal/porcelain at 17, 16; amalgam at 15 and at 13 buccal aspect; composite at 13. (CE) Cement excess; (DM) deficient margin; (OHM) overhanging margin; (OCM) overcontoured margin; (OC) open contact

might, in turn, find that the use of wood points is being impeded or even prevented by partially or totally occluded interproximal spaces and that dental floss is becoming caught or shredded during interdental cleaning. Laboratory processed cast metal and porcelain restorations may also have over- or under-extended margins and impinge on embrasure spaces. Each of these reflect primarily an inadequate clinical examination of the restoration prior to cementation. Occasionally, the failure to remove excess cement might also create problems.

Avoidance of iatrogenic factors

Prevention of problems due to restorations is obviously preferable and depends on a combination of careful cavity margin preparation, an awareness of tooth surface morphology with respect to potential problem sites, effective wedging of matrix bands, the possible use of rubber dam to completely isolate the tooth for improved operative conditions and visibility and, finally, close examination of margins upon completion. Where imperfections of restorative materials do occur, these should be carved or trimmed appropriately at the time. Similarly, the marginal fit and coronal contour of laboratory processed restorations must always be checked very carefully and rectified prior to cementation, even at the expense of remaking the restoration.

Placing restoration margins within the gingival sulcus should, as a general rule, also be avoided whenever possible. Fortunately, the concept of subgingival extension for caries prevention is no longer held to be true. The gingival sulcus need therefore be invaded only where demanded by aesthetics and in the management of subgingival caries (which are examined here) and where subgingival coronal fractures have occurred and which will be considered later.

Anterior crown margins

The clinical dilemma of supra- or subgingival crown margins is best avoided by simply advising patients

of the risks involved. Many will then accept a slight aesthetic compromise in the interests of gingival health, especially as the supragingival placement of crown margins need not necessarily be displeasing. Indeed, where there is good marginal adaptation, contouring and shading of porcelain crowns, the porcelain to tooth junctions can be virtually invisible and so no different from any other tooth. With bonded crowns the problem of appearance is harder to solve without placing the margin just into the gingival sulcus. An additional problem is caused by discoloured dentine of non-vital teeth which causes an unsightly dark line at the junction of crown and root. The level of the lip when the patient smiles will also do much to influence any decision regarding the appearances.

Where subgingival margins are unavoidable, tooth preparation should extend to only 0.5 mm apical to the gingival crest. Great care must be taken at all stages not to traumatize the tissues, especially when they are thin and knife-edged, lest gingival recession ensues (see Chapter 21). The patient should however always be warned at the outset that the gingiva may still recede and reveal the crown margin. No attempt should be made to gain greater subgingival extension at preparation, in the hope of delaying exposure of the margins for longer in the event of recession, as this usually proves to be counter-productive. This is because of not only the increased risks of gingival operative trauma, but also the difficulties of accurate impression technique at the less accessible tooth preparation margins and of finishing and assessing the fit of such more deeply placed margins. Most importantly effective plaque control is impossible.

Specific advice in plaque control, preferably with a single tufted brush, is essential following the fitting of crowns. The patient must ensure that the bristles actually reach any subgingival crown margins, but do not inadvertently scratch the tissues, for this might lead to recession. A similarly careful use of dental floss is advocated for the approximal surfaces. Initially, the patient's efforts are best assessed fairly frequently to ensure that marginal health is being maintained.

Subgingival caries

The risk of a plaque-induced marginal gingivitis, following restoration of caries extending into the gingival sulcus, can be minimized by ensuring high technical standards and subsequent plaque control. However, where marginal inflammation and detachment occurs, gingival recession may follow exposing the restoration margin and resolving the problem. The alternative of the pre-restorative surgical exposure of the subgingival margin of the carious lesion does exist, but seldom finds favour with patients when it achieves the same ultimate effect! Where, on the other hand, access for tooth restoration is impeded by the gingivae, the offending tissue should be dealt with first, by surgical resection or apical repositioning (depending on the features of the case) with or without bone removal (see later). Where this surgery would be simplified by inflammatory resolution, an interim restoration is often indicated to protect the pulp or for aesthetic reasons. These topics are discussed next.

Restorations in the presence of pockets

Treatment sequence

Individual sites frequently require both restorative and periodontal therapy, so that two closely related but separate problems exist. The combination of problems encountered might, however, sometimes dictate that a tooth is extracted instead and should be resolved before processing further. (See also Chapter 26.)

The sequence of treatment is simply dictated by basic practical considerations. Firstly, when pain is being experienced this is obviously treated first. Secondly, patient functional comfort and aesthetic needs usually dictate a predilection for the restorative aspects of combined therapy. Thirdly, the technically simpler exercise is best dealt with first. Fourthly, that aspect of therapy with the least favourable prognosis (usually furcation involvement or endodontic complications) is preferably resolved before committing the patient to other treatment. In all instances the dental and periodontal status of the rest of the mouth must also be considered.

Operative measures

Pulpal pain

Pulpal symptoms demand the insertion of either a sedative dressing or the appropriate pulpal therapy, which need not be considered here. Placement of this dressing might be interfered with by bleeding and tissue proliferation into the tooth surface defect. Isolation of the tooth with rubber dam is sometimes possible, but elsewhere the expediency of removing

the offending tissue electrosurgically, or by simple heat cauterization is advocated.

Asymptomatic dental lesions

Inaccessible carious defects are best left untreated pending gingival inflammatory resolution following root surface debridement and the appropriate oral hygiene instructions. Plaque retentive features of defective restorations are corrected as described in Chapter 11. With tissue shrinkage the dental lesion becomes more accessible, and cavity preparation and restoration insertion become possible without the complication of gingival bleeding.

Persistent gingival inflammation

Where patient cooperation in plaque control is questionable so that little inflammatory resolution is expected, or where the patient's demand for immediate restorative treatment does not allow for the requisite inflammatory resolution, expedient restorative therapy is indicated. That is, restoration is carried out in the best possible manner under the prevailing adverse conditions, using amalgam or tooth-coloured materials and, where necessary, laboratory processed acrylic crowns and bridges fitted as semi-permanent restorations. These will not only satisfy most functional and aesthetic needs, while further attempts are made at gaining tissue marginal health, but can also be readily improved upon or replaced when conditions allow.

Uncertain periodontal prognosis

There are several advantages to the expedient approach outlined above and, not least, its applicability to other situations necessitating complex restorative care, but having a questionable long-term periodontal prognosis as with furcation involvement or endodontic complications. In the first place continuous reassessment, as consistently advocated in this text, is still possible. This then allows for any modifications necessary to the initially conceived treatment plan as dictated by changing circumstances and findings. In addition, the provisional restorations fitted give the patient the opportunity of assessing in practical terms the relative merits of the proposed treatment. This may then either be endorsed or perhaps, a simpler and more economical alternative treatment objective be decided upon. This prolonged clinical re-evaluation period may often also provide the cue for improved patient cleaning efforts and thereby a better prognosis.

In cases of uncertain prognosis where the continued presence of semipermanent restorations is no longer feasible technically nor acceptable to the patient, little alternative exists but to provide

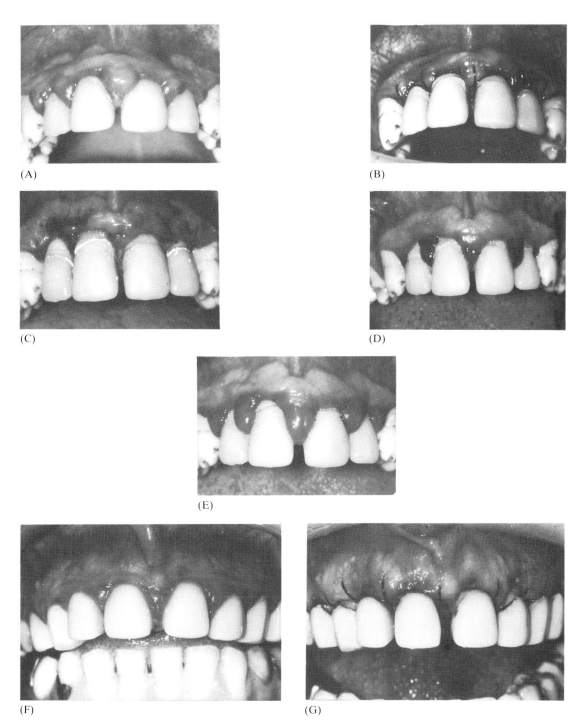

Figure 24.2 (A) Pre-restorative pocket correction about provisional acrylic crowns in 18-year-old man with poor oral hygiene. (B) Tissue resected and flaps sutured to expose former subgingivally located margins. (C) Healing at 1 week. (D) 1 month and (E) 6 month presentation-persistent plaque induced inflammation associated with tissue proliferation and almost total gingival relapse. (F) Replacement of aesthetically unacceptable longstanding acrylic crowns sought by 22-year-old woman. Patient unaware of poor crown margins or significance of related gingival inflammation – note mandibular gingival health. (G) Pockets resected and surgical flaps sutured – crown margins exposed but not corrected lest debris contaminated surgical field.

366

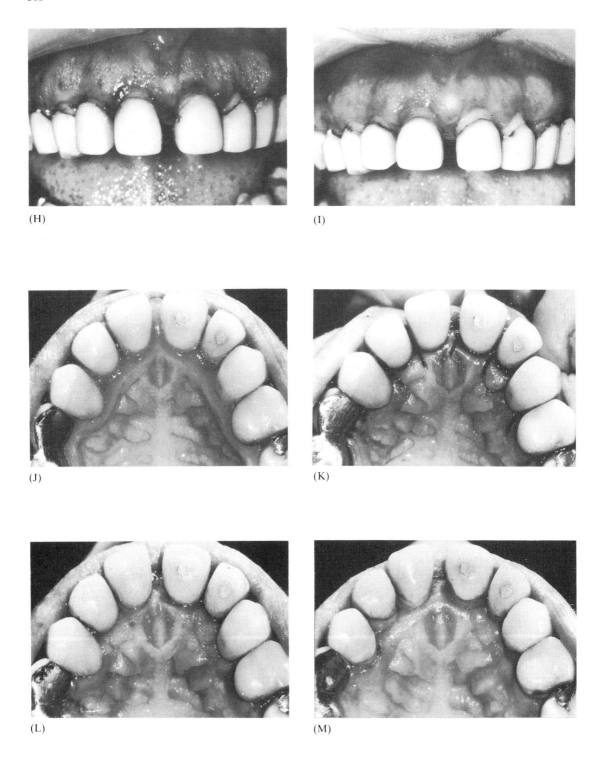

(H)

(I)

(J)

(K)

(L)

(M)

Figure 24.2 (*cont.*) (H) Healing at 1 week when crown margins reduced to facilitate plaque control. (I) 2 weeks postoperative – note recontoured crown margins. (I–M) Palatal views – (J) pre-operatively, (K) sutured, (L) 1 week and (M) 2 week healing.

more permanent restorations. Surgical exposure of the shoulders of the proposed preparations together with optimal pocket elimination should, however, be carried out first as shown in Figure 24.2 (B). It might, in retrospect, then be argued that this surgical intervention would have been simpler at the outset in these cases. Although this is difficult to counter on technical grounds, the principle of achieving optimal plaque control in the future interests of the dentition remains paramount and so justifies the therapeutic approach advocated. This is well illustrated in Figure 24.2 (A–D) where in spite of the regular use of a chlorhexidine mouthwash for a 6-month post-surgical period, a recurrent gingival inflammatory overgrowth developed. On the other hand, in those instances where this surgical therapy is rejected by the patient, restoration must be carried out under the existing adverse conditions of the marginal periodontal status.

Defective complex restorations

Where replacement of existing complex cast metal and porcelain restorations is necessary, several other problems arise. Firstly, the patient is seldom prepared to delay treatment for many months pending the outcome of gingival response therapy and which might, in any case, be affected adversely by plaque retention of the existing defective restorations. Secondly, it is frequently not possible to rectify these plaque retentive defective margins particularly when located interproximally. Thirdly, if left unattended and surgical therapy is instituted, the roughened edges of the restorations hamper not only surgical instrumentation and suturing, but may also sometimes interfere with post-surgical oral hygiene. The use of a chlorhexidine mouthwash post-surgically does not always compensate adequately for ineffective cleaning, as shown above.

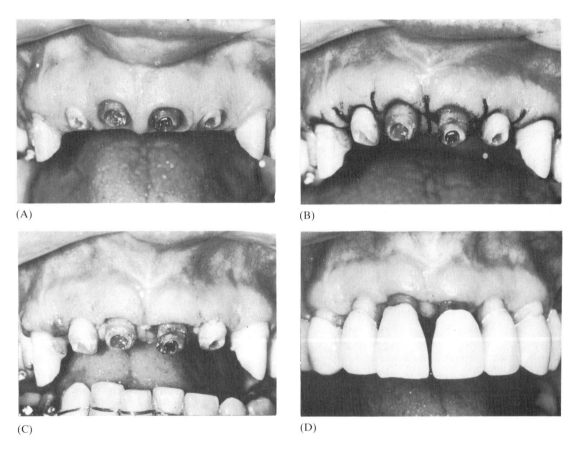

(A)　(B)

(C)　(D)

Figure 24.3 (A) Pathological drifting in 35-year-old woman corrected orthodontically. Temporary splints removed to facilitate pre-restorative pocket resection. (B) Flaps sutured. (C) 1 week and (D) 4 weeks postoperatively. Coronal reconstruction fitted after 6 months. (E) Presentation at 1 year – note supragingival margins. (F–J) Right maxillary quadrant views – (F) presurgical, (G) sutured, (H) 1 week, (I) 4 weeks and (J) 1 year postoperative. (K–N) Palatal views – (K) presurgical, (L) sutured.

369

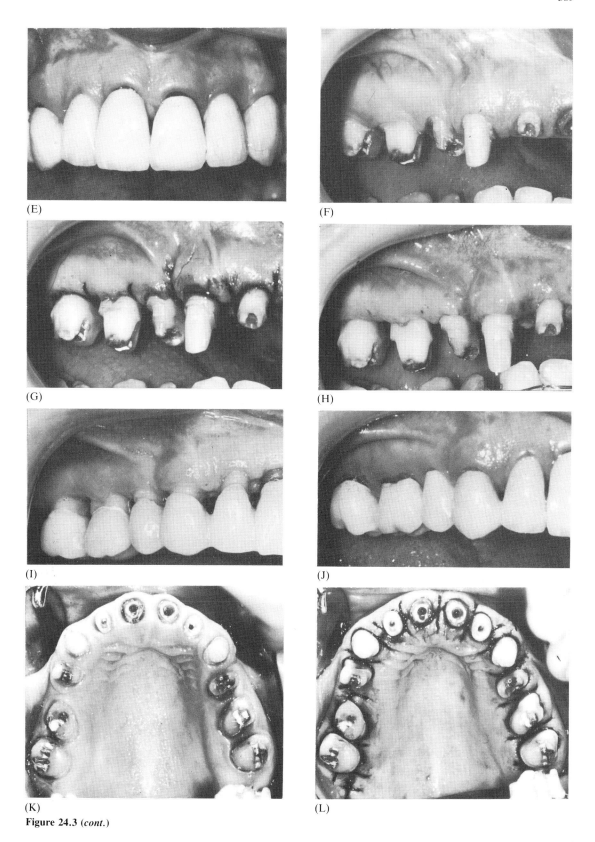

(E)

(F)

(G)

(H)

(I)

(J)

(K)

(L)

Figure 24.3 (*cont.*)

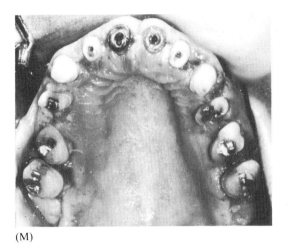

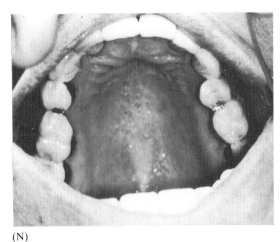

(M)   (N)

Figure 24.3 (*cont.*) (M) 1 week and (N) 1 year postoperative (Restorative treatment by courtesy Department of Conservation, Royal Dental Hospital). See also Figure 26.6

The above problems can be overcome in two ways. In the one, semi-permanent acrylic restorations are fitted at the outset and surgical correction of the pockets then carried out, having removed the restorations at operation for better access and to simplify surgery (Figure 24.3. See also Figure 16.20). In the other, the technical surgical inconvenience of the adverse restorations is tolerated and then corrected as necessary following surgery (Figure 24.2 F–M). This is best delayed at least until after suture removal rather than at completion of surgery, lest the debris contaminates the wound. Those restoration margins that are located at some distance coronal to the post-surgical gingival margins and which do not impede cleaning, need not be altered. The chosen solution will be dictated by the features of the case and individual operator preference.

Complex restorations and interceptive pocket surgery

Pre-restorative surgical intervention is sometimes warranted for pockets at sites that might be expected, time permitting, to respond favourably to gingival response therapy alone. The rationale for this is that the appearance of any crowns fitted in the presence of such pocketing would be spoilt by the gingival recession anticipated. Surgery would help to safeguard the ultimate gingival margin position and minimize the risk of any subsequent recession or that following any necessary correction of detached marginal tissue (Figure 24.2 N–T and see also

Figure 11.7). Similarly, where a removable prosthesis is incorporated into complex treatment, functional comfort will not be compromised by the development of spacing between the prosthesis and the mucosa as a result of gingival recession.

In summary, the great cost of prosthodontic therapy, coupled with the extensive treatment times and patient discomfort is such that the early establishment of an optimal dentogingival relationship is an essential prerequisite to treatment. Indeed, such prerestorative preparation for the comparatively few individuals able to undergo such complex prosthodontic therapy, remains one of the few positive indications for elective pocket surgery. The need for careful treatment planning and discussion with the patient (before therapy) is implicit in these cases.

Timing of permanent restorations

In individuals demanding optimal aesthetic results the fitting of crowns is best delayed for 3–4 months after surgery to allow the marginal tissue position to stabilize. The margins of prematurely fitted crowns might otherwise become exposed by normal, albeit not totally predictable, post-surgical gingival shrinkage. The optimal time has, surprisingly, yet to be established by controlled investigations but an interval of not less than 3 months is recommended. In contrast, where no aesthetic considerations exist, as in the posterior part of the arch (see Figure 24.3) and at the lingual and palatal aspects elsewhere, the treatment can be commenced as soon as the patient wishes. However, as the teeth in most surgical fields usually remain tender for some weeks post-surgically, most operators choose to delay further treatment until after that. This assumes that adequate provisional restorations are in place or that the existing modified restorations are aesthetically and functionally acceptable. (See also Chapter 34 – Prerestorative periodontal surgery.)

Periodontal surgery to expedite restorative dentistry

The problem

The surgical removal of healthy periodontal tissues is sometimes necessary to facilitate restorative treatment. The indications are: (a) where caries extends subgingivally and prevents adequate shoulder preparation, (b) cusp fracture lines extend below the gingival margin, (c) the mechanical retention of any proposed restorations and/or prostheses is inadequate, and, finally (d) the displeasing aesthetics of short or uneven clinical crown lengths following extensive attrition and erosion.

The difficulties of tooth restoration following both subgingival caries and cusp fracture lines that extend subgingivally are similar although are somewhat more complex in the latter (Figure 24.4 A–J). Thus, in the first place, gingival bleeding following the removal of the fractured portion interferes with subsequent visibility and techniques. Secondly, an adequate finishing line to the tooth preparation is neither readily established nor clearly recorded during impression techniques, whilst the application of any matrix band is often impossible. Thirdly, bone must be removed where the fracture extends apical to the crestal bone. Finally, gingival proliferation over the exposed root surface is frequently encountered when the fractured coronal fragment segment has been lost prior to attendance.

An essentially comparable technical situation exists where clinical crown lengths, reduced by

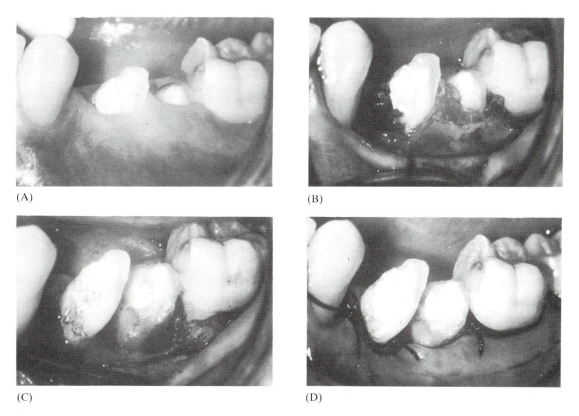

(A)

(B)

(C)

(D)

Figure 24.4 Coronal fractures – Pre-restorative technique. (A) Traumatic fracture 34, 35, 36. (B) Flap reflection and exposure of coronal remnants. (C) Bone removed to lengthen clinical crowns. (D) Flaps apically repositioned and sutured.

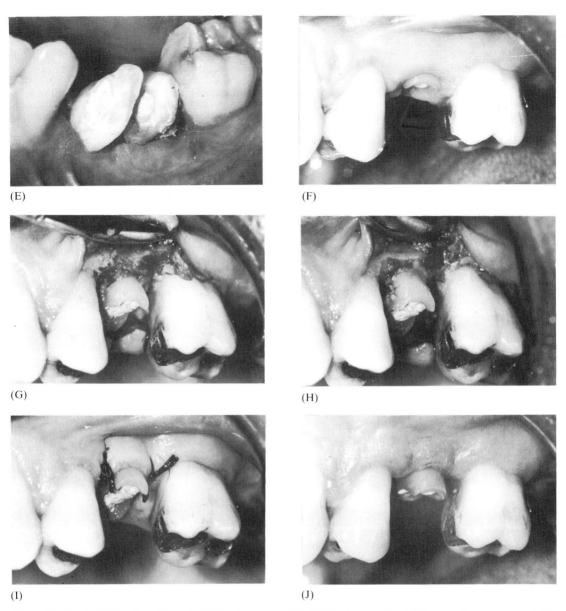

(E)

(F)

(G)

(H)

(I)

(J)

Figure 24.4 (*cont.*) (E) Healing at 1 week. (F) Fractured crown 25. (G) Root exposed and (H) supporting bone removed for crown lengthening. (I) Flaps sutured. (J) Healing at 1 week

occlusal attrition and erosion (Figure 24.6 K), or the crowns are inherently small, compromise the retention of any proposed restoration. The necessary increase in the clinical crown length is greatly facilitated by the need to eliminate any co-existing pocketing, for the twin objectives are achieved coincidentally. This is also true of the correction of chronic gingival hyperplasia (e.g. Figures 15.21, 15.22 and 16.12), for restorative purposes (e.g. Figures 15.17 and 24.3) or to enhance retention of

removable prostheses (e.g. Figures 16.22 and 16.23).

Clinical crown lengthening in the presence of pocketing involves detached tissues and the appropriate surgical techniques have already been described in Chapters 15 and 16. In contrast, the sacrifice of sound supporting tissue, often including bone, is required for crown lengthening in periodontal health. The surgical exercise represents an extension of simple pocket surgery, but is technically more difficult and invariably results in greater postoperative symptoms. The technique for crown lengthening described below is also applicable to the pre-restorative management of cusp fractures and subgingival caries.

Clinical crown lengthening

The surgical principles

The apical repositioning and indirect resection techniques are utilized according to the location of the surgical site. These techniques provide routine access to crestal bone for assessment *in situ* and any necessary removal of bone for the crown lengthening required or for root face and shoulder preparation elsewhere. In the latter, a minimum of 2 mm of sound root surface coronal to crestal bone should be the aim. Although the methods of bone removal and the precautions are described in Chapter 19, the technique is advocated primarily for crown lengthening purposes and so it (Figure 24.5 A–A3) and

the appropriate instruments are illustrated here (Figure 24.5 B, C and D). The furcation morphology can also be assessed with respect to future plaque control measures and restorative treatment planning. Where necessary, root resection could also be undertaken at this stage although, as indicated in Chapter 18, this might best be deferred to a later date.

The surgical flap should extend as far laterally as necessary to satisfy the individual aesthetic demands of each case. The flap margin is then finally repositioned apically or resected as required, so as to just cover crestal bone (Figure 24.5 A3). Suturing is required and a periodontal dressing generally necessary following apical repositioning. The clinical surgical sequences are shown in Figures 24.6–24.8.

Where provisional crowns removed to expedite surgery are recemented, the excess Temp-Bond (Kerr Manufacturing Corporation, Romulus, MI 48174, USA) cementing material tends to flow over the surgical flap margins. This does then sometimes

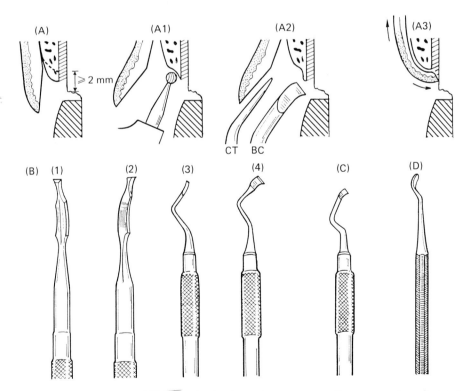

Figure 24.5 Bone removal. (A) Flap reflection for *in situ* assessment of bone removal required (≥2 mm). (A1) Dental bur used for gross reduction leaving (A2) thin plate for removal with Cavitron TFI-3 Tip (CT), bone chisel (BC) as shown, or hand instrument to minimize risk of damage to tooth surface. (A3) Flap apically repositioned (or resected as necessary elsewhere) for crown lengthening. (B) Ochsenbein (Hu Friedy, Chicago, IL 60618, USA), chisels No. 1–4. (C) Rhodes (Hu Friedy, Chicago, IL 60618, USA), 36/37 chisel. (D) Cumine (Ash Instrument Div. Dentsply Ltd, Gloucester, UK), 152 scaler

374

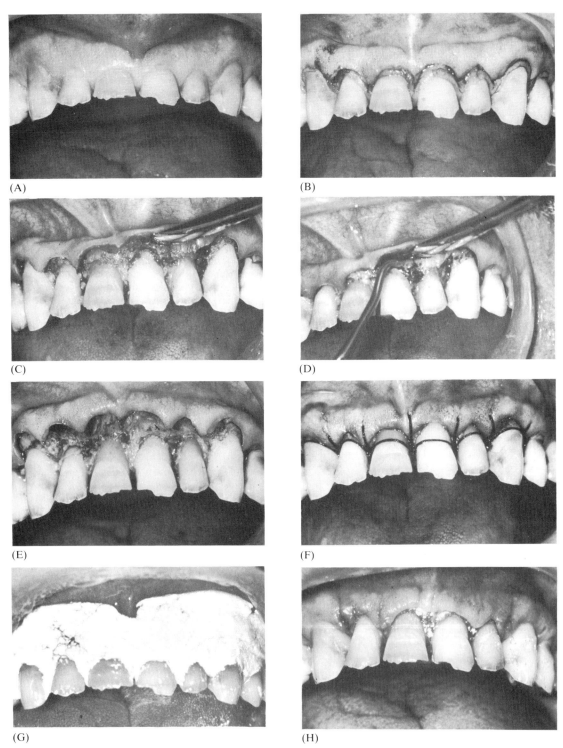

(A)

(B)

(C)

(D)

(E)

(F)

(G)

(H)

Figure 24.6 Cosmetic and functional restoration of marked incisal attrition and erosion. (A) Initial presentation in middle aged male. (B) Surgical flap preparation. (C) Flap reflection. Resection crestal bone required. (D) Bone removal with cumine scaler shown at 21. (E) Bone removal completed. (F) Flap apically repositioned and sutured. (G) Stabilizing dressing. (H) Healing at 1 week. Note mucosal displacement from dressing with bony denudation at 21.

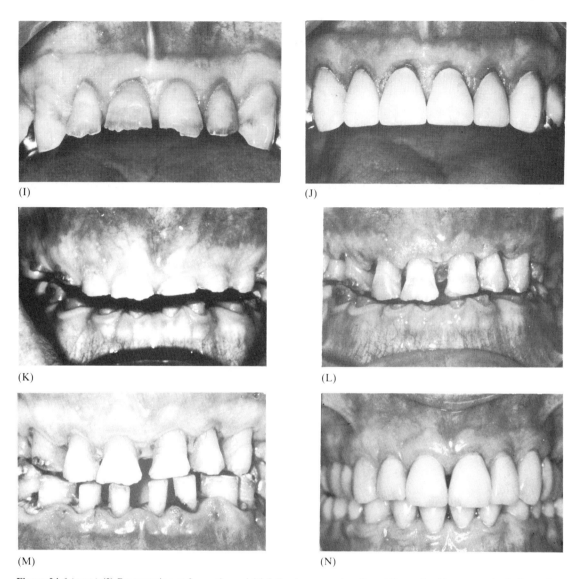

Figure 24.6 (*cont.*) (I) Presentation at 3 months and (J) following reconstruction at 9 months. Note supragingival margins. (K) Gross wear both arches in 32-year-old man. (L) 1 week postoperative in maxilla, (M) 1 week postoperative in mandible and 3 weeks in maxilla. (N) Crowns fitted at 1 year. (Restorative treatment by courtesy of Department of Conservation, Institute of Dental Surgery)

serve as an effective substitute for a periodontal dressing for flap fixation although it can be readily used in combination with any dressing necessary. In any event the attempted removal of the excess material may, at this stage, interfere with flap adaptation and so is best avoided. As the suture thread obviously becomes incorporated in the Temp-Bond in such cases, post-surgical suture removal should be preceded by simply cracking and dislodging the material with an ultrasonic scaler.

The greater postoperative pain experienced in crown lengthening cases is probably related to a combination of the trauma of removing sound supporting bone coupled with the longer operating time than routine pocket surgery. The patient must therefore be warned lest undue concern be aroused.

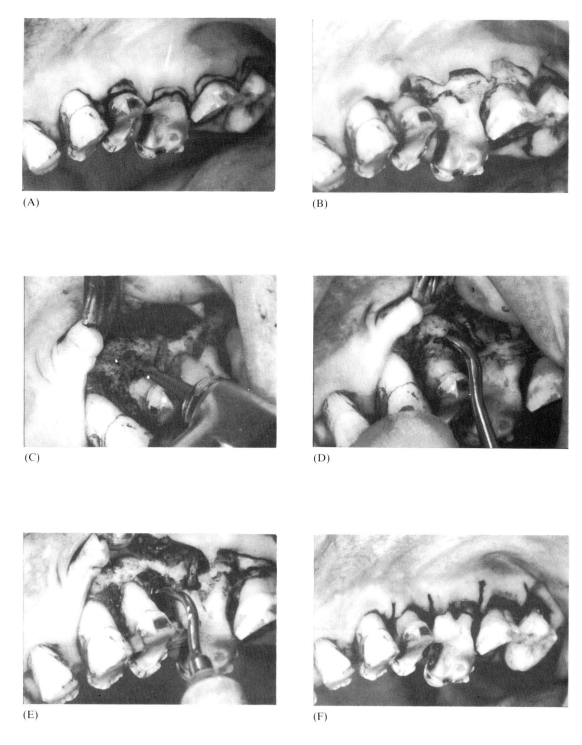

(A)

(B)

(C)

(D)

(E)

(F)

Figure 24.7 Crown lengthening technique. (A) Initial presentation of same patient as in Figure 24.6 (K) showing exaggerated scalloped outline incision. (B) Flap reflected, cervical wedge tissue removed and crestal bone exposed. (C) Thick subcrestal buccal and corresponding interdental bone reduction with bur. (D) Residual thin buccal bone removed with Cumine scaler and (E) that interdentally with Cavitron TFI-10 tip. Bone in 26 furcation preserved. (F) Flap apically repositioned and sutured. Note minor flap margin to crestal bone inconsistencies.

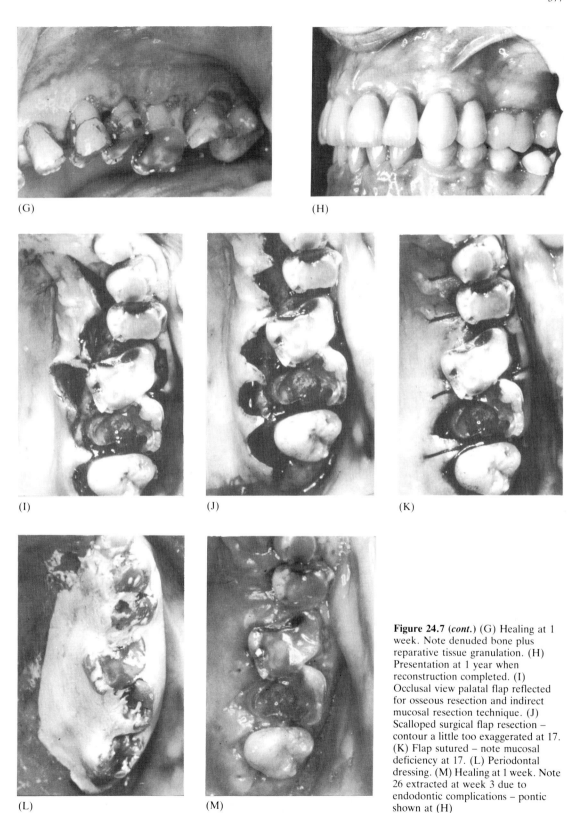

Figure 24.7 (*cont.*) (G) Healing at 1 week. Note denuded bone plus reparative tissue granulation. (H) Presentation at 1 year when reconstruction completed. (I) Occlusal view palatal flap reflected for osseous resection and indirect mucosal resection technique. (J) Scalloped surgical flap resection – contour a little too exaggerated at 17. (K) Flap sutured – note mucosal deficiency at 17. (L) Periodontal dressing. (M) Healing at 1 week. Note 26 extracted at week 3 due to endodontic complications – pontic shown at (H)

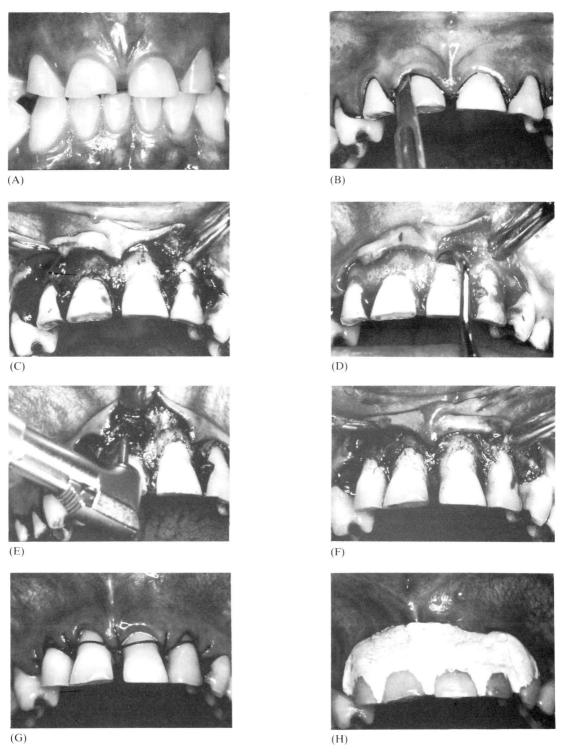

(A)   (B)

(C)   (D)

(E)   (F)

(G)   (H)

Figure 24.8 (A) Crown lengthening prior to provision of crowns for displeasing extensive incisal wear 12, 11, 21, 22 in 32-year-old man. (B) Crevicular incision with papillary filletting. (C) Flap reflection – note bony dehiscence at 22. (D) Bone removal with chisel and (E) with bur. (F) Clinical crown heights adequate – flap apically repositioned. (G) Suturing. (H) Periodontal dressing critical.

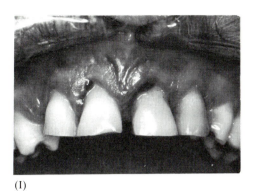

(I)

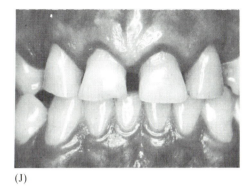

(J)

Figure 24.8 (*cont.*) (I) 1 week postoperative – note granulation at margins of 11, 21 possibly derived from residual periodontal ligament tissue? (J) Presentation at 6 months totally acceptable to patient so restorative plan abandoned

Alternative operative options

Soft tissue resection, by an external bevel gingivectomy or electrosurgical techniques, is best avoided in these cases. Although undoubtedly simpler technical exercises, neither can provide postoperative mucosal tissue coverage of bone when, as is so often the case, bone removal is found to be necessary. Any such bone denudation will in turn lead to a painful, irreversible postoperative loss of attachment. The use of electrosurgery close to bone will, in addition, frequently result in extensive bony necrosis.

Furcation involvement

Where surgical detachment would expose molar root furcations as shown in Figure 24.7 E, the potential periodontal hazards must be weighed carefully against the restorative benefits. Fortunately, such involvement is seldom necessary but, where inevitable, usually occurs in subjects who have sustained little attachment loss in the past so apparently being 'resistant' to periodontal breakdown. In other words, deliberate furcation exposure might be tolerated with minimal ill-effects. This situation does, however, demand controlled researched investigation.

Fixed bridgework

Where the operative field lies adjacent to an edentulous zone restored by a fixed bridge pontic, the surgical production of greater crown length in particular, but also even routine pocket correction can be difficult. Poor access and close apposition of the pontics to the mucosa complicates both flap

preparation and subsequent flap management. The difficulties are, however, readily overcome by common-sense modifications of the surgical techniques described in Chapters 14 to 17. The particular technique used depends on whether reduction of the edentulous ridge zone is also required or not. Thus, when preservation of ridge mucosa is desirable, or is already of physiological thickness, the inverse bevel papillectomy technique (Figure 24.9 A) is used. When aesthetics are unimportant, and the best possible access for future plaque control at abutment units is critical, then the edentulous site resection technique is indicated (Figure 24.9 B–D). The appropriate technical modifications are now described.

Papillectomy technique

Where the ridge mucosal form is being maintained, the related bridge pontics are simply regarded as standing teeth. Inverse bevel incisions are first made at the facial and oral aspects of the abutment teeth. These are continued as 'crevicular' incisions about the adjacent tooth pontics and then extended apically as oblique relieving incisions as shown in Figure 24.9 (A1 and A2). The two papillary flaps are reflected and filletted as necessary (Figure 24.9 A3 and A4). The exposed cervical wedge tissue located between the abutment tooth and its adjacent pontic is then separated from the contiguous ridge mucosa by deepening the facial and oral pontic 'crevicular' incisions with a Swann Morton No. 11 or 13 blade until they meet under the pontic. The, thus, isolated tissue can then be curetted away and the operation completed as described before.

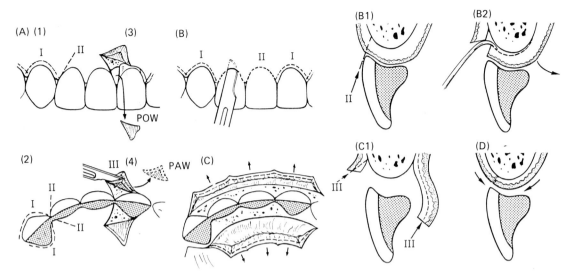

Figure 24.9 Pocket reduction adjacent to bridge pontics. Bridge shown with abutment tooth crowns at 13, 21 and pontics 12, 11. (A1–A4) Labial and occlusal views of inverse bevel papillectomy technique for pockets at 13 mesial and 21 distal aspects, (A1 and 2) 13 inverse bevel (I) incision and adjacent pontic zone oblique relieving (II) incisions. (A3) Next stage of papillary flap reflection shown at 11 revealing thick buccal papillary form and isolating the pontic zone cervical wedge (POW) tissue for removal. (A4) Papillary tissue filletting (III) incisions with No. 15 blade are then carried out as shown at 21 mesiobuccal aspect with discarded papillary wedge tissue (PAW) ghosted and shown completed at palatal aspect prior to flap coaptation. (B and B1) Where subpontic ridge mucosal reduction is also necessary, buccal crevicular type relieving (II) incisions are made about the pontic cervical margins. (B2) Minimal buccal flap elevation, blunt dissection of subpontic ridge mucosa and palatal mucoperiosteal flap reflection. (C and C1) Reflected buccal and palatal flaps for filletting (III) along dotted lines. (D) Flap coaptation following correction of any overlapping tissue (by resection or buccal apical repositioning)

Mucosal ridge reduction

The linear incision of the edentulous site technique advocated elsewhere, can obviously not be made along the crest of the mucosal ridge, for this is inaccessible. The incision is made instead at the facial or oral aspect of the pontics, representing crevicular incisions. The location is dictated by, firstly, the mucosal thickness and contour coupled with the ease of flap reflection and displacement from under the pontics; secondly, the access available for subsequent filletting. Thus, for example, the form of the ridge mucosa shown in Figure 24.9 (B1) precludes deflection of the tissue buccally from under the pontics. Accordingly, the 'linear crevicular' incision is made buccally and the flap reflected from under the pontics to the palatal aspect instead. Filletting in this case would also be reasonably easy from the palatal aspect (see also Figure 24.10).

The 'linear crevicular' incision follows the scalloped cervical margin contour of the pontic(s) (Figure 24.9 B and B1) having made the necessary incisions at the abutment teeth. The buccal flap is reflected and filletted, and the ridge mucosa thus exposed under the pontics, freed from its underlying bone by blunt dissection, using a fine scaler from the buccal aspect (Figure 24.9 B2). The flap is then eased out palatally from under the pontic and deflected into a vertical posture (Figure 24.9 C and C1). Following the appropriate thinning the ridge flap is manipulated back into place over the bone and, having corrected of any overlapping excess (Figure 24.9 D), the flaps are sutured.

In those instances where the ridge mucosa is oedematous and/or hyperplastic and is uneven in thickness, as in a denture hyperplasia, neither mucosal flap reflection nor filletting is accomplished easily. Postoperative mucosal necrosis and ulceration is therefore not uncommon in these situations, and when external bevel resection should preferably be considered instead (see Chapter 16).

Cosmetic considerations

Where a displeasing uneven marginal gingival contour exists at maxillary anterior teeth at which

381

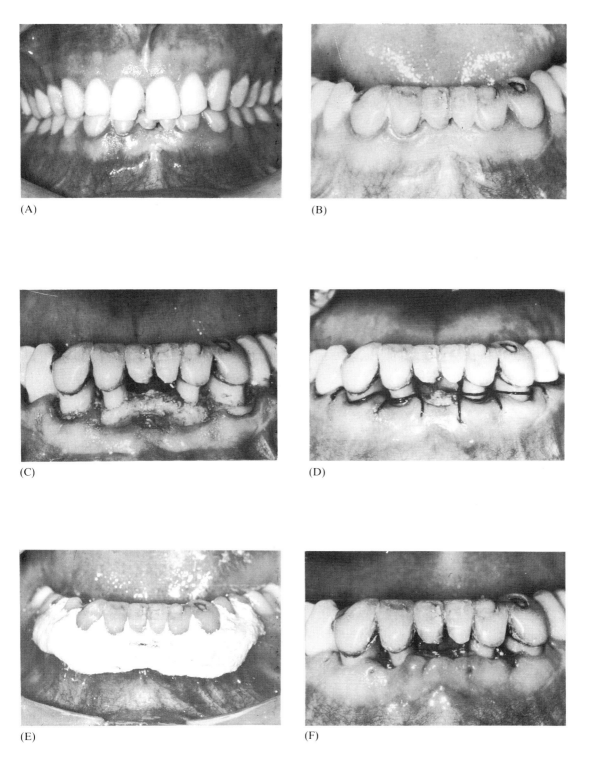

(A)

(B)

(C)

(D)

(E)

(F)

Figure 24.10 (A) Replacement worn acrylic bridge indicated in 32-year-old man. Initial presentation. (B) Presurgical. (C) Surgical flaps reflected and pontic zone tissue filletted. Some crestal bone reduction was necessary. (D) Flaps apically repositioned and sutured. Bony denudation under pontics inevitable. (E) Periodontal dressing to maintain flap displacement. (F) 1 week postoperative – optimal flap positioning has not been maintained.

382

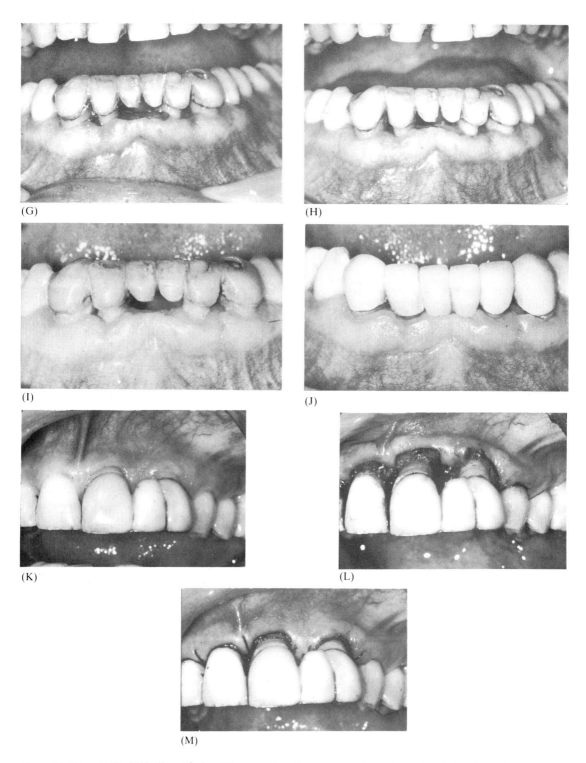

(G)

(H)

(I)

(J)

(K)

(L)

(M)

Figure 24.10 (*cont.*) (G–I) Healing at 2, 4 and 8 weeks. Note tissue regeneration at bony denudation sites. (J) Bridge fitted at 6 months – note residual gingival deformity 32, 33. (Bridge by courtesy Department of Conservation, Royal Dental Hospital, London). (K) Crown lengthening adjacent to bridge pontic in 38-year-old woman. Initial presentation. (L) Pontic zone tissue displaced labially for filletting. (M) Flap sutured.

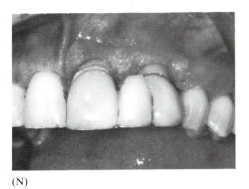

(N)

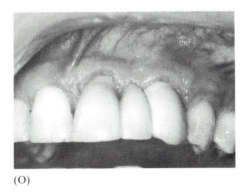

(O)

Figure 24.10 (*cont.*) (N) Healing at 1 week. (O) Replacement bridge fitted at 3 months (See also Figure 26.5)

crowning is contemplated, surgical gingival recontouring is indicated. Depending on the features of the case, this is carried out by the apical repositioning or direct inverse bevel resection.

Apical surgery and the periodontal tissues

The surgical flap reflected to gain access to the apical lesion must be designed so as to compromise neither healing of the lesion nor the integrity of periodontal tissue. It is, therefore, necessary to consider the design and management of the surgical flap in itself and in relationship to the underlying bone and the supracrestal attachment, in both health and in the presence of pocketing. The problem of combined periodontal–endodontic lesions, in which the periodontal and pulpal disease communicate, will then also be considered.

Surgical flap design

There are several possible options to the position of the flap outline incision (Figure 24.11). The first is a horizontal or vertical incision made directly over the discharging mucosal sinus (Figure 24.11 AII and G), as when establishing surgical drainage. The mucosal breach then spans the surgical bony access cavity and the related flap edges become unsupported post-surgically. The importance of this is that should the submucosal blood clot break down, ischaemic mucosal necrosis ensue post-surgically, or more especially, the apical endodontic seal be inadequate, an irreparable epithelialized mucosal fenestration communicating with the root apex would result, and lead to gingival recession as well, as shown in Figure 21.5 (C and D).

The post-surgical complications cited above can be avoided by ensuring that the incision always lies over bone, either apical to or coronal to the endodontic lesion. In the former vestibular mucosal site (Figure 24.11 AI and G), the horizontal semilunar incision should be located about 10 mm apical to the lesion. The resulting surgical flap preparation demands greater surgical finesse than elsewhere, and although some difficulty can arise in flap retraction coronally whilst simultaneously retracting the lip or cheek, very good access to the apical lesion accrues. This type of incision is best suited to situations where apical surgery has to be repeated when the risk of post-surgical mucosal fenestration appears to be especially high. It should also be considered where gingival recession might follow crevicular incisions.

The alternative coronally situated, so-called submarginal incision, should be located about 10 mm from the lesion and be situated ideally within keratinized tissue (Figure 24.11 AIII and G). The incision should, however, avoid the 3–4 mm of marginal tissue lest the supracrestal attachment be damaged. A horizontal incision with oblique relieving cuts sometimes offers better access, so may be preferred to the semilunar outline incision.

Submarginal incisions may encounter two potential hazards. The first is the involvement of bony fenestrations (as depicted in Figure 24.11 H) or dehiscences when the flap margin would lie over periodontal ligament rather than bone. This carries the risk of mucosal fenestration with root surface exposure in the event of post-surgical complications (see also Figure 21.5). The incision is therefore best avoided when bony deficiencies are suspected by the presence of readily observed undulating root forms coupled with a thin overlying mucosa. The second relates to periodontal pocketing, for supracrestal attachment involvement is likely with all but modest

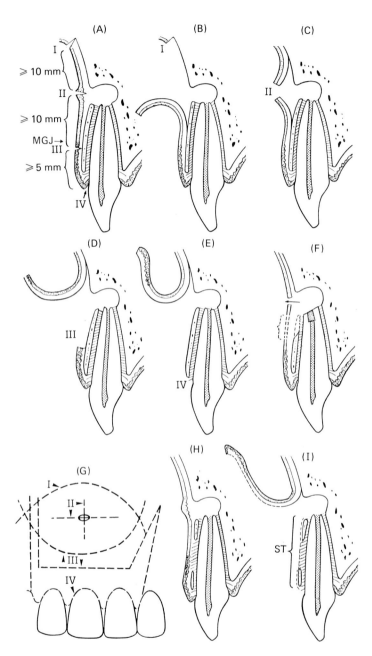

Figure 24.11 Flap design for periapical surgery – periodontal health. (A and G) Incision may be located (I) apical, (II) over, (III) coronal to the endodontic sinus within keratinized tissue (note mucogingival junction – MGJ) or (IV) within the gingival crevice. Optional use of semilunar or linear type II incision and of vertical and oblique relieving incisions at 13, 12 and 21, 22 respectively. (B–E) Full thickness flap reflection following each incision type. (F) Failed apical surgery with persistent sinus (arrowed) and possible complications (broken lines) of mucosal and/or bony necrosis leading to mucosal fenestration and root exposure. (H) Submarginal type III incisions avoided where bony deficiencies are suspected and when (I) type IV incision coupled with split-thickness (ST) flap dissection best carried out instead

attachment losses, whilst elsewhere perforation of the pocket wall is inevitable, as shown in Figure 24.12 (B). These complications are considered further below.

The last possible location of the incision is at the gingival margin within an intact gingival sulcus (Figure 24.11 AIV and G) or into any pocket space (Figure 24.12 C). Relieving incisions (Figure 24.11 G) are necessary, resulting in a triangular-shaped flap for the unilateral incision and a trapezoidal-shaped flap where bilateral relieving incisions are made. The latter type flap is more readily retracted and supported during operation, so provides better access and minimizes stretching of the tissues. *Note*: The traditional oblique nature of relieving incisions is designed to maximize the surgical flap vasculature. However, as most of the mucosal blood vessels run vertically, the use of vertical relieving incisions

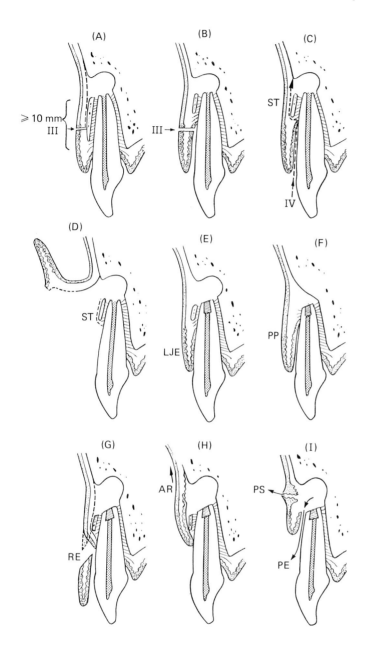

Figure 24.12 Flap design for periapical surgery – periodontal pocketing. (A) Submarginal incisions used only where length of remaining periodontal attachment exceeds 10 mm to avoid (B) pocket wall perforation. (C) Crevicular type IV incision indicated with preferably split-thickness (ST) flap dissection. (D) Flap reflection with periosteal retention. (E) Optimal healing with long junctional epithelium (LJE), but slight crestal bone loss. (F) Persistent pocket (PP) with further loss of bone, some attachment loss and epithelial migration. (G) Technical possibility of co-existing pocket elimination by tissue resection (RE) but (H) apical repositioning (AR) contraindicated. (I) Post-surgical complications with persistent sinus (PS) and development of combined periodontal–endodontal lesion (PE)

instead would be unlikely to compromise the flap. In addition, the possible involvement of bony dehiscences and fenestrations would be eliminated (see also Chapter 17).

Influence of pocketing

Provided that the remaining periodontal attachment, measured by the distance between the base of the pocket and the apical lesion, is more than about 10 mm a submarginal incision, as shown in Figure 24.10 (A) is permissible. With greater periodontal destruction a crevicular-type incision within the pocket space is made instead (Figure 24.12 C). Pocket wall perforation could precipitate ischaemic necrosis and a painful sloughing of the marginal tissue or, less critically, result in post-surgical epithelialization from both the oral and pocket aspects and a mucosal fenestration.

Mucosal flap management

Full thickness mucoperiosteal flaps are reflected by blunt dissection (Figure 24.11). This minimizes the risk of inadvertent mucosal perforation, particularly of the friable tissue associated with any discharging sinus, and which might lead to painful flap necrosis and possible mucosal fenestration. The importance of post-surgical mucosal integrity thus outweighs the disadvantages of the surgical exposure of bone (see Chapter 19), although where bony deficiencies are suspected, split-thickness dissection might best maintain the integrity of the remaining bone and the related periodontal ligament tissue (Figure 24.11 I). Similarly, with markedly reduced periodontal support a split-thickness flap over the remaining supporting bone is prudent, mucosal thickness permitting (Figure 24.12 C and D). This is designed to minimize the traumatic effects of flap reflection itself and of bone exposure during apical surgery and in turn, to safeguard the integrity of the underlying periodontal ligament. The risk of irreversible bony necrosis coupled with some loss of attachment does nevertheless still exist under even optimal healing conditions, as depicted in Figure 24.12 (E).

On completion of the apical surgery the periodontally involved root surfaces are carefully debrided, taking care not to damage the supracrestal attachment, and the flap sutured back into position using interrupted sutures. Relieving incisions are not sutured so as to permit drainage and minimize postoperative swelling. Where pocketing has necessitated the use of crevicular incisions, the pocket wall component to the flap is sutured back into its presurgical position, in anticipation of optimal healing with pocket closure coupled with the development of a long junctional epithelium (Figure 24.12 E) (see also below). On the other hand, the pocket may persist and indeed even be deeper, following further loss of attachment (Figure 24.12 F).

Sequence of apical and pocket surgery

Where both apical and periodontal lesions existing at a tooth demand surgical correction, the former should, as a rule, be treated first as a separate exercise, so as to avoid compromising the remaining periodontal support. That is, only when the apical lesion has resolved should surgical correction of residual pocketing be attempted. The importance of this clinical sequence is reflected in the possible consequences of combined surgical therapy shown in Figure 24.12 (G–I).

In the first place, while the pocket wall might simply be cut away, vestibular morphology permitting, by inverse bevel resection (Figure 24.12 G), the additional surgical trauma could further compromise the underlying bony blood supply and lead

to mucosal ischaemic necrosis and sloughing. The alternative of apical repositioning (Figure 24.12 H), presents similar hazards plus the added possible complication relating to the management of the epithelialized pocket lining. Any attempted removal of pocket epithelium, in the interests of optimal healing over the bone, could in turn precipitate mucosal necrosis, whilst its retention might not only retard healing of the flap to the underlying bone and periodontal attachment but also deny these tissues the optimal benefits of mucosal connective tissue coverage in the early post-surgical healing phase. In summary, in each situation cited, an unnecessary risk of post-surgical complications coupled with further attachment loss arises. Even worse, should the apicectomy itself fail, an epithelialized communication between pocket and the root apex might develop giving rise to a combined periodontal–endodontic lesion with or without a persistent labial sinus (Figure 24.12 I). For these reasons, pocket reduction surgery should preferably not be carried out in conjunction with apical surgery.

Combined periodontal–endodontal lesions

The nature of the problem

A periodontal pocket that communicates with an endodontic lesion is referred to as a combined periodontal–endodontal lesion. This may come about in three ways:

(1) periodontal breakdown with secondary pulpal involvement (Figure 24.13 C);
(2) pulpal necrosis with secondary periodontal involvement (Figure 24.13 A and B);
(3) co-existing periodontal and pulpal lesions that enlarge and then merge to become 'true' combined lesions (Figure 24.13 D).

The essential feature of these lesions is that of periapical infection following pulpal necrosis. This should always be treated first, although where a radiographically sound root filling is already in place, it is difficult to judge whether the endodontic component is significant and so necessitates a repeat of endodontic treatment. The resulting clinical dilemma is of some prognostic importance, for the primary apical endodontic lesion that tracks coronally and drains at the gingival margin so masquerading as a localized pocket (Figure 24.13 B), appears to have a more favourable outlook (as illustrated by the cases shown in Figure 24.14) than a plaque-induced periodontal pocket extending to the root apex would suggest.

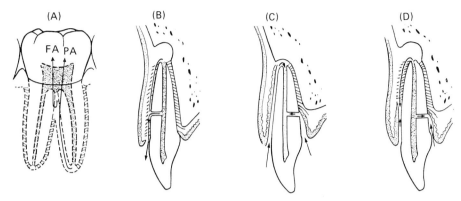

Figure 24.13 Combined periodontal–endodontal lesions possible paths of discharge. (A) Non-vital molar pulp with discharge stemming from furcation accessory canal (FA) or periapical (PA) lesion via periodontal ligament space. (B) Similar pattern possible from labial accessory canal or labial aspect of root when associated with developmental bony deficiency. (C) Vital pulp involved by buccal periodontal attachment loss extending to root apex or palatal accessory canal exposure resulting in pulpal necrosis. (D) Non-vital pulp inflammatory discharge coronally from periapical or palatal accessory canal lesions, communicating with co-existing progressive periodontal disease and establishing true combined lesion

The pathogenesis of combined lesions

In the first mechanism, a plaque-induced periodontal breakdown involves the pulp of a tooth by either exposing lateral or furcation accessory pulp canals or extending to the root apex (Figure 24.13 C) with the development of a retrograde pulpal infection and necrosis (see also Figure 18.11 L). In the second, the local periodontal tissue morphology, as for example that shown in Figure 24.13 (B), influences the path of inflammatory drainage from pulpal necrosis. The inflammatory exudate may stem from either the apical lesion itself, especially at molar teeth as shown in Figures 24.13 (A) and 24.14 (A), or an accessory canal, or from endodontic complications, such as instrumental root perforation and root fractures. Each leads to a coronally directed destruction of the periodontal attachment and presents ultimately as, and simulates, a localized plaque-induced periodontal pocket. Finally, true combined lesions result from the variable pattern of drainage of pulpal lesions communicating with the pocket bases of co-existing plaque-induced periodontal breakdown (Figure 24.13 D) as suggested by the case shown in Figure 24.14 (E).

The diagnostic implications

The presentation of an isolated extensive periodontal lesion at a heavily restored tooth with a suspect pulpal status, or a tooth with an existing root canal filling in an otherwise periodontally sound or only minimally diseased dentition, is likely to be of primarily endodontic origin (see Figure 24.14 A). Whereas, if similar periodontal pockets exist elsewhere in the mouth as shown in Figure 24.14 (E), the primary origins of the problem at a heavily restored tooth is less easily established. Thus, this might either be periodontal or endodontic in nature or indeed simply represent a true combined lesion. This is when diagnosis depends very much on the availability of previous detailed clinical records. In each of these instances, however, a primary endodontic component obviously can only be considered when the pulp is clearly non-vital as judged by routine clinical and radiographic findings, radiographic evidence of an inadequate root filling with radiolucencies either apically or in relation to an accessory canal, or alternatively an endodontic perforation or a root fracture. When, on the other hand, a satisfactorily root filled tooth with no associated radiolucencies is associated with a pocket extending to the root apex, this should be regarded and treated initially as a periodontal lesion as in Figure 18.10 (G).

The apparently true combined lesions at root furcations of endodontically treated molars pose a special diagnostic problem. This is because the radiographic and clinical presentation of any such suspected primarily endodontic lesion is no different from that of plaque-induced periodontal furcation involvement, whilst any accessory canal that might be incriminated can rarely be identified until it is actually filled by orthograde endodontic measures. As a rule of thumb, where the lesion is localized to a single unit, primary pulpal origin should be assumed

388

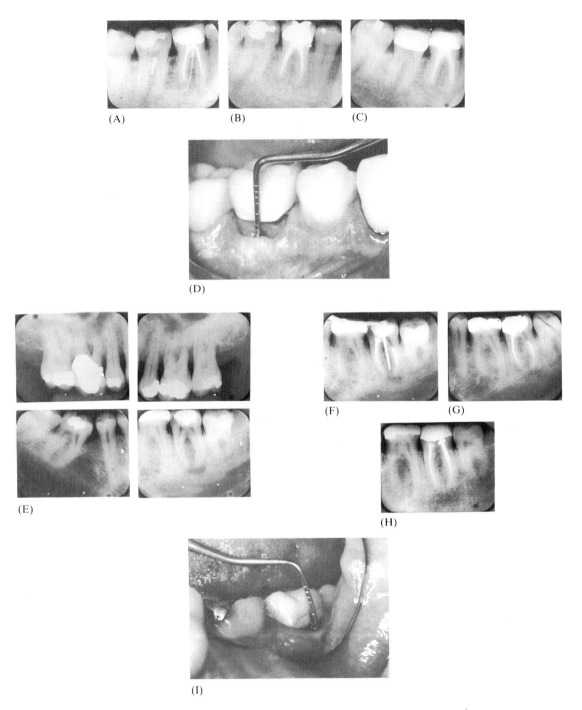

Figure 24.14 Combined periodontal–endodontal lesions. (A) Endodontically treated 46 associated with isolated buccal furcation pocket with gutta percha point inserted. Passes to distal root despite mesial radiolucency. Primary endodontic lesion diagnosed. Radiographic findings at (B) 6 months and (C) 4 years following endodontic treatment. (D) Minimal probing depth at 4 years. (E) Suspected true combined lesion at 37. Obvious apical endodontic lesion discharging via buccal furcation pocket space, but diagnostic dilemma in view of plaque-induced attachment loss with extensive furcation involvement at maxillary molars. Endodontic treatment carried out. Pocket persisted for (F) 6 months (probe in place) but then gradually reduced to 4 mm by (G) 18 months as the apical radiolucency resolved. (H) Radiographic and (I) clinical findings after 3 years. (Endodontics by courtesy Mr C. J. R. Stock)

and the appropriate endodontic therapy reinstituted in the first instance, whereas the finding of multiple periodontal furcation involvements at other molar teeth would suggest that the problem is rather more likely to be of primarily periodontal origin and should be treated as such. On the other hand, it should be realized that whatever the pathogenesis of the lesion, once optimal access for plaque control has been established (see Chapter 18), the then supragingival location of the furcation space itself means that any co-existing endodontal component is no longer of much clinical importance.

The practical implications

High levels of oral hygiene and careful subgingival root surface debridement are essential in all cases, but the outcome cannot be ensured until any suspected endodontic component has been satisfactorily treated. The appropriate endodontic measures should therefore always be instituted at the outset and the situation reassessed at intervals. In some instances the pocket heals spontaneously by, presumably, a combination of new attachment and a long junctional epithelium, for no such histological data are available. A clinical pocket closure was observed in the cases shown in Figure 24.14 (D and I). Where, however, no improvement occurs following repeated debridement over a period of 4–6 months, surgical reattachment as for any localized persistent pocket may be indicated.

The decision whether to attempt treatment at combined lesions of questionable origin, should be determined by the likely success of the endodontic component of this treatment, the coronal restorative requirements of both the tooth in question and the neighbouring teeth, and the predictability of periodontal therapy. Furthermore, the possibly detrimental effects of any periodontal surgical intervention itself and, in the event of failure, of the persistent periodontal lesion upon the neighbouring teeth must not be overlooked. These considerations should therefore be fully discussed with the patient and a practical solution evolved (see also Chapter 26). In many instances the extent and thus financial implications of combined therapy, coupled with its unpredictability is such that tooth extraction is elected as and when symptoms dictate. The facility to carry out root resection (*cf.* Chapter 18) at the outset instead, as shown in Figure 18.11 (L), or indeed after attempted, but abortive, therapy should not be discounted.

In conclusion, whilst the pathogenesis and differential diagnosis of combined lesions may be complicated, once diagnosed the clinical problem is essentially quite straightforward. That is, an endodontic lesion simply exists and is associated with an extensive periodontal pocket and, whilst the former is often amenable to therapy, the latter problem proves to be the ultimate barrier to success in many instances. (See also Chapter 30 – Accessory furcation canals and endodontic–periodontic lesions.)

Removable prostheses and the periodontium

Any understanding of the traditionally-held adverse effects of prostheses on the periodontal tissues demands a clear division between those effects attributable purely to the prosthesis itself, and that of any co-existing plaque-induced marginal disease. These are discussed below but the reader is referred elsewhere for details of the other potentially detrimental effects of prostheses with respect to caries, alveolar bony resorption and monilial mucosal lesions. The management of situations where removable prosthesis must be worn following pocket corrective surgery will also be dealt with. (See also Chapter 34 – Removable prostheses and the periodontium.)

Prostheses in gingival health

Well designed and constructed partial dentures will, in themselves, not compromise the integrity of either the marginal gingivae or the periodontal attachment. Similarly, when such prostheses are first fitted, the risk of an irreversible tissue damage occurring from traumatic marginal gingival ulceration associated with minor technical defects is invariably averted by prompt, professional attention being sought. Thus it is only when the patient perseveres despite the pain, that a traumatic loss of marginal tissue is sustained. The resulting gingival recession is then not unlike that following toothbrush trauma. Similar lesions developing on the attached gingiva could be followed by mucosal fenestration and then gingival recession as described, for example, in deep overbites (see Figure 21.12), although where the tissue is thicker an adaptive gingival hyperplasia is more likely. The above tissue reactions should therefore be regarded merely as adaptive changes to physical trauma and, provided that subsequent denture stability is ensured, no further damage should be expected. In summary, the provision of satisfactory partial dentures in the presence of periodontal health will not compromise dentogingival integrity.

Poorly designed, primarily tissue supported partial dentures, especially of the free-end saddle-type in the mandible, are, in contrast, liable to damage the supracrestal periodontal attachment. Thus, such dentures gradually become displaced down the lingual tooth and gingival surface inclines, physically detaching even healthy intact marginal gingivae ('gum stripping') and leading to progressive gingival recession. Mucosal fenestration might also occur under lingual bars at sites associated with developmental bony deficiencies. Any associated alveolar resorption under the denture saddles will aggravate the situation. This problem occurs much less frequently in the maxilla because of the inherently thicker palatal mucosa and the support of the palatal vault for the prosthesis.

Prostheses and the development of gingivitis

The initial gingival discomfort sometimes experienced when any partial denture is first fitted, might conceivably inhibit oral hygiene efforts and, in combination with inadequate denture hygiene, lead to the onset of a plaque-induced marginal gingivitis. The resulting gingival bleeding and tenderness with subsequent toothbrushing may then set up a vicious cycle, but this can be readily broken by early diagnosis and the institution of good oral hygiene.

It is not clear whether the physical presence of the denture itself induces a marginal tissue oedema (swelling) or will aggravate a pre-existing plaque-induced marginal inflammation. If so, the provision of a relief area between the denture base and the gingival margin would preclude any such traumatic effect, but this would soon be nullified by a plaque-induced inflammatory oedema (see Chapter 34 – Plaque-retentive potential). The role of plaque accumulation within the intrinsically porous nature of acrylic with its high level of water absorption, on the onset and perpetuation of marginal inflammation can, however, not be discounted. Although metal-based dentures appear to be less prone to this phenomenon, the finding of an oral monilia-induced denture-sore mouth in the palate, is generally attributed to microbial retention upon and within the micro-irregularities of the denture base fitting surface. A comparable effect might then reasonably be expected to also operate upon the marginal gingivae, making it difficult to differentiate between the possible causes of marginal inflammation associated with a prosthesis. Whatever these origins, it is also not clear whether any relationship exists between the keratinized gingival inflammatory reaction itself and that of plaque-induced intra-crevicular inflammation.

Finally, a hyperplastic marginal gingivitis, with or without a denture-sore mouth-type palatal mucosal hyperplasia, is sometimes observed in children wearing removable orthodontic appliances. Although the appliance itself might be incriminated where marginal gingival health has apparently existed prior to orthodontic therapy, the frequently indifferent oral hygiene levels in these individuals would not support this. This is, in turn, demonstrated by the finding of gingival inflammation at sites unrelated to the appliance and also of inadequate appliance hygiene because effective cleaning has possibly been avoided lest the appliance distorts or breaks. Indeed, it seems more likely that a previously undiagnosed existence of gingivitis will have only become apparent to the operator with the development of the more obvious clinical signs of disease associated with appliance therapy, and to which it is then erroneously attributed. This demands further investigation.

Prostheses in established disease

The incidence of plaque-induced marginal disease is such that the majority of individuals first fitted with partial dentures will not only be suffering from the disease, but some of the teeth being replaced will have been lost as a result of past disease. In addition, the variable and unpredictable clinical presentation of periodontal disease makes it difficult to isolate any potentially detrimental superimposed effects of a partial denture upon the tissues. Thus, in some cases, there might be no signs of disease yet, in others, combinations of marked gingival inflammatory hyperplasia and recession and extensive attachment loss and pocketing are observed. Finally, although the prosthesis might be expected to modify the clinical presentation of pre-existing disease, merely by its physical presence against already inflamed tissue and by its predisposition to greater plaque retention, its influence upon the pattern of attachment loss, is still not clear. These important issues will be examined further.

Increased gingival inflammation

This potential stems from a minor physical irritation from the newly fitted prosthesis inhibiting an already ineffective oral hygiene, greater plaque accummulation between the tissues and the prosthesis, and possibly microbial contamination of the prosthetic base material, each of which have been considered above.

Gingival hyperplasia

Although palatal hyperplasia is not uncommon in long-standing partial denture wearers it is by no means inevitable, for it does not seem to occur where marginal tissue health has been maintained. The possibility of a co-existing chronic monilial inflammatory hyperplasia has already been considered. The effect of marginal tissue proliferation (i.e. false pocketing) is to complicate plaque control and predispose to loss of attachment.

Gingival recession

Recession in partial denture wearers, might simply be a coincidental finding of co-existing chronic periodontal disease or result from physical displacement of detached tissues by poorly supported dentures. The latter effect is especially likely considering the facility with which inflamed gingival tissue may be physically displaced. Such dentures could, in addition, produce a gradual pressure necrosis of the marginal tissues and following a merger of the pocket lining and gingival epithelial surfaces, present as recession. Finally, frank perforation of pocket wall tissue may also be encountered as shown in Figure 21.5 (G) resulting ultimately in gingival recession.

Extensive periodontal attachment loss

While this finding at denture-bearing sites might suggest that the prosthesis is responsible, there are several other possible explanations. Firstly, lingual and palatal attachment levels are frequently worse than at the facial aspects. This is presumably because the former are rather less accessible to plaque control. Secondly, comparable attachment levels often exist at both denture and non-denture bearing sites, excluding any possible prosthetic influence. Indeed, in the former, the associated pocket depths might actually be shallower because of gingival recession and when it might even be argued that dentures are advantageous. Thirdly, the findings could be purely coincidental, simply reflecting the variable pattern of periodontal disease in the past. Each of these possibilities do, however, demand further investigation (*cf.* Chapter 34 – The potential for damage).

Denture design

Individuals requiring functional or aesthetic replacement of missing teeth frequently present with persistent periodontal disease despite treatment efforts. Indeed, the extractions leading to prosthetic replacement may have been one operator's solution to periodontal disease, or possibly the result of the patient's apparently questionable interest in dental health (see also Chapter 26). The possibility that the provision of partial dentures in these cases might lead to greater plaque retention and, in turn, aggravate the marginal lesion and so hasten the loss of the dentition presents quite a clinical dilemma.

Denture design is of some importance in that the greater the marginal gingival coverage the more likely is the plaque retention in those with poor oral hygiene. Cast metal skeleton-type, as opposed to acrylic, prostheses would therefore seem to be preferable, especially as the added benefits of tooth support are more readily incorporated. However, this type of denture is very much more expensive and is not readily modified to accommodate any changes in gingival contour or further tooth loss occurring during its expected lifespan. Accordingly, before constructing such prostheses some consideration should be given to the feasibility of optimal pocket reduction surgery as shown in Figures 16.22 and 16.23. In addition, prosthetic extraction of units with questionable prognosis should also be contemplated or, alternatively, the denture designed so that their subsequent loss can be accommodated. The denture could, on the other hand, be simply but expensively replaced as and when necessary.

The obvious alternative in any questionable situations is to fit instead acrylic-based dentures which can be readily and inexpensively modified as necessary. In practice, this option is frequently exercised, patient tolerance of such dentures being surprisingly good especially when some form of occlusal support and clasping is incorporated. However, the influence of progressive bone resorption at deteriorating dentate sites on the future prosthetic needs, must be weighed up against the patient's current prosthetic requirements with respect to aesthetics, comfort and function. Similarly, where progressive disease and total tooth loss is inevitable, the potentially detrimental effects of less than ideal dentures upon the edentulous bony ridges, with respect to future full dentures must not be overlooked. Unfortunately, little documented data exist upon which to base such assessments.

Restoration of edentulous spaces

The aforementioned dilemma does, in turn, revolve about the need to replace missing units. It does appear that aesthetic needs are paramount, for extensive studies in The Netherlands have revealed that the majority of the subjects actually removed partial dentures at meal times, although these were normally worn throughout the day. Furthermore, the few remaining natural anterior units constituted a functional dentition and replacement of posterior units was frequently not necessary for adequate function. Where, on the other hand, replacement is required and the long-term risks of partial dentures deemed unacceptable, the feasibility of overdentures instead or even a dental clearance and full dentures must be considered. This decision will depend on a combination of the individual patient's aesthetic and functional needs, existing and future restorative requirements and, not least, the economic implications. These issues are considered further in Chapter 26 and represent a steadily greater challenge to the profession with the ever-increasing proportion of ageing dentate patients in the community. (See also Chapter 34 – The risks of non-replacements.)

Fixed or removable prostheses

There would, in the interests of oral hygiene, seem to be some merit in providing partial dentures for less cooperative and disinterested patients and fixed bridgework for others. That is, in the former, plaque control could be maintained more readily because the prosthesis can be removed, although this advantage might be partially offset by the potential for increased plaque retention by the denture. It might, on the other hand, equally be argued that fixed prostheses would be preferable in these individuals, so as to limit the plaque-retentive potential to only those few teeth used as bridge abutments. This question too demands further investigation. The economic argument would, however, be against placing expensive fixed prostheses in people who show little inclination to care for their mouths. (See also Chapter 34 – Fixed various removable prostheses.)

Prosthetic management following pocket surgery

Care must be taken not to displace the sutured flaps, when a prosthesis is seated back into position following pocket surgery (see Chapter 16). Any mucosal blanching associated with insertion of the prosthesis signifies surgical oedema and the risk of impending ischaemic necrosis of the flap, and when the appliance is, preferably, not worn or worn as little as possible until the initial swelling has subsided. The presence of a dressing itself may create similar problems, so should be avoided unless positively required for flap apposition, to occlude large spaces between the denture fit surface and the post-surgical mucosal contour, or to aid retention of the denture. The pressure effect can be minimized by using a soft mix of Coe-pak. This is applied to the teeth as normal when a skeleton-type denture is involved (see Figure 16.14) and, elsewhere, to the denture base itself as if it were being relined, and then inserted immediately (Figure 16.21).

The denture-cum-dressing should be left in place until suture removal. When earlier removal of the denture is attempted the adherent dressing material not only distorts, complicating re-insertion, but also causes any incorporated sutures to be pulled out, possibly disturbing healing. Consequently where, as with an obturator, periodic removal of the prosthesis is necessary, the following options are available. In the first, the fit surface is generously coated with petroleum jelly, to minimize the chances of the Coe-pak sticking to it and the dressing applied to the teeth as usual. Once the material has hardened, the excess, which has squeezed out from around the appliance is scraped away, and the appliance carefully removed. Any material becoming displaced from the teeth in the process is patted back into place, the appliance again coated with petroleum jelly and re-seated and removed several times as necessary until quite free.

In the other option, petroleum jelly is first applied to the sutures and the necks of the teeth before seating the appliance, laden with Coe-pak, into position. The excess material and especially that being squeezed out from between the teeth is then carefully removed while the Coe-pak is still setting. Once set, the appliance is withdrawn and those remaining parts of the still pliable material that had extended interproximally or into undercuts and so have become distorted, trimmed away with a scalpel from the (in effect) relined prosthesis. Any other partially displaced or distorted material on the edges of the fit surface is first patted back into place, coated with petroleum jelly and the appliance then reseated and removed as described above.

The sutures and dressing are best removed after about 4–5 days, for this appears to reduce post-surgical discomfort. A further dressing/relining of Coe-pak is applied as and when necessary for retention and patient comfort. The denture can, in fact, be relined repeatedly in this way during postoperative healing and tissue maturation period, pending the provision of either a more permanent relining or a replacement prosthesis. The latter should however preferably be delayed for at least a couple of months.

25

Acute periodontal problems

The problem
Pain on toothbrushing
Pain on interdental cleaning

Pain on chewing
Painful gums
Wisdom tooth pain — third molar problems

The problem

Plaque-induced periodontal disease is a typical example of chronic inflammation which is characterized by sites of tissue breakdown occurring alongside those of repair. The destructive phases apparently occur only at fairly infrequent intervals and then only for short duration bursts. It is only at these active times, when the inflammatory reaction may become heightened (acute inflammation), that any discomfort or pain is likely to be experienced. Consequently, the disease is generally free of distressful symptoms.

The differential diagnosis of pain arising from periodontal disease seldom presents much difficulty. The various possible causes are considered here, not as individual entities but in terms of their typical presenting complaints, although it must be appreciated that the subjective perception of pain is such that great variation should be expected to occur between patients experiencing similar conditions. Moreover, complaints of painful gums often prove to be related to the teeth instead.

Pain on toothbrushing

Gingival trauma and inflammation

This can occur both in disease and in gingival health. In disease, pain or at least discomfort is to be expected during any toothbrushing that makes contact with the more vulnerable inflamed marginal gingivae. This is widely attributed by patients to naturally tender gums and so is not often complained of. However, this complaint should be anticipated as a result of the initially more enthusiastic and effective brushing following oral hygiene instruction, and the patient should be forewarned. It may also occur subsequently when conscientious brushing has not been maintained but is recommended just before periodontal review appointments! The symptoms tend not to persist after brushing and are invariably associated with bleeding from within the gingival crevices, which resolves any diagnostic difficulties. In some instances a residual gingival tenderness may also be complained of. The clinical presentation of a plaque-induced marginal inflammation with superimposed gingival abrasions which are very sensitive to gentle probing and which may cause bleeding is diagnostic of toothbrush trauma. These lesions may, however, often also present as gingival ulceration making the diagnosis more difficult (see also below).

In gingival health the pain on brushing is most frequently due simply to toothbrush trauma. Thus, scratches or abrasions on the gingival margins and attached gingiva may be encountered (see Figure 8.7 A). The frequently resulting ulcer (i.e. a mucosal breach with an inflammatory or necrotic tissue bed) is by far the commonest cause of gingival ulceration. (It is worth noting that apthous-type ulcers which, in turn, represent the commonest type of oral ulcer do not occur on keratinized tissue – see also 'Painful Gums'.) These ulcers are very painful to the touch and may bleed on probing (the bleeding in these instances occurring from lesions on the surface of the gingiva rather than from within the gingival crevice as above) and tend to sting in response to acidic dietary constituents. The ulcer itself is readily identified by its uneven reddish-grey surface appearance and the irregularly reddened periphery.

The use of a new toothbrush, an over-enthusiastic technique or accidental damage from the brush-head are most commonly responsible for these traumatic gingival lesions. An intentional brushing (or even massaging) of the gingivae with the toothbrush, due to misunderstanding, is sometimes at fault. The presence of cervical tooth surface abrasion and areas of localized gingival recession (see Figure 8.7 A) so commonly attributable to over-vigorous toothbrushing, corroborate the diagnosis. Careless or excessively forceful use of toothpicks, dental floss and interproximal brushes will, as might be expected, also cause gingival ulceration (see Figure 8.8 B and C). These lesions are, however, easily diagnosed for their outlines conform closely to the contact areas with the causative device (see also 'Pain on interdental cleaning').

Finally, existing plaque-induced inflammatory gingival tenderness will be increased when the tissues have been traumatized during professional cleaning. Gingival abrasions can be produced by rotating polishing brushes in particular and the over-enthusiastic use of hand instruments, whilst ultrasonic tips may burn the adjacent marginal tissues. The complaint of such symptoms following treatment is, in part, an indictment of operator technique and reassessment of instrumentation methods may be indicated.

Traumatic gingival ulcers heal uneventfully over a period of 7–10 days. Symptomatic relief may be provided by the use of antiseptic (e.g. chlorhexidine) mouth rinses or the application of proprietary antiseptic topical anaesthetic gels or occlusive type protective ointments. The choice of medicament appears to be fairly subjective. (*cf.* Chapter 21 – Influence of deep overbites on disease – management of the problem.)

Dentinal sensitivity

Pain experienced on cleaning, whether by brush, toothpick or floss, is often due to dentinal hypersensitivity, but misinterpreted by the patient as being of gingival origin. The finding of gingival recession and exposed root surfaces or coronal surface abrasion is highly suggestive of sensitive dentine. Confirmation is by the comparable pain produced by stimulating these tooth surfaces by probing or extremes of temperature. Symptoms of dentinal sensitivity tend to be periodic in nature and are frequently related to dietary acidic fruits and drinks (*cf.* Chapters 8, 10, 24 and 25).

The presence of patent dental tubules seems to be important in hypersensitivity; these are thought to allow penetration of bacterial plaque products to either irritate the pulp or reduce pain thresholds to other stimuli. The exposure of accessory canals in furcations or other lateral pulp canals, in instances of more extensive periodontal breakdown, will initially also evoke a comparable dentinal hypersensitivity. A retrograde pulpitis developing via a periodontally involved root apex may also present in this way. Diagnosis of accessory canals is extremely difficult, especially when the teeth are heavily restored, and depends on a process of elimination (*cf.* Chapters 18 and 30 – Accessory furcation canals and endodontic–periodontic lesions).

Dentinal hypersensitivity uncomplicated by pulpal infection, is well controlled by the use of both standard fluoride and specific desensitizing dentifrices, fluoride mouth rinses and the professional application of fluoride preparations. Acidic dietary constituents should also be avoided and any gastric regurgitation countered. Where symptoms do persist they may be followed by pulpal inflammation and pulp extirpation may be unavoidable, although, in practice, this rarely proves to be necessary.

Pain on interdental cleaning

Pain may also be experienced from minor abrasions caused by the over-enthusiastic use of interdental cleaning devices at healthy sites, or merely their physical contact with inflamed interdental tissue. Interdental root surface sensitivity is often misinterpreted as gingival pain. Limited visibility can sometimes make it difficult to distinguish between minor traumatic ulceration and plaque-induced tissue inflammation. However, where pain persists and intensifies over a period of a day or so, is accompanied by gingival 'itchiness' plus free or even spontaneous bleeding, an unpleasant metallic taste and halitosis, then an acute necrotizing gingivitis is diagnosed. This condition is considered further below.

Pain on chewing

Pain can be caused by the mere physical presence of food at inflamed tissue sites, its impaction by an opposing tooth against the gingiva or into open interdental contacts. Pain can be elicited by simply chewing food or by occlusal contacts, be they functional or parafunctional.

Gingival pain

Pain is inevitable when hard crusty foods, apples, etc. come into contact with or, more so, become impacted against plaque-induced inflamed or traumatically ulcerated gingiva, and so is readily diagnosed. The tissues in deep incisal overbites (*cf.* Chapter 21) and that overlying an erupting or impacted third molar (see below – Wisdom tooth pain) are especially vulnerable in this respect. The latter too is readily diagnosed (pericoronitis) and represents a combination of a plaque-induced marginal gingivitis and pericoronal folliculitis which, as in deep overbites, is then complicated by a secondary direct trauma to the swollen tissues from the opposing tooth. The direct tooth to soft tissue contact is the major cause of pain experienced, for relief follows directly when the offending opposing cusps are trimmed or the tooth itself is removed. The periodontal implications of third molars are considered later in this chapter.

When impaction of food into open contact points causes pain, this is unlikely to be due to the food impaction between the teeth itself, rather its effect upon a pre-existing interdental tissue inflammation as described above. Similarly, where the initial physical separation of the teeth is tolerated by the patient and the impacted food not removed, the onset of symptoms subsequently can be attributed to the effects of the co-existing long-standing retained bacterial plaque.

A dull nagging pain in the gums about upper molar teeth aggravated by chewing and thermal changes and associated with buccal and palatal mucosal tenderness over the root apices, but with no obvious dental or periodontal abnormalities, is suggestive of maxillary sinusitis. Further confirmatory clinical tests are indicated.

Tooth contact pain

Pain produced on biting, or pressing against a tooth as during cleaning, may be of either periodontal or pulpal origin. Establishment of pulp status is therefore critical to diagnosis. Periodontal type pain is most commonly due to an inflammatory exacerbation within a related pocket. A recently inserted high restoration, a history of extrinsic trauma or the presence of a fractured tooth may also be responsible. The tooth may become increasingly tender to touch (periostitic), appear 'high' to the bite (suggestive of tooth extrusion and premature contact with the opposing teeth) and feel loose. This may be followed by a more persistent gingival pain and swelling. Finally where, in addition, radiographic findings reveal extensive loss of supporting bone even at a single aspect of the tooth and the pulp is vital, diagnosis of a lateral periodontal abscess is most likely. This should also be assumed where pulp vitality test responses are equivocal so that the complaint is initially treated as being of periodontal origin.

When, on the other hand, the pulp is clearly non-vital, with or without radiographic findings of any apical change or of any root filling in place, differential diagnosis can be more difficult for both apical endodontic and lateral periodontal lesions

might then exist. In addition, the possibility of a primarily causative fractured root cannot be excluded (see below). The gingiva and adjacent alveolar mucosa may be swollen and exquisitely tender. Pus might discharge from the associated pocket or from a sinus at the centre of the mucosal swelling. Facial swelling and lymphadenopathy may also be evident. Insertion of a gutta percha endodontic point into the pocket, or any inflammatory sinus track present, is often helpful in distinguishing between periodontal and endodontic lesions when examined radiographically. Similarly, opening the pulp chamber of a non-root-filled tooth or the removal of an obviously defective root filling, which results in pus discharge and an immediate feeling of relief, is indicative of an apical abscess irrespective of any associated periodontal lesion. Surgical drainage of a periapical abscess may also be achieved by incising the mucosal swelling, but need not be considered further here. Extraction is often indicated (*cf.* Chapter 26), but there may be a possibility of dealing with both the endodontic and then the periodontal components (*cf.* Chapter 24).

Management

A periodontal abscess is drained via the pocket following root surface debridement, by a surgical incision of the pocket wall or by the excision of the pocket wall itself. The methods available depend on the severity and extent of the inflammation which will limit the possibility of effective local anaesthetic.

Where local infiltrations or mandibular block anaesthesia is contra-indicated, the swelling is anaesthetized directly by inserting the needle tangentially and only very superficially into its most prominent point. The smallest amount of solution causing mucosal blanching is injected, and Swann Morton No. 15 blade then thrust vertically into the swelling to release the pus (Figure 25.1 A–C). When, however, complete anaesthesia can be achieved a simultaneous surgical drainage and pocket reduction should be considered. Thus, an inverse bevel incision to conserve tissue is made at the abscess site (Figure 25.1 D–L) or, where located interdentally, facial and oral papillectomy type incisions are made instead. The cervical wedge tissue incorporates the acutely inflamed tissue which is removed following minimal flap reflection. The root surfaces are then carefully instrumented and the flap loosely sutured.

Palliative occlusal adjustment to relieve pressure on the tooth is often indicated. Where difficulty in anaesthesia exists, the very tender mobile tooth is carefully supported with the fingers or with suitably adapted impression compound to avoid causing further pain by tooth displacement during grinding. Hot saline mouth rinses are prescribed, together

396

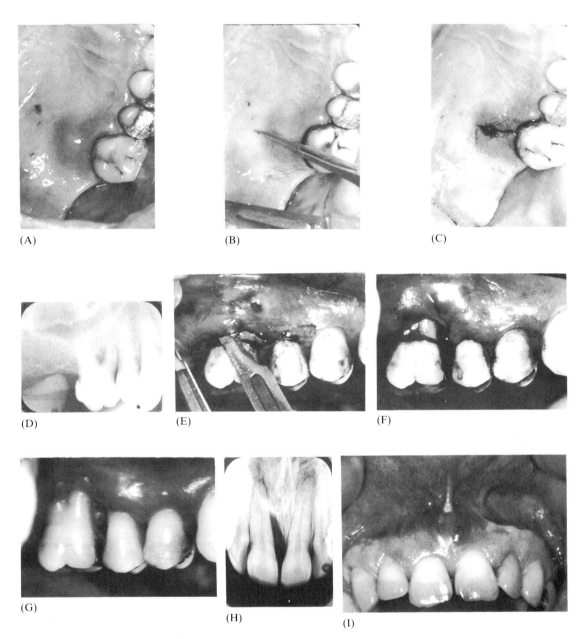

(A)

(B)

(C)

(D)

(E)

(F)

(G)

(H)

(I)

Figure 25.1 (A) Lateral periodontal abscess at localized palatal pocket on vital tooth. (B) Surgical drainage by vertical incision with No. 15 blade (C) extending to gingival margin. (D) Radiograph periodontal abscess involving mesial and buccal furcations of first molar. (E) Inverse bevel incision (F) Flap loosely sutured on completion of surgical drainage and root debridement. (G) Healing at 6 weeks. (H) Radiograph of extensive localized mesial pocket at 11 at vital tooth – apical thickening result of associated increased mobility. (I) Labial swelling from acute abscess on presentation.

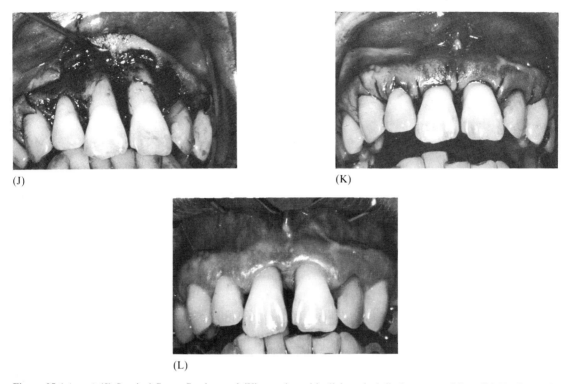

(J)

(K)

(L)

Figure 25.1 (*cont.*) (J) Surgical flap reflection and (K) suturing with slight apical displacement of flap. (L) Healing at 6 months – note tissue recession

with appropriate antibiotics where necessary. Upon resolution of the acute phase, any endodontic treatment is completed in conjunction with routine periodontal therapy.

In the absence of pocketing, pain at a non-vital tooth with or without any mucosal tenderness or swelling and which is non-root-filled or poorly filled and has an obvious apical radiolucency, is readily diagnosed as an apical lesion and need not be considered here. Where, however, the periapical zone appears normal on a radiograph of an adequately root-filled heavily restored tooth, the possible existence of a root fracture or root perforation should be suspected. This will be supported by the localized nature of the tooth tenderness and mobility and the radiographic findings of a wider periodontal ligament space (Figure 25.2 A). In addition, movement might be detected between the margin of the restoration and the root surface within the gingival sulcus at the fracture site. The situation is, however, not always so clear cut, because longer-standing root fractures

may often masquerade as a localized periodontal pocket and, as such, present as combined periodontal–endodontic lesion. Root fractures at obviously periodontally involved teeth can also be very difficult to diagnose, because the signs and symptoms are so similar. Indeed it is often only by reflecting a gingival flap and inspecting the root *in situ*, that the fracture can be detected. In some instances the offending root section can simply be removed (see also Chapter 24), but extraction of the tooth is frequently necessary.

Finally, exquisite pulpal type pain that lingers for some minutes after being initiated by tooth-to-tooth contact, in the presence of a normal periodontal support or apparently asymptomatic pocketing, at a tooth with no caries or defective restoration or cervical root surface exposure, is highly suggestive of a cracked tooth involving the pulp chamber. Although the periodontal ligament is inevitably traumatized during forced displacement of the fractured lesser component, the major and overriding source of pain is pulpal irritation.

398

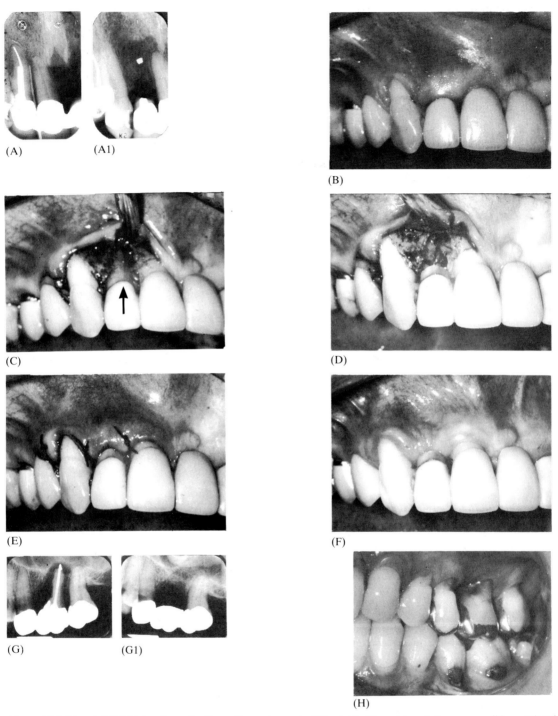

Figure 25.2 (A and A1) Initial and post-healing radiographs – note GP point in 12 mesial pocket space, possibly associated with root fracture. Tooth is an abutment to a bridge which the patient is anxious to retain. (B) Initial presentation with buccal swelling. (C) Surgical flap revealed (arrowed) vertical fracture line. (D) Root sectioned and removed in stages (*cf.* Figure 18.8) to preserve bony support. Small segment of metal post had become displaced and lodged in apical part of extraction socket – noted on post-healing radiograph (A1). (E) Flap sutured. Note unavoidable flap displacement at 11. (F) Healing at 15 months. (G) Radiograph of combined lesion and (G1) 9-month post-resection healing 26. (H) Patient presented with acute abscess (I).

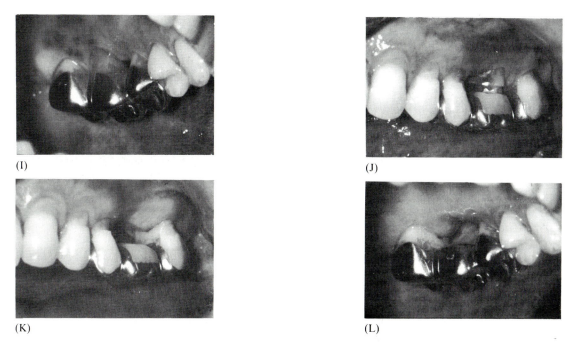

(I) (J)

(K) (L)

Figure 25.2 (*cont.*) (I) Abscess pointing palatally. Mesiobuccal root had been resected and 25, 26, 27 splinted 1 year previously. (J) Remaining fused roots sectioned from crown as shown; then small buccal flap reflected to facilitate removal. (K and L) Buccal and palatal views of healing at 9 months

Painful gums

The patient's complaint of painful ulceration between the teeth causing cratering between the related papillae, is consistent with a diagnosis of acute necrotizing gingivitis (ANG). This may involve only a few interdental sites or be more widespread (Figure 25.3 A–C). The ulcer base is formed by a greyish slough with a well delineated reddened margin, and bleeds readily when touched or even spontaneously, leading to the formation of blood clots about the teeth. The ulcers might enlarge over the interdental papillae and extend along the adjoining gingival margins as shown in Figure 25.3 (D) destroying the gingival form and producing a flattened or even a reverse scalloped gingival contour. Lymphadenitis is a fairly consistent finding, whilst with the more flamboyant form, fever and malaise will often be present. The acute phase usually subsides spontaneously but recurrent bouts may occur, or more rarely a low grade condition persist.

The condition, also variously called 'acute ulcerative gingivitis', 'Vincent's gingivitis' and 'trench mouth' to name a few, is not commonly encountered nowadays so need not be considered in any length here (*cf.* Chapter 4). It does appear to be predisposed to by a plaque-induced marginal disease, smoking and emotional stress and, more recently, HIV infection. The distinctive clinical features allow it to be diagnosed readily and it is amenable to routine periodontal treatment. The acute phase responds rapidly to metronidazole 200 mg thrice daily for 3 days. The traditional emphasis on surgical correction of the altered gingival form *per se* is not often warranted (Figure 25.3 D–F) (see also Chapter 31 – The treatment of intrabony defects – physiological form), although any underlying periodontal defects are treated on their individual merits.

The sudden onset of gingival pain preceded by a sore throat, marked regional lymphadenopathy and fever are fairly classic features of an acute herpetic gingivostomatitis (AHG). Indiscriminate and irregularly distributed painful ulceration of both gingivae and oral mucosa occurs. The gingivae become very inflamed overall, warranting the description of a pangingivitis (Figure 25.3 G). Gingival bleeding is uncommon but will occur should ANG supervene, presenting some diagnostic confusion (Figure 25.3 I). However, the finding of oral mucosal ulceration, the pattern of the gingival ulceration and the pangingivitis in AHG, are sufficiently distinctive for differential diagnostic purposes (Figure 25.3 I and

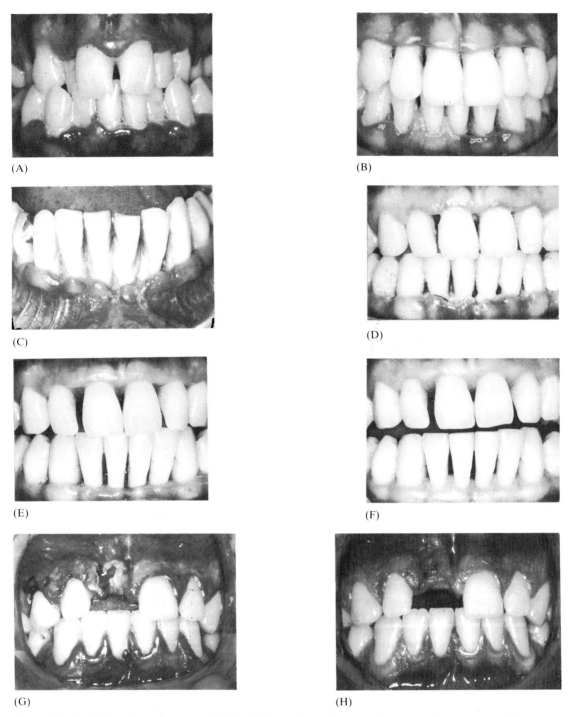

Figure 25.3 (A–F) Variable presentation of ANG. (A) Isolated interdental papillary ulceration extending slightly over adjacent margins. Superimposed upon chronic gingivitis in teenager. (B) Recurrent subacute bouts sustained in maxilla but at only localized sites in mandible with loss of scalloped gingival form. (C) Similar but more extensive destruction at mandibular anterior units associated with chronic periodontal breakdown (same case as in Figure 9.1 O). (D) Recurrent acute episode. (E) Tissue response to plaque control and root surface debridement alone at 6 weeks and (F) 6 months. Note tissue remodelling. (G) AHG in 24-year-old man – pangingivitis and gingival ulceration especially under prosthesis. (H) Ulceration healed at 1 week.

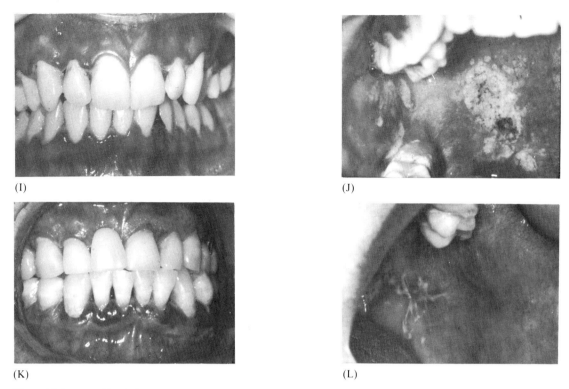

(I)   (J)

(K)   (L)

Figure 25.3 (*cont.*) (I) ANG superimposed upon AHG in 28-year-old man. Note bleeding associated with papillary ulceration and (J) extensive ulceration of soft palate and buccal mucosa. (K) Erosive lichen planus masquerades as plaque-induced lesion. Note (L) buccal mucosal striations

J). Furthermore AHG is most commonly encountered in children whilst ANG has a predeliction for older age groups, although as illustrated here, AHG should not be discounted in adulthood. The condition is self-limiting within 10–14 days (see Figure 25.3 H), but symptomatic relief is provided by a tetracycline mouthwash four times daily. The contents of a single 250-mg capsule are dissolved in a dessertspoon of warm water, rinsed for 1 min. and then swallowed. This is best avoided in children because of the risk of staining during tooth calcification. A chlorhexidine mouthwash is also helpful, as in all such conditions, to compensate for the patient's inability to clean.

Gingival 'rawness' in adults, suggestive of toothbrush trauma and persistent inflammation despite careful cleaning, is most commonly due to erosive lichen planus (Figure 25.3 K). The characteristic mucosal striations of the condition may be noted on adjacent gingivae and on the buccal mucosa (Figure 25.3 L). There are several other conditions (including drug reactions), some locally acting but the majority manifestations of systemic disorders that might also be encountered, albeit rarely, and these should not be ruled out. The reader is referred to oral medicine texts for further details.

Wisdom tooth pain – third molar problems

The periodontal problems involving third molars occur mainly in the mandible. These problems concern, first and foremost, the difficulties of disease control at the erupted functional tooth and, even more so at any impacted tooth and the related distal aspect of the second molar; secondly, pericoronitis and its potential influence on the distal periodontal attachment of the second molar; thirdly, the influence of impacted teeth on periodontal surgical pocket elimination at the adjacent second molar; lastly, the effects of the surgical removal of impacted teeth on the distal periodontal support of the second molar. (See also Chapter 31 – Third molar post-extraction healing.)

Disease control

The local tissue anatomy at the back of both arches impedes plaque control and precludes surgical pocket elimination at third molar teeth (*cf.* Chapters 20 and 21). The associated difficulties of disease control at the interproximal sites between the third and second molars might then in turn compromise the distal periodontal support of the second molar. Extraction of third molars might therefore be preferable in all such instances, although where for any reason a poor prognosis already exists at the second molar, its retention as a potential distal abutment is indicated instead.

Plaque control is virtually impossible between the partially erupted impacted third molar tooth (Figure 25.4 C1) and its associated second molar so that the existence of some disease is inevitable. It is, however, not clear whether the impaction site itself on the distal aspect of the second molar is more susceptible to attachment loss in established disease as shown in Figure 25.4 (C, C1 and C2). Thus, the pathogenesis of plaque-induced disease might be influenced by the lack of periodontal supporting bone at the site, coupled with the possibly damaging effect of the crown of the impacting tooth upon the second molar distal support. The former thesis would not be supported by the fact that broadly comparable situations of an absence of bone at developmental bony dehiscences, are no more vulnerable to plaque-induced periodontal destruction than elsewhere (*cf.* Chapter 31 – The nature of bony defects). The latter possibility might be significant with respect to the occasional finding of root resorption at the second molar and the finding that the essential prerequisite for root resorption elsewhere is that of necrosis of the periodontal ligament (see Chapter 31 – The role of bone in new attachment).

On the other hand, a localized attachment loss at the distal aspect of second molars is not an uncommon finding following the removal of impacted third molars (Figure 25.4 B1 and C3 and 25.5 H). Furthermore, these losses are often greater than

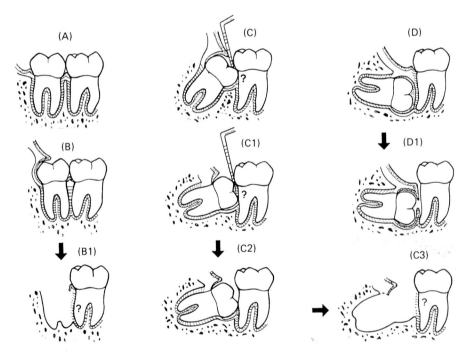

Figure 25.4 Lower third molar problems. (A) Normally positioned tooth with ideal interproximal relationship to second molar. (B) Disto-angular impaction with close root apposition and no interproximal bone. (C) High mesio-angular and (C1) near horizontal impactions related to supracrestal attachment at second molar. (D) Horizontal impaction not communicating with oral cavity and associated with intact second molar distal attachment. Note potential for pericoronitis at (C) and (D) with secondary damage to second molar distal periodontal ligament resulting in attachment loss. Close contact at impaction site precludes assessment by probing of any secondary attachment loss as at (C and C1), as well as the possibility of a primary plaque-induced attachment loss at second molar leading to pericoronitis and combined pericoronal–periodontal pocket as at (C2 and D1). Removal of third molar (B1 and C3) exposes second molar distal root surface periodontal ligament with risk (?) of necrosis and attachment loss in event of post-extraction healing complications. Note problem of establishing both pre- and post-extraction probing attachment levels at second molar distal aspect

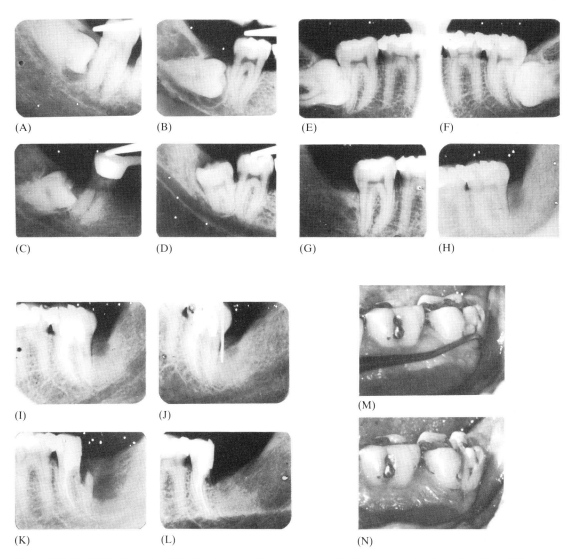

Figure 25.5 (A–D) Radiographs of third molar impactions associated with clinical signs of pericoronitis. (A and B) Horizontal impactions (A) with possible and (B) without distal attachment loss at second molars. (C) Mesio-angular impaction with extensive distal pocket. (D) Disto-angular impaction with possible distal pocket. (E and F) Pre-extraction views of horizontal impactions with pericoronitis plus possible distal attachment loss. At 6 months (G) optimal healing but (H) extensive pocket apparent at second molar as a complication of, or its pre-existence merely confirmed by, extraction. (I–L) Radiographic sequence of management of second molar pocket, shown at (H): (I) endodontic therapy and occlusion of entire access cavity with amalgam. (J) Probing depth (K) coronal hemisection avoiding damage to furcation prior to removal of distal root segment (L) healing at 1 year when residual coronal spicule trimmed down. (M–R) Clinical sequence of hemisection technique: (M) Probing depth. (N) Tooth hemisection cut avoiding furcation.

those occurring elsewhere in the mouth, suggesting a greater predisposition to plaque-induced periodontal destruction at these sites. There is, however, another explanation which is that attachment loss has been sustained as a result of extraction itself, and as such, represents a post-surgical complication (see below). This is, however, not readily assessed because of the difficulties of establishing, by clinical probing (Figure 25.4 C and C1) or radiographically, the attachment levels at the second molar while the impacted tooth is still present, and even following its removal (Figure 25.4 B1 and C3). The comparable difficulty of assessing attachment levels at closely approximated roots within periodontally involved molar furcations has already been cited (Chapter 18).

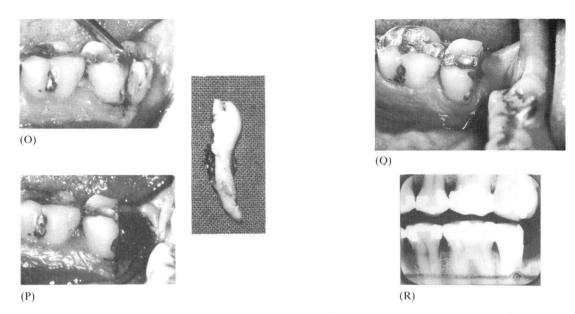

(O)

(P)

(Q)

(R)

Figure 25.5 (*cont.*) (O) Distal part fractured away with elevator and (P) crown and root components removed separately – shown on right. (Q) Healing at 1 year. Existing amalgam restoration still satisfactory and remained so, as shown on (R) bitewing radiograph at 10 years

Pericoronitis

This occurs most commonly during normal tooth eruption, but is of greater clinical relevance when occurring at erupted third molars associated with vestibular mucosal tissue impaction and, more especially, impacted teeth (Figure 25.4 B and C). The condition develops from plaque accumulation within the pericoronal follicular remnants and/or from physical trauma from the opposing tooth; each may operate as an exciting or an aggravating factor or sometimes even together. The pericoronal tissue about any partially erupted tooth does in practical terms represent a pericoronal pocket within which periodic acute inflammatory exacerbations are to be expected.

Recurrent pericoronal lesions might compromise the distal periodontal support of the second molar in two ways. Firstly, by discouraging local plaque control measures and so predispose to loss of attachment as elsewhere. The other involves tissue destruction during episodes of pericoronitis of not only the perifollicular tissue, but also the adjacent periodontal ligament of the second molar as depicted in Figure 25.4 (C1 and C2). This particular mechanism of periodontal destruction cannot be readily substantiated, and the extent of this tissue damage would depend primarily on the nature of the impaction. It is, however, equally possible that the opposite situation of a progressive destruction of the pericoronal tissues stems from a primary plaque-induced loss of attachment at the second molar instead, as shown in Figure 25.4 (D1). The practical difficulties of clinical probing and of radiographic interpretation complicates the diagnostic differentiation between each possibility.

Surgical pocket elimination

The position of the impacted third molar tooth frequently thwarts effective pocket surgery at the distal aspect of the second molar as is evident from Figure 25.4 (C and D). It is only at the deepest horizontal impaction that normal distal periodontal tissue morphology might exist. Even then, surgical flap preparation and adaptation will inevitably involve the third molar perifollicular tissue. Furthermore, any resulting communication between the pocket base and the pericoronal space will predispose to pericoronal infections. Pockets extending in between the impacting surfaces can obviously not be eliminated nor the root surface debrided; although surgical reduction of the pocket space, if not the entire perifollicular space, may still be possible coronal to the impaction site.

In summary, pocket correction at the distal aspect of second molars, in the presence of asymptomatic totally embedded impacted third molars as at Figure 25.4 (D) is best avoided, for this will not only fail to achieve its objective but may also even establish a communication between the oral cavity and the hitherto uninfected pericoronal space and, in turn, predispose to pericoronitis and its sequelae. Where, however, symptoms of pericoronitis and/or periodontitis as at Figure 25.4 (C2 and D1) demand surgical intervention, the difficulties of pocket elimination dictate that the removal of one or other tooth is preferable. This decision should depend primarily on the prognosis of the second molar and the clinical problems associated with surgical removal of the impacted tooth. For example, where an extensive distal attachment loss already exists or could follow a complicated surgical extraction (see below), extraction of the second molar should be considered, although hemisection of the tooth and removal of only the distal component is sometimes feasible, as shown in Figure 25.5 (I–R). In either event, the impacted tooth might then also be extracted via the improved access, or more simply, retained and kept under observation. Each situation must be considered individually (see Figure 25.5 A–D).

Effects of surgical extraction

Significant attachment loss on the distal surface of the second molar (Figure 25.4 B1 and C3 and Figure 25.5 H) may be observed following surgical removal of impacted third molars (see Chapter 31). There are several possible reasons for this, but periodontal ligament necrosis would seem to be the essential prerequisite to epithelial downgrowth. This might simply be the result of physical trauma sustained by the periodontal ligament during surgical operation, post-surgical ischaemia following surgical interference of the related mucoperiosteum and bone, or delayed healing associated with post-extraction infection ('dry socket'). On the other hand, as stated above, the removal of the impacted tooth might merely have allowed recognition of a pre-existing and previously undiagnosed loss of attachment.

In conclusion, the optimal method of handling impacting and impacted third molars demands further examination in well designed clinical research studies but, until then, any potential problems are best circumvented by early diagnosis and removal of impacting third molars to minimize the risk of post-extraction complications. The asymptomatic deeply impacted third molar is best retained, lest the inevitably greater surgical extraction trauma damages the support of the second molar. Optimal plaque control at such second molars is also critical to obviate the insurmountable complications following involvement of the impacted tooth in periodontal breakdown.

26

Prognosis

The problem

Current knowledge dictates that disease can be prevented at the outset by a high standard of plaque control. Similarly in established disease, further loss of attachment can be checked, where the patient is willing and able to clean effectively. While it follows that periodontal health is dependent upon patient cooperation and cleansability of the dento-epithelial junction, the essentially comparable mean data of the outcomes of both surgical and non-surgical periodontal therapy (see Chapter 29 – Evaluation of modified Widman flap type technique) suggest that, in many instances, optimal dentogingival morphology might not be critical to checking attachment losses. Furthermore, where disease has been arrested following surgical pocket elimination therapy the favourable outcome might not necessarily have been due to surgical therapy itself. That is, disease might have been arrested prior to surgery, having been the result of effective root surface debridement carried in preparation for pocket surgery or having been due simply to the patient's greater oral hygiene efforts stemming from the surgical experience itself. Finally, the possibility of a spontaneous remission phase in disease activity, unrelated to therapy, cannot be discounted. Each of these possibilities demands further, and more carefully controlled, investigation.

It is apparent from clinical experience and limited reported data (see Chapter 29 – Evaluation of different surgical methods), that in a very small number of instances, despite rigid adherence to oral hygiene and optimal surgical results, further inexorable loss of attachment ensues. It is at present not possible to identify these susceptible individuals prospectively or the particular sites likely to be affected by this inexplicable deterioration. The management of these cases constitutes a major challenge and obviously requires much further investigation. In contrast, instances where the prerequisites for periodontal health are not satisfied persistent disease is to be expected. This therapeutic failure may be due on the one hand, to the patient failing to clean properly despite an amenable dentogingival morphology, or on the other, the surgical objectives being thwarted by the pattern of periodontal breakdown and root morphology.

The persistent marginal inflammation resulting from the patient's shortcomings will, in many instances, be accompanied by insignificant attachment losses that do not appear to threaten the dentition and so not constitute a therapeutic problem. Where, however, appreciable degrees of attachment loss have been sustained and further losses are likely, periodic professional cleaning, with or without a surgical component, may compensate adequately for the shortcomings in supragingival plaque control. However, where in these cases and where optimal surgical results have not been possible and periodic effective subgingival debridement is precluded, the sites must be regarded as being untreatable in the strictest sense of the word. This is not to say that tooth loss is inevitable or that extraction is indicated, rather that it has to be accepted that ideal treatment objectives cannot be achieved.

The practical implications of the, fortunately, unusual situations of unexpected loss of attachment and the not uncommon finding of possibly untreatable units in clinical practice must be examined further. In addition, the management of the

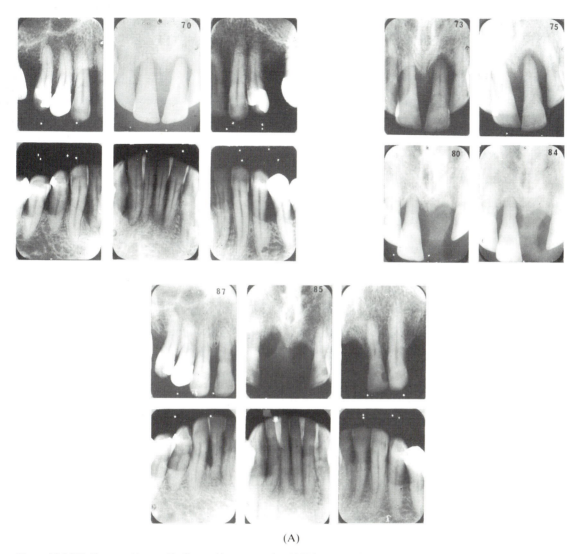

(A)

Figure 26.1 (A) 48-year-old man. Radiographic presentation 1970 (see also Figure 19.4 C and 23.1 J). Progressive attachment loss expected at 11, 21 but exfoliation 21 and 11 occurred 1975 and 1985 (see below) respectively. Note 1987 status and loss of 24 following pulpitis.

apparently uncooperative patient who fails to clean effectively despite repeated advice and regular attendance, and the seemingly disinterested individual who only attends for symptomatic treatment will also be considered.

Inexplicable deterioration

Research workers in Gothenburg (see Chapter 29) have observed further attachment losses in a small number of sites in a small proportion of a group of patients treated and then maintained by a careful regime over a 14-year period. The patients were selected for this longitudinal investigation because of their willingness to maintain high standards of plaque control and to undergo therapy which created totally cleansable dentogingival morphology. This included multiple extractions, root resections and coronal reconstructions followed by regular maintenance care (see Chapters 30 – The efficacy of therapy and 34 – The dilemma of tooth replacement). It was concluded that periodontal disease is a site-specific disorder that recurs quite unpredictably in even well maintained individuals.

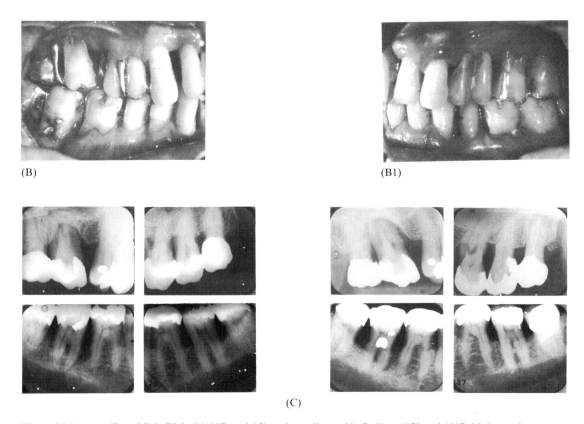

(B)   (B1)

(C)

Figure 26.1 (*cont.*) (B and B1) Clinical (1987) and (C) molar radiographic findings 1970 and 1987. Molar pocket surgery (1972). Despite furcation involvement and other localized areas of destruction little further deterioration occurred apart from at 17 combined lesion (developed 1985 but remained asymptomatic). Note 18, 17 and 26, 27, 28 had been linked with cast restorations to overcome food packing in 1964.

Note: This incomplete series of radiographs shown here and in Figures 26.2–26.7 reflect the patient's understandable reluctance at review appointments to have other than clinically necessary views taken

This phenomenon has been observed by the author in a number of cases in clinical practice, although only a few have received a comparable complex prosthodontic care (e.g. Figures 26.6 and 26.7). These cases and others, examples of which are illustrated in Figures 26.1–26.5, have maintained almost consistently high standards of oral hygiene, have been subjected to pocket elimination surgery and have received meticulous professional cleaning at 3–6-monthly intervals. In addition, root morphology and tooth position could not be incriminated as contributory factors in progressive breakdown. Similarly, the plaque-retentive problems of recurrent pocketing have not been prominent features in these cases, because the attachment losses at these readily cleansable situations have been accompanied by gingival recession. The possible influence of professional cleaning itself, coupled with diligent intrasulcular miniscrub and dental floss oral hygiene practices on the progressive loss of attachment cannot be dismissed (see Chapter 29 – Clinical implications), but cannot be reconciled with the uneven pattern of deterioration that occurred. It must, however, be stated that in some individuals further attachment losses were sustained as might have been expected at some molar furcations, but this did not occur in any consistent fashion. Indeed some sites appeared to be remarkably resistant to further disease.

It is now appropriate to consider situations at which extensive furcation involvement or uneven patterns of breakdown would suggest progressive attachment loss to be inevitable. Yet, it is apparent that in some instances this does not occur or only

409

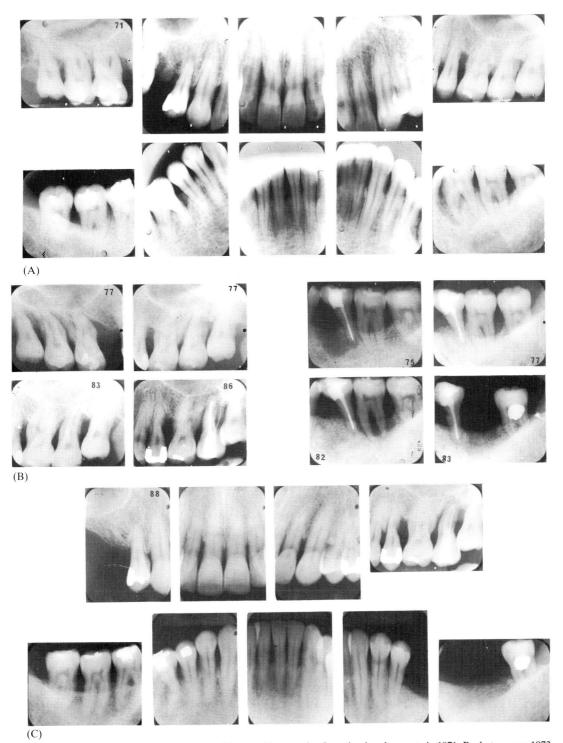

(A)

(B)

(C)

Figure 26.2 (A–C) Radiographs of a 32-year-old man with extensive furcation involvements in 1971. Pocket surgery 1973. However, inconsistent pattern of progressive deterioration occurred at isolated sites shown through to 1983 despite further localized surgical intervention. Mesial root 36 resected 1975 and tooth exfoliated in 1984. 18, 17, 16 removed during 1978. Distobuccal root 27 resected 1987. Presentation in 1988 shown below. Note favourable response to therapy anteriorly, 48, 47, 46, 38 and 25, 26, 28

410

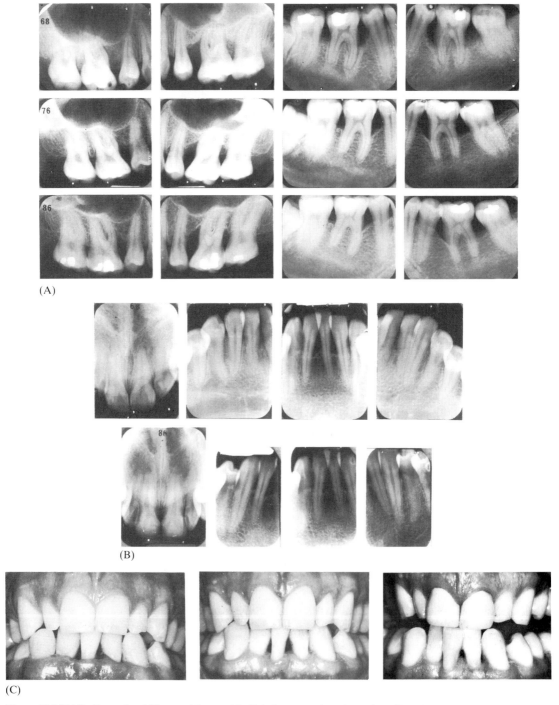

(A)

(B)

(C)

Figure 26.3 (A) Radiographs of 22-year-old man with clinical presentation of post-juvenile periodontitis at first molars and mandibular incisors. Gingival therapy followed by pocket elimination surgery at molars in 1969 and then periodic subgingival debridement over next 18 years to 1986. Note widened periodontal ligament spaces associated with initial supracrestal inflammation and mobility (1968). No obvious radiographic or clinical probing attachment loss sustained during maintenance phase. (B) Radiographs of incisors at 1968 and 1986. (C) Initial clinical presentation (1968). Note gingival response at lower anteriors by 1970 maintained to 1986. Crowns at 11, 21 following accidental coronal tooth fractures

does so at a rate that is consistent with retaining the tooth in satisfactory function and comfort for many years (*cf.* Tolerable levels of disease – Chapter 10).

Untreatable units

The management of untreatable tooth sites depends on several variables but should first and foremost reflect the wishes of the patient. This, in turn, demands a clear understanding, by both the patient and operator, of the overall nature of the problem. Thus, special attention must be paid to patient and dentist attitudes to tooth loss, the rate of periodontal destruction, risk of compromising adjacent units, risk of acute symptoms, systemic hazards, restorative and endodontic needs and prosthetic implications of tooth loss.

Patient attitude to tooth loss

The patient should be encouraged to express frank opinions about the aesthetic, functional and psychological consequences of tooth loss, as final decisions about these factors cannot be decided upon on the patient's behalf. Thus, the patient may be quite prepared to tolerate, as a lesser evil, periodic bouts of pain associated with advanced disease (e.g. Figure 23.4 B). They may also be prepared to modify eating habits to avoid discomfort at mobile teeth (e.g. Figure 23.1 I, L, N and O) or to ignore the poor appearance of drifted teeth (e.g. Figures 23.1 I and 23.2 O) than to lose a tooth. Only where tooth loss is deemed preferable and extraction actually requested by the patient should this option be exercised.

Dentist attitude to extraction

This is influenced by a number of factors whose relative importance will vary from operator to operator. The most important follows from the operator's undergraduate training and the expectations from clinical practice. The pattern of dental practice in which the new graduate commences work and then becomes accustomed to, plus aspirations for operative treatment are all major modifying influences. Economic factors will also dictate treatment together with the perceived difficulties or inconvenience to the operator of retaining teeth. The latter is well illustrated by the common practice of extracting several adjacent teeth that have sustained comparable or greater periodontal destruction, even though symptoms are being complained of only at a single unit. The purpose of this might be, for example, to minimize the need to modify periodically existing partial dentures, when subsequent extraction of these other questionable teeth becomes necessary. Another reason may be

professional convenience, in an endeavour to reduce the likelihood of unscheduled attendance by the patient in pain and thereby, avoiding disruption of an orderly professional appointment system. Such an extraction philosophy revolves primarily about operator, rather than patient, needs.

Rate of attachment loss

Periodontal breakdown is no longer regarded as being slowly progressive but phasic, with relatively short bursts of destruction. The pattern of attachment loss at any particular site can, moreover, not be predicted with any reliability, although as a crude rule of thumb the previous attachment loss does gives some indication of the likely prognosis. Thus, the chances of tooth loss during the patient's natural lifespan might be greater where, for example, half the periodontal support has been lost by the mid-twenties than by middle age. Nevertheless, having instituted the optimal level of plaque control in such cases, it is necessary to re-evaluate periodically any suspect sites over a period of some years before the likely pattern of breakdown can be judged. Even then, the long-term outlook can still not be established with any degree of confidence, because under these conditions, as shown in the clinical case presentations Figure 26.1–26.7, some sites may undergo further deterioration at any stage whilst others remain stable.

Effect on neighbouring units

The presence of an extensive deteriorating condition affecting an untreatable tooth might eventually compromise the contiguous periodontal support of an adjacent tooth (see Figure 23.4 B). In addition, in the event of an acute abscess developing, incidental damage might occur to the supporting bone and periodontal attachment at neighbouring teeth, although there is little documentary support for this assumption. These tissues are, however, likely to be damaged by any attempted surgical corrective therapy at the untreatable tooth. Extraction should therefore be given serious consideration in such instances and more especially where interproximal furcations of adjacent maxillary molars are involved (e.g. Figure 26.5 A and B). The removal of an untreatable tooth may not only provide better access for plaque control but also obviate the need for more complex furcation therapy.

Acute symptoms

Considering how frequently extensive loss of attachment is observed in clinical practice, the development of periodontal abscesses and secondary acute pulpal involvement is not that common (e.g. see

412

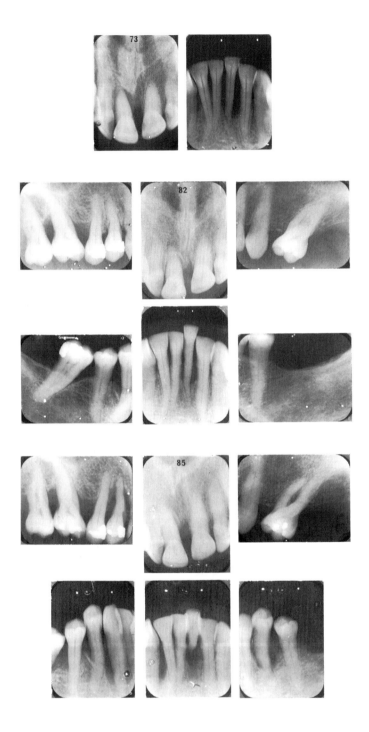

Figure 26.4

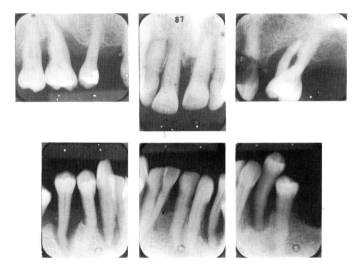

Figure 26.4 Radiographs of 73-year-old woman in 1982 through to 1987. See also Figure 23.2 (M–R). Initial presentation of incisors (in 1973) also shown for completeness here. An inexplicable pattern of rapid attachment loss occurred at several isolated sites in presence of generally good oral hygiene efforts bearing in mind patient's age. Yet note apparent improvement at 11 and minimal involvement elsewhere. Note space closure following fracture and non-replacement of composite bridge at 31. Artefact at 23 in 1987

Figures 23.4 B and 26.1 C). When these acute conditions do occur they are generally dealt with quite readily (*cf.* Chapter 25), although in some instances the associated complications may necessitate emergency surgical drainage or even tooth extraction under general anaesthesia. The added pain, mental stress and potential hazards of this more complex treatment to the patient should be considered. Also the availability of the professional expertise necessary to cater for such problems must not be forgotten and in appropriate circumstances prophylactic extraction should be carried out instead. Consideration might be given to the provision of a course of antibiotics in some cases, to be retained by the patient should acute symptoms develop at times when access to professional care might not be feasible.

Systemic hazards

Patients 'at risk' (e.g. rheumatic fever, cardiac valvular disease, etc.) should not be exposed to the additional hazards of bacteraemia, with its potential complications, in the endeavour to preserve untreatable units and the removal of such teeth should be considered instead. On the other hand, the potential systemic risks must be carefully weighed up against the individual patient's subjective perception of the consequences of tooth loss, whilst always ensuring

that any risk to life overrules every other consideration. Consultation with the patient's physician is essential to resolve any doubt in these cases.

Restorative needs

Where complex restorative and/or endodontic treatment is necessary at any suspect tooth, extraction should be a considered option. This is especially so, when combined periodontal and endodontal lesions exist, because the outcome of treatment is insufficiently predictable to justify the extensive and expensive operative measures required. Similarly, where soundly supported neighbouring teeth require complex restoration, extraction of the untreatable units and replacement with a fixed bridge, which is comparatively predictable, might be considered. On the other hand, where complex restorations are already in place and bridge work would necessitate their premature replacement, the patient might prefer to accept the possible hazards of retaining suspect units. Finally, where such a unit is an abutment of complex fixed bridge work, it may be possible to resect the involved root thus creating an additional pontic (Figure 26.6 D and see also Figure 25.2). This is only possible if the remaining abutments still provide sufficient support.

In cases where a partial denture is first contemplated the extraction of untreatable teeth prior to

414

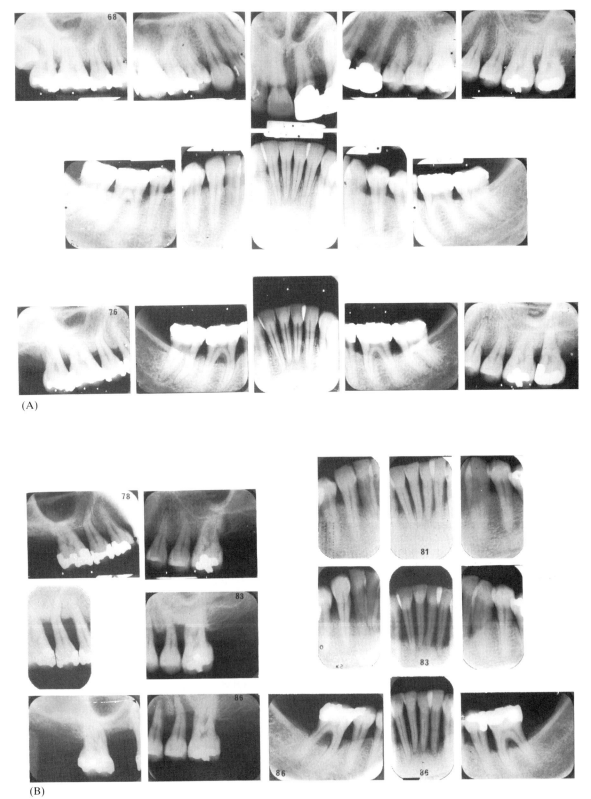

(A)

(B)

Figure 26.5

415

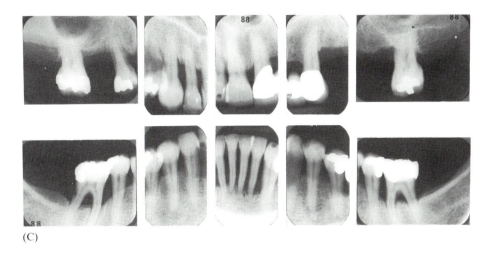

(C)

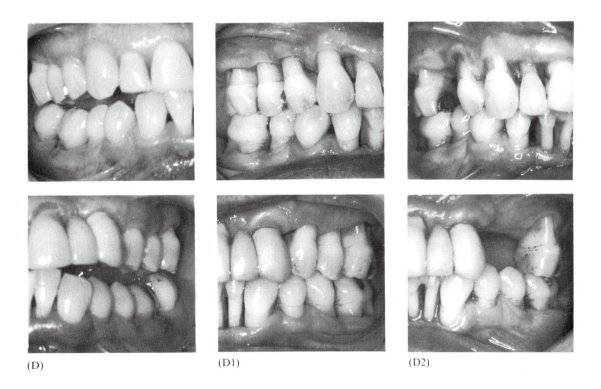

(D)   (D1)   (D2)

Figure 26.5 (A) Radiographic presentation of a 37-year-old woman in 1968 through to 1976. (See also Figure 23.2 G–I.) 17, 16, 26, 27 and 47, 46 pocket surgery and removal 18 in 1969. 17 and 27 then removed (1977) in deference to 16, 26. (B) Findings (1978–1986) optimal healing 16, 26 distal aspects but progressive deterioration 42, 41, 31, 32, and at 15, 24, 25 and 46, 36 (despite further pocket surgery) with loss of 15 (1985). Unopposed 47, 37 removed (1984) to simplify plaque control 46, 36. Presentation (C) radiographically (1988) and clinically (D) in 1978, (D1) 1983 and (D2)1988.

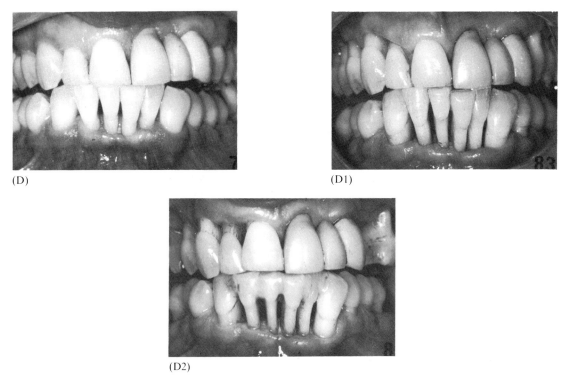

(D) (D1)

(D2)

Figure 26.5 (*cont.*) (D) Clinically in 1978, 1983 and 1988

denture construction is often indicated, or alternatively the facility for subsequent additions to the denture planned. Similarly, extraction may be the treatment of choice when it is not possible to modify the proposed denture to make such additions.

Future prosthetic implications

Progressive loss of periodontal attachment is accompanied by alveolar bone resorption. Retention of untreatable periodontally involved teeth might then reasonably be expected to carry the risk of greater alveolar bony ridge reduction to the detriment of the support of any future denture. On the other hand, alveolar resorption also occurs following tooth extraction. It cannot, however, be predicted whether extraction or retention would retain the best alveolar support. This, then, adds to the dilemma of the optimal handling of untreatable units.

The benefits perceived by the patient, of retaining questionable teeth for a longer time, must in all instances be carefully weighed up against the possibly greater difficulties likely to be encountered when a denture is ultimately fitted because of the, then, smaller remaining edentulous ridge. The

added factor of the patient being that much older at that stage and so possibly being less adaptable to such innovations must also be considered. Finally, the feasibility of extracting all but a few strategically placed teeth with the best support, for endodontic treatment and preparation to support an over-denture might also be considered in suitable cases. Thus, each case must be evaluated individually, the advantages and disadvantages of the possible options carefully explained to the patients and their appropriate wishes and needs then carried out. These important issues all demand controlled investigations.

Conclusions

The prognosis of untreatable teeth depends not only on a number of local factors but also the attitudes of the patient and operator to the problem. It is, therefore, not possible to simply state that any such tooth should be treated in one particular way; rather each situation must be considered on its individual merits and the treatment selected reflect primarily the informed wishes of the patient. The operator will then find that the combination of the generally

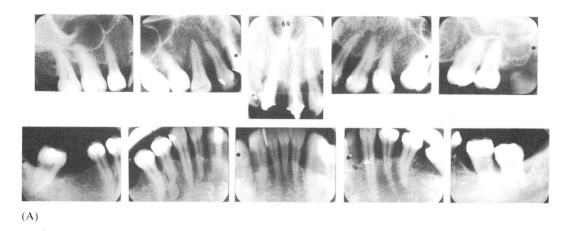

(A)

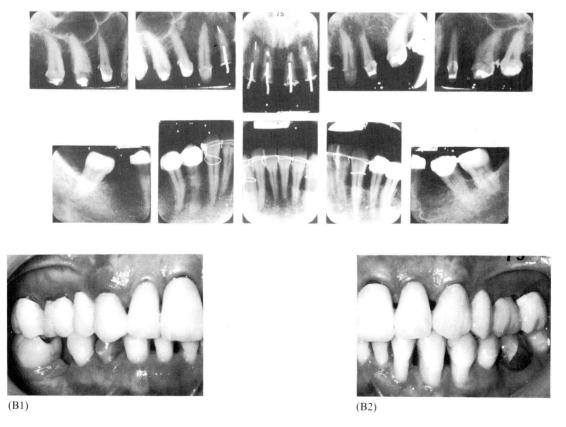

(B1)   (B2)

Figure 26.6 (A) Radiographic presentation in 1969 of 30-year-old woman with pathological drifting and varying degrees of breakdown. (B) Radiographs post-orthodontic realignment followed by full mouth pocket elimination surgery (see also Figure 24.3) completed 1975. (B1 and B2) Coronal reconstruction fitted 1977.

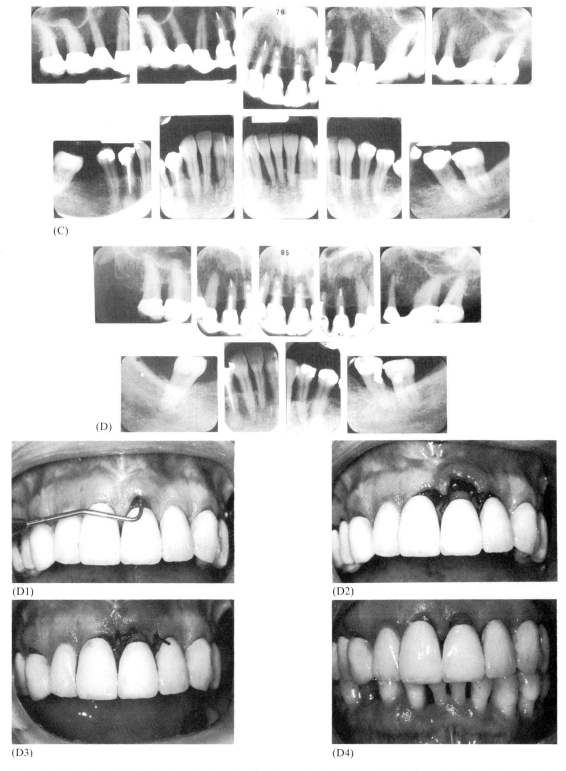

Figure 26.6 (*cont.*) (C) By 1979 further deterioration despite good oral hygiene with development (D and D1) combined lesion at 21 in 1985 necessitating (D2 and D3) root resection in 1986. (D4) Healing at 1 year.

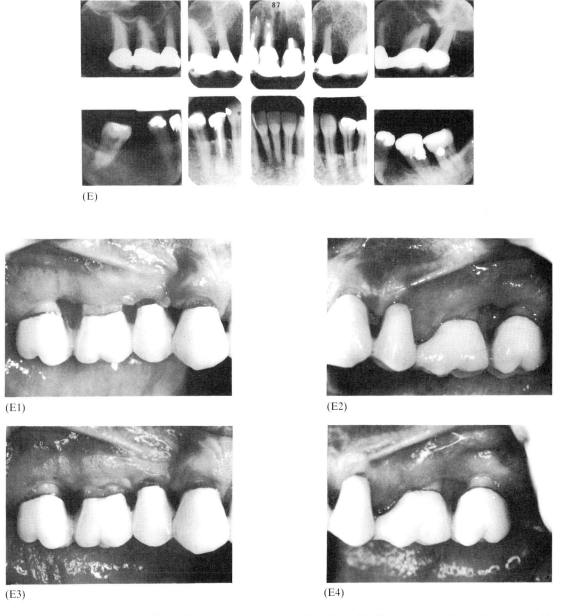

(E)

(E1)   (E2)

(E3)   (E4)

Figure 26.6 (*cont.*) (E, E1 and E2) Rapid breakdown then occurred at 17, 16, 26, 27 with acute periodontal abscesses with equivocal pulpal status during 1987. Surgical reduction of extensive interdental pockets carried out. (E3 and E4) Healing at 9 months – interdental tissue regrowth. Note patient declined endodontic therapy at asymptomatic 24 and 37

420

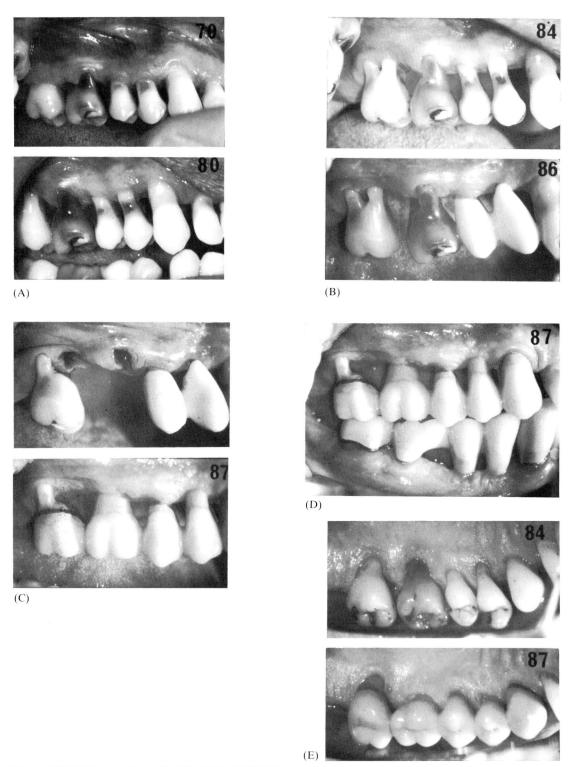

Figure 26.7 (A) 32-year-old man 17–13 in 1970 and 1980. (See also Figure 18.11 A.) 16 distobuccal root resection (1976). (B) 1984–1986 when 14 extracted and replaced with provisional bridge. (C) 16 progressive breakdown – extracted and 17 mesiobuccal root resected. Bridge 17–13 fitted 1987. (D) Buccal occlusion of bridges with (E) palatal views 1984 and 1987.

421

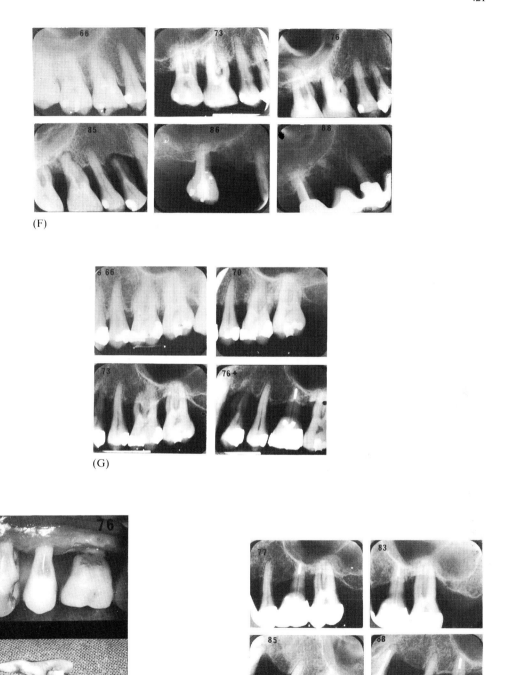

Figure 26.7 (cont.) (F) Radiographs of 17–14 from 1966–1986. (G) Radiographs 24–27 (1966–1976) and (I) 1977–1988. 26 buccal roots resected 1974. (H) Clinical presentation (1976) prior to removal bi-rooted 24 and

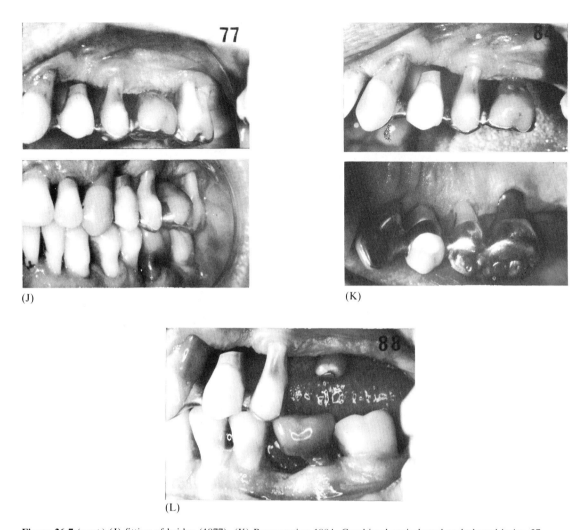

(J)

(K)

(L)

Figure 26.7 *(cont.)* (J) fitting of bridge (1977). (K) Presentation 1984. Combined periodontal endodontal lesion 27 mesiopalatal aspect – extraction 1982. (L) 1988 – following horizontal supragingival fracture 26 palatal root.

very slow overall rate of attachment loss, the infrequency with which lateral periodontal abscesses or secondary pulpal complications develop and necessitate professional intervention, the very gradual increase in mobility sustained, the acceptable functional and aesthetic aspects and, most importantly, the patient's understanding and tolerance of the problems of questionable units, are such that extraction is most often rejected and, in many instances, the teeth will be retained for many years, as shown in Figures 26.1–26.5. On the other hand, periodontal breakdown may in some instances progress very rapidly leading to early loss of teeth as shown in Figure 23.1 (M–Q).

The optimal management of these questionable teeth will then depend on several factors. First, the highest standard of supragingival plaque control possible should be demanded in an effort to retard

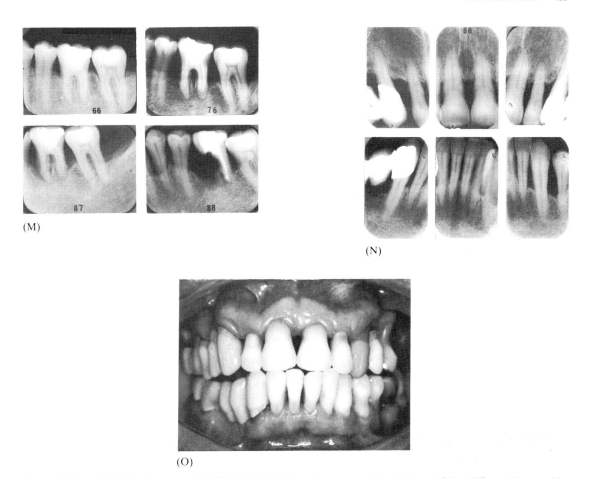

Figure 26.7 (*cont.*) (M) Radiographs of 35–37 (1966–1988). Development combined lesion at 36 in 1987 – not improved by endodontic therapy. 36 mesial root resection 1988. Note sites of more rapid breakdown can be attributed to root form but little detectable change at lower molar furcations. (N) Radiographic and (O) clinical presentation anteriorly 1988 (Restorations by courtesy of Mr P. J. Russell)

the subgingival microbial repopulation following professional cleaning at these sites (see Chapter 28 – The significance of residual pockets). Secondly, physical disruption of the subgingival flora is attempted by the most careful subgingival debridement possible. This should be carried out initially at about 2–3-monthly intervals and the effects then evaluated to determine the subsequent frequency of instrumentation. The possibility of introducing chemotherapeutic agents locally to inhibit microbial repopulation and suppress the bacterial pathogenic potential, and so retard the overall rate of disease, should also be considered (*cf.* Chapter 35). Thirdly, as the success of professional cleaning at these sites is so dependent upon the accessibility of the subgingival root surface, further surgical pocket reduction and optimal exposure of root furcations in conjunction with, if necessary, root resection may be justified in some instances (see Figure 26.7). It is, however, important in these instances that the patient fully understands the reasons for this further surgery.

The case presentations in Figures 26.1–26.7 demonstrate many of the features considered above. It must be stressed that each patient maintained almost consistently high standards of plaque control, complied rigidly with regular recall regime for professional cleaning, and acceded to surgical pocket therapy as dictated by the treatment rationale expounded in the text. It must also be reiterated that the facility of adjunctive complex prosthodontic (including endodontic) options in these cases have for the most part, been precluded by limited financial resources. Furthermore, the pattern of breakdown observed could, in most instances, be attributed to plaque retention sites associated with root form but has also been inexplicable in a few cases. On the other hand, numerous comparatively inaccessible sites appeared to remain remarkably resistant to further attachment losses in the light of previous destruction sustained. It should be noted that the lack of full-mouth radiographic surveys, in some instances, here reflects the understandable unwillingness of the patients to have any unnecessary radiographs taken.

Uncooperative patients

In any dental practice there will be a proportion of patients whose response to repeated advice on oral hygiene, careful supervision and periodic professional cleaning will be disappointing. While the associated pattern of disease might, as in any patient, range from gingivitis alone to gingivitis plus extensive loss of attachment, only those in the latter extreme would seem to present a problem to the operator. The natural inclination is to brand the above patients as uncooperative but this is not always justified, as will be borne out by the record of frequency of attendance for periodontal care, coupled with the not uncommon finding of extensive restorative treatment. There are a number of possible factors that could be responsible for these apparent inconsistencies in behaviour.

(1) Patients may assume that the process of merely attending at regular intervals for professional care will, by itself, prevent tooth loss. Thus, the responsibility for maintaining periodontal health and for repairing any damage sustained is delegated to the dentist. This presumably stems from the long-established biannual dental checkup and restorative treatment regime operated by the profession. Some blame must also attach to the limited impact of the emphasis on self-care with the application of preventive measures by the patient (*cf.* Chapters 6 and 7).

(2) A conviction that the existing periodontal disease will not threaten the dentition is encapsulated in the view that the 'loss of teeth affects other people not me'. On the other hand, the existing overall pattern of attachment loss might be such that it does pose a risk to the dentition overall or, alternatively, the sites of significant destruction may be localized to only a few areas that are considered unimportant by the patient. The patient might therefore consider that neither personal nor professional evasive action would appear necessary.

(3) Perhaps there is a lack of confidence that periodontal disease can be arrested and that tooth loss is inevitable. This leads to a fatalism that can see little point in treatment that is evidently unable to alter the pattern of tooth loss significantly. Indeed, the individual's personal record coupled with experience of others of tooth loss, despite extensive treatment efforts in the past, will unfortunately often endorse this belief.

(4) The patient's expectations for his teeth might be no more than that of a reasonably comfortable functional and aesthetically pleasing dentition. Consequently, periodic bleeding and tenderness associated with cleaning or even a bad taste and perhaps halitosis (especially in those indifferent to personal body odours) might be considered as insignificant. This is particularly so when the periodic professional cleaning appears to clear up these relatively minor symptoms until the next routine visit. Moreover, these symptoms might constitute less of an inconvenience to the patient than the self-discipline of regular thorough personal oral hygiene efforts. The risk of losing a few teeth as a result of indifferent cleaning might also be allotted a low level of priority because their loss might not even be disabling, but where necessary could be replaced quite simply by the dentist. In fact such prosthetic replacement of missing teeth might be quite acceptable to the patient. In summary, these patients would see little merit in the troublesome maintenance of good oral hygiene to avert something that will ultimately not constitute a problem anyway.

(5) A failure of communication between patient and operator might frequently be responsible. Thus the patient might not have appreciated the nature of disease and the all-importance of plaque control or understood the mechanics of effective cleaning. There are, in turn, several possible reasons for this:
   (a) Apprehension and fear arousal by the clinical environment of the dental surgery

would constitute a powerful distraction for most individuals whilst attempting to grasp oral hygiene instructions. Previous experience would dictate that the surgery is concerned with operative treatment, rather than advice about the nature and treatment of a condition which has not been mentioned before or not recalled by the individual. Finally, some patients may simply interpret this advice as an innovative method of chair-side reassurance prior to unpleasant operative therapy, and so dismiss it as irrelevant chat. The use of a non-clinical environment instead for advice might obviate these problems (*cf.* Chapters 6 and 7).

(b) Conflicting methods of oral hygiene represent a major hurdle to understanding. Thus, advice from previous dentists or hygienists, information gained from the media or peer group advice is often at variance with present advice given, leading to confusion and also a possible lack of confidence or even mistrust.

(c) Individual capacity to assimilate advice and to grasp the pure mechanics of oral hygiene varies. Some patients simply forget much of what has been said or totally misinterpret it. This is unfortunately not always appreciated by clinicians because of the common failure to encourage any feedback from the patient (*cf.* Chapters 6 and 7). As an example, a patient might not recall or might even deny that a specific cleaning technique, clearly recorded in the clinical records, has ever been advocated.

It is difficult to judge the receptive capacity of each patient, but it is apparent that most of what has been said at the start of consultation is remembered and progressively less thereafter. The most important things might therefore best be dealt with first and, in questionable cases, details spread over several successive appointments. There can be no correct method and that used ultimately will be dictated by operator experience and assessment of the likely capacity of each patient to absorb advice. In any event it is necessary to check periodically the patient's understanding and practical performance.

(d) The personalities of patient and operator might clash, and the potentially sensitive and personal implications of a dirty mouth be resented by some patients. Alternative approaches must, therefore, be evolved for each different personality type likely to be encountered. Once again, the technique used by each operator will reflect what best suits his own and his patients' perceived needs, and it would be presumptive to attempt to impose a particular approach here. The old adage 'You can't win them all' is important here and where failure is suspected, the approach can either be modified quickly or the patient be given the option of seeking the advice of and treatment from another clinician. The patient will however often seize the initiative and not return.

(6) Limited manual dexterity may be a real problem and, while rarely presenting much difficulty anteriorly, may defy effective cleaning at the more complex multi-rooted posterior units.

(7) The cost to the patient in terms of money, time and the discomfort of active treatment might represent too great a sacrifice, becoming a subconscious barrier to a total commitment to plaque control. Thus, some patients may have certain preconceived threshold levels of treatment complexity. This might, in some instances, even represent a hidden barrier to achieving the requisite standard of oral hygiene to justify surgery, so as to avoid surgery as a treatment option.

There can be no panacea for the handling of these situations. Rather, each must be discussed frankly and honestly with the patient and a mutually acceptable practical solution worked out. Several possible options should be considered.

In the first, a trial period of more frequent professional cleaning and closer monitoring of the patient's efforts might be rewarded by an improved marginal tissue status. The reason for this improvement might not be clear, but could be either the professional cleaning itself or the motivational impact of the regime. This can only be assessed by trial and error in each case.

Secondly, where it is perceived that the patient is not prepared to negotiate relatively inaccessible subgingival root surfaces, pocket reduction surgery to simplify future access would not seem unreasonable.

Thirdly, periodontal surgical intervention has been claimed by some to be a powerful motivation to improved oral hygiene. This is apparently true for some individuals, for whom test case surgery would be appropriate.

Finally, surgical reduction of pocketing to prolong the longevity of the dentition would be warranted where it can be shown that overall rates of destruction are related directly to actual pocket depths. There is however as yet little documentary support for this. Surgery is probably also warranted as a delaying tactic in those cases with a tendency for periodontal abscesses, that might otherwise necessitate extraction.

The disinterested patient

Patients with obviously dirty, uncared-for mouths may present with marked gingival inflammation yet minimal attachment loss. While there would seem to be no cause for alarm on periodontal grounds in these instances, there could be social reasons including personal freshness for improved periodontal care. The patient might therefore be made aware of the condition and its potential consequences, and if acceptable the appropriate advice and treatment could be given.

Individuals who attend only when in pain, be it periodontal, pulpal or periapical, must be advised of the nature of disease and appropriate instructions in plaque control and diet be given. This advice will, in many instances, go unheeded, the patient being concerned about neither poor oral hygiene nor the resulting disease. The removal of the offending tooth is usually requested and the patient not seen again until further pain necessitates it. Sometimes the prophylactic removal of other similarly involved but asymptomatic units may also be requested. The patient then becomes progressively more edentulous and ultimately demands total clearance of the remaining teeth, regardless of status, and the provision of full dentures.

Conclusion

It is at present not possible to predict the outcome of disease in any individual, although certain trends may be evident in some cases. It is clear that the prognosis of each tooth and the dentition as a whole is dictated by a multiplicity of factors and it is the responsibility of the operator to make the patient aware of these and to discuss the various treatment options. Dental therapy thus revolves about patient understanding of the problem(s), the desire to control, if not eliminate, the causative factors and the operator's ability to satisfy the corrective operative measures. The technical difficulties of the latter, coupled with the frustrating influence of the periodontal tissue morphology and, not least, the economic aspects of the associated prosthodontic requirements, will inevitably determine the choice of therapy in any one case, but without necessarily ensuring the ultimate outcome. This is well illustrated in the clinical cases presented in Figures 26.1–26.7 and is considered further in the next chapter.

27

Maintenance therapy

The enigma of maintenance
True maintenance therapy

Continuation therapy
Conclusion

The enigma of maintenance

The patient might reasonably expect that following surgical therapy periodontal health will be achieved and then readily maintained. This is because periodontal surgery tends to be equated in the patient's mind with the ultimate resolution of the problem, and that the surgically corrected dento-gingival morphology is amenable to primary preventative plaque control measures. This would then constitute maintenance care in the true sense of the word. However, whilst conceptually valid, in practice some form of follow-up professional treatment is frequently found to be necessary in some parts of the mouth, representing what is best regarded as continuation therapy. This, in turn, is synonymous with gingival response therapy and implies that maintenance of health cannot simply be assumed following surgical therapy.

Continuation therapy is necessary following attempted pocket elimination surgery, when totally cleansible dentogingival morphology has not been achieved. This will have been due primarily to the characteristically uneven pattern of destruction and the involvement of complex periodontal morphology. It must however be stressed that the lack of ideal dentogingival morphology is not followed inevitably by progressive disease, although it does imply increased risk. The difficulty of identifying deteriorating sites with any certainty does, of course, still exist. Careful post-surgical examination and documentation is therefore necessary, although the likely location of these suspect sites can usually be anticipated from previous findings recorded during both non-surgical and surgical phases of treatment.

The success of both true maintenance and of continuation therapy remains highly dependent upon the individual patient's own efforts of plaque control. Comparatively few individuals appear capable of maintaining consistently the levels of control required. Regular professional supervision and where necessary, compensatory professional cleaning, may be able to overcome this deficiency, although its feasibility will be dictated very much by the availability of local professional and financial resources. The practical aspects of true maintenance and continuation therapy are, for descriptive purposes here, considered separately.

True maintenance therapy

This is applicable to the totally cleansible units following gingival response therapy or simple pocket surgery and also, in those few instances of complex pocket surgery where root resections or extraction of 'non-treatable' teeth, in conjunction with any necessary prosthodontic reconstructions have been possible. In the former category, the dentogingival morphology presents no difficulties in plaque control, and periodontal health can be ensured by simply maintaining the high standards of oral hygiene already achieved, which needs no further comment.

Successful maintenance is apparently also likely in the latter more complex situations, for the now classic Scandinavian investigations (see Chapter 29 – Post-surgical maintenance), have demonstrated that further disease can almost invariably be checked regardless of the extent of breakdown. The key factor for success appeared to be motivated individuals willing and able to carry out a high standard of oral hygiene. It must also be realized that plaque control in these individuals will have been rather simpler and less time consuming than elsewhere by virtue of fewer remaining teeth. Furthermore, the potentially more susceptible units will have been removed, so possibly predicating a more favourable outcome of therapy. However, even so, further breakdown was observed after a decade, at isolated sites in some of these patients.

Patients undergoing surgery are best reviewed at least every 4–6 weeks initially, and the appropriate advice in oral hygiene given as necessary. Then, depending on the individual patient's ability to maintain gingival health subsequent appointments are made at longer intervals (see Chapter 29). Professional tooth cleaning is undertaken traditionally at each maintenance review appointment. It is by no means clear that the objective of plaque-free dentogingival junctions is actually achieved, for this is rarely checked by using a disclosing agent. The importance of such professional cleaning in the maintenance of health might therefore be questioned and even more so, where a high standard of plaque control is already being maintained between visits.

The respective influences of home care and professional cleaning have been put in perspective by the findings of another Scandinavian investigation. A group of subjects, selected randomly from a recall programme following periodontal therapy, received professional cleaning at monthly intervals at contralateral quadrants over a 1 year period. No attempt was made to influence the participants' cleaning habits. Periodontal health was maintained at all quadrants, indicating that factors other than mechanical professional cleaning were responsible. The possible motivational impact on oral hygiene habits gained by merely participating in the study and the possible influence of the meticulous recall system on patient behaviour were cited. Where, on the other hand, effective home care is not consistently practised, as shown by recurrent marginal inflammation, professional cleaning would presumably be advantageous. This is supported by other investigations (see Chapter 29). Professional cleaning might then not only compensate for the patient's failings and remove calculus deposits impeding plaque removal but also possibly stimulate better efforts.

There are several practical implications of these studies on maintenance therapy. In the first place, the operator might best function primarily as a professional supervisor and only thereafter as a professional cleaner. Secondly, the motivational impact of periodic attendance itself might ultimately prove to be more important in the maintenance of periodontal health than any psychological, physical or biological benefits of professional cleaning. Thirdly, it is not as yet clear whether maintenance is best conducted by the periodontist, the referring general practitioner or their respective hygienists. This choice should be dictated by the personal requirements and expectations of individual patients. Fourthly, there can be no universally applicable maintenance regime. The frequency and content of professional reviews will ideally reflect the informed wishes of the patient, the levels of plaque control practised and the need for further root surface instrumentation based on the clinical status of the tissues. This, in turn, makes the final demand; that is periodic careful clinical examination and documentation of attachment levels by site is essential lest further breakdown goes undetected. Thus, as stated above, further destruction might still occur unpredictably at some sites even in well maintained subjects.

Continuation therapy

This might be required at only a few isolated sites in some individuals, whilst in others the therapy might involve many more sites. These sites are likely to be located at the initially deepest localized pockets, where an uneven pattern of destruction has been sustained and, more especially, at root furcation involvement. These unavoidable surgical failures will, therefore, have resulted from the variations of periodontal tissue form and root anatomy encountered at operation, thwarting the surgical objective of totally cleansible dentogingival junctions. The patient must be advised that surgery has not been completely successful and that the problems of plaque control, at these persistent pocket sites, are essentially no different from those experienced before operation. These pockets will however be invariably shallower than before and fewer in number, the root furcations be rather more accessible and hopefully, a more careful debridement of the associated subgingival root surfaces have been carried out at the time of operation.

A chart indicating the location of the suspect sites should be provided to guide the patient and the appropriate advice in cleaning given, as in gingival response therapy. The interspace-type brush is most useful in these situations, while patent root furcations are best negotiated with interproximal brushes. Subgingival irrigation with chlorhexidine might also be considered (*cf.* Chapter 35). Periodic professional tooth cleaning is also undertaken as in gingival response therapy, and although the optimal frequency cannot be clearly defined, based on rates of subgingival bacterial repopulation (*cf.* Chapter 28), it should be initially at about 2–3-monthly intervals. The tissue response to this debridement is then assessed in terms of subgingival bleeding and probing depths. Where improvement is observed over a series of appointments, longer intervals should be considered, but this should always be dictated by the needs of the least responsive sites. On the other hand, a more frequent regime should be instituted where no improvement is elicited. If signs of disease still persist and progressive destruction appears inevitable, then a further attempt at corrective surgery should be considered although in most instances the patient will choose instead to accept the situation. The management of these seemingly untreatable sites has been considered in the previous chapter.

Finally, it is instructive to reflect upon the frequency with which post-surgical pocketing persists at the initially deepest pocket sites in any surgical field. This residual pocketing is often comparable to that present initially, at other shallower pocket sites, for which surgery had also been considered necessary. The practical implications are that continuation therapy, then necessary at such residual pocket sites is permissible following attempted surgical intervention, but not before it. This presumably also forms the basis of the student's plaintive plea that residual pockets of any particular depth following surgical treatment may be maintained by subgingival debridement, yet those of a similar depth prior to surgery will have represented an indication for surgical intervention! There might however be some truth in this assumption, because attachment levels are often maintained at such post-surgical sites. There are several possible reasons for this.

(1) the effective root surface debridement undertaken at surgery followed by a high standard of supragingival plaque control;
(2) the improved access to the subgingival plaque front during continuation therapy as a result of surgical pocket reduction (as opposed to the intended elimination);
(3) progressive destruction may have already been checked prior to surgery by gingival response type therapy as suggested by the comparable clinical responses reported following both surgical and non-surgical therapy (*cf.* Chapters 28 and 29);
(4) the disease process might have entered a spontaneous phase of remission that is independent of any professional administrations; and, finally
(5) deterioration could be continuing but be incapable of detection by current clinical methods.

Indeed, each of the five possibilities cited might be applicable in different situations in the same individual. This once again highlights the difficulties of deciding when to intervene surgically as discussed in Chapter 13. This dilemma is considered further in Part III.

Conclusion

Periodontal health can be maintained following the creation, by whatever means, of a cleansible morphology combined with effective patient home-care. This then represents true maintenance care. However in the many instances that these conditions are not achieved disease is liable to progress. Perseverence with continuation therapy, which is represented by gingival response therapy, is therefore chosen in the hope that the rate of disease will be slowed down as much as possible and the longevity of the dentition prolonged. This might then constitute a tolerable level of disease (*cf.* Chapter 10).

Part III The scientific basis of therapy

28

The role of surgery:
I The clinical implications of surgical access for debridement

Introduction
Nature of the root surface
The assessment of adequate debridement
Instruments for debridement

Difficulties of subgingival instrumentation
Assessment of the need for surgical access
Management following surgical debridement
The significance of residual pockets

Introduction

The case for 'blind' versus 'open' debridement

The increasing trend towards the surgical exposure of periodontally involved root surfaces to facilitate proper instrumentation (Pihlström *et al.,* 1981; Axelsson and Lindhe 1981 a; Frandsen, 1983), stems from the difficulties experienced with 'blind' subgingival instrumentation of the root surfaces. This implies a rationale based on operative expediency rather than established biological need. The latter contention is endorsed by the similarity of the reported reductions in mean probing depths and maintenance of mean attachment levels following 'blind' subgingival root surface instrumentation alone and when compared with 'open' instrumentation in conjunction with modified Widman flaps (MWF) (Pihlström *et al.,* 1981, 1983; Hill *et al.,* 1981; Lindhe *et al.,* 1982 a, 1984; Isidor *et al.,* 1984 a; Westfelt *et al.,* 1985; Lindhe and Nyman, 1985; Isidor and Karring, 1986; Ramfjord *et al.,* 1987).

The rationale for surgical exposure

The above investigations indicate that 'blind' debridement can be effective. Accordingly, the rationale for the surgical exposure of root surfaces, in order to expedite effective debridement, demands closer examination. It is paradoxical that, while the efficacy of debridement can be assessed retrospectively, there are no reliable criteria for judging this at the time of surgical instrumentation (Poole *et al.,* 1984; Eaton *et al.,* 1985). A variety of different

aspects affecting access for debridement need to be examined. These are the nature of the periodontally involved root surface, the assessment of the adequacy of debridement, the instruments used for debridement, the technical difficulties of subgingival debridement, assessing the outcome of debridement, case management following surgical debridement and, finally, the significance of residual pockets.

Nature of the root surface

Plaque, calculus and cementum changes

The periodontally involved root surface is characterized by three features. The first is bacterial plaque (*cf.* Chapter 4) which may be loosely or firmly adherent, as described by Fine *et al.* (1978 a), or calcified, thus becoming calculus and constituting the next feature (Review: Mandel and Gaffar, 1986). Neither need be considered further here. The third is best described as cementum contamination from the toxic products of bacterial plaque and substances derived from inflammation (Review: Daly *et al.,* 1979). This requires closer examination.

Cemental contaminants

It is known that the subgingival flora elaborate lytic enzymes and possess noxious cellular constituents and produce cytotoxic substances (Review: Listgarten, 1987) (*cf.* Chapters 4 and 5). The tissue destructive potential and antigenic activities of these substances have the ability to produce the various inflammatory and destructive changes of the disease. Of the noxious substances cited, endotoxin (lipopolysaccharide-[LPS]) derived from the cell walls of Gram-negative organisms, has been considered a major factor in the pathogenesis of the disease and has been subject to much investigation (Review: Daly *et al.*, 1980). It also serves as an indicator of both the likely distribution of other noxious substances and of the efficacy of root surface instrumentation (see below).

Cytotoxic potential of cementum

The possibility that periodontally involved cementum could exert a cytotoxic effect upon the periodontal tissues was first proposed by Hatfield and Baumhammers (1971). This was endorsed by the finding that the cementum was toxic to cell cultures (Aleo *et al.*, 1974, 1975). These workers introduced the term 'cementum bound' LPS, which implied the absorption of LPS by periodontally involved cementum, but could not exclude the presence of LPS associated with plaque trapped within cemental surface imperfections, such as resorption lacunae (Sottosanti and Garrett 1975; Smukler and Tagger, 1976; Waerhaug, 1978 a). Daly *et al.* (1980) thus suggested that the term 'cementum-associated' LPS might be more appropriate. Other workers concluded that LPS was adsorbed onto, or penetrated, the cementum (Jones and O'Leary, 1978; Nishimine and O'Leary, 1979). Fine *et al.* (1980) in turn claimed that endotoxin penetrated deeply into cementum on the basis of the identification of the ketodeoxyoctonic acid (KDO), a carbohydrate unique to endotoxin, in root surface eluates.

Histological assessment of periodontally involved cementum revealed microbial deposits in surface defects (see above) and within defects at the cemento–dentinal junction (Daly *et al.*, 1982). In addition, these workers observed the penetration of microorganisms and their deposits (possibly including LPS) to a depth of about $10\,\mu m$ beneath the cementum surface ('subsurface bacterial contamination') in the absence of any surface defects. Together, these findings suggest that the removal of at least a superficial layer of periodontally involved cementum could be necessary during root surface instrumentation.

Superficial toxicity of cementum

An alternative view is presented by Nakib *et al.* (1982), demonstrating that endotoxin adheres only weakly to the tooth surface and can be brushed away. They further showed that cemental penetration by LPS is precluded by its comparatively large molecular size, in relation to the small pore size of

the highly mineralized surface layer of the cementum. This view was confirmed by Ito *et al.* (1985) who demonstrated that only minimal amounts of endotoxin, or an endotoxin-like substance, appears to be present within cementum, the bulk of this substance being associated with surface accretions. In this context mineralized surface coating, probably identical in origin to dental cuticle has been observed in scanning electron microscopic investigations of root surfaces exposed by periodontal disease (Eide *et al.*, 1983, 1984). This coating appears to stem principally from the adsorption of components of the gingival inflammatory exudate onto the root surface. The cytotoxic potential of periodontally involved cementum might therefore be related to exogenous cytotoxic substances being incorporated within this surface coating and would, thereby, question the rationale for removal of tooth substance as an essential part of root surface debridement (Lie and Leknes, 1985). This has in turn been endorsed by subsequent research findings on the distribution of root surface associated LPS (see below).

Distribution of lipopolysaccharide (LPS)

The distribution of LPS in relation to periodontally involved root surfaces has been subject to much investigation. Early findings indicated that the LPS content of the essentially superficial loosely-adherent plaque (which could be removed with a stream of water) was greater than that of the remaining more firmly adherent plaque (Fine *et al.*, 1978 a and b). The juxtaposition of this superficial plaque to the pocket wall would thus facilitate LPS diffusion into the tissues, and is consistent with correlations shown between endotoxin levels in gingival exudates and the clinical and histological degrees of gingival inflammation (Simon *et al.*, 1969, 1970, 1971). This finding has been endorsed by Shapiro *et al.* (1972), using the limulus lysate assay (LLA) (Levin and Bang, 1964) which is generally considered to be the most sensitive test for bacterial LPS (Yin *et al.*, 1972). A positive LLA can however also be induced by a number of other substances including thrombin, thromboplastin, ribonucleic acids and ribonuclease (Elin and Wolff, 1973).

The possibility of false positive findings has been circumvented by using LLA in conjunction with a technique of affinity chromatography (Wilson *et al.*, 1986). These workers positively identified for the first time the presence of LPS in pooled samples of root surface eluates. The distribution of LPS on roots of extracted periodontally diseased teeth was then assessed by assaying pooled samples of eluates derived from gentle washing (loosely adherent plaque), brushing (firmly adherent plaque), and from root surface material stripped with a dental bur to a depth of 1 mm (Moore *et al.*, 1986). Less than

1% of LPS demonstrated in this way, was located within the root surface cementum itself, a finding endorsed by Hughes and Smales (1986) in an immunohistochemical investigation. A subsequent *in vitro* investigation (Maidwell-Smith *et al.*, 1987) assessed the total LPS levels in eluates derived from individual teeth. The observations suggested the likely presence of LPS in relation to all periodontally involved root surfaces, a finding supported by McCoy *et al.* (1987). However, wide variations were found between different teeth which might in turn simply reflect the episodic nature of disease (Socransky *et al.*, 1984) or that the role of LPS in disease has been overrated (Nakib *et al.*, 1982). In this respect, Slots and Dahlen (1985) have shown no obvious correlation between LPS properties and periodontopathic potential.

The merits of cementum removal

The superficial and loosely associated nature of the bulk of bacterial endotoxin within periodontal pockets is probably true for other exogenous cytotoxic substances (Nakib *et al.*, 1982). This is supported by the finding of a similar pattern of healing in an animal model, following root surface polishing alone at operation versus exposed cementum removal with diamond burs (Nyman *et al.*, 1986). This has since been confirmed in humans (Nyman *et al.*, 1988). However, it is not clear to what extent any such polishing might also remove possibly contaminated superficial root material (Moore *et al.*, 1986) and so contribute to healing. It has been shown, for example, that 3–4 µm of enamel may be removed during polishing with a rubber cup and pumice paste for only 30 seconds (Vrbic *et al.*, 1967). Finally, growing belief as to the superficial location of cytotoxic substances has been reinforced by the finding that periodontally involved roots debrided *in vitro*, with only 15 carefully executed hand instrument strokes to ensure overlapping instrumentation on each root surface, was sufficient to remove all but minute amounts of LPS (Cheetham *et al.*, 1988). An equally effective debridement has been demonstrated in an *in vitro* ultrasonic instrumentation of less than 20 seconds duration per root surface of teeth having minimal amounts of clinically discernible deposits of calculus (Smart, 1987).

Conclusions

The emphasis placed upon the deliberate removal of the cementum by root planing remains highly questionable. Furthermore, the clinical improvements observed following traditional root planing (removal of cementum) might be due simply to the concomitant elimination of microbial and other

exogenous toxic products adjacent to the cementum, rather than to the intentional removal of cementum itself. Unfortunately, the difficulties of differentiating clinically between 'clean' and supposedly 'diseased' root surfaces, for assessing the adequacy of debridement, remains a major hurdle.

The assessment of adequate debridement

Root surface smoothness

Traditionally, the creation of a glassy smooth root surface is taken to indicate the completion of 'blind' root planing. Despite this, residual calculus is often present (Review: O'Leary, 1986 and more recently, Caffesse *et al.*, 1986; Saglie *et al.*, 1986; Buchanan and Robertson, 1987). As this residual calculus has also been observed following 'open' surgical root planing (Waerhaug, 1978 b; Caffesse *et al.*, 1986; Buchanan and Robertson, 1987) the finding of root surface smoothness, judged by the use of explorer tips, is not a reliable indicator of root surface characteristics (Jones *et al.*, 1972; Jones and O'Leary, 1978; Rabbani *et al.*, 1981). Unfortunately, no alternative exists to the use of this somewhat subjective tactile parameter at the time of non-surgical instrumentation, although it is surprising how little attention has been devoted by the proponents of open surgical debridement, as to whether the primary objective of root surface cleanliness has actually been achieved.

Site vision with surgical access

Adequate surgical exposure enhances access for root surface instrumentation (Eaton *et al.*, 1985; Caffesse *et al.*, 1986; Buchanan and Robertson, 1987). It is, however, of only limited value for any direct visual assessment of its efficacy, for although residual stained calculus deposits can be seen, it is impossible to discriminate visually between instrumented and uninstrumented root surfaces. This also applies to the plaque front at the bottom of the pocket, which is the same colour as tooth tissue (Waerhaug, 1978 b). In addition, the associated bleeding will tend to mask the field of operation whilst the interproximal root surfaces and those related to furcation involvements or intrabony defects are often obscured because of the adjacent root or bone form.

Disclosing residual plaque deposits

Some clinicians have advocated the use of disclosing agents at the time of operation (after Waerhaug, 1975). This technique was investigated by Eaton *et al.* (1985 a and b). These workers first showed in an *in vitro* investigation that non-furcated periodontally involved root surfaces could be planed with curettes so that no staining could be produced by a 2% gentian violet solution. This apparent root surface cleanliness could, however, not be reproduced in the subsequent *in vivo* component of the investigation carried out at the buccal aspects of anterior teeth (Eaton *et al.*, 1985 b). 'Open' surgical root planing was, nevertheless, more effective than 'blind' subgingival root planing and would thereby support the use of surgical access for root surface instrumentation. However, the comparable clinical response to either method reported previously, coupled with the greater difficulties imposed by the relationships of interproximal root surfaces or of root morphology and the apparent lack of total cleanliness achieved here following each method, suggests that the residual stained material may not be important clinically. Furthermore that efforts to achieve non-stainable root surfaces by root planing might represent over-instrumentation.

Microscopic evidence

The nature of surfaces instrumented *in vitro* has been clarified by a scanning electron microscopic investigation (Poole *et al.*, 1984). Surfaces that could not be stained with gentian violet were consistently shown to be devoid of cementum (i.e. were comprised of dentine), whereas cementum and any accretions were always stained, thus supporting the light microscopical findings of Eaton *et al.* (1985b). The unstainable areas of dentine achieved by careful root planing were, however, shown to accept stain following deliberate roughening and thereby necessitating caution in the interpretation of the finding of root surface staining immediately after instrumentation. This has been endorsed by the results of an *in vivo* investigation (Breininger *et al.*, 1987) in which the majority of stained deposits were shown, by scanning electron microscopic examination, to be composed of adherent fibrin and instrumentation debris. Together these findings confirm the difficulties of establishing clinically when total root surface cleanliness, that is, free of plaque and accretions, has been achieved and judging precisely when all the cementum has been removed without sustaining an unnecessary loss of dentine. Furthermore, the time expended in producing non-stainable (namely cementum-free) surfaces in this *in vitro* investigation reinforced the earlier clinical findings that total cementum removal is not feasible clinically (O'Leary and Kafrawy, 1983).

Conclusions

It can be concluded that as the traditional efforts at removing allegedly contaminated cementum will also remove the entire surface of the periodontally involved root together with its accretions, the clinical benefits of root planing may simply be due to the latter. Accordingly, the clinical success of root surface instrumentation may not depend on the removal of cementum *per se* but on a less extensive, but thorough, degree of surface instrumentation. Such a debridement regime highlights the importance of ensuring that instrument strokes totally overlap each other, for any incompletely instrumented surfaces are liable to result in a more rapid bacterial recolonization (Waerhaug, 1978).

Instruments for debridement
Evaluation

Investigations of instrumentation carried out on extracted roots, by macroscopic, light microscopic or scanning electron microscopic techniques demonstrate a broadly comparable efficacy for both hand instruments and ultrasonic devices in the removal of subgingival calculus (Torfason *et al.*, 1979; Hunter *et al.*, 1984; Gellin *et al.*, 1986; Breininger *et al.*, 1986). There is rather less consensus about cementum removal but with the majority view finding curettes to be more effective (Review: O'Leary, 1986). Ultrasonics may also result in greater surface roughness (e.g. Hunter *et al.*, 1984), attributable in part to the degree of pressure used and the power setting of the unit (Lie and Leknes, 1985). In contrast, the findings of Pearlman (1982) reveal that under optimal operating conditions, ultrasonic devices are capable of planing cementum to a smooth dentinal surface.

The traditionally claimed importance of concluding ultrasonic subgingival instrumentation with hand curettes because of incomplete removal of cementum and the surface roughness produced by these devices (Reviews: Suppipat, 1974; Brown *et al.*, 1987), is questionable. The former objective has, as discussed previously, yet to be substantiated. Subgingival root surface roughness might in turn be expected to influence bacterial recolonization and rates of plaque formation. However, it was found to be insignificant with respect to junctional epithelial adaptation (Waerhaug, 1956 a and b), the development of gingival inflammation (Rosenberg and Ash, 1974), or healing following subgingival instrumentation by both hand instruments and ultrasonics (Torfason *et al.*, 1979) and modified Widman flap surgery (Khatiblou and Ghodssi, 1983). In addition, comparable clinically evaluated gingival responses have been demonstrated following both hand and ultrasonic methods at both moderately deep (Torfason *et al.*, 1979; Badersten *et al.*, 1981; Leon and Vogel, 1987) and deep pockets (Badersten *et al.*, 1984 a; Oosterwaal *et al.*, 1987). In this context investigations by Lie and Leknes (1985), Gelling *et al.* (1986) and Loos *et al.* (1987) on the newer generation lower vibration frequency air turbine scalers suggest they are efficient alternatives to their ultrasonic competitors.

The roughness sustained from any instrumentation might however be associated with an unnecessary loss of tooth substance, the resulting exposure of dentinal tubules leading to hypersensitive surfaces and ultimately possible pulpal damage. The damaging potential of the low speed rotating diamond points and the Roto-Pro instrument (Ellman) specially designed for calculus removal has been evaluated (e.g. Meyer and Lie, 1977; Lie and Meyer, 1977) with a consensus view that these devices should be avoided.

Ultrasonics and hand instruments have been shown to be equally effective in subgingival plaque removal (Thornton and Garnick, 1982; Leon and Vogel, 1987; Oosterwaal *et al.*, 1987). Indeed Breininger *et al.* (1987) showed both methods of instrumentation to be highly effective in bacterial debridement of subgingival root surfaces. The ease with which the high frequency vibration (see Suppipat, 1974) coupled with the cavitational cleansing activity of the ultrasonic device coolant fluid (Walmsley *et al.*, 1984, 1988) removes supragingival plaque, exogenous tooth surface staining and accretions against that of hand instruments might also favour its use subgingivally. Adherent subgingival accretions, including the mineralized surface coatings (Eide *et al.*, 1984), might similarly be removed in this way. This has been endorsed by the series of *in vitro* investigations by Poole *et al.* (1984), Eaton *et al.* (1985), Smart (1987) and Cheetham *et al.* (1988). This facility might in turn explain the favourable clinical responses reported following ultrasonic subgingival debridement and would, more importantly, favour its use at less accessible pocket sites and within root furcations as shown by Leon and Vogel (1987).

Choice of instrumentation

This should be influenced primarily by individual operator preference and patient reaction. A consensus in favour of ultrasonic instrumentation by both patients and operators was reported by Suppipat (1974). The preference by operators has also been endorsed by Eaton *et al.* (1985) and Oosterwaal *et al.* (1987). This could be influenced by instrumentation taking less time with ultrasonics than with hand instruments (Suppipat, 1974; Torfason *et al.*, 1979; Badersten *et al.*, 1981; Oosterwaal *et al.*, 1987). In addition, hand instrumentation appears to demand a very much greater degree of operator skill and effort to ensure that each surface being instrumented is not only scraped clean, but that instrumentation strokes do overlap each other (Waerhaug, 1978 b).

Air–powder cleansing

The possible use of the recently introduced air–powder abrasive polishing technique (e.g. Prophy-Jet) for root surface debridement during periodontal surgery must also be considered. The efficacy of this technique in the removal of supragingival stain and plaque is well established (e.g. Weaks *et al.*, 1984; Berkstein *et al.*, 1987), while Atkinson *et al.* (1984) have demonstrated *in vitro* their considerable potential for the debridement of diseased root surfaces and in particular within root furcations. However, Boyde (1984) has shown that air polishing of cementum removed at least 160 μm/min, whilst Atkinson *et al.* (1984) have reported values for removal rates about eight times higher. The abrasivity of the Prophy-Jet device on root surfaces has been shown in *in vitro* investigations to be less than that of hand curettes in the removal of supragingival stain (Berkstein *et al.*, 1987), and of pumice in a rubber cup (Galloway and Pashley, 1987), but it can still cause clinically significant losses of tooth structure if used excessively. This risk coupled with the risks of surgical emphysema following the reflection of a surgical flap and that of possibly implanting powder or any powder residue upon the adjacent periodontal ligament, bone and mucosa (Newman *et al.*, 1985), must obviously be clearly established before its routine use during periodontal surgery can be recommended. In this context, Mishkin *et al.* (1986) concluded that the incidental gingival irritation caused during its use supragingivally was not of any clinical significance. There is also a considerable risk of damage to certain restorative materials (Patterson and McLundie, 1984) which must not be overlooked.

Conclusion

Pending the outcome of further investigation it is clear that the removal of the root surface associated materials rather than the root surface itself should become the most important objective of instrumentation. That is, ideally, instruments and techniques for root cleaning surfaces should remove plaque, calculus and bacterial components from the cementum surface with no sacrifice of tooth substance, and aim to avoid the production of any surface roughness (Lie and Leknes, 1985). The barriers to doing so during non-surgical, gingival response-type therapy, as advocated in Part II, are now considered.

Difficulties of subgingival instrumentation
Factors affecting access

Root surface instrumentation may be impeded by the pocket wall tissue itself, the extent and pattern of pocketing, the root morphology and tooth position in the arch. The operator's attitude and the patient's reactions to treatment are also a major consideration. Each should be examined further.

Tooth position and form

Tooth position appears to be of least importance as demonstrated in several investigations. In the first place no differences have been found in the amounts of residual calculus on non-furcated root surfaces of anterior and posterior teeth following subgingival scaling and root planing alone (Rabbani *et al.*, 1981) and scaling and root planing, with and without periodontal flap surgery (Caffesse *et al.*, 1986). In contrast, Buchanan and Robertson (1987) have reported that surgical scaling and root planing were more effective at an anterior teeth than at the non-furcated aspects of posterior teeth. It is of interest that approximal root surfaces were more readily instrumented than the facial and lingual aspects, in accordance with the observations of Stambough *et al.* (1981). Secondly, the findings of Lindhe *et al.* (1982 a, 1984), Pihlström *et al.* (1984) and Nordland *et al.* (1987) indicate that flat surface sites of molars and of non-molar teeth respond equally well to subgingival debridement. Thirdly, residual deposits of calculus following subgingival debridement have been observed most commonly at the cemento–enamel junctions, reflecting retention factors unrelated to tooth position (Caffesse *et al.*, 1986). On the other hand, Caffesse and co-workers also sometimes observed residual deposits within root surface concavities, grooves and within furcation areas, consistent with the findings of Waerhaug (1980), Stambough *et al.* (1981) and Saglie *et al.* (1987). This has in turn been endorsed by the results of clinical investigations. For example, Badersten *et al.* (1985 c) reported a greater frequency of sites with further attachment loss following non-surgical debridement of non-molar teeth to be associated with root surface fissures, concavities and furcations (and also intra-osseous defects). The clinical failure was attributed to either inadequate subgingival debridement because of an inability to instrument these sites properly, or to poor gingival adaptation at these root surface depressions during healing which allowed recolonization. Similarly Nordland *et al.* (1987) showed a poorer response to debridement at molar furcation sites than elsewhere. These findings thus support current clinical impressions that complex root morphology at molars and at many maxillary first premolars, complicate, if not preclude professional cleaning, even under optimal surgical conditions (Lindhe and Nyman, 1987; Ramfjord, 1987).

Influence of pocket depths

The relevance of pocket depth *per se* in subgingival instrumentation is contentious, although it is widely accepted that the deeper the pocket the more difficult will be the removal of plaque and calculus (Lövdal *et al.*, 1961; Waerhaug, 1978 b; Rabbani *et al.*, 1981; Stambough *et al.*, 1981; Caffesse *et al.*, 1986; Saglie *et al.*, 1986; Buchanan and Robertson, 1987). These workers have claimed that adequate debridement can only be ensured to a subgingival depth of about 5 mm and that surgical intervention is indicated for deeper pockets. The feasibility of effective debridement within such limits has moreover been clearly demonstrated (Tagge *et al.*, 1975; Hughes and Caffesse, 1978; Helldén *et al.*, 1979; Torfason *et al.*, 1979; Morrison *et al.*, 1980; Cercek *et al.*, 1983; Preber and Bergström, 1985).

On the other hand depths up to 7 mm can also be successfully negotiated (Listgarten *et al.*, 1978). In addition, Badersten *et al.* (1984 a), concluded that there was no certain magnitude of pockets, at least at non-furcated surfaces that would preclude adequate debridement. The facility to carry out such debridement is also supported by the fact that 'blind' root planing is as effective as 'open' root planing when the latter is carried out in conjunction with modified Widman flap surgery in subjects with moderately advanced disease (Pihlström *et al.*, 1981 and 1983; Hill *et al.*, 1981; Lindhe *et al.*, 1982 and 1984; Isidor *et al.*, 1984; Westfelt *et al.*, 1985; Lindhe and Nyman, 1985; Isidor and Karring, 1986; Ramfjord *et al.*, 1987).

Factors associated with pocket depth

Several factors other than pocket depth *per se*, might also influence the efficacy of subgingival debridement. These are first, the tough fibrous nature of the pocket wall tissue itself and, even more so, the bony walls of any associated intrabony defects, impede instrument manipulation and preclude any displacement of the instrument shank necessary to avoid interference from clinical crown contours or when negotiating complex root forms. Secondly, pain produced during subgingival inflammation will inhibit the operator and the use of, for example, local anaesthesia may be unacceptable or inconvenient. Thirdly, the more extensive root surface involvement associated with deeper pocketing demands a greater expenditure of operator time and effort. This may not be fully appreciated and so not exercised. In addition, the operator's attitude towards such difficulties, or subconscious bias instilled by traditional teaching, may prejudice the outcome of subgingival debridement in preference to a surgical approach. Unfortunately, although each of these factors have been referred to in the literature (e.g. Waerhaug, 1978 b; Stambough *et al.*, 1981; Saglie *et al.*, 1986; O'Leary, 1986; Badersten *et al.*, 1987), none is readily measurable and so not subject to any controlled investigation. This in turn complicates any analysis of their relative importance in the management of disease. Badersten *et al.* (1987 a) did however conclude that the 24-month outcome of plaque control and debridement of proximal surfaces of non-molar teeth is not influenced by the severity of the initial soft tissue or bony lesions. This has been endorsed by the 48-month findings (Badersten *et al.*, 1987 b) based on 87% of the teeth initially treated.

Operator effort and effect of repeated debridement

The favourable clinical responses to subgingival debridement referred to above may have been due to a combination of more diligent and time-consuming efforts of the clinicians operating under the special conditions of the experimental protocols. For example, between 5–8 h was devoted by Hill *et al.* (1981) and Pihlström *et al.* (1981) to non-surgical debridement and oral hygiene instruction. This has, incidentally, represented more than twice the number of hours of active treatment when compared with that performed surgically (Lindhe *et al.*, 1982). In addition, the operators may have possessed particular skills for subgingival instrumentation, although the importance of operator variability appears to be small (Badersten *et al.*, 1985 a). Thus, negligible differences were observed when assessing the effects of ultrasonic subgingival debridement under local anaesthesia at single rooted teeth with pockets of up to 11 mm, carried out by an experienced periodontist and five individual hygienists with varying professional experience. The time spent on each tooth ranged from 9 to 12 min, whereas in a previous study (Badersten *et al.*, 1984 b) similar clinical results were obtained following an average instrumentation time of 5 min per tooth. Gellin *et al.* (1986) have in turn reported that an average of 90 min per half mouth was necessary to achieve clinically smooth root surfaces.

The possibility that the cumulative effect of repeated subgingival instrumentation at intervals represents an overall effective debridement cannot be discounted. That is, the clinical consequences of incomplete subgingival debridement described by Waerhaug (1978 a) and attributed to non-overlapping instrument strokes and to root surface features (Waerhaug, 1978 b), may have been averted by further debridement at sites displaying persistent signs of subgingival inflammation as advocated in Part II. On the other hand, it has been shown that the significant clinical improvements following a single thorough subgingival debridement (Proye *et al.*, 1982) can be maintained over a 4-month evaluation period (Caton *et al.*, 1982) and moreover be as effective as three repeated debridements in a total period of 9 months (Badersten *et al.*, 1984 b). While this can be interpreted to mean that

an adequate debridement was accomplished initially and that repeated instrumentation was of limited value, it is impossible to draw any firm conclusions because of the difficulties of assessing the efficacy of debridement carried out in each situation.

Chemotherapeutic options

The feasibility of the supplementary or even the alternative use of non-mechanical methods of detoxifying periodontally involved root surfaces should not be overlooked. For example, the attachment of junctional epithelium to calculus deposits, indistinguishable from that occurring elsewhere on tooth surfaces, was attributed by Listgarten and Ellegaard (1973) to the inhibiting effect of chlorhexidine gluconate on plaque formation and a possible concomitant lowering of calculus toxicity. Accordingly, chemotherapeutic measures include the local application of antiseptics (e.g. chlorhexidine) or the more specialized use of antibiotics (e.g. tetracycline, metronidazole, etc.) as described in Chapter 35, and other agents, like 2% sodium desoxycholate and human plasma fraction Cohn IV (Wirthlin *et al.*, 1981; Wirthlin and Hancock, 1982), citric acid (Daly, 1982), EDTA and sodium hypochlorite (Sarbinoff *et al.*, 1983; Lasho *et al.*, 1983), detergent substances (Blomlöf *et al.*, 1987) and mixtures of sodium bicarbonate, sodium chloride and hydrogen peroxide (e.g. Rosling, 1983; Rosling *et al.*, 1986; Greenwell *et al.*, 1985; Pihlström *et al.*, 1987; Wolff *et al.*, 1987). The possibility that the mere physical application of these substances serves to remove residual minute areas of plaque missed by previous mechanical debridement or any dispersed bacteria after instrumentation (Wirthlin and Hancock, 1982) can also not be excluded.

Other considerations

There are other possible explanations for the comparable healing reported after different methods of debridement. In the first place, it is possible that neither the expenditure of time nor effort in root surface debridement has actually been necessary in these investigations and that similar results would have been achieved by a much lesser and simpler superficial root surface cleaning alone, as suggested by the findings of Nyman *et al.* (1986), Moore *et al.* (1986), Smart (1987) and Cheetham *et al.* (1988). Secondly, the improved supragingival plaque control achieved in all but a few clinical investigations, namely those of Knowles *et al.* (1979), Pihlström *et al.* (1981), Ramfjord *et al.* (1982), might have influenced the destructive potential of the subgingival flora (see below) so reducing the relative importance of the different (namely surgical or non-surgical) methods of root surface instrumentation.

Finally, the methods of data analysis may be significant. For example, the use of mean values will mask any marked individual variations in probing attachment levels occurring at site-specific lesions (Socransky *et al.*, 1984). This possibility was demonstrated by Lindhe and Nyman (1985) who examined the data by the use of frequency distributions. Thus, while average recordings of clinical parameters revealed comparable results, the frequency of sites with pockets exceeding 6 mm, which bled on probing, was greater following non-surgical than surgical therapy. Similarly, the lack of longitudinal information about disease activity in the subjects suggests that sites in remission may dilute the measured effect of the therapeutic response. Findings by Goodson (1986) indicate that inactive sites might constitute a large proportion of those being investigated creating a major swamping effect on the results.

Conclusion

It may be reasonable to conclude that given sufficient time be it at a single or successive appointments, a reasonably dextrous operator, anaesthesia where necessary and a cooperative patient, all subgingival root surfaces can be adequately instrumented, root morphology permitting. This implies that, root morphology aside, the need for surgical access for debridement depends more on individual operator and patient preferences than to features of the pocketing *per se*. This is reinforced by the comparable clinical responses to both blind and open root debridement. This, coupled with the demonstration of only minute amounts of cytopathic substances within periodontally involved cementum itself, raises doubts about the validity of traditional concepts of root surface management. Thus, the clinical improvements observed following root surface instrumentation may be due simply to the concurrent removal of overlying root surface accretions and bacterial plaque rather than so-called diseased cementum. Less exacting methods of subgingival root surface debridement may therefore suffice. The clinical implications are far reaching and form the basis of the continuous assessment approach to therapy described in Part II.

Clinical implications

Subgingival instrumentation should aim at root surface cleanliness equivalent to the removal of supragingival coronal accretions and staining during routine professional cleaning. Ultrasonic devices would seem to be preferable in the hands of most operators and at most sites. Only where, despite repeated conscientious efforts in plaque control by both patient and operator, subgingival inflammation is consistently noted at any site, should reflection of a surgical flap to create better access be considered. However, neither the optimal stage at which this is done nor the clinical criteria, upon which this decision is based, have been clearly determined.

Reflection of facial and oral surgical flaps provides optimal access to the related root surfaces, but not the interproximal root surfaces. This necessitates either sacrificing the interdental tissue following the initial flap reflection or their incorporation within one or other surgical flap. Post-surgical interdental cratering is inevitable with the first option and liable to occur elsewhere due to tissue necrosis (*cf.* Chapters 14 and 16) with an outcome that is inconsistent with the surgical objective of access for debridement. Furthermore, the replacement of the flaps in their former positions on completion of root surface debridement, will recreate difficulties for subsequent subgingival debridement because of possible persistent pockets, the very existence of which necessitated surgical intervention in the first place. This is even more applicable at sites involving furcation morphology. Accordingly, surgical intervention should preferably be directed at ensuring future instrumentation, that is pocket elimination plus, where necessary, the appropriate correction of furcation morphology. The evidence in support of this is considered in Chapter 29.

Assessment of the need for surgical access

General considerations

Assessment of disease progression as an indication for surgical intervention, and indeed in maintenance care, has been focused primarily on the clinical characteristics of periodontitis. Increasing attention is, however, being devoted to immunological responses with respect to both peripheral blood antibody profiles and local tissue markers, and to microbiological monitoring. In addition the influence of the natural progression of disease and of the individual patient susceptibility and age upon these assessments cannot be overlooked.

Currently, the most important clinical assessments are of bleeding on probing, probing pocket depths and probing attachment levels and of radiographic presentations. Gingival bleeding is universally accepted as an indicator of gingival inflammation (Reviews: Greenstein, 1984; Polson and Goodson, 1985 and see also Lindhe *et al.*, 1978; Brecy *et al.*, 1987; Ericsson *et al.*, 1987) but its relationship to disease progression is unclear. Similarly, observed changes in attachment levels may only indicate past destruction and not differentiate between stable and progressive periodontal lesions (Reviews: Goodson, 1986; Lindhe *et al.*, 1986; Kornman, 1987). Accordingly, as pointed out by Badersten (1985 d) 'any therapist who elects to institute supplementary surgical therapy following re-evaluation based upon clinical signs of bleeding, suppuration and indeed deep residual probing depths, should be aware that he may be treating residual symptoms of disease rather than the disease itself.'

Bleeding and suppuration and disease progression

The diagnostic sensitivity of bleeding on probing is poor, for the chances of it actually being associated with actively diseased sites are low (Haffajee *et al.*, 1983; Badersten *et al.*, 1985 d; Vanooteghem *et al.*, 1987). Similarly, the diagnostic specificity is poor, because bleeding could even be detected at sites with no active disease. Lang *et al.* (1986) have observed, however, that sites which bled on probing at four successive maintenance appointments had a 30% chance of loss of attachment, whereas sites which bled on only one visit or not at all had less than a 3% chance of losing attachment. Disappearance of the sign of bleeding on probing in periodontitis must be regarded as beneficial, since it is associated with diminution of connective tissue inflammatory infiltrate (Lindhe *et al.*, 1986) and increased amounts of collagen which is in turn manifested clinically as pocket closure (Lindhe *et al.*, 1982 a, 1984). Indeed, the findings of Harper and Robinson (1987) suggest that the absence of diminishing probing depths following subgingival debridement is a more sensitive method than bleeding changes in identifying refractory sites in deep periodontal pockets (see below). Finally, the results of other investigations suggest that the bleeding/plaque ratio in an individual may be regarded as a prognostic indicator for the degree of experimentally induced gingival inflammation (Abbas *et al.*, 1986) and for periodontal breakdown (Van der Velden *et al.*, 1986).

Suppuration also does not reflect active destructive periodontal disease activity (Haffajee *et al.*, 1983; Badersten *et al.*, 1985 d) but rather only the accumulation of dead and dying polymorphs, bacteria, tissue breakdown products and fluid exudate. As such it is the biological defence reaction to a tissue insult and does not indicate the succcess or failure of that defence. Thus, the predictability value of suppuration in identifying a deteriorating site was shown by Badersten *et al.* (1985 d) to be, at best, only 1 out of 3, but was improved to 1 out of 2 when occurring with bleeding. Gingival crevicular fluid has long been associated with inflammation (Review: Polson and Goodson, 1985) and its

components may yet prove to be useful as diagnostic indicators (Reviews: Fine and Mandell, 1986; Kornman, 1987).

Probing and disease progression

The periodontal probe is used to measure periodontal pocket depth and periodontal attachment levels, but is associated with a number of problems (Reviews: Listgarten, 1980; Polson and Goodson, 1985).

Probing difficulties

The factors affecting reproducibility of probing attachment level measurements have been evaluated by Badersten *et al.* (1984 c). In the first place, accuracy can be no better than and ± 0.5 mm by estimating between calibration intervals. Secondly, recordings may be complicated by the frequent lack of distinct fixed reference points and of parallax error. The former can be resolved by using soft acrylic onlays (e.g. Badersten *et al.*, 1984 c; Isidor *et al.*, 1984 b; Watts, 1987), as in clinical trials, but these are probably uneconomic for routine clinical practice. Electronic probing devices have been developed which automatically determine the cemento–enamel junction (Jeffcoat *et al.*, 1986) or the occlusal or incisal surface of the tooth (Birek *et al.*, 1987) as fixed reference points and utilize a controlled pressure probing force. The risk of inconsistent probing forces in clinical practice and the establishment of inter-examiner reproducibility is readily obviated by the use of such controlled pressure probes (Review: Polson and Goodson, 1985) as shown, for example, by Kalkwarf *et al.* (1986) and McCulloch *et al.* (1987).

There are also difficulties in standardization of probe design in view of the many different types available and in probing position and angulation (Watts, 1987). The latter relate, in particular, to the deflective contour of root or crown and of physical closure of pocket spaces associated with inflammatory resolution which restrict the probing path (Badersten *et al.*, 1987). Finally, patient cooperation and tolerance are critical to accurate measurement.

Inflammation and probing

The presence of an inflammatory infiltrate in the gingival connective tissue and the apical extension of this infiltrate will influence the results of probing assessments (see Listgarten, 1980; Polson and Goodson, 1985). Thus, when the tissues subjacent to pocket epithelium are infiltrated with inflammatory cells, the probe usually penetrates beyond the apical extension of the dentogingival epithelium resulting in an over-estimation of true levels of attachment. Conversely, when the inflammatory infiltrate resolves as a result of therapy, the probe tip will, in most cases, not reach the apical termination of the epithelium so leading to an under-estimated recording. The practical implication is that reduced probing depths may only represent the resolution of inflammatory lesions rather than gains in attachment (e.g. Lindhe *et al.*, 1982 a, 1984).

Effect of data analysis

There has in recent years been much discussion on statistical interpretation of probing measurements (Review: Imrey, 1986). Furthermore the variability inherent in repeated probing measurements necessitates establishing a threshold measurement. The 'critical probing depth', or 'tolerance' has to be beyond the expected variability in the probing technique (see Haffajee and Socransky, 1986; Lindhe *et al.*, 1986), for one to be confident that a true loss of attachment has actually occurred. Thus, for example, in a long-term evaluation of periodontal treatment, Isidor and Karring (1986) regarded only attachment losses of more than 2 mm as valid indicators of destruction.

The pattern of progressive disease

The chances of actually detecting true increases in probing attachment levels at any one site are small. This is because chronic inflammatory periodontal disease appears not to be the generalized slowly progressive condition as traditionally believed, but to progress as acute exacerbations followed by periods of remission involving a number of site specific lesions (Socransky *et al.*, 1984). That is, various numbers of sites in an individual's mouth may be affected at some stage of the disease process at any one time, undergoing only brief bursts of destruction resulting in significant probing attachment level losses over relatively short periods of time.

Goodson *et al.* (1982) have, for example, shown in a group of 22 untreated patients with existing periodontal pockets, that only 5.7% of 1155 sites, monitored at monthly intervals for 1 year, became deeper. Moreover, a variable pattern of deterioration was observed, with some sites deepening progressively while others only deepened at the end of the monitoring period. Similarly, in 64 adults with untreated moderate disease monitored over a 6-year period, significant attachment losses (>2 mm) were observed in only 12% of all sites examined (Lindhe *et al.*, 1983 a). Once again a variable pattern was observed, with only a third of the sites deteriorating in the first 3-year period showing any further loss, while about half of those sites showing no loss in the first period did so in the second 3 years. In the same study another 36 adults with untreated advanced disease, demonstrated 3.2% of sites with attachment losses (>2 mm) over 1 year.

It is of interest that similar patterns of destruction have also been reported at single rooted teeth during a 2-year assessment of non-surgical periodontal treatment in 33 subjects (Badersten *et al.*, 1985 c). Probing attachment loss (>1 mm) was demonstrated in 4.9% of the 1368 sites examined when compared to baseline. Data analysis by scatter diagrams and regression analysis revealed a gradual linear deterioration in 73% of sites. The majority of the other sites sustained initial early losses followed by stable measurements, while the remaining few exhibited undulating changes.

Conclusion

The above findings highlight the difficulties of establishing incremental attachment loss over comparatively short time intervals. This reinforces the need for long periods of assessment (*cf.* Chapter 12) during which periodic careful probing attachment level measurements are recorded. Even then, when a loss of attachment is recorded there is no way of determining if it is progressive. Conversely, where no changes are evident, deterioration or gain may yet follow. Only where incremental attachment losses are consistently observed may progressive periodontal disease activity be confirmed.

Other methods

Radiographic quantification of crestal bone levels has for long been used in treatment planning (Review: Lang and Hill, 1977). The different methods of reading radiographs have been compared (Albander and Abbas, 1986) and the absolute technique (Albander *et al.*, 1985) shown to be preferable. The use of more sophisticated radiological techniques, such as computer-assisted subtraction radiography (e.g. Gröndahl *et al.*, 1983; Gröndahl and Gröndahl, 1983; Hausmann *et al.*, 1985; Hausmann *et al.*, 1986; Gröndhal *et al.*, 1987) and radiodensitometric analysis (e.g. Ortman *et al.*, 1985; Payot *et al.*, 1987), for measuring bone destruction have much to offer. Similarly, the use of microbiological techniques for monitoring periodontal flora and the assessment of immunological responses detected in peripheral blood, tissue biopsies and crevicular fluid as indications of progressive periodontal destruction appear to be promising (Chapter 4, Polson and Goodson, 1985; Goodson, 1986; Kornman, 1987 and see also Shenker, 1987). However, in order to establish any definite association with progressive periodontal destruction, these parameters must first be correlated with other clinical criteria which measure disease activity.

Individual susceptibility

Disease and lifespan

The net effect of periodic losses of attachment on the overall rate of attachment loss in terms of the retention of a functional dentition during the individual's natural lifespan should also be considered. This will be closely related to both the natural history of disease as well as its 'unnatural history' (Greene, 1986), in which the process is disturbed by patient homecare and professional intervention.

Individual variation

Some patients are more susceptible to periodontal destruction than others, whilst the extent of involvement in each individual can vary widely, independent of treatment (Hirschfeld and Wasserman, 1978; Axelsson and Lindhe, 1978 and 1981; Selikowitz *et al.*, 1981; Lindhe and Nyman, 1984; Buckley and Crowley, 1984; Baelum *et al.*, 1986; Listgarten, 1986). As an example of a group without periodontal care, Löe *et al.* (1986) have demonstrated three subgroups of a unique Sri Lankan population. The analysis was based on attachment losses and tooth mortality rates with teeth being lost due to spontaneous exfoliation or digital removal. The subgroups comprised individuals ($\approx 8\%$) with rapid progression of periodontal disease, those ($\approx 81\%$) with moderate progression, and a group ($\approx 11\%$) who exhibited no progression of periodontal disease beyond gingivitis. Other investigations following periodontal treatment have revealed that recurrent disease occurs in relatively few individuals and that the bulk of the affected surfaces observed occurred in fewer still (Hirschfeld and Wasserman, 1978; Selikowitz *et al.*, 1981; Lindhe and Nyman, 1984).

Age and disease

The influence of the patient's age on the response to treatment and the predisposition to recurrent disease should also be considered (Review: Van der Velden, 1984). It was concluded by Lindhe *et al.* (1985) that the age of patients with moderately or advanced periodontal destruction did not influence either healing or the incidence of recurrent disease, although this finding is at variance with that reported by Abbas et al. (1984).

Supragingival plaque levels

The influence of supragingival plaque levels on progressive periodontal attachment losses is unclear (Review: Kornman, 1986). Some studies have demonstrated more rapid deterioration in individuals with poorer oral hygiene (Suomi *et al.*, 1971;

Löe *et al.*, 1978; Axelsson and Lindhe, 1978, 1981). Others have found little periodontal destruction despite a high prevalence of gingival inflammation (Listgarten, 1986; Reddy, 1985). Improved plaque levels from toothbrushing alone have been shown by Chawla *et al.* (1975) to be of little benefit in curing gingivitis or checking attachment losses, but toothbrushing was effective when combined with periodic scaling. Similarly, Listgarten *et al.* (1978), Hellden *et al.* (1979) and Lindhe *et al.* (1983 b and c) demonstrated that improved supragingival plaque measures had little effect on probing attachment levels. Limited improvements in clinical probing depths, due primarily to reduced gingival inflammation, have however been demonstrated following improved oral hygiene by Tagge *et al.* (1975), Tabita *et al.* (1981), Cercek *et al.* (1983) and Badersten *et al.* (1984 a), although some gain in clinical attachment has also been observed (Müller *et al.*, 1986).

Some relationship does appear to exist between supragingival and subgingival microbial activities. Subgingival bacterial recolonization following debridement occurs more rapidly with ineffective supragingival plaque control (Mousques *et al.*, 1980; Magnusson *et al.*, 1984) although no such differences were observed by Lavanchy *et al.* (1987). Recolonization following periodic subgingival debridement may also be averted by supragingival cleaning alone (Badersten *et al.*, 1984 a; Lindhe *et al.*, 1984). Furthermore, significant reductions in subgingival anaerobes have resulted from frequent professional removal of supragingival plaque alone in humans (Smulow *et al.*, 1983) and in monkeys (Siegrist and Kornman, 1982). Similarly, Müller *et al.* (1986) observed a shift in the composition of the subgingival microflora to that associated with relatively healthy periodontal conditions following periodic supragingival professional cleaning alone. However the possible influence of the repeated sampling of the subgingival flora cannot be ruled out. In contrast, others (Listgarten *et al.*, 1978; Kho *et al.*, 1985; Beltrami *et al.*, 1987) have shown that in humans, improved supragingival plaque control measures alone have little effect on microbiological parameters.

Conclusion

Caution must be exercised in the interpretation of the traditional clinical methods of detecting progressive disease to support surgical intervention for the purposes of both proper debridement and for pocket elimination. Until totally reliable and practical indicators of destructive disease activity have been developed, the dilemma of when to intervene surgically will continue to be resolved by the clinical impressions and priorities of individual operators.

This must be coupled with the patients' understanding of the problem and their attitude to treatment as emphasized by Pihlström *et al.* (1983).

Where surgical access for debridement is decided upon, residual probing depths will frequently persist. This is due to incomplete pocket closure and the limited gingival recession expected following this type of surgery. The subsequent management of these sites will now be considered.

Management following surgical debridement

Evaluation

Any evaluation of post-surgical debridement therapy must of necessity be based primarily upon findings following modified Widman flap (MWF) surgery with which all but two of the controlled clinical investigations on surgical debridement (Svoboda *et al.*, 1984; Lindhe and Nyman, 1985), have been associated. Such a comparison is in order because surgical flap reflection to gain access for instrumentation and its subsequent replacement is essentially the same as the MWF procedure. Furthermore, the technical difference represented by the intentional removal of the pocket epithelium in the latter appears to be of little consequence because of the rapid re-epithelialization that follows. This results in a situation very similar to that following surgical access therapy as in the Kirkland flap where the epithelium is retained (Svoboda *et al.*, 1984 and Lindhe and Nyman 1985).

The maintenance regimes

The nature of post-surgical maintenance depends on the dentogingival relationships achieved. Sites with minimal probing depth attributed to the establishment of a long junction epithelium, pocket closure or marginal gingival recession, are maintained as any normal healthy dentogingival junction and require no further comment here. Whereas, sites with residual probing depths due to a failure of pocket closure demand more specific measures. The extent of the need for any subgingival instrumentation is however not always made clear from the literature when examining how the various maintenance regimes are implemented.

Long-term studies

Routine supra- and subgingival prophylaxis was carried out three to four times per year by Hill *et al.* (1981) and Pihlström *et al.* (1983), the latter demanding cleaning to the best of a hygienist's ability during 1-h appointments. In contrast, after an initial intensive regime of 2-weekly professional cleaning (ad modum Axelsson and Lindhe, 1974). Lindhe *et al.* (1984) instituted three to four monthly bouts of professional cleaning between 6 and 24 months, but then avoided further subgingival instrumentation during the subsequent professional cleaning until completion of the study at 5 years. Isidor and Karring (1986) in turn performed subgingival scaling in conjunction with professional cleaning at each recall appointment over the last 4 years of a 5-year investigation period. The recalls were scheduled at 3-monthly intervals in the second year and 6-monthly thereafter. A 3-monthly regime was also adopted by Ramfjord *et al.* (1987) over a 5-year assessment period.

Short-term studies

A 2-weekly cleaning regime (ad modum Axelsson and Lindhe, 1974), was utilized by Isidor *et al.* (1984) and Westfelt *et al.* (1985) over 6 months, and by Lindhe and Nyman (1985) during the initial 3 months, followed by 3-monthly prophylaxis up to 1 year. Westfelt *et al.* (1985) specifically avoided subgingival instrumentation altogether during the maintenance phase because of previous studies which showed that an optimal postoperative standard of supragingival plaque control is the decisive factor in proper healing and tissue maturation following healing (Rosling *et al.*, 1976 a, b; Nyman *et al.*, 1977).

Influence of oral hygiene

The importance of a high standard of supragingival plaque control following surgical debridement has been demonstrated by Lindhe *et al.* (1984). Virtually no signs of recurrent disease occurred in individuals with a high frequency of plaque-free tooth surfaces following effective root surface debridement. Conversely, those with a low frequency of plaque-free tooth surfaces demonstrated a high frequency of sites showing inflammation and additional losses of attachment. This has, however, been questioned by the findings of Ramfjord *et al.* (1982, 1987) and Pihlström *et al.* (1983). Clinical success accrued from periodic professional supra- and subgingival cleaning alone without any improvement in pre-treatment supragingival plaque indices. This has been endorsed in another investigation in which the number of sites deteriorating did not correlate with the levels of self-performed oral hygiene (Isidor and Karring, 1986). These workers thus concluded that subgingival plaque removal is an important factor in arresting the progression of periodontitis in patients not maintaining a high standard of oral hygiene. Furthermore, it was suggested that abstention from subgingival scaling might have been responsible for the recurrent disease observed by Lindhe *et al.* (1984) (see above). This does in turn imply that adequate access has existed for this periodic subgingival cleaning and does in addition question the need for surgical access at the outset. Indeed the findings by Ramfjord *et al.* (1987) indicate that although sites requiring retreatment during the maintenance phase were derived mainly from non-surgically treated sites, the results of additional blind debridement were as effective as further surgical measures.

Technique in perspective

The investigations on surgical debridement would seem to support the efficacy of the MWF technique in averting further attachment losses; this, despite the presence in many instances of residual probing depths that were similar to those existing before operation and which might be expected to preclude further effective subgingival debridement during the post-surgical observation periods. The comparable findings with non-surgical blind debridement throughout these investigations must however be kept in perspective. This suggests that the actual technique used for debridement is less important than the efficiency of the root instrumentation but does also assume that adequate access exists for this. On the other hand, in each of the investigations the possibility of spontaneous remissions in disease activity being misinterpreted as clinical success following treatment should not be discounted.

The significance of residual pockets

Microbial repopulation

Residual pockets following surgical debridement may be associated with persistent subgingival inflammation which suggests bacterial recolonization. This might stem from either residual subgingival sources, following incomplete debridement (Waerhaug, 1978 b), or by apical proliferation from supragingival sources (Magnusson *et al.*, 1984). Thus it has been shown that, in the presence of a high standard of supragingival plaque control, significant repopulation can be averted for 6 months following subgingival instrumentation (Braatz *et al.*, 1985; MacAlpine *et al.*, 1985). Whereas, with ineffective oral hygiene, bacterial recolonization is very much more rapid and will develop within a few months (Mousques *et al.*, 1980; Magnusson *et al.*, 1984). This endorses not only the critical role of the patient in therapy and of not intervening surgically until control of reasonably accessible plaque has been demonstrated, as prescribed in Part II, but also of gaining optimal pocket elimination in the interests of subsequent debridement, whenever pocket surgery is undertaken.

Residual bacteria

The importance of residual bacterial flora for subgingival repopulation following periodontal surgery is supported by the fact that totally effective root surface debridement may not always be achieved (Eaton *et al.*, 1985). Furthermore, the findings of Westfelt *et al.* (1983), revealed smaller gains in clinical attachment in subjects maintained on a chlorhexidine mouthwash following MWF surgery, than those who received supra- and subgingival professional cleaning, ad modum Axelsson and Lindhe (1974). Thus, as chlorhexidine rinsing is unlikely to have any influence subgingivally (Flötra *et al.*, 1972), any recurrence of inflammation in the deeper portion of the pockets will most likely have occurred from subgingival recolonization arising from residual deposits. This repopulation may nevertheless be checked by periodic subgingival debridement coupled with a high standard of oral hygiene during the early phase of maintenance, followed by supragingival plaque control measures alone (Lindhe *et al.*, 1984). Implicit in this early phase of the maintenance regime is adequate access to the subgingival root surfaces. This is, as noted above, even more critical when oral hygiene is inadequate, for recolonization control is then dependent upon periodic subgingival debridement (Ramfjord *et al.*, 1982, 1987; Pihlström *et al.*, 1983, 1984; Isidor and Karring 1986).

Post-surgical control

The evidence for the role of subgingival root surface debridement during postoperative maintenance care is equivocal. If disease control depends ultimately upon recurrent subgingival debridement then the rationale for the surgical component of treatment must be questioned. That is, if these sites can be negotiated following surgery would they not also have been accessible prior to surgery? It does therefore seem that the decision to intervene surgically must ultimately be dictated by the individual operator's discretion (Ramfjord *et al.*, 1987) rather than objective parameters. It must be conceded that some marginal tissue shrinkage (gingival recession) does occur following surgical debridement (Badersten *et al.*, 1984 a, b; Isidor *et al.*, 1984 a; Lindhe *et al.*, 1987). This results in some decrease in post-surgical probing depths with respect to debridement. The extent of these residual probing depths is related to the presurgical pocket depths (e.g. Knowles *et al.*, 1979; Pihlström *et al.*, 1981, 1983; Isidor *et al.*, 1984 b). It should however be re-emphasized that while somewhat greater pocket reductions are usually achieved initially following attempted surgical pocket elimination, these are not maintained over long time periods (Hill, 1981; Pihlström, 1981, 1983; Lindhe *et al.*, 1982 a; Ramfjord, 1987).

Root morphology

The difficulties related to root morphology encountered during maintenance debridement may also prove to be insurmountable. The likelihood of residual subgingival colonies being present following root surface debridement exists even with the benefit of surgical access at the comparatively inaccessible furcations (Waerhaug, 1980; Stambough *et al.*, 1981; Saglie *et al.*, 1986 and see also Chapter 29). Subgingival repopulation would then seem to be inevitable because of the difficulties of negotiating these sites during maintenance care as stressed by Ramfjord *et al.* (1987).

Conclusion

Where the development of a reasonably accessible dentogingival morphology is likely following surgical debridement, then blind root surface debridement will probably be as effective and would be the treatment of choice. Where probing depths greater than about 5 mm would remain following surgical debridement, difficulties with subsequent subgingival debridement similar to those which necessitated surgical access at the outset should be anticipated. Surgical pocket elimination by apical repositioning or resection of the flap should therefore be carried out instead. Finally, surgical access for debridement should only be considered where the uneven pattern of breakdown prevents or precludes pocket elimination at the most severely affected sites and when pocket reduction must be accepted as a compromise.

29

The role of surgery:
II The choice of surgical technique and
post-surgical maintenance

The surgical options

There are three basic options in soft tissue pocket surgery. The first is to gain surgical reattachment of the detached tissue as described in Part II. This procedure is for practical purposes, synonymous with the curettage technique (see below), raising access flaps for root surface debridement (Lindhe *et al.*, 1982), the modified Widman flap (MWF) (Ramfjord and Nissle, 1976), the Kirkland flap (e.g. (Lindhe and Nyman, 1985), the gingival fibre retention technique (Levine, 1972) and the excisional new attachment procedure (ENAP) (Yukna, 1976). These procedures are referred to collectively as pocket correction. The other two options aim in turn to eliminate the pocket by resecting the detached tissue (gingivectomy) or, alternatively, by displacing this tissue apically (apically repositioned flap) as described in Part II (see also Kieser, 1974 and Review: Kakehashi and Parakkal, 1982).

The above suprabony pocket management techniques are also applicable in the presence of intrabony pocketing and where the non-supporting bony component of such pocketing is amenable to comparable surgical options. Thus, bony regeneration within the defect (bone fill) represents surgical reattachment. This healing is, in common with its suprabony soft tissue counterpart, rarely accompanied by a new connective tissue attachment between cementum and bone (new attachment) (see Chapter 31). Instead a long junctional epithelium becomes interposed. Resection of the non-supporting bone (osteoectomy) is in turn analgous to suprabony

pocket elimination by external bevel gingivectomy (see Chapter 14).

While the above classification is useful for descriptive and teaching purposes, the clinical application is less clear cut. This is because the variable pattern of periodontal breakdown encountered in any surgical field necessitates the use of several different surgical methods. Moreover the inevitable overlapping of these methods coupled with the risk of jeopardizing the contiguous less involved tissues in the pursuit of the objectives at individual sites, means that compromise technical solutions are frequently imposed. The resulting difficulties of deciding upon the appropriate surgical method are greatly simplified by the flexibility of the surgical approach advocated in Part II.

Influence on clinical investigations

The variable pattern of disease in any one mouth also hampers the clinical investigation of any pocket elimination technique by precluding its precise execution in all parts of the surgical field to eliminate any pocket. Thus, neither complete resection of the pocket nor the requisite apical repositioning is physically possible at sites with uneven attachment losses resulting in a surgical reattachment relationship instead. Similarly, even in the MWF technique the intended flap positioning might not be achieved and the flap become displaced apically, so that, in many instances, the differences between the immediate post-surgical outcomes of the techniques become quite small. These difficulties have been considered in some detail in Chapters 14 and 17.

The operative difficulties cited above also complicate the interpretation of clinical investigations by presenting some difficulties, not least of which relates to the above cited operative problems. It is also not easy to extract and compare, or coordinate the findings from the various studies because of differences in experimental design. These differences may involve the initial disease severity, the operational sites (i.e. split mouth or whole mouth), molar and non-molar teeth, the use of control sites or not, the inclusion and length of postoperative evaluation periods, levels of pre- and post-surgical plaque control and its supervision, or of the nature and frequency of professional cleaning. In addition, it is difficult to connect grouped data, relating to initial pocket depths, to individual clinical cases having various combinations of pocket depths. The problems related to the methods of data analysis and presentation have been described previously (Chapter 28). Finally, misleading or inaccurate terminology with respect to surgical procedures undertaken, means that it is not always clear precisely what has been carried out nor what influence this might have had on the surgical outcome. In particular, the term modified Widman flap (MWF) is loosely ascribed to several pocket reduction-type techniques and, to compound matters, is rarely performed as described originally by Ramfjord and Nissle (1974). The latter shortcoming is undoubtedly due to the technical difficulties encountered in carrying out this technique. It would be instructive to consider these difficulties here and also the role of tissue curettage which features as one of the treatment modalities in several of the non-surgical and surgical therapy comparative investigations.

The modified Widman flap

The technical difficulties

The initial inverse bevel incision made at the facial and oral aspects to excise the epithelialized pocket lining is not possible interproximally. Any effort to do so inevitably results in total destruction of interdental tissue and the development of an interdental soft tissue crater. This then precludes post-surgical tissue adaptation as intended. The exaggerated surgical scalloping advocated to facilitate closer interproximal flap adaptation, is seldom achieved at the molar teeth and especially within approximal root surface concavities. Even where successful there is a high risk of necrosis of the resulting inevitable narrow finger-like parts of the flap and in turn post-surgical interdental cratering. Close interproximal flap adaptation may, however, be achieved anteriorly because of the labiolingual

dimensions of the teeth (*cf.* Chapters 14–16). The secondary crevicular incisions extending down to the crestal bone, intended to preserve the supracrestal periodontal attachment to the root surface, are not readily achieved when pocket depths are unequal and even more so within bony defects. This also applies to the final horizontal incision coronal to the crestal bone designed to free the cervical wedge tissue whilst preserving the supracrestal attachment. Difficulty does incidentally also arise in the gingival fibre retention technique (Levine, 1972).

The surgical outcome

The difficulties experienced are such that the immediate operative oucome of the MWF is not unlike that following the technically simpler surgical reattachment technique as described in Part II. Furthermore, the surgical objectives of both techniques are the same so that the MWF is not advocated as an operative technique, although the frequent finding of the term modified Widman flap in the literature necessitates its use in the subsequent review for consistency.

Tissue curettage

Introduction

A general definition of curettage has been given as 'The removal of granulation tissue growths or other material from the wall of a cavity or other surface' (Jablonski, 1982). In periodontal therapy the terms gingival curettage, subgingival curettage, root curettage or simply curettage are frequently encountered. Gingival curettage relates to the soft tissue pocket wall and subgingival curettage to the tissue between the apical end of the epithelial attachment and the alveolar crest (Grant *et al.,* 1979; Ramfjord and Ash, 1979; Carranza, 1984). The practical differences between them is, however, not clear cut for gingival curettage is likely to include inadvertently some subgingival curettage. The single term subgingival curettage is used here. The use of the term curettage is not explicit and that in relation to root surfaces is misleading and best replaced by root surface instrumentation or subgingival debridement (Lindhe *et al.,* 1982).

Subgingival curettage has been advocated for resolving a persistent gingivitis, reducing pockets, encouraging a more rapid healing, debriding pockets presurgically, treating periodontal abscesses and for use during periodontal maintenance therapy (Grant *et al.,* 1979; Ramfjord and Ash, 1979; Manson, 1980; Goldman and Cohen, 1980; MacPhee and Cowley, 1981; Carranza, 1984). It is also sometimes recommended as a non-definitive procedure in cases where more complex surgical techniques are contraindicated owing to the patient's age, systemic disorders or psychological problems (Grant *et al.*, 1979; Carranza, 1984).

The technique aims to create a surgical wound surface which is adapted closely to the debrided root surface with the expectation of the development of a new connective tissue attachment. This rarely occurs (see below) although pocket closure is achieved with or without the development of a long junctional epithelium. Pocket closure may however also follow root surface debridement alone as described in Chapter 28 and in Part II (Gingival response), warranting closer examination of the subgingival curettage technique and its effects.

The rationale

Removal of noxious products

The intentional debridement of the pocket wall to remove debris, toxic products and sloughing tissue (Review: Ramfjord and Ash, 1979) is reasonable. However, this appears to be an inevitable accompaniment of subgingival root surface instrumentation alone (Ramfjord and Kiester, 1954; Moskow, 1962; Schaffer *et al.*, 1964; O'Bannon, 1964) and more especially from the additional flushing effect of any ultrasonic scaling device used (Review: Brown *et al.*, 1987). Haemorrhage and inflammatory exudate following root surface instrumentation may also provide flushing, although this can be enhanced by deliberate curettage by virtue of the resulting more marked inflammatory infiltrate (Stahl *et al.*, 1971 and Lopez and Belvederessi, 1977).

Bacterial invasion

Bacterial invasion of pocket epithelium has been shown in some cases of advanced adult and juvenile type periodontitis (Review: Saglie and Elbaz, 1983; and more recently Slots and Genco, 1984; Manor *et al.*, 1984; Saglie *et al.*, 1985, 1987; Pertuiset *et al.*, 1987) and in animal models (Allenspach-Petrzilka and Guggenheim, 1983; Sanavi *et al.*, 1985). On the other hand, the findings may be explained by bacterial translocation into the tissues (Listgarten, 1986; Liakoni *et al.*, 1987 a, b; Saravanamuttu, 1987), as is evidenced by the common occurrence of bacteraemias following professional instrumentation. Ericsson *et al.* (1987) have in turn failed to demonstrate bacterial invasion in experimental periodontitis. The removal of any invaded tissue or that containing bacteria might yet prove necessary in some cases and so warrant subgingival curettage, but this requires further investigation.

Removal of epithelium

The rationale for the removal of the epithelialized pocket lining and the elimination of the epithelial

rete ridge structure is questionable. Thus, once the epithelium has been removed it reforms rapidly (Review: Smith and Echeverri, 1984), whilst the rete ridges may undergo spontaneous involution following root debridement alone (Waerhaug, 1955; Lindhe *et al.*, 1978). In addition, a long junctional epithelium rather than a new connective tissue attachment invariably results (Caton and Zander, 1979), although some new attachment may occur at the apical aspect of the healed wound (Caton *et al.*, 1980) and at small 'windows' within the long junctional epithelium (Caton and Zander, 1979). It is therefore fortunate that the long junctional epithelial adhesion has been shown to be no more vulnerable to plaque-induced disease than a normal dentogingival attachment (Magnusson *et al.*, 1983; Beaumont *et al.*, 1984; Stahl and Froum, 1986). The existence of pocket epithelium can, in turn, be assumed to be of little clinical importance in surgical therapy other than following flap apical repositioning (see below), when it may impede healing, although there is as yet no documentary support for this.

Creation of surgical wound

The creation of a surgical wound by curettage neither enhances the rate nor the quality of healing compared with that following root debridement alone, as measured by reductions of gingival inflammation or of pocket depths, or by increases of clinical attachment levels (Ainslie and Caffesse, 1981 a and b; Hill *et al.*, 1981; Echeverria and Caffesse, 1983). Furthermore, the surgical removal of granulation tissue in conjunction with root debridement, did not improve healing when compared with root debridement alone carried out via Kirkland-type access flaps (Lindhe and Nyman, 1985). This has been endorsed by Smith *et al.* (1987).

The operative technique

Tissue removal

This is usually performed with sharp hand curettes commencing at the bottom of the pocket progressively dissecting away epithelium and inflamed connective tissue until a firm mature collagen surface is detected. There is no consensus view as to how effectively this can be achieved (Review: Smith and Echeverri, 1984). In most instances some epithelium is retained and the junctional epithelium is invariably disrupted with a risk of a further loss of attachment.

Site accessibility

The technique is performed readily only at the accessible facial and oral aspects where external digital pressure against the detached gingiva (considered essential to counteract the force of the curetting strokes) can be applied. This in turn is not possible interproximally because of the use of instrumentation compounded by the confined space and the limited mesiodistal dimensions of the interdental tissue septum. Attempted curettage leads almost inevitably to tissue perforation and possibly even total disruption of the septum and the creation of an interdental crater at completion of operation. Even where this is avoided, close apposition of the remaining interdental septal tissue to the adjacent tooth surfaces is technically impossible (see Figure 14.3), thereby thwarting the surgical objective.

Alternative methods of tissue removal

Ultrasonic devices have been shown to be effective for the removal of pocket epithelium but are less so for connective tissue (Nadler, 1962; Sanderson, 1965). The heat generated apparently leads to coagulation of the tissue which is then removed by the mechanical action of the vibrating instrument point and the cavitational effect of the cooling water spray.

   Surgical excision of the pocket wall tissue with an inverse bevel incision is utilized in the essentially comparable techniques of the excisional new attachment procedure (ENAP) (Yukna, 1976) and the modified Widman flap (MWF) (Ramfjord and Nissle, 1974). However, Litch *et al.* (1984) revealed that pocket epithelium cannot be removed consistently with either crestal or subcrestal inverse bevel incisions. Similarly, removal of interdental tissue epithelium is even less likely, short of total excision of the tissue septum and creation of an interdental crater.

   Chemical curettage has been recommended (Review: Smith and Escheverri, 1984), but its use is limited by the unpredictable extent of epithelium removal and the potential for uncontrolled tissue destruction. This appears not to be the case with the use of sodium hypochlorite and citric acid (Kalwarf *et al.*, 1982), following which healing is similar to that occurring after mechanical curettage (Vieira *et al.*, 1982). In another investigation (Forgas and Gound, 1987) the technique failed to enhance the effects of scaling and root planing alone.

Root surface instrumentation

Whatever technique is used for subgingival curettage the associated root surfaces are always instrumented, clouding any assessment of the relative roles of each operative component. Indeed, Manson (1980) concluded that ' . . . it is likely that the tissue changes that take place after subgingival curettage are very little different from the tissue changes after

an efficient scaling', while Ramfjord (1980) stated 'It is not known if soft tissue curettage adds anything to the results of scaling and root planing' and subsequently (Ramfjord *et al.*, 1987) that 'deliberate soft-tissue curettage does not seem to enhance the results of scaling and root planing'. Unfortunately, assessment is further complicated by the fact that an element of inadvertent soft tissue curettage is, as noted above, inevitable during root surface instrumentation. The extent of the tissue removal will be influenced by the degree of inflammation, the operator's care and dexterity, the depth of instrumentation and, as pointed out by Isidor *et al.* (1984), whether or not local anaesthesia is used. However the fact that local anaesthesia is so rarely necessary for subgingival debridement implies that minimal inadvertent subgingival curettage is sustained during gingival response therapy (see Part II). In addition, comparable clinical results have been achieved with root debridement alone and that supplemented by subgingival curettage (Ainslie and Caffesse, 1981 a and b; Hill *et al.*, 1981; Echeverria and Caffesse, 1983), further questioning the role of this technique.

Conclusion

The additional tissue trauma and postoperative discomfort sustained by the patient as a result of subgingival curettage is not warranted in the light of the similar clinical improvements observed with root surface debridement alone. The favourable response to subgingival curettage can therefore be attributed primarily to the associated subgingival root surface instrumentation. Furthermore, the use of local anaesthesia, so necessary for subgingival curettage, may in some instances permit more effective root surface debridement by eliminating pain and enhancing access by the associated slight deflection of pocket wall tissue from the teeth. Tissue curettage obviously reduces the physical bulk of the pocket wall and so leads to a more rapid pocket reduction (gingival recession), whilst the surgical exercise itself might motivate some to higher standards of plaque control and thereby enhanced healing. Finally, it must be conceded that the inadvertent removal of microorganisms possibly present within the soft tissue pocket wall could be critical to healing, and as such, constitute an indication for the technique.

Evaluation of modified Widman flap type technique

Controlled investigations

Numerous controlled investigations have been carried out where the MWF used in conjunction with root debridement is compared with 'blind' subgingival debridement alone (Hill *et al.*, 1981; Pihlstrom *et al.*, 1981, 1983; Lindhe *et al.*, 1982 a, 1984; Isidor *et al.*, 1984; Westfelt *et al.*, 1985; Lindhe and Nyman, 1985; Isidor and Karring, 1986 and Ramfjord *et al.*, 1987). Whitehead and Watts (1987) compared the short-term effect of the MWF with Keyes' method of non-surgical therapy. Both methods have been shown to be equally effective when judged by mean levels of attachment, pocket depth and gingival inflammation. Although individual differences do exist between these investigations they have several findings in common.

Attachment levels

Loss of attachment was sustained at the shallowest pocket sites (<3 mm) with both methods. The exception to this was the study by Hill *et al.* (1981) who found no change at non-surgical sites. These minute losses do not however appear to represent a threat to the future maintenance of the dentition (Lindhe, 1982 a; Ramfjord *et al.*, 1987). Slight gains in attachment have been reported at both initially moderate (4–6 mm) and deep (>7 mm) pocket sites. These gains were greater with non-surgical therapy at the moderate sites and following surgical therapy in the deeper sites but with two inconsistent findings with respect to 4–6 mm sites following surgery. Greater attachment gains were recorded by Lindhe *et al.* (1982 a) whilst Hill *et al.* (1981) observed loss of attachment. The superiority of surgical methods at the deepest sites was not maintained over longer time periods although that of non-surgical debridement was still maintained at shallower sites (Ramfjord *et al.*, 1987). In this context Badersten *et al.* (1987 b) noted that many of the probing attachment gains recorded during the 24 months after blind debridement at initially deeper sites, were lost over the following 24 months.

Lindhe *et al.* (1982 b) used regression analysis to determine the critical probing depths at which shallow sites would lose, and deeper ones gain, clinical attachment. This proved to be 2.9 mm for the former and 4.2 mm for the latter. These findings were taken to mean that patients having a large number of sites with shallow probing depths should preferably be treated conservatively, whilst situations with predominantly deep pockets, might best be treated surgically. Using frequency distributions, Lindhe and Nyman (1985) revealed that non-surgical techniques resulted in a larger number of pockets exceeding 6 mm and that the majority of these bled on probing to the base of the pockets. Comparisons based on mean data however revealed no differences between surgical and non-surgical treatments.

Pocket depths

Significant pocket reductions were achieved by both surgical and non-surgical methods at sites initially 4–6 mm deep. A difference in favour of surgery failed to be maintained consistently over the evaluation periods. Greater reductions were achieved, regardless of treatment method, with the deeper initial pocket depths.

Influence of plaque control

Clinical improvements were dependent upon high levels of patient plaque control in all but one of the above studies (Pihlstrom *et al.*, 1981), failing which deeper probing depths and further attachment losses occurred. In addition Ramfjord (1987) has shown that periodic prophylaxis may prevent loss of clinical attachment over long periods of time in patients with less than perfect oral hygiene.

Uncontrolled investigations

There have been a few uncontrolled longitudinal investigations on surgical reattachment techniques at sites with moderate pocket depth. Raeste and Kilpinen (1981) and Axelsson and Lindhe (1981) evaluated the MWF technique over periods of 4 and 6 years respectively, while in a 5-year study, Yukna and Williams (1980) assessed the excisional new attachment procedure (ENAP). The ENAP is in effect a subgingival curettage (SGC) carried out by surgical excision. Significant pocket reductions were achieved but with attachment levels essentially unaltered.

Evaluation of different surgical methods

Uncontrolled investigations

It has been shown that the progression of disease even in the advanced stages can be prevented by surgical therapy in patients willing and able to maintain plaque-free dentitions (Lindhe and Nyman, 1975). Pocket elimination was carried out by resection or apical repositioned flap (ARF) and furcation therapy used as dictated by the features of the case. Optimal plaque control was then maintained ad modum Axelsson and Lindhe (1974). The effects were first reported after 5 years (Linde and Nyman, 1975), then 8 years (Nyman and Lindhe, 1979) and finally at 14 years (Lindhe and Nyman, 1984). The mean values for post-surgical probing depths, attachment levels and bone heights did not alter significantly throughout the evaluation periods, although individual site analysis (Lindhe and Nyman, 1984) revealed that a small number of sites in a few patients sustained substantial attachment losses. This supports the findings of Hirschfeld and Wasserman (1978) from a retrospective analysis over an average period of 22 years on 600 patients treated according to the surgical dictates at the time. Most individuals were found to be 'well maintained' but a few exhibited 'extreme down-hill' patterns of attachment loss. Together, these investigations reinforce recent concepts that disease is a site-specific disorder (Socransky *et al.*, 1984), which evidently develops and progresses in a few apparently unpredictable sites in a small minority of vulnerable individuals, rather than being a generalized phenomenon affecting most periodontal patients. More importantly, it appears that recurrent disease might occur in a similarly unpredictable fashion in spite of the creation of totally cleansible dentogingival morphology (Lindhe and Nyman, 1984) and elsewhere, following more conventional therapy (Hirschfeld and Wasserman, 1978) and non-surgical debridement alone (Badersten *et al.*, 1987 b). This should therefore be borne in mind in any assessment of treatment procedures.

Controlled investigations

Split mouth experimental designs have been used in several investigations of different durations. These are grouped for convenience into long-term and short-term (less than 1 year) studies. The increasing trend towards the latter short-term studies reflects the growing realization that tissue alterations resulting from surgical therapy are completed within the first 6 months (Rosling *et al.*, 1976 a and b; Pihlström *et al.*, 1981; Lindhe *et al.*, 1982 a) whilst those occurring thereafter are the result of recurrent disease or subsequent instrumentation or both (Lindhe *et al.*, 1982 a, 1984).

Long-term studies

The effects of surgical pocket elimination (ARF and resection), and subgingival curettage (SGC) coupled with root planing were assessed by Ramfjord *et al.* (1968). Subsequently, the MWF was included as an additional surgical method and the findings reported at intervals of up to 8 years (Ramfjord *et al.*, 1973, 1975, 1987; Knowles *et al.*, 1979). A similar investigation was carried out over a 2-year period by Hill *et al.* (1981), but included scaling and root planing alone in one quadrant. Rosling *et al.* (1976 a) and Rosling (1983) in turn evaluated the effects of the ARF and the MWF, with and without removal of bone, and gingivectomy without bone removal followed by an optimal oral hygiene regime over 2- and 6-year periods respectively. Waite (1976) compared the effects of conventional gingivectomy

with non-surgical debridement over a period of 1 year. The effects of MWF, the reverse bevel flap and that of root planing under local anaesthesia have been evaluated over a 5-year period (Isidor and Karring, 1986), whilst Meador *et al.* (1985) assessed the effectiveness of these techniques carried out in clinical practice, based upon a retrospective analysis after an interval of over 7 years.

Short-term studies

There have been a number of 4–6 month evaluation period investigations. Zamet (1975) evaluated SGC, MWF and ARF with osseous recontouring; Smith *et al.* (1980) open flap curettage (a resective technique) with ARF plus osseous surgery; Isidor *et al.* (1984) compared root planing (under local anaesthesia) with MWF and ARF; while Lindhe and Nyman (1985) did so with MWF and the modified Kirkland flap (Kirkland, 1931). Finally, Westfelt *et al.* (1985) compared scaling and root planing alone with scaling and root planing combined with a gingivectomy procedure and with both MWF and ARF, each with and without bone recontouring.

The findings

In the short-term studies the same degree of pocket reduction has been reported regardless of the surgical methods used, although this result was found to be at the expense of slight losses in clinical attachment levels (Zamet, 1975; Smith *et al.*, 1980). In the other investigations, attachment losses were sustained at only the shallowest sites, gains occurring elsewhere. The findings of the longer-term investigations reveal significant pocket reductions irrespective of technique, although once again slight losses in attachment were sustained at the shallow pocket sites. Elsewhere attachment levels were either maintained or improved with non-surgical methods effecting the most favourable outcome at moderate pocket sites. The greatest clinical attachment gains were located at the initially deepest pocket sites, with the MWF being superior to the other surgical techniques in achieving these gains.

The clinical improvements have as elsewhere (see above), depended on high standards of oral hygiene in all but one study (Ramfjord *et al.*, 1982, 1987) in which compensatory periodic professional cleaning appears to have sufficed. This majority finding is endorsed by the fact that periodontal surgery in the presence of ineffective cleaning has resulted not only in recurrent pocketing but more importantly, significant attachment losses (Nyman *et al.*, 1977). The critical role of the patient in therapy, as advocated in Part II, is thus reinforced.

Clinical implications

The comparable outcomes of pocket reduction and pocket elimination surgery in these investigations must be explained. The possible factors relate to the variable pattern of disease, the difficulties of the appropriate flap positioning and of data analysis are discussed earlier. The clinical changes relating to attachment losses and gains and of pocket reductions are examined here.

Post-surgical healing and attachment losses

The problem

The tissue alterations resulting from surgical therapy are completed within the first 6 months as noted above; any subsequent attachment losses should be attributed to either recurrent disease or the result of repeated subgingival instrumentation (Lindhe *et al.*, 1982 a, 1984). This in turn implies that surgical access for debridement is an effective means of controlling disease activity for at least 6 months and that any recurrent disease is the result of difficulties of subgingival debridement at residual pocket sites. This would add support to the recommendation in Part II that optimal pocket reduction, if not elimination, be attempted when any pocket surgery is undertaken.

Instrumentation damage

The possible influence of periodic subgingival instrumentation on periodontal attachment levels is reflected in the consistent finding of attachment losses at the initially shallow pocket sites, whilst gains occurred at the deep sites (Knowles *et al.*, 1979; Pihlström *et al.*, 1981, 1983; Lindhe *et al.*, 1982; Isidor *et al.*, 1984; Westfelt *et al.*, 1985 and Ramfjord *et al.*, 1987). This is also true, with some minor variations between studies, following non-surgical debridement (Badersten *et al.*, 1981, 1984 a and b, 1987 a; Hill *et al.*, 1981; Lindhe *et al.*, 1982 a and b; Pihlström *et al.*, 1983). The comparatively superficial location of the supracrestal attachment at these sites predisposes to inadvertent trauma. Any such mechanical wounding and detachment of supracrestal fibres from cementum may, as shown by Lindhe *et al.* (1982 c), result in a reparative repopulation of the root surface by junctional epithelial cells which prevents a connective tissue reattachment. It should also be emphasized that the risks of trauma might be increased by the use of local anaesthesia during debridement at any site (Isidor *et al.*, 1984 a and Westfelt *et al.*, 1985). The benefits of avoiding local anaesthesia during subgingival debridement as advocated in Part II, is thus emphasized.

Site location

The fact that losses occurred mainly at buccal aspects may also be explained by the thinner tissue morphology at these sites (Claffey and Shanley, 1986) rendering them more vulnerable to the effects of instrumental trauma. In addition, the possible role of toothbrush damage to the marginal gingival tissues cannot be discounted (Badersten *et al.*, 1985 c, 1987 a), for similar patterns of attachment loss have also been observed following oral hygiene measures alone (Cercek *et al.*, 1983).

The predominant location of sites displaying attachment losses at the facial and oral aspects may also reflect the technical ease of probing at those sites. Greater precision in probing is likely at shallow, accessible and readily visible sites (Badersten *et al.*, 1984 c), with a bias towards lesser probe penetration elsewhere at which the inflammatory resolution and improved tissue tones (pocket closure) will offer greater resistence to periodontal probing (Magnusson and Listgarten, 1980), and thereby give the erroneous impression of more favourable attachment levels (Lindhe *et al.*, 1986). Thus, in reality attachment losses might be sustained quite commonly yet only be detected easily at the shallowest sites. Furthermore, the facial and oral periodontal tissue morphology appears to be inherently most susceptible to attachment losses following surgical flap procedures (*cf.* Chapter 31, Osseous therapy) and which may therefore be unrelated to pocket depth *per se*. Finally, remodelling of attachment levels around the tooth during healing ('levelling' – Fleszar *et al.*, 1980) may also be involved, affecting mostly the facial and oral aspects.

Gains in clinical attachment

These might simply be due to inflammatory resolution, as implied above, and so only reflect altered quality rather than quantity of the soft tissue attachment (Lindhe *et al.*, 1982 a; Isidor *et al.*, 1984 a; Westfelt *et al.*, 1985 and Badersten *et al.*, 1987 a). Significant gains in connective tissue attachment have yet to be demonstrated (*cf.* Chapter 31, Osseous therapy). Thus, for example, the mean gains in attachment of 3 mm reported at 7–12 mm sites (Knowles *et al.*, 1980) may merely represent 'pocket closure' or at best a long junctional epithelium. On the other hand, unaltered attachment levels might only reflect an imperceptibly slow rate of disease. It can also mean that disease activity has been either arrested prior to surgery by non-surgical debridement or had entered a spontaneous phase of remission at the time of operation and so not be the result of surgical intervention itself (*cf.* Chapter 28).

Pocket reductions

There was an unexpected finding that the mean pocket reductions achieved at the initially deepest pocket sites (7–12 mm), were not only as little as 4 mm, but were also similar for both pocket elimination and pocket correction techniques (Knowles *et al.*, 1979 and Ramfjord *et al.*, 1987). The reductions observed at 4–6-mm sites were proportionally somewhat better. This apparent failure of pocket elimination surgery may however be explained by the frequently uneven distribution of the initially deepest sites within the chosen surgical fields and the physical constraints imposed on surgery by adjacent shallower pockets. This limiting influence is most evident when the deepest pockets are located interdentally, and at which there is also a strong tendency for coronal tissue proliferation leading to restoration of papillary form (Van der Velden, 1982). It must in this context also be appreciated that non-resective surgical methods result in some marginal tissue recession (e.g. Badersten *et al.*, 1984 a; Westfelt *et al.*, 1985) thereby rendering more likely comparable clinical outcomes of the different surgical methods (Lindhe and Nyman 1987; Lindhe *et al.*, 1987). This in turn means that similar degrees of root surface exposure may occur regardless of the surgical, or indeed non-surgical, treatment methods.

Conclusion

The findings reinforce the difficulties encountered in surgically eliminating isolated deep pockets and those associated with uneven patterns of breakdown. A surgical compromise accepting reattachment is frequently enforced because the alternatives, of sacrificing supporting tissue at the less involved neighbouring units or of costly complex furcation therapy, to eliminate the pocket are rejected as too great a penalty in many cases (*cf.* Chapter 34 – Restorative/prosthetic implications). Whilst this surgical compromise fails to satisfy the initial surgical objective of pocket elimination, the opportunity for improved root surface debridement at operation and that facilitated by the modest pocket reduction achieved may together simplify, if not ensure the subsequent control of disease (*cf.* Chapter 27 – Continuation therapy). It is also apparent that where pocket elimination has not been achieved, post-surgical attachment levels are not dependent upon either the type of surgical procedure employed or the degree of pocket reduction ultimately achieved. This in turn suggests that the outcome of an elective technique of surgical access for more effective debridement will be similar to that achieved by the intentional but abortive attempt at pocket elimination *per se*. Furthermore, provided that progressive periodontal destruction

actually existed at the time of operation (something that is not readily demonstrated), the post-surgical clinical improvements with respect to attachment levels, must be attributed to the root surface debridement at surgery coupled with that carried out periodically during the post-surgical maintenance phase. The relative importance of the latter component does however remain unclear. Accordingly where problems of such subgingival debridement are anticipated and aesthetics permit, these are minimized, as advocated in Part II, by optimal pocket reduction (namely attempted pocket elimination) whenever surgery is undertaken.

Influence of root morphology

The abundant references within the literature concerning the specific management of root furcation involvement are reviewed in Chapter 30. The relevance of root morphology to the outcome of surgical therapy and to maintenance care will be considered here, although it must be realized that effective longitudinal evaluation is limited by the difficulties of reproducible clinical and radiographic measurements. Most clinicians do however agree that the furcation area does constitute the main therapeutic problem. This is reflected in, for example, the observation that subgingival scaling invariably failed to remove the related bacterial deposits and that attachment loss within the furcations was more advanced than on the flat surfaces of the teeth (Waerhaug, 1980). On the other hand, it is apparent that furcation involvement does not necessarily condemn the tooth to a poor prognosis as shown by the long-term findings of Ross and Thompson (1978, 1980) and Hirshfeld and Wasserman (1978). Ramfjord *et al.* (1980) concluded that despite the rather less pocket reductions and attachment level gains achieved at maxillary molars and bicuspids than elsewhere, the prognosis is good for the treatment of periodontal pockets in all areas of the mouth although subsequent observations (Ramfjord *et al.*, 1987), indicated otherwise.

The traditional assumption that the prognosis for single-rooted teeth is better than for teeth with furcation involvement, stems primarily from the technical difficulties of plaque control and of plaque elimination. Thus, Lindhe *et al.* (1982 a) and Pihlström *et al.* (1984) demonstrated greater pocket reductions although comparable attachment gains at non-molar than molar teeth. This may simply be due to difficulties in stabilizing the surgical flap at the back of the mouth rather than problems peculiar to root morphology *per se*, as cited by Lindhe and co-workers. In addition, Halazonetis *et al.* (1985) reported a greater frequency of recurrent pocketing 3 years post-surgically at molars, particularly in the maxilla, than at other teeth.

The influence of the attitude of the individual patient and operator towards the preservation or extraction of such teeth must not be overlooked, but is unfortunately not easily determined. Thus, whilst retrospective evaluations of tooth loss following comprehensive periodontal care by McFall (1982) and Goldman *et al.* (1986) have demonstrated the greater vulnerability of molars on account of furcation involvement, the possibility of operator variability in treatment planning has also been cited. Similarly the finding that tooth loss (mainly molars) was sustained only in erratic attenders over a 5-year maintenance period following periodontal therapy (Wilson *et al.*, 1987), might only reflect a professional bias in the management of those apparently less interested patients (*cf.* Chapter 26, Prognosis). Data on bone loss in subjects following periodontal therapy without frequent periodontal maintenance care (De Vore *et al.*, 1986), also suggests that molars are at greater risk than other units.

Conclusion

Further investigations are necessary to clarify these issues, but on balance it does seem that whenever surgery involving molar teeth is contemplated the attempted elimination of the pocket is preferable to minimize future problems of furcation debridement. This is in accord with the treatment principles in Part II, but accepts the frequent need for compromise on pragmatic grounds.

Post-surgical maintenance

The high level of plaque control traditionally advocated by periodontists is very demanding and is often not sustained by the patient. Moreover, the economic factors and limitations of professional manpower restrict the availability of the associated frequent professional cleaning and supervision of oral hygiene behaviour. The basis for this approach to maintenance therapy and the feasibility of less regimented regimes are examined here.

Optimal oral hygiene levels

It has been well established that periodontal health can be maintained both from the outset (Axelsson and Lindhe, 1981 b) and by a high standard of oral hygiene associated with frequent professional cleaning (Lindhe and Nyman, 1975; Nyman *et al.*, 1975; Rosling *et al.*, 1976; Axelsson and Lindhe, 1981 a; Lindhe *et al.*, 1982 a). On the other hand, despite optimal oral hygiene levels, significant attachment losses were encountered subsequently (Lindhe and Nyman, 1984) in a small number of sites in a few patients of a large group monitored over a 14-year period. The reasons for the deterioration are not

clear and must be attributed to the site specificity of disease (Socransky *et al.*, 1984) being apparently independent of plaque levels. This requires further investigation.

The 2-weekly professional cleaning proposed and tested by Axelsson and Lindhe (1974) was designed to ensure optimally low levels of plaque for the purposes of clinical research. This has however been misinterpreted by many clinicians and resulted in the imposition of similarly rigid maintenance regimes as essential prerequisites to health without establishing their necessity. Indeed, as referred to in Chapter 28, the relative importance of the respective separate roles of the patient's efforts and of professional cleaning *per se* has yet to be clearly identified. In this context, Glavind (1977) conducted a split-mouth crossover investigation on the effects of monthly professional cleaning at contralateral quadrants over a maintenance period of 1 year. No difference in gingival health was observed between experimental and control quadrants, indicating that factors other than professional cleaning were responsible. The motivational impact of participating in the study was cited as the most likely reason in this one study. In another investigation, Westfelt *et al.* (1983) concluded that high standards of oral hygiene are more critical than frequency of recall to the maintenance of periodontal health, although a higher frequency of plaque-free surfaces resulted from more frequent recall appointments.

The influence of the patients' own concern in maintaining periodontal health is reinforced by the findings of Raeste and Kilpinen (1981). Highly significant reductions in pocket depths and only minimal mean losses of attachment were observed over a 4-year maintenance period in subjects who, following MWF surgery, had been referred back to their own dentist for maintenance care. The implied lack of a regular recall system and professional cleaning, were compensated for by the good levels of oral hygiene. These were attributed to the tooth cleaning instructions repeated regularly during the long initial phase of the treatment and a strong patient motivation to save the teeth. In another investigation (Johansson *et al.*, 1984), subjects were referred back to their own dentists with a prescribed maintenance care programme following non-surgical treatment. Periodontal health was maintained over a 3-year period, in spite of the fact that the levels of compliance, both professionally and individually, were considerably less than that traditionally recommended.

Söderholm *et al.* (1982) and Söderholm and Egelberg (1982) have concluded that comprehensive maintenance programmes may be unnecessary and may furthermore not increase the effects of basic plaque control instruction given during active periodontal therapy.

The consensus view taken from these studies does

therefore seem to indicate that individuals able to maintain high levels of cleaning are likely to establish optimal conditions for healing regardless of the frequency of professional supervision and cleaning.

Unaltered oral hygiene levels

The results of some long-term post-surgical studies (e.g. Pihlström *et al.*, 1981; Morrison *et al.*, 1982) and endorsed by Ramfjord (1987), would, at first sight, appear to oppose the above view. They show that mean attachment levels and pocket reductions were not significantly influenced by unimproved (Pihlström *et al.*, 1981) or variable (Morrison *et al.*, 1982) oral hygiene levels. In the latter investigation responses did however tend to be more favourable in patients with good than with poor oral hygiene (Ramfjord *et al.*, 1982). This suggests that under such circumstances, clinical success can be assured by 3–6 monthly professional supra- and subgingival cleaning and that this not only inhibits the re-establishment of a complex pathogenic subgingival flora (*cf.* Chapter 28), but also compensates for inadequacies in the patients' supragingival plaque control. This is supported by findings by Isidor and Karring (1986).

Poorly controlled oral hygiene levels

The control subjects in two surgical studies referred to above, were recalled for 6-monthly professional cleaning (Nyman *et al.*, 1975) or referred back to the referring dentist for maintenance care (Axelsson and Lindhe, 1981 a) over 2- and 6-year observation periods respectively. This meant that carefully supervised post-surgical maintenance regimes were not carried out. In another investigation (Nyman *et al.*, 1977), cleaning was advised upon only once before pocket surgery and not again over a 2-year post-surgical observation period. Becker *et al.* (1984) in turn, presented the findings on 44 patients, who failed to attend for maintenance care over a period of about 5 years following periodontal therapy including pocket reduction surgery. In each of these investigations periodontal health was not maintained and further breakdown with some tooth loss was sustained. This trend is reinforced by the greater recurrence of pockets over a 3-year assessment period in subjects with poor rather than with good oral hygiene (Halazonetis *et al.*, 1985), and the increased bone loss sustained in association with infrequent maintenance care following periodontal therapy (De Vore *et al.*, 1986).

In examining this evidence it should be appreciated that the presence of obvious clinical signs of gingival inflammation does not mean that attachment losses are inevitable (Listgarten *et al.*, 1985; Reddy *et al.*, 1985). Similarly, that the persistence of

a mild recurrent gingivitis during a 3-monthly maintenance recall regime was not found to affect pocket depths or attachment levels significantly (Morrison *et al.*, 1982).

Clinical implications

Recurrent disease appears to be related to a combination of patient oral hygiene efforts, the rate of subgingival plaque formation plus its pathogenicity and the tissue susceptibility. It is difficult to reconcile the relative influence of these variables with the marked differences observed between individuals and between different sites in the same mouth. However, it is apparent that with good oral hygiene and gingivae that are free of inflammation following professional cleaning, subgingival plaque reforms less rapidly and reaches its pathogenic potential more slowly. The opposite is also true if oral hygiene is poor and the gingival tissues are inflamed (Goh *et al.*, 1986). Neither the susceptibility to reinfection nor the microbiological pathogenicity can at present be evaluated reliably. Whilst some idea of the likely host response may be gained from the extent of attachment loss already sustained at any site and the patient's age, Abbas *et al.* (1984) and Lindhe *et al.* (1985) have failed to demonstrate consistent relationships (Review: Van der Velden, 1984).

Conclusion

No clear message about the optimal frequency of maintenance visits can be gained from existing studies. Recommendations for recall prophylaxis must therefore be based on individual patient requirements with an emphasis on total flexibility. Furthermore, the practical and economic aspects of any recall system must be kept in perspective and be tailored to the circumstances of each case as advocated in Chapter 27 (Maintenance therapy). Finally, whether care is provided by the periodontist, the referring dentist or an hygienist under the guidance of the clinician must be a matter of individual preference provided always that good levels of communication are maintained.

References

Abbas, F., Van der Velden, U. and Hart, A. A. M. (1984) Relation between wound healing after surgery and susceptibility to periodontal disease. *J. Clin. Periodontol.* **11**, 221–229

Abbas, F., Van der Velden, U., Hart, A. A. M. Moorer, W. R., Vroom, T. M. and Scholte, G. (1986) Bleeding/plaque ratio and the development of gingival inflammation. *J. Clin. Periodontol.* **13**, 774–782

Ainslie, P. T. and Caffesse, R. G. (1981a) A biometric

evaluation of gingival curettage (I). *Quintessence Int.* **5**, 519–527

Ainslie, P. T. and Caffesse, R. G. (1981b) A biometric evaluation of gingival curettage (II). *Quintessence Int.* **6**, 609–614

Albandar, J. M. and Abbas, D. K. (1986) Radiographic quantification of alveolar bone level changes. *J. Clin. Periodontol.* **13**, 810–813

Albandar, J. M., Abbas, D. K., Waerhaug, M. and Gjermo, P. (1985) Comparison between standardized periapical and bitewing radiographs in assessing alveolar bone loss. *Comm. Dent. Oral Epid.* **13**, 222–225

Aleo, J. J., de Renzis, F. A., Farber, P. A. and Varboncoeur, A. P. (1974) The presence and biologic activity of cementum-bound endotoxin. *J. Periodontol.* **45**, 672–675

Aleo, J. J., de Renzis, F. A. and Farber, P. A. (1975) *In vitro* attachment of human gingival fibroblasts to root surfaces. *J. Periodontol.* **46**, 639–645

Allenspach-Petrzilka, G. E. and Guggenheim, B. (1983) Bacterial invasion of the periodontium; an important factor in the pathogenesis of periodontitis? *J. Clin. Periodontol.* **10**, 609–617

Atkinson, D. Ross, Cobb, C. M. and Killoy, W. J. (1984) The effect of an air-powder abrasive system on *in vitro* root surfaces. *J. Periodontol.* **55**, 13–18

Axelsson, P. and Lindhe, J. (1974) The effect of a preventive programme on dental plaque, gingivitis and caries in schoolchildren. Results after one and two years. *J. Clin. Periodontol.* **1**, 126–138

Axelsson, P. and Lindhe, J. (1978) Effect of controlled oral hygiene procedures on caries and periodontal disease in adults. *J. Clin. Periodontol.* **5**, 133–151

Axelsson, P. and Lindhe, J. (1981a) The significance of maintenance care in the treatment of periodontal disease. *J. Clin. Periodontol.* **8**, 281–294

Axelsson, P. and Lindhe, J. (1981b) Effect of controlled oral hygiene procedures on caries and periodontal disease in adults. *J. Clin. Periodontol.* **8**, 239–248

Badersten, A., Nilveus, R. and Egelberg, J. (1981) Effect of nonsurgical periodontal therapy. I. Moderately advanced periodontitis. *J. Clin. Periodontol.* **8**, 57–72

Badersten, A., Nilveus, R. and Egelberg, J. (1984a) Effect of nonsurgical periodontal therapy. II. Severely advanced periodontitis. *J. Clin. Periodontol.* **11**, 63–76

Badersten, A., Nilveus, R. and Egelberg, J. (1984b) Effect of nonsurgical periodontal therapy. III. Single versus repeated instrumentation. *J. Clin. Periodontol.* **11**, 114–124

Badersten, A., Nilveus, R. and Egelberg, J. (1984c) Reproducibility of probing attachment level measurements. *J. Clin. Periodontol.* **11**, 475–485

Badersten, A., Nilveus, R. and Egelberg, J. (1985a) Effect of non-surgical periodontal therapy. IV. Operator variability. *J. Clin. Periodontol.* **12**, 190–200

Badersten, A., Nilveus, R. and Egelberg, J. (1985b) Effect of non-surgical periodontal therapy. V. Patterns of probing attachment loss in non-responding sites. *J. Clin. Periodontol.* **12**, 270–282

Badersten, A., Nilveus, R. and Egelberg, J. (1985c) Effect of non-surgical periodontal therapy. VI. Localisation of sites with probing attachment loss. *J. Clin. Periodontol.* **12**, 351–359

Badersten, A., Nilveus, R. and Egelberg, J. (1985d) Effect of non-surgical periodontal therapy. VII. Bleeding, suppuration and probing depth in sites with probing attachment loss. *J. Clin. Periodontol.* **12**, 432–440

Badersten, A., Nilveus, R. and Egelberg, J. (1987a) Effect of non-surgical periodontal therapy. VIII. Probing attachment changes related to clinical characteristics. *J. Clin. Periodontol.* **14**, 425–432

Badersten, A., Nilveus, R. and Egelberg, J. (1987b) Four-year observations of basic periodontal therapy. *J. Clin. Periodontol.* **14**, 438–444

Baelum, V., Fejerskov, O. and Karring, T. (1986) Oral hygiene, gingivitis and periodontal breakdown in adult Tanzanians. *J. Periodont. Res.* **21**, 221–232

Beaumont, R. H., O'Leary, T. J. and Kafrawy, A. H. (1984) Relative resistance of long junctional epithelial adhesions and connective tissue attachments to plaque-induced inflammation. *J. Periodontol.* **55**, 213–223

Becker, W., Becker, B. E. and Berg, L. E. (1984) Periodontal treatment without maintenance. A retrospective study in 44 patients. *J. Periodontol.* **55**, 505–509

Beltrami, M., Bickel, M. and Baehni, P. C. (1987) The effect of supragingival plaque control on the composition of the subgingival microflora in human periodontitis. *J. Clin. Periodontol.* **14**, 161–164

Bergenholtz, A. (1972) Radectomy of multirooted teeth. *J. Am. Dent. Assoc.* **85**, 870–875

Berkstein, S., Reiff, R. L., McKinney, J. F. and Killoy, W. J. (1987) Supragingival root surface removal during maintenance procedures utilizingan air-powder abrasive system or hand scaling. *J. Periodontol.* **58**, 327–330

Birek, P., McCulloch, C. A. G. and Hardy, V. (1987) Gingival attachment level measurements with an automatic periodontal probe. *J. Clin. Periodontol.* **14**, 472–477

Björn, A.-L. and Hjort, P. (1982) Bone loss of furcated mandibular molars. A longitudinal study. *J. Clin. Periodontol.* **9**, 402–408

Blomlöf, L., Lindskog, S., Appelgren, R., Jonsson, B., Weintraub, A. and Hammarström, L. (1987) New attachment in monkeys with experimental periodontitis with and without the removal of the cementum. *J. Clin. Periodontol.* **14**, 136–143

Boyde, A. (1984) Air-polishing effects on enamel, dentine, cement and bone. *Br. Dent. J.* **156**, 287–291

Braatz, L., Garrett, S., Claffey, N. and Egelberg, J. (1985) Antimicrobial irrigation of deep pockets to supplement non-surgical periodontal therapy. II. Daily irrigation. *J. Clin. Periodontol.* **12**, 630–638

Brecy, M. C., Schlegel, K., Gehr, P. and Lang, N. P. (1987) Comparison between histological and clinical parameters during human experimental gingivitis. *J. Periodont. Res.* **22**, 50–57

Breininger, D. R., O'Leary, T. J. and Blumenshine, R. V.

H. (1987) Comparative effectiveness of ultrasonic and hand scaling for the removal of subgingival plaque and calculus. *J. Periodontol.* **58**, 9–18

Brown, F. H., Lubow, R. M. and Cooley, R. L. (1987) A review of applied ultrasonics in periodontal therapy. *J. West. Soc. Periodontol.* **35**, 53–60

Buchanan, S. A. and Robertson, P. B. (1987) Calculus removal by scaling/root planing with and without surgical access. *J. Periodontol.* **58**, 159–163

Buckley, L. A. and Crowley, M. J. (1984) A longitudinal study of untreated periodontal disease. *J. Clin. Periodontol.* **11**, 523–530

Caffesse, R. G., Sweeney, P. L. and Smith, B. A. (1986) Scaling and root planing with and without periodontal flap surgery. *J. Clin. Periodontol.* **13**, 205–210

Carranza, F. A. Jr (1984) *Glickman's Clinical Periodontology.* 6th Edition, pp. 773–778. W. B. Saunders Company, Philadelphia

Caton, J., Nyman, S. and Zander, H. (1980) Histometric evaluation of periodontal surgery. II. Connective tissue attachment levels after four regenerative procedures. *J. Clin. Periodontol.* **7**, 224–231

Caton, J., Proye, M. and Polson, A. (1982) Maintenance of healed periodontal pockets after a single episode of root planing. *J. Periodontol.* **53**, 420–424

Caton, J. G. and Zander, H. A. (1979) The attachment between tooth and gingival tissues after periodic root planing and soft tissue curettage. *J. Periodontol.* **50**, 462–466

Cercek, J. F., Kiger, R. D., Garrett, S. and Egelberg J. (1983) Relative effects of plaque control and instrumentation on the clinical parameters of human periodontal disease. *J. Clin. Periodontol.* **10**, 46–56

Chawla, T. N., Nanda, R. S. and Kapoor, K. K. (1975) Dental prophylaxis procedures in control of periodontal disease in Lucknow (Rural) India. *J. Periodontol.* **46**, 498–503

Cheetham, A. H., Wilson, M. and Kieser, J. B. (1988) Root surface debridement – an *in vitro* assessment. *J. Clin. Periodontol.* **15**, 288–292

Claffey, N. and Shanley, D. (1986) Relationship of gingival thickness and bleeding to loss of probing attachment in shallow sites following non-surgical therapy. *J. Clin. Periodontol.* **13**, 654–657

Current Procedural Terminology (1977) 4th Edition. American Academy of Periodontology, Chicago

Daly, C. G. (1982) Anti-bacterial effect of citric acid treatment of periodontally diseased root surfaces *in vitro. J. Clin. Periodontol.* **9**, 386–392

Daly, C. G., Kieser, J. B., Corbet, E. F. and Seymour, G. J. (1979) Cementum involved in periodontal disease: a review of its features and clinical management. *J. Dent.* **7**, 185–193

Daly, C. G., Seymour, G. J. and Kieser, J. B. (1980) Bacterial endotoxin: a role in chronic inflammatory periodontal disease? *J. Oral Pathol.* **9**, 1–15

Daly, C. G., Seymour, G. J., Kieser, J. B. and Corbet, E. F. (1982) Histological assessment of periodontally involved cementum. *J. Clin. Periodontol.* **9**, 266–274

De Vore, C. H., Duckworth, J. E., Beck, F. M., Hicks, M. J., Brumfield, F. W. and Horton, J. E. (1986) Bone loss following periodontal therapy in subjects without frequent periodontal maintenance. *J. Periodontol.* **57**, 354–359

Eaton, K. A., Kieser, J. B. and Baker, R. (1985a) Assessment of plaque by image analysis. *J. Clin. Periodontol.* **12**, 135–140

Eaton, K. A., Kieser, J. B. and Davies, R. M. (1985b) The removal of root surface deposits. *J. Clin. Periodontol.* **12**, 141–142

Echeverria, J. J. and Caffesse, R. G. (1983) Effects of gingival curettage when performed 1 month after root instrumentation. A biometric evaluation. *J. Clin. Periodontol.* **10**, 277–286

Eide, B., Lie, T. and Selvig, K. A. (1983) Surface coatings on dental cementum incident to periodontal disease. *J. Clin. Periodontol.* **10**, 157–171

Eide, B., Lie, T. and Selvig, K. A. (1984) Surface coatings on dental cementum incident to periodontal disease. (II) Scanning electron microscopic confirmation of a mineralized cuticle. *J. Clin. Periodontol.* **11**, 565–575

Elin, R. and Wolff, S. (1973) Nonspecificity of the Limulus amebocyte lysate test: Positive reactions with polynucleotides and proteins. *J. Infect. Dis.* **128**, 349–352

Ericsson, I., Lindhe, J., Liljenberg, B. and Persson, A.-L. (1987) Lack of bacterial invasion in experimental periodontitis. *J. Clin. Periodontol.* **14**, 478–485

Fine, D., Tabak, L., Oshrain, H., Salkind, A. and Siegel, K. (1978a) Studies in plaque pathogenicity. I. Plaque collection and Limulus lysate screening of adherent and loosely adherent plaque. *J. Periodont. Res.* **13**, 17–23

Fine, D., Tabak, L., Salkind, A. and Oshrain, H. (1978b) Studies in plaque pathogenicity. II. A technique for the specific detection of endotoxin in plaque samples using the Limulus lysate assay. *J. Periodont. Res.* **13**, 127–133

Fine, D. H. and Mandel, I. D. (1986) Indicators of periodontal disease activity: an evaluation. *J. Clin. Periodontol.* **13**, 533–546

Fine, D. H., Morris, M. L., Tabak, L. and Cole, J. D. (1980) Preliminary characterization of material eluted from the roots of periodontally diseased teeth. *J. Periodont. Res.* **15**, 10–19

Fleszar, T. J., Knowles, J. W., Morrison, E. C., Burgett, F. G., Nissle, R. R. and Ramfjord, S. P. (1980) Tooth mobility and periodontal therapy. *J. Clin. Periodontol.* **7**, 495–505

Flötra, L., Gjermo, P., Rölla, G. and Waerhaug, J. (1972) A 4-month study on the effect of chlorhexidine mouth washes on 50 soldiers. *Scand. J. Dent. Res.* **80**, 10–17

Forgas, L. B. and Gound, S. (1987) The effects of antiformin-citric acid chemical curettage on the microbial flora of the periodontal pocket. *J. Periodontol.* **58**, 153–158

Frandsen, A. (1983) Periodontal surgery: Objectives and indications. In *Textbook of Periodontology,* 1st Edition. (Ed. Lindhe, J.) pp. 353–357. Munksgaard, Copenhagen

Galloway, S. E. and Pashley, D. H. (1987) Rate of

removal of root structures by the use of the Prophy-Jet device. *J. Periodontol.* **58**, 464–469

Gellin, R. G., Miller, M. C., Javed, T., Engler, W. O. and Mishkin, D. J. (1986) The effectiveness of the Titan-Sonic scaler versus curettes in the removal of subgingival calculus. *J. Periodontol.* **57**, 672–680

Genco, R. J. and Slots, J. (1984) Host responses in periodontal diseases. *J. Dent. Res.* **63**, 441–451

Glavind, L. (1977) Effect of monthly professional mechanical tooth cleaning on periodontal health in adults. *J. Clin. Periodontol.* **4**, 100–106

Goh *et al.* (1986) Gingival inflammation and plaque formation. *Br. Dent. J.* **161**, 165–169

Goldman, H. M. and Cohen, D. W. (Ed.) (1980) *Periodontal Therapy,* 6th Edition, pp. 441–443. C. W. Mosby Company, St Louis

Goldman, M. J., Ross, I. R. and Goteiner, D. (1986) Effect of periodontal therapy on patients maintained for 15 years or longer. A retrospective study. *J. Periodontol.* **57**, 347–353

Goodson, J. M. (1986) Clinical measurements of periodontitis. *J. Clin. Periodontol.* **13**, 446–455

Goodson, J. M., Tanner, A. C. R., Haffajee, A. D., Sornberger, G. C. and Socransky, S. S. (1982) Patterns of progression and regression of advanced destructive periodontal disease. *J. Clin. Periodontol.* **9**, 472–481

Grant, D. A., Stern, I. B. and Everett, F. G. (1979) *Periodontics in the tradition of Orban and Gottlieb,* 5th Edition, pp. 621–624 and 631. C. W. Mosby Company, St Louis

Greene, J. C. (1986) Discussion: natural history of periodontal disease in man. *J. Clin. Periodontol.* **13**, 441–444

Greenstein, G. (1984) The role of bleeding upon probing in the diagnosis of periodontal disease: a literature review. *J. Periodontol.* **55**, 684–688

Greenwell, H., Bakr, A., Bissada, N., Debanne, S. and Rowland, D. (1985) The effect of Keyes' method of oral hygiene on the subgingival microflora compared to the effect of scaling and/or surgery. *J. Clin. Periodontol.* **12**, 327–341

Gröndahl, H.-G. and Gröndahl, K. (1983) Subtraction radiography for thediagnosis of periodontal bone lesions. *Oral Surg. Oral Med.* **55**, 208–213

Gröndahl, H.-G., Gröndahl, K. and Webber, R. L. (1983) A digital subtraction technique for dental radiography. *Oral Surg. Oral Med.* **55**, 96–102

Gröndahl, K., Gröndahl, H. G., Wennström, J. and Heijl, L. (1987) Examiner agreement in estimating changes in periodontal bone from conventional and subtraction radiographs. *J. Clin. Periodontol.* **14**, 74–79

Haffajee, A. D. and Socransky, S. S. (1986) Attachment level changes in destructive periodontal diseases. *J. Clin. Periodontol.* **13**, 461–472

Haffajee, A. D., Socransky, S. S. and Goodson, J. M. (1983) Clinical parameters as predictors of destructive periodontal disease activity. *J. Clin. Periodontol.* **10**, 257–265

Halazonetis, T. D., Smulow, J. B., Donnenfeld, O. W.

and Mejias, J. E. (1985) Pocket formation 3 years after comprehensive periodontal therapy. A retrospective study. *J. Periodontol.* **56**, 515–521

Hamp, S.-E., Nyman, S. and Lindhe, J. (1975) Periodontal treatment of multirooted teeth. Results after 5 years. *J. Clin. Periodontol.* **2**, 126–135

Harper, D. S. and Robinson, P. J. (1987) Correlation of histometric, microbial and clinical indicators of periodontal disease status before and after root planing. *J. Clin. Periodontol.* **14**, 190–196

Hatfield, C. G. and Baumhammers, A. (1971) Cytotoxic effects of periodontally involved surfaces of human teeth. *Arch. Oral Biol.* **16**, 465–468

Hausmann, E., Christersson, L., Dunford, R., Wikesjö, U., Phyo, J. and Genco, R. J. (1985) Usefulness of subtraction radiography in the evaluation of periodontal therapy. *J. Periodontol.* **56**, (Suppl. I), 4–7

Hausmann, E., Dunford, R., Wikesjö, U., Christersson, L. and McHenry, K. (1986) Progression of untreated periodontitis as assessed by subtraction radiography. *J. Periodont. Res.* **21**, 716–721

Hellden, L. B., Listgarten, M. A. and Lindhe, J. (1979) The effect of tetracycline and/or scaling on human periodontal disease. *J. Clin. Periodontol.* **6**, 222–230

Hill, R. W., Ramfjord, S. P., Morrison, E. C., Appleberry, E. A., Caffesse, R. G., Kerry, G. J. and Nissle, R. R. (1981) Four types of periodontal treatment compared over two years. *J. Periodontol.* **52**, 655–662

Hirschfeld, L. and Wasserman, B. (1978) A long-term survey of tooth loss in 600 treated periodontal patients. *J. Periodontol.* **49**, 225–237

Horning, G. M., Cobb, C. M. and Killoy, W. J. (1987) Effect of an air-abrasive system on root surfaces in periodontal surgery. *J. Clin. Periodontol.* **14**, 213–220

Hughes, T. P. and Caffesse, R. G. (1978) Gingival changes following scaling, root planing and oral hygiene. A biometric evaluation. *J. Periodontol.* **49**, 245–252

Hughes, F. J. and Smales, F. C. (1986) Immunohistochemical investigation of the presence and distribution of cementum-associated lipopolysaccharides in periodontal disease. *J. Periodont. Res.* **21**, 660–667

Hunter, R. K., O'Leary, T. J., Kafrawy, A. H. (1984) The effectiveness of hand versus ultrasonic instrumentation in open flap root planing. *J. Periodontol.* **55**, 697–703

Imrey, P. B. (1986) Considerations in the statistical analysis of clinical trials in periodontitis. *J. Clin. Periodontol.* **13**, 517–528

Isidor, F. and Karring, T. (1986) Long-term effect of surgical and non-surgical periodontal treatment. A 5-year clinical study. *J. Periodont. Res.* **21**, 462–472

Isidor, F., Karring, T. and Attström, R. (1984a) The effect of root planing as compared to that of surgical treatment. *J. Clin. Periodontol.* **11**, 669–681

Isidor, F., Karring, T. and Attström, R. (1984b) Reproducibility of pocket depth and attachment level measurements when using a flexible splint. *J. Clin. Periodontol.* **11**, 662–668

Ito, K., Hindman, R. E., O'Leary, T. J. and Kafrawy, A. H. (1985) Determination of the presence of root-bound endotoxin using the local Shwartzman phenomenon (LSP). *J. Periodontol.* **56**, 8–17

Jablonski, S. (1982) *Illustrated Dictionary of Dentistry.* W. B. Saunders & Company, Philadelphia

Jeffcoat, M. K., Jeffcoat, R. L., Jens, S. G. and Captain, K. (1986) A new periodontal probe with automated cemento-enamel junction detection. *J. Clin. Periodontol.* **13**, 276–280

Johansson, L.-A., Öster, B. and Hamp, S.-E. (1984) Evaluation of cause-related periodontal therapy and compliance with maintenance care recommendations. *J. Clin. Periodontol.* **11**, 689–699

Jones, S. J., Lozdan, J. and Boyde, A. (1972) Tooth surfaces treated in situ with periodontal instruments. Scanning electron microscopic studies. *Br. Dent. J.* **132**, 57–64

Jones, W. A. and O'Leary, T. J. (1978) The effectiveness of in vivo root planing in removing bacterial endotoxin from the roots of periodontally involved teeth. *J. Periodontol.* **49**, 337–342

Kakehashi, S. and Parakkal, P. F. (1982) Proceedings from the state of the art workshop on surgical therapy for periodontitis. *J. Periodontol.* **53**, 475–501

Kalkwarf, K. L., Tussing, G. J. and Davis, M. J. (1982) Histologic evaluation of gingival curettage facilitated by sodium hypochlorite solution. *J. Periodontol.* **53**, 63–70

Kalkwarf, K. L. Kaldahl, W. B. and Patil, K. D. (1986) Comparison of manual and pressure-controlled periodontal probing. *J. Periodontol.* **57**, 467–471

Khatiblou, F. A. and Ghodssi, A. (1983) Root surface smoothness or roughness in periodontal treatment. A clinical study. *J. Periodontol.* **54**, 365–367

Kho, P., Smales, F. C. and Hardie, J. M. (1985) The effect of supragingival plaque control on the subgingival microflora. *J. Clin. Periodontol.* **12**, 676–686

Kieser, J. B. (1974) An approach to periodontal pocket elimination. *Br. J. Oral Surg.* **12**, 177–195

Kirkland, O. (1931) The suppurative periodontal pus socket: its treatment by modified flap operation. *J. Am. Dent. Assoc.* **18**, 1462–1470

Knowles, J., Burgett, F., Morrison, E., Nissle, R. and Ramfjord, S. (1980) Comparison of results following three modalities of periodontal therapy related to tooth type and initial pocket depth. *J. Clin. Periodontol.* **7**, 32–47

Knowles, J. W., Burgett, F. G., Nissle, R. R., Shick, R. A., Morrison, E. C. and Ramfjord, S. P. (1979) Results of periodontal treatment related to pocket depth and attachment level. Eight years. *J. Periodontol.* **50**, 225–233

Kornman, K. S. (1986) The role of supragingival plaque in the prevention and treatment of periodontal diseases. *J. Periodont. Res. Suppl.* 5–22

Kornman, K. S. (1987) Nature of periodontal diseases: Assessment and diagnosis. *J. Periodont. Res.* **22**, 192–204

Lang, N. P. and Hill, R. W. (1977) Radiographs in periodontics. *J. Clin. Periodontol.* **4**, 16–28

Lang, N. P., Joss, A., Orsanic, T., Gusberti, F. A. and

Siegrist, B. E. (1986) Bleeding on probing. A predictor for the progression of periodontal disease? *J. Clin. Periodontol.* **13**, 590–596

Larson, C., Ribi, E., Milner, K. and Lieberman, J. (1960) A method for titrating endotoxic activity in the skin of rabbits. *J. Exp. Med.* **111**, 1–20

Lasho, D. J., O'Leary, T. J. and Kafrawy, A. H. (1983) A scanning electron microscope study of the effects of various agents on instrumented periodontally involved root surfaces. *J. Periodontol.* **54**, 210–220

Lavanchy, D. L., Bickel, M. and Baehni, P. C. (1987) The effect of plaque control after scaling and root planing on the subgingival microflora in human periodontitis. *J. Clin. Periodontol.* **14**, 295–299

Leon, L. E. and Vogel, R. I. (1987) A comparison of the effectiveness of hard scaling and ultrasonic debridement in furcations as evaluated by differential dark-field microscopy. *J. Periodontol.* **58**, 86–94

Levin, J. and Bang, F. (1964) The role of endotoxin in the extracellular coagulation of Limulus blood. *Bull. Johns Hopkins Hosp.* **115**, 265–274

Levine, H. L. (1972) Periodontal flap surgery with gingival fiber retention. *J. Periodontol.* **43**, 91–98

Liakoni, H., Barber, P. and Newman, H. N. (1987a) Bacterial penetration of pocket soft tissues in chronic adult and juvenile periodontitis cases – an ultrastructural study. *J. Clin. Periodontol.* **14**, 22–28

Liakoni, H., Barber, P. and Newman, H. N. (1987b) Bacterial penetration of the pocket tissues in juvenile/post juvenile periodontitis after the presurgical oral hygiene phase. *J. Periodontol.* **58**, 847–855

Lie, T. and Leknes, K. N. (1985) Evaluation of the effect on root surfaces of air turbine scalers and ultrasonic instrumentation. *J. Periodontol.* **56**, 522–531

Lie, T. and Meyer, K. (1977) Calculus removal and loss of tooth substance in response to different periodontal instruments. A scanning electron microscope study. *J. Clin. Periodontol.* **4**, 250–262

Lindhe, J. and Nyman, S. (1975) The effect of plaque control and surgical pocket elimination on the establishment and maintenance of periodontal health. A longitudinal study of periodontal therapy in cases of advanced disease. *J. Clin. Periodontol.* **2**, 67–79

Lindhe, J. and Nyman, S. (1984) Long-term maintenance of patients treated for advanced periodontal disease. *J. Clin. Periodontol.* **11**, 504–514

Lindhe, J. and Nyman, S. (1985) Scaling and granulation tissue removal in periodontal therapy. *J. Clin. Periodontol.* **12**, 374–388

Lindhe, J. and Nyman, S. (1987) Clinical trials in periodontal therapy. *J. Periodont. Res.* **22**, 217–221

Lindhe, J., Parodi, R., Liljenberg, B. and Fornell, J. (1978) Clinical and structural alterations characterizing healing gingiva. *J. Periodont. Res.* **13**, 410–424

Lindhe, J., Westfelt, E., Nyman, S., Socransky, S. S., Heijl, L and Bratthall, G. (1982a) Healing following surgical/non-surgical treatment of periodontal disease. A clinical study. *J. Clin. Periodontol.* **9**, 115–128

Lindhe, J., Socransky, S. S., Nyman, S., Haffajee, A. and

Westfelt, E.(1982b) 'Critical probing depths' in periodontal therapy. *J. Clin. Periodontol.* 9, 323–336

Lindhe, J., Nyman, S. and Karring, T. (1982c) Scaling and root planing in shallow pockets. *J. Clin. Periodontol.* 9, 415–418

Lindhe, J., Haffajee, A. D. and Socransky, S. S. (1983a) Progression of periodontal disease in adult subjects in the absence of periodontal therapy. *J. Clin. Periodontol.* 10, 433–442

Lindhe, J., Liljenberg, B., Adielsson, B. and Börjesson, I. (1983b) Use of metronidazole as a probe in the study of human periodontal disease. *J. Clin. Periodontol.* 10, 100–112

Lindhe, J., Liljenberg, B. and Adielsson, B. (1983c) Effect of long-term tetracycline therapy on human periodontal disease. *J. Clin. Periodontol.* 10, 590–601

Lindhe, J., Westfelt, E., Nyman, S., Socransky, S. S. and Haffajee, A. D. (1984) Long-term effect of surgical/non-surgical treatment of periodontal disease. *J. Clin. Periodontol.* 11, 448–458

Lindhe, J., Socransky, S. S., Nyman, S., Westfelt, E. and Haffajee, A. (1985) Effect of age on healing following periodontal therapy. *J. Clin. Periodontol.* 12, 774–787

Lindhe, J., Socransky, S. S. and Wennström, J. (1986) Design of clinical trials of traditional therapies of periodontitis. *J. Clin. Periodontol.* 13, 488–497

Lindhe, J., Socransky, S. S., Nyman, S. and Westfelt, E. (1987) Dimensional alteration of the periodontal tissues following therapy. *Int. J. Periodont. Rest. Dent.* 2, 9–21

Listgarten, M. A. (1980) Periodontal probing: what does it mean? *J. Clin. Periodontol.* 7, 165–176

Listgarten, M. A. (1986) Pathogenesis of periodontitis. *J. Clin. Periodontol.* 13, 418–425

Listgarten, M. A. (1987) Nature of periodontal diseases: pathogenic mechanisms. *J. Periodont. Res.* 22, 172–178

Listgarten, M. A. and Ellegaard, B. (1973) Electron microscopic evidence of a cellular attachment between junctional epithelium and dental calculus. *J. Periodont. Res.* 8, 143–150

Listgarten, M. A., Lindhe, J. and Hellden, L. (1978) Effect of tetracycline and/or scaling on human periodontal disease. Clinical, microbiological and histological observations. *J. Clin. Periodontol.* 5, 246–271

Listgarten, M. A., Schifter, C. C. and Laster, L. (1985) 3-year longitudinal study of the periodontal status of an adult population with gingivitis. *J. Clin. Periodontol.* 12, 225–238

Litch, J. M., O'Leary, T. J. and Kafrawy, A. H. (1984) Pocket epithelium removal via crestal and subcrestal scalloped internal bevel incisions. *J. Periodontol.* 55, 142–148

Löe, H., Anerud, A., Boysen, H. and Smith, M. (1978) The natural history of periodontal disease in man. The rate of periodontal destruction before 40 years of age. *J. Periodontol.* 49, 607–620

Löe, H., Anerud, A., Boysen, H. and Morrison, E. (1986) Natural history of periodontal disease in man. *J. Clin. Periodontol.* 49, 607–620

Loos, B., Kiger, R. and Egelberg, J. (1987) An evaluation of basic periodontal therapy using sonic and ultrasonic scalers. *J. Clin. Periodontol.* 14, 29–33

Lopez, N. and Belvederessi, M. (1977) Subgingival scaling with root planing and curettage. Effects upon gingival inflammation: A comparative study. *J. Periodontol.* 48, 354–362

Lövdal, A., Arno, A., Schei, O. and Waerhaug, J. (1961) Combined effect of subgingival scaling and controlled oral hygiene on the incidence of gingivitis. *Acta Odontol. Scand.* 19, 537–555

MacAlpine, R., Magnusson, I., Kiger, R., Crigger, M., Garrett, S. and Egelberg, J. (1985) Antimicrobial irrigation of deep pockets to supplement oral hygiene instruction and root debridement. I. Bi-weekly irrigation. *J. Clin. Periodontol.* 12, 568–577

McCoy, S. A., Creamer, H. R., Kawanami, M. and Adams, D. F. (1987) The concentration of lipopolysaccharide on individual root surfaces at varying times following *in vitro* root planing. *J. Periodontol.* 58, 393–399

McCulloch, C. A. G., Birek, P. and Hardy, V. (1987) Comparison of gingival attachment level measurements with an automated periodontal probe and a pressure-sensitive probe. *J. Periodont. Res.* 22, 348–352

McFall, W. T. Jr. (1982) Tooth loss in 100 treated patients with periodontal disease. A long-term study. *J. Periodontol.* 53, 539–549

MacPhee, T. and Cowley, C. (1981) *Essentials of Periodontology and Periodontics.* 3rd Edition, pp. 263–266. Blackwell Scientific Publications, Oxford

Magnusson, I. and Listgarten, M. A. (1980) Histological evaluation of probing depth following periodontal treatment. *J. Clin. Periodontol.* 7, 26–31

Magnusson, I, Runstad, L., Nyman, S. and Lindhe, J. (1983) A long junctional epithelium – a locus minoris resistentiae in plaque infection? *J. Clin. Periodontol.* 10, 333–340

Magnusson, I., Lindhe, J., Yoneyama, T. and Liljenberg, B. (1984) Recolonization of a subgingival microbiota following scaling in deep pockets. *J. Clin. Periodontol.* 11, 193–207

Maidwell-Smith, M. A., Wilson, M. and Kieser, J. B. (1987) Endotoxin content of individual periodontally-involved teeth. *J. Clin. Periodontol.* 14, 453–454

Mandel, I. D. and Gaffar, A. (1986) Calculus revisited. A review. *J. Clin. Periodontol.* 13, 249–257

Manor, A., Lebendiger, M., Shiffer, A. and Tovel, H. (1985) Bacterial invasion of periodontal tissues in advanced periodontitis in humans. *J. Periodontol.* 55, 567–573

Manson, J. D. (1980) *Periodontics.* 4th Edition, pp. 136–137. Henry Kimpton, London

Meador, H. L., Lane, J. J. and Suddick, R. P. (1985) The long-term effectiveness of periodontal therapy in a clinical practice. *J. Periodontol.* 56, 253–258

Meyer, K. and Lie, T. (1977) Root surface roughness in response to periodontal instrumentation studied by combined use of microroughness measurements and scanning electron microscopy. *J. Clin. Periodontol.* **4**, 77–91

Mishkin, D. J., Engler, W. O., Javed, T., Darby, T. D., Cobb, R. L. and Coffman, M. A. (1986) A clinical comparison of the effect on the gingiva of the prophy-jet and the rubber cup and paste techniques. *J. Periodontol.* **57**, 151–154

Moore, J., Wilson, M. and Kieser, J. B. (1986) The distribution of bacterial lipopolysaccharide (endotoxin) in relation to periodontally involved root surfaces. *J. Clin. Periodontol.* **13**, 748–751

Morrison, E. C., Ramfjord, S. P. and Hill, R. W. (1980) Short-term effects of initial, nonsurgical periodontal treatment (hygienic phase). *J. Clin. Periodontol.* **7**, 199–211

Morrison, E. C., Ramfjord, S. P., Burgett, F. G., Nissle, R. R. and Shick, R. A. (1982) The significance of gingivitis during the maintenance phase of periodontal treatment. *J. Periodontol.* **53**, 31–34.

Moskow, B. S. (1962) The response of the gingival sulcus to instrumentation: a histological investigation. I. The scaling procedure. *J. Periodontol.* **33**, 282–291.

Mousques, T., Listgarten, M. A. and Phillips, R. W. (1980) Effect of scaling and root planing on the composition of the human subgingival microbial flora. *J. Periodont. Res.* **15**, 144–151

Müller, H. P., Hartmann, J. and Flores-de-Jacoby, L. (1986) Clinical alterations in relation to the morphological composition of the subgingival microflora following scaling and root planing. *J. Clin. Periodontol.* **13**, 825–832

Nadler, H. (1962) Removal of crevicular epithelium by ultrasonic curettes. *J. Periodontol.* **33**, 220–225

Nakib, N. M., Bissada, N. F., Simmelink, J. W. and Goldstine, S. N. (1982) Endotoxin penetration into root cementum of periodontally healthy and diseased human teeth. *J. Periodontol.* **53**, 368–378

Newman, P. S., Silverwood, R. A. and Dolby, A. E. (1985) The effects of an airbrasive instrument on dental hard tissues, skin and oral mucosa. *Br. Dent. J.* **159**, 9–12

Nishimine, D. and O'Leary, T. J. (1979) Hand instrumentation versus ultrasonics in the removal of endotoxins from root surfaces. *J. Periodontol.* **50**, 345–349

Nordland, P., Garrett, S., Vanooteghem, R., Hutchens, L. H. and Egelberg, J. (1987) The effect of plaque control and root debridement in molar teeth. *J. Clin. Periodontol.* **14**, 231–236

Nyman, S. and Lindhe, J. (1979) A longitudinal study of combined periodontal and prosthetic treatment of patients with advanced periodontal disease. *J. Periodontol.* **50**, 163–169

Nyman, S., Rosling, B. and Lindhe, J. (1975) Effect of professional tooth cleaning on healing after periodontal surgery. *J. Clin. Periodontol.* **2**, 80–86

Nyman, S., Lindhe, J. and Rosling, B. (1977) Periodontal surgery in plaque-infected dentitions. *J. Clin. Periodontol.* **4**, 240–249

Nyman, S., Sarhed, G., Ericsson, I., Gottlow, J. and Karring, T. (1986) The role of 'diseased' root cementum for healing following treatment of periodontal disease. *J. Periodont. Res.* **21**, 496–503

Nyman, S., Westfelt, E., Sarhed, G. and Karring, T. (1988) Role of 'diseased' root cementum in healing following treatment of periodontol disease. A clinical study. *J. Clin. Periodontol.* **15**, 464–468

O'Bannon, J. Y. (1964) The gingival tissues before and after scaling the teeth. *J. Periodontol.* **35**, 69–80

O'Leary, T. J. (1986) The impact of research on scaling and root planing. *J. Periodontol.* **57**, 69–75

O'Leary, T. J. and Kafrawy, A. H. (1983) Total cementum removal: a realistic objective? *J. Periodontol.* **54**, 221–226

Oosterwaal, P. J. M., Matee, M. I., Mikx, F. H. M., van't Hof, M. A. and Renggli, H. H. (1987) The effect of subgingival debridement with hand and ultrasonic instruments on the subgingival microflora. *J. Clin. Periodontol.* **14**, 528–533

Ortmann, L. F., Dunford, R., McHenry, K. and Hausmann, E. (1985) Subtraction radiography and computer assisted densitometric analysis of standardized radiographs – a comparison study with ^{125}I absorptiometric. *J. Periodont. Res.* **20**, 644–651

Patterson, C. J. W. and McLundie, A. C. (1984) A comparison of the effects of two different prophylaxis regimes *in vitro* on some restorative dental materials. *Br. Dent. J.* **157**, 166–170

Payot, P., Haroutunian, B., Pochon, Y., Herr, P., Bickel, M. and Cimasoni, G. (1987) Densitometric analysis of lower molar interradicular areas in superposable radiographs. *J. Clin. Periodontol.* **14**, 1–7

Pearlman, B. A. (1982) Ultrasonic root planing. *Aust. Dent. J.* **27**, 109–116

Pertuiset, J. H., Saglie, F. R., Lofthus, J., Rezende, M. and Sanz, M. (1987) Recurrent periodontal disease and bacterial presence in the gingiva. *J. Periodontol.* **58**, 553–558

Pihlström, B. L., Ortiz-Campos, C. and McHugh, R. B. (1981) A randomized four-year study of periodontal therapy. *J. Periodontol.* **52**, 227–242

Pihlström, B. L., McHugh, R. B., Oliphant, T. H. and Ortiz-Campos, C. (1983) Comparison of surgical and nonsurgical treatment of periodontal disease. A review of current studies and additional results after 6½ years. *J. Clin. Periodontol.* **10**, 524–541

Pihlström, B. L., Oliphant, T. H. and McHugh, R. B. (1984) Molar and nonmolar teeth compared over 6½ years following two methods of periodontal therapy. *J. Periodontol.* **55**, 499–504

Pihlström, B. L., Wolff, L. F., Bakdash, M. B., Schaffer, E. M., Jensen, J. R., Aeppli, D. M. and Bandt, C. L. (1987) Salt and peroxide compared with conventional oral hygiene. *J. Periodontol.* **58**, 291–300

Polson, A. M. and Goodson, J. M. (1985) Periodontal diagnosis. Current status and future needs. *J. Periodontol.* **56**, 25–34

Poole, S. J., Kieser, J. B., Boyde, A., Jones, S. J. and Reid, S. A. (1984) Recent developments in SEM shed light on root planing. J. Dent. Res. **63**, 497 (IADR Abstr. 70)

Preber, H. and Bergström, J. (1985) The effect of non-surgical treatment on periodontal pockets in smokers and non-smokers. *J. Clin. Periodontol.* **13**, 319–323

Proye, M., Caton, J. and Polson, A. (1982) Initial healing of periodontal pockets after a single episode of root planing monitored by controlled probing forces. *J. Periodontol.* **53**, 296–301

Rabbani, G. M., Ash, M. and Caffesse, R. G. (1981) The effectiveness of subgingival scaling and root planing in calculus removal. *J. Periodontol.* **52**, 119–123

Raeste, A. M. and Kilpinen, E. (1981) Clinical and radiographic long-term study of teeth with periodontal destruction treated by a modified flap operation. *J. Clin. Periodontol.* **8**, 415–423

Ramfjord, S. P. (1980) Root planing and curettage. *Int. Dent. J.* **30**, 93–100

Ramfjord, S. P. (1987) Maintenance care for treated periodontitis patients. *J. Clin. Periodontol.* **14**, 433–437

Ramfjord, S. P. and Ash, M. M. (1979) Periodontology and Periodontics. 1st Edition, pp. 521–525. W. B. Saunders Company, Philadelphia

Ramfjord, S. P. and Kiester, G. (1954) The gingival sulcus and the periodontal pocket immediately following scaling of teeth. *J. Periodontol.* **25**, 167–176

Ramfjord, S. P. and Nissle, R. R. (1974) The modified Widman flap. *J. Periodontol.* **45**, 601–607

Ramfjord, S. P., Nissle, R. R., Shick, R. A. and Cooper, Jr., H. (1968) Subgingival curettage versus surgical elimination of periodontal pockets. *J. Periodontol.* **39**, 167–175

Ramfjord, S. P., Knowles, J. W., Nissle, R. R., Shick, R. A. and Burgett, F. G. (1973) Longitudintal study of periodontal theory. *J. Periodontol.* **44**, 66–77

Ramfjord, S. P., Knowles, J. W., Nissle, R. R., Burgett, F. G. and Shick, R. A. (1975) Results following three modalities of periodontal therapy. *J. Periodontol.* **46**, 522–526

Ramfjord, S. P., Knowles, J. W., Morrison, E. C., Burgett, F. G. and Nissle, R. R. (1980) Results of periodontal therapy related to tooth type. *J. Periodontol.* **51**, 270–273

Ramfjord, S. P., Morrison, E. C., Burgett, F. G., Nissle, R. R., Shick, R. A., Zann, G. J. and Knowles, J. W. (1982) Oral hygiene and maintenance of periodontal support. *J. Periodontol.* **53**, 26–30

Ramfjord, S. P., Caffesse, R. G., Morrison, E. C., Hill, R. W., Kerry, G. J., Appleberry, E. A., Nissle, R. R. and Stults, D. L. (1987) Four modalities of periodontal treatment compared over 5 years. *J. Clin. Periodontol.* **14**, 445–452

Reddy, J., Parker, J. R., Africa, C. W. and Stephen, L. X. G. (1985) Prevalence and severity of periodontitis in a high fluoride area in South Africa. *Comm. Dent. Oral Epidemiol.* **13**, 108–112

Rosenberg, R. M. and Ash, M. M. Jr. (1974) The effect of root roughness on plaque accumulation and gingival inflammation. *J. Periodontol.* **45**, 146–150

Rosling, B. (1983) Periodontally treated dentitions: their maintenance and prognosis. *Int. Dent. J.* **33**, 147–151

Rosling, B., Nyman, S., Lindhe, J. and Jern, B. (1976a) The healing potential of the periodontal tissues following different techniques of periodontal surgery in plaque-free dentitions. A 2-year clinical study. *J. Clin. Periodontol.* **3**, 233–250

Rosling, B., Nyman, S. and Lindhe, J. (1976b) The effect of systematic plaque control on bone regeneration in infrabony pockets. *J. Clin. Periodontol.* **3**, 38–53

Rosling, B. G., Slots, J., Webber, R. L., Christersson, L. A. and Genco, R. J. (1983) Microbiological and clinical effects of topical subgingival antimicrobial treatment on human periodontal disease. *J. Clin. Periodontol.* **10**, 487–514

Rosling, B. G., Slots, J., Christersson, L. A., Gröndahl, H. G. and Genco, R. J. (1986) Topical antimicrobial therapy and diagnosis of subgingival bacteria in the management of inflammatory periodontal disease. *J. Clin. Periodontol.* **13**, 975–981

Ross, I. F. and Thompson, R. H. Jr. (1978) A long-term study of root retention in the treatment of maxillary molars with furcation involvement. *J. Periodontol.* **49**, 238–244

Ross, I. F. and Thompson, R. H. Jr. (1980) Furcation involvement in maxillary and mandibular molars. *J. Periodontol.* **51**, 450–454

Saglie, F. R., Carranza, F. A. Jr. and Newman, M. G. (1985) The presence of bacteria within the oral epithelium in periodontal disease. I. A scanning and transmission electron microscopic study. *J. Periodontol.* **56**, 618–624

Saglie, R. and Elbaz, J. (1983) Bacterial penetration into the gingival tissue in periodontal disease. *J. West Soc. Periodont. Periodont. Abstr.* **31**, 85–93

Saglie, F. R., Johansen, J. R. and Feo, M. F. (1986) Tooth surfaces after scaling and root planing: Stereomicroscopic and scanning electron microscopic studies. *Compend. Contin. Educ. Dent.* **7**, 494–506

Saglie, F. R., Pertuiset, J. H., Rezende, M. T., Sabet, M. S., Raoufi, D. and Carranza, F. A. Jr. (1987) Bacterial invasion in experimental gingivitis in man. *J. Periodontol.* **58**, 837–846

Sanavi, F., Listgarten, M. A., Boyd, F., Sallay, K. and Nowotny, A. (1985) The colonization and establishment of invading bacteria in periodontium of ligature-treated immunosuppressed rats. *J. Periodontol.* **56**, 273–280

Sanderson, A. D. (1965) Gingival curettage by hand and ultrasonic instruments. A histologic comparison. *J. Periodontol.* **37**, 279–290

Saravanamuttu, R. (1987) Bacterial invasion of the periodontium in chronic periodontitis: the role of surgical contamination. *Br. Dent. J.* **162**, 68–72

Sarbinoff, J. A., O'Leary, T. J. and Miller, C. H. (1983) The comparative effectiveness of various agents in detoxifying diseased root surfaces. *J. Periodontol.* **54**, 77–80

Schaffer, E. M., Steude, G. and King, D. (1964) Healing

of periodontal pocket tissues following ultrasonic scaling and hand planing. *J. Periodontol.* **35**, 140–148

Selikowitz, H.-S., Sheiham, A., Albert, D. and Williams, G. M. (1981) Retrospective longitudinal study of the rate of alveolar bone loss in humans using bite-wing radiographs. *J. Clin. Periodontol.* **8**, 431–438

Shapiro, L., Lodato, F. M. Jr., Courant, P. R. and Stallard, R. E. (1972) Endotoxin determinations in gingival inflammation. *J. Periodontol.* **43**, 591–596

Shenker, B. J. (1987) Immunologic dysfunction in the pathogenesis of periodontal diseases. *J. Clin. Periodontol.* **14**, 489–498

Siegrist, B. and Kornman, K. S. (1982) The effect of supragingival plaque control on the composition of the subgingival microbial flora in ligature-induced periodontitis in the monkey. *J. Dent. Res.* **7**, 936–941

Simon, B. I., Goldman, H. M., Ruben, M. P. and Baker, E. (1969) The role of endotoxin in periodontal disease. I. A reproducible, quantitative method for determining the amount of endotoxin in human gingival exudate. *J. Periodontol.* **40**, 695–701

Simon, B. I., Goldman, H. M., Ruben, M. P. and Baker, E. (1970) The role of endotoxin in periodontal disease. II. Correlation of the quantity of endotoxin in human gingival exudate with the clinical degree of inflammation. *J. Periodontol.* **41**, 81–86

Simon, B. I., Goldman, H. M., Ruben, M. P. and Baker, E. (1971) The role of endotoxin in periodontal disease. III. Correlation of the amount of endotoxin in human gingival exudate with the histologic degree of inflammation. *J. Periodontol.* **42**, 210–216

Simon, B. I., Goldman, H. M., Ruben, M. P., Broitman, S. and Baker, E. (1972) The role of endotoxin in periodontal disease. IV Bacteriologic analyses of human gingival exudate as related to the quantity of endotoxin and clinical degree of inflammation. *J. Periodontol.* **43**, 468–475

Slots, J. and Dahlen, G. (1985) Subgingival microorganisms and bacterial virulence factors in periodontitis. *Scand. J. Dent. Res.* **93**, 119–127

Slots, J. and Genco, R. J. (1984a) Microbial pathogenicity. *J. Dent. Res.* **63**, 412–421

Slots, J. and Genco, R. J. (1984b) Host responses. *J. Dent. Res.* **63**, 441–451

Smart, G. J. (1987) Ultrasonic root surface debridement *in vitro*. MSc Thesis, University of London

Smith, B. A. and Echeverri, M. (1984) The removal of pocket epithelium: a review. *J. West Soc. Periodont. Periodont. Abstr.* **32**, 45–59

Smith, B. A., Echeverri, M. and Caffesse, R.G (1987) Mucoperiosteal flaps with and without removal of the pocket epithelium. *J. Periodontol.* **58**, 78–85

Smith, D. H., Ammons, W. F. Jr. and van Belle, G. (1980) A longitudinal study of periodontal status comparing osseous recontouring with flap curettage. I. Results after 6 months. *J. Periodontol.* **51**, 367–375

Smukler, H. and Tagger, M. (1976) Vital root amputation. A clinical and histological study. *J. Periodontol.* **47**, 324–330

Smulow, J. B., Turesky, S. S. and Hill, R. G. (1983) The effect of supragingival plaque removal on anaerobic bacteria in deep periodontal pockets. *J. Am. Dent. Assoc.* **107**, 737–742

Socransky, S. S., Haffajee, A. D., Goodson, J. M. and Lindhe, J. (1984) New concepts of destructive periodontal disease. *J. Clin. Periodontol.* **11**, 21–32

Söderholm, G. and Egelberg, J. (1982) Teaching plaque control. II. 30-minute versus 15-minute appointments in a three-visit program. *J. Clin. Periodontol.* **9**, 214–222

Söderholm, G., Nobreus, N., Attström, R. and Egelberg, J. (1982) Teaching plaque control. I. A five-visit versus a two-visit program. *J. Clin. Periodontol.* **9**, 203–213

Sottosanti, J. S. and Garrett, J. S. (1975) A rationale for root preparation – a scanning electron microscopic study of diseased cementum. *J. Periodontol.* **46**, 628–629

Stahl, S., Weiner, J. M., Benjamin, S. and Jamada, L. (1971) Soft tissue healing following curettage and root planing. *J. Periodontol.* **42**, 678–684

Stahl, S. S. and Froum, S. (1986) Histological evaluation of human intraosseous healing responses to the placement of tricalcium phosphate ceramic implants. *J. Periodontol.* **57**, 211–217

Stambough, R. V., Dragoo, M., Smith, D. M. and Carasali, L. (1981) The limits of subgingival scaling. *Int. J. Periodont. Rest. Dent.* **1**, 31–41

Suomi, J. D., Greene, J. C., Vermillion, J. R., Doyle, J., Chang, J. J. and Leatherwood, E. C. (1971) The effect of controlled oral hygiene procedures on the progression of periodontal disease in adults: results after third and final year. *J. Periodontol.* **42**, 152–160

Suppipat, N. (1974) Ultrasonics in periodontics. *J. Clin. Periodontol.* **1**, 206–213

Svoboda, P. J., Reeve, C. M. and Sheridan, P. J. (1984) Effect of retention of gingival sulcular epithelium on attachment and pocket depth after periodontal surgery. *J. Periodontol.* **55**, 563–566

Tabita, P. V., Bissada, N. F. and Maybury, J. E. (1981) Effectiveness of supragingival plaque control on the development of subgingival plaque and gingival inflammation in patients with moderate pocket depth. *J. Periodontol.* **52**, 88–93

Tagge, D. L., O'Leary, T. J. and El-Kafrawy, A. H. (1975) The clinical and histological response of periodontal pockets to root planing and oral hygiene. *J. Periodontol.* **46**, 527–533

Thornton, S. and Garnick, J. (1982) Comparison of ultrasonic to hand instruments in the removal of subgingival plaque. *J. Periodontol.* **53**, 35–37

Torfason, T., Kiger, R., Selvig, K. A. and Egelberg, J. (1979) Clinical improvement of gingival conditions following ultrasonic versus hand instrumentation of periodontal pockets. *J. Clin. Periodontol.* **6**, 165–176

Van der Velden, U. (1982) Regeneration of the interdental soft tissues following denudation procedures. *J. Clin. Periodontol.* **9**, 455–459

Van der Velden, U. (1984) Effect of age on the periodontium. *J. Clin. Periodontol.* **11**, 281–294

Van der Velden, U., Abbas, F. and Winkel, E. G. (1986)

Probing considerations in relation to susceptibility to periodontal breakdown. *J. Clin. Periodontol.* **13**, 894–899

Vanooteghem, R., Hutchens, L. H., Garrett, S., Kieger, R. and Egelberg, J. (1987) Bleeding on probing and probing depth as indicators of the response to plaque control and root debridement. *J. Clin. Periodontol.* **14**, 226–230

Vieira, E. M., O'Leary, T. J. and Kafrway, A. H. (1982) The effect of sodium hypochlorite and citric acid solutions on healing of periodontal pockets. *J. Periodontol.* **53**, 71–80

Vrbic, V., Brudevold, F. and McCann, H. G. (1967) Acquisition of fluoride by enamel from fluoride pumice pastes. *Helv. Odont. Acta* **11**, 21–26

Waerhaug, J. (1956a) Enamel cuticle. *J. Dent. Res.* **35**, 313–322

Waerhaug, J. (1956b) Effect of rough surfaces upon gingival tissue. *J. Dent. Res.* **35**, 323–325

Waerhaug, J. (1975) A method of evaluation of periodontal problems on extracted teeth. *J. Clin. Periodontol.* **2**, 160–168

Waerhaug, J. (1978a) Healing of the dento-epithelial junction following subgingival plaque control. I. As observed in human biopsy material. *J. Periodontol.* **49**, 1–8

Waerhaug, J. (1978b) Healing of the dento-epithelial junction following subgingival plaque control. II. As observed on extracted teeth. *J. Periodontol.* **49**, 119–134

Waerhaug, J. (1980) The furcation problem. Etiology, pathogenesis, diagnosis, therapy and prognosis. *J. Clin. Periodontol.* **7**, 73–95

Waite, I. M. (1976) A comparison between conventional gingivectomy and a non-surgical regime in the treatment of periodontitis. *J. Clin. Periodontol.* **3**, 173–185

Walmsley, A. D., Laird, W. R. E. and Williams, A. R. (1984) A model system to demonstrate the role of cavitational activity in ultrasonic scaling. *J. Dent. Res.* **63**, 1162–1165

Walmsley, A. D., Laird, W. R. E. and Williams, A. R. (1988) Dental plaque removal by cavitational activity during ultrasonic scaling. *J. Clin. Periodontol.* **15**, 539–543

Watts, T. (1987) Constant force probing with and without a stent in untreated periodontal disease: the clinical reproducibility problem and possible sources of error. *J. Clin. Periodontol.* **14**, 407–411

Weaks, L. M., Lescher, N. B., Barnes, C. M. and Holroyd, S. V. (1984) Clinical evaluation of the Prophy-Jet as an instrument for routine removal of tooth stain and plaque. *J. Periodontol.* **55**, 486–488

Westfelt, E., Nyman, S., Lindhe, J. and Socransky, S. (1983) Use of chlorhexidine as a plaque control measure following surgical treatment of periodontal disease. *J. Clin. Periodontol.* **10**, 22–36

Westfelt, E., Nyman, S., Socransky, S. and Lindhe, J. (1983) Significance of frequency of professional tooth cleaning for healing following periodontal surgery. *J. Clin. Periodontol.* **10**, 148–156

Westfelt, E., Bragd, L., Socransky, S. S., Haffajee, A. D., Nyman, S. and Lindhe, J. (1985) Improved periodontal conditions following therapy. *J. Clin. Periodontol.* **12**, 283–293

Whitehead, S. P. and Watts, T. L. P. (1987) Short-term effect of Keyes' approach to periodontal therapy compared with modified Widman flap surgery. *J. Clin. Periodontol.* **14**, 599–604

Wilson, M., Moore, J. and Kieser, J. B. (1986) Identity of limulus amoebocyte lysate-active root surface materials from periodontally involved teeth. *J. Clin. Periodontol.* **13**, 743–747

Wilson, T. Jr. (1987) Compliance. A review of the literature with possible applications to periodontics. *J. Periodontol.* **58**, 706–714

Wilson, T. G. Jr., Glover, M. E., Malik, A. K., Schoen, J. A. and Dorsett, D. (1987) Tooth loss in maintenance patients in a private periodontal practice. *J. Periodontol.* **58**, 231–235

Wirthlin, M. R. and Hancock, E. B. (1982) Regeneration and repair after biologic treatment of root surfaces in monkeys. II. Proximal surfaces posterior teeth. *J. Periodontol.* **53**, 302–306

Wirthlin, M. R., Hancock, E. B. and Gaugler, R. W. (1981) Regeneration and repair after biologic treatment of root surfaces in monkeys. I. Facial surfaces maxillary incisors. *J. Periodontol.* **52**, 729–735

Wolff, L. F., Pihlström, B. L., Bakdash, M. B., Schaffer, E. M., Jensen, J. R., Aeppli, D. M. and Bandt, C. L. (1987) Salt and peroxide compared with conventional oral hygiene. *J. Periodontol.* **58**, 301–307

Yin, E., Galanos, C., Kinsky, S., Bradshaw, R., Wessler, S., Lüderitz, O. and Sarmiento, M. (1972) Picogram-sensitive assay for endotoxin: gelation of Limulus polyphemus blood cell lysate induced by purified lipopolysaccharides and Lipid A from Gram-negative bacteria. *Biochim. Biophys. Acta* **261**, 284–289

Yukna, R. A. (1976) A clinical and histologic study of healing following the excisional new attachment procedure in rhesus monkeys. *J. Periodontol.* **47**, 701–709

Yukna, R. A. and Williams, J. E. (1980) Five-year evaluation of the excisional new attachment procedure. *J. Periodontol.* **51**, 382–385

Zamet, J. S. (1975) A comparative clinical study of three periodontal surgical techniques. *J. Clin. Periodontol.* **2**, 87–97

30

Furcation involvements

Susceptibility to breakdown
The efficacy of therapy
Post-resection implications

Accessory furcation canals and
   endodontic–periodontic lesions
References

There are a number of aspects of teeth that should be considered where the root furcation is involved by attachment destruction. These are the clinical impression that multirooted units are more prone to periodontal breakdown, the effectiveness of the various forms of treatment of furcation involvement, the apparent problems of hypermobility and tooth fracture affecting teeth following root resection, the stability of root resected teeth in prosthodontic therapy, and finally combined endodontic–periodontic lesions associated with furcation accessory canals.

The reader is also referred to the extensive reviews of the management of furcation involvement by Newell (1981) and Saadoun (1985).

Susceptibility to breakdown

It has long been assumed that bi- or trifurcated teeth are more prone to periodontal breakdown. In this respect, Masters and Hoskins (1964), among others, have cited cervical enamel projections into the furcations leading to localized weaker periodontal attachments as predisposing factors (see also Hou and Tsai, 1987). Similarly, bifurcation ridges of dentine or cementum between the roots, where plaque can accumulate, have also been incriminated (Everett et al., 1958; Burch and Hulen, 1974).

Furcated teeth are located at the back of the mouth where plaque control is understandably more difficult which might reasonably explain any predisposition to disease at furcation sites. In addition, the greater incidence of plaque-induced disease interproximally than elsewhere would increase the

likelihood of furcation involvement, at least in the maxilla, and would, as such, represent the effect rather than the cause of involvement. The predominantly interproximal location of maxillary molar furcations might in turn account for the observation that furcation involvement was three times more frequent in maxillary than in mandibular molars (Ross and Thompson, 1980). Larato (1975) found that a high proportion of furcation defects at maxillary and mandibular molars were associated with the close proximity of the furca to the cemento-enamel junctions. This relationship has also been shown (in the mandible) by Volchansky and Cleaton-Jones (1978), Tal (1982 a and b) and Tal and Lemmer (1982). Once exposed to the microflora, the furcation morphology does complicate both plaque removal and root surface instrumentation (Abrams and Trachtenberg, 1974; Bower, 1979 a and b; Waerhaug, 1980; Gher and Vernino, 1980). The findings of Booker and Loughlin (1985) show this to be equally applicable to maxillary first premolars. These difficulties become progressively greater as further breakdown involves the complex shapes of the root surface concavities, as described in Chapter 18.

The traditional incrimination of occlusal forces in the development of furcation lesions (e.g. Youdelis and Mann, 1965; Staffileno, 1969) was questioned by Waerhaug (1980), for increased mobility was found to be only a very late and an inconsistent symptom. Furthermore, the obvious premature occlusal contacts, mobility and pain, observed in all cases of furcation periodonal abscesses could be explained readily by the secondary inflammatory extrusion of the tooth.

In conclusion, the aetiology of the furcation lesion appears no different from anywhere else but once established is undoubtedly more difficult to treat because of the furcation morphology itself.

The efficacy of therapy

The management of incipient furcation involvement by reshaping the adjacent tooth surfaces and bone to attain physiological contours and enhance access for plaque control, was first suggested by Goldman (1958). This 'furcation operation' (Hamp *et al.*, 1975) technique was later combined with the lateral repositioned mucoperiosteal flap (Goldman *et al.*, 1968) as a means of 'sealing off' the inter-radicular furcation involvement. The elimination of the totally involved furcation, by amputating a root (root resection) appears to have been first described by Farrar (1884) as cited by Klavan (1975). Messinger and Orban (1954) are however generally credited with having rekindled the major interest in the root resection technique which has since been described by many (for Reviews see Newell, 1981; Saadoun, 1985; Green, 1986). Hemisection, as described by Black (1915), represents an extension of the root resection technique, in that the overlying crown is also removed to produce a single rooted unit (Abrams and Trachtenberg 1974). Tunnel preparation to open the furcation for inter-radicular plaque removal has also been described (Saxe and Carmen, 1969), but has rather limited clinical applications. Finally, the principle of guided tissue regeneration (*cf.* Chapter 31) in the more conservative management of furcation involvement appears to be most promising, as shown by the findings of Pontoriero *et al.* (1988, 1989). Similarly, the technique of acid conditioning in conjunction with flap coronal positioning (Martin *et al.*, 1988; Gantes *et al.*, 1988) warrants further investigation.

The indications for retaining or extracting teeth with involved furcations have been the subject of some discussion (e.g. Basabara, 1969), most authors being somewhat pessimistic and advocating extraction on the basis of rather vague generalizations (e.g. Saxe and Carmen, 1969). Others have in turn advocated extraction to preserve the periodontal health of adjacent teeth (Arvins, 1961), especially where these would make good prosthetic abutments (Everett and Stern, 1969; Grant *et al.*, 1979) and to simplify overall treatment in relation to expected benefits and to facilitate future plaque control (Nyman and Lindhe, 1976). Goldman and Cohen (1980) advocated early removal of these hopeless teeth in deference to the neighbouring units and lest the patient postponed the necessary prosthodontic treatment to the detriment of the entire dentition. Prichard (1979), on the other hand, stated that such teeth should not be extracted merely on the evidence of extensive furcation involvement.

The above opinions will be put into a clearer perspective by examining the findings of the available clinical investigations. In the first of these, Hamp *et al.* (1975) extracted 44% of a total of 310 multirooted teeth with furcation involvement during presurgical therapy. This was based on several criteria including the extent of the destruction involving the apical portion of the periodontal ligament, the limited perceived benefits of these units to the overall treatment plan, or because the furcation would never be readily cleansible. An example of the latter would be at maxillary first premolars with furcations located too far apically. In addition, practically all third molars and half of the second molars involved were also extracted as these were considered too difficult to clean properly. Of the 175 teeth that were retained, 18% were only root planed, 28% had furcation operations, 50% had root resections and the remaining 4% (7 units) had tunnel preparations. The 5-year postoperative evaluation revealed that only 16 of the retained units had pocket depths exceeding 3 mm. The clinical success achieved was ascribed to the total elimination of plaque retention areas and the high standard of plaque control and professional care maintained.

Hirschfeld and Wasserman (1978) presented the findings on 600 patients re-examined an average of 22 years after active periodontal therapy and maintenance care in accordance with prevailing views. The furcation involved teeth were treated with the expectation of reducing pocket depths rather than eliminating them, and only 17 root amputations were performed. Of the 1464 teeth (10.7% of total units) with furcation involvements at the outset, 460 were lost, of which 240 occurred in only one-sixth of the patients. These patients were, however, deemed to have rates of periodontal deterioration classed as being 'extreme downhill'. In contrast, in the well maintained group only 19.3% of the molars were eventually lost, compared with 84.4% and 69.9% for the 'extreme downhill' and 'downhill' groups respectively. In each instance it was the maxillary molars that gave the poorer response and there appeared to be little difference attributable to periodontal surgery. It is also noteworthy that in all groups the disease process observed often followed a pattern of irregularly shaped cycles of destruction. Thus, some advanced cases responded well for over 20 years but then many teeth were lost while others were shown to remain stable for years, interspaced with sporadic periods of destruction. This finding appears to support the recently expressed hypotheses of periodontal breakdown (Socransky *et al.*, 1984).

Ross and Thompson (1978) evaluated the 'functional survival', (i.e. that the 'tooth is functioning efficiently in a healthy state and without pain') of

387 maxillary molars in 100 patients treated over periods ranging from 5 to 26 years. An 88% survival was shown, despite the fact that many units had at least one root with 50% or less of bone support before commencing treatment. Specific therapy for this group involved only soft tissue surgery (with considerable emphasis on improving occlusal function), but in no instance was root amputation, hemisection or even furcation operation carried out. Of the 46 (12%) teeth that were ultimately lost, 25 were retained for significant periods of between 6 and 18 years. These findings, coupled with those of another study on 615 maxillary and mandibular molars in 72 patients over a similar time span (Ross and Thompson, 1980) suggest that the traditionally held view of the poor prognosis of molars with furcation involvement is not justified. While furcation involvement is important, it should not by itself condemn a tooth to extraction. This conclusion has been supported by the findings of Ramfjord *et al.* (1980) and Pihlström *et al.* (1984) (*cf.* Chapter 29).

Langer *et al.* (1981) reported a 38% failure of 100 root resected units during a 10-year observation period although few occurred in the initial 5 years. Most failures were due to endodontic or restorative problems, especially in the mandible, even though the primary reason for treatment was progressive periodontal breakdown.

Björn and Hjort (1982) presented data based on orthopantomographic and bitewing radiographic appearances of the inter-radicular bony septa of mandibular molars in 221 individuals treated routinely over a 13-year period. Only 9% of the molars with furcation involvement were lost during the observation period. However, as other areas of the dentitions had also deteriorated, it was concluded that furcation involvement *per se* had evidently not played a dominant part in tooth loss.

Most recently, Payot *et al.* (1987) reported on the effects over 1 year of subgingival curettage, modified Widman flap surgery and furcation osteoplasty and furcationplasty on mandibular molars with degrees 1 and 2 furcation involvements. Significant pocket reductions were achieved with furcationplasty alone. Although there were no changes in probing attachment levels, significant bony alterations were observed by quantitative radiodensitometric analysis, thus questioning the accuracy of routine probing measurements. Nordland *et al.* (1987) demonstrated that molar furcation sites respond less favourably to root surface debridement than molar flat surface sites and non-molar sites over a 2-year assessment period. However, with the increasingly widespread use of ultrasonic instruments in clinical practice more effective debridement (Leon and Vogel, 1987) and scaling (Matia *et al.*, 1986) within the furcation areas should be forthcoming.

Two other studies might also be considered here,

although restorative and endodontic problems were the main reasons for treatment. In the first, Bergenholtz (1972) described a method for resection of one or more roots of multirooted teeth (radectomy) with and without the related part of the crown; a total of 45 radectomies performed on 40 patients who were observed for periods of up to 11 years. In the other study, Erpenstein (1983) reported on the findings over 1–7 years (mean 3 years) on 34 hemisected molars. The teeth treated were predominantly mandibular molars and 22 were used as bridge abutments. The overall findings of these investigations indicated that the prognosis for teeth after a radectomy and hemisection is good, the risk of periodontal failure very small and that these teeth may function as sound abutments for bridges.

In conclusion, it does appear that the outlook at molars with involved furcation areas (there being insufficient data relating to maxillary first premolars) is rather more favourable than has been thought traditionally and as such constitutes the basis for the compromise therapy advocated in Chapter 18. However, where root resections are undertaken the possible restorative and occlusal implications and not least the endodontic considerations must not be overlooked. The latter need not be considered further here.

Post-resection implications

Coronal restorative needs

Tradition holds to the view that teeth are more likely to fracture following endodontic therapy and that this complication can be averted by a suitable restoration (see Ross, 1980). These beliefs stem mainly from the loss of internal dentine both during the creation of access and endodontic instrumentation, but also from the decreased moisture content (e.g. Helfer *et al.* (1972) who demonstrated 9% less moisture) and the resulting brittleness of pulpless teeth. However, Ross (1980) questioned the justification for the use of internal supporting devices (posts) and complete coverage restorations to protect endodontically treated teeth from fracture. Nearly two-thirds of 220 treated teeth in 102 subjects, observed over a 5-year period, had endodontics therapy only, yet no evidence of fracture of any tooth was found. The limited data provided in this study precludes further analysis.

The loss of tooth material associated with root resections might be expected to weaken the tooth further and necessitate complex restoration. However in unpublished data, the author has observed over a period of 5–14 years (mean 7 years), only one instance of tooth fracture through the furcation and in four cases fracture of the unsupported remaining coronal tooth material, out of a total of 35 root resected molars (31 maxillary) at which no specific cusp protected coronal restoration had been provided (*cf.* Chapter 18). Further investigations are required to clarify the position but these are likely to be hampered by the difficulties of obtaining non-restored control units. This difficulty stems from the traditional provision of full cuspal coverage in the restoration of such teeth together with the removal of the remaining tooth material overlying any resected root (hemisection) in most instances. There have been numerous descriptions of this type of treatment (Rosen and Gitnick, 1964, 1969; Basaraba, 1969; Abrams and Trachtenberg, 1974; Nyman *et al.*, 1975; Highfield, 1978; Nyman and Lindhe, 1979; Appleton, 1980). Another investigation problem is the obvious economic need to incorporate the design of any restoration of such root resected teeth into overall treatment planning. This then raises the additional question of occlusal function and mobility of these teeth with reduced radicular support.

Mobility

The possible consequences of increased tooth mobility following root resections have not been evaluated adequately, due to the frequency with which the remaining root(s) have either been splinted or used as bridge abutments. However, in a retrospective analysis on 24 root resected maxillary molars which had neither been splinted nor supported in any way (although there was some occlusal adjustment), Klavan (1975) reported the development of increased mobility over a period of 3 years in only three instances. It was concluded that splinting of teeth following root amputation is not always necessary. Similarly, Erpenstein (1983) revealed that only one of 24 root resected maxillary molars, that had not been splinted or incorporated into bridges or removable partial dentures, showed any sign of increased mobility.

The above findings are consistent with the author's clinical observations at such maxillary molars and indeed also at mandibular molars, but at which it must be stressed, marginal tissue health had been maintained (*cf.* Chapter 18). Resected lower molars are in contrast most often splinted to prevent drifting or rotation, although this may instead merely reflect the effect of the associated restorative requirements at the site. In this context, the observations of Erpenstein (1983) confirm that hemisected teeth, and those with markedly reduced periodontal support, may be used as fixed bridge abutments (Nyman *et al.*, 1975). This does however demand the reconstruction of a stable occlusion and a high standard of plaque control (Lindhe and Nyman, 1975).

Vital root resection

It is generally held that the root canal therapy is an integral part of, and is mandatory for, successful root amputation. When amputation is pre-planned, endodontics precedes surgery to establish whether successful endodontic therapy is possible, and also for convenience. However, where the need to resect a root can only be confirmed at operation, immediate resection at that stage has been advocated (Basaraba, 1969; Abrams and Trachtenberg, 1974). The exposed pulp is dressed with zinc oxide–eugenol or calcium hydroxide paste and endodontic treatment postponed to a later and more convenient time. On the other hand, Smukler and Jagger (1976) and Jagger and Smukler (1977) have shown that exposed healthy vital pulps remained without symptoms for a 2-week period even when not dressed following root amputation. It may therefore be feasible to delay any elective endodontic therapy for some weeks until after periodontal surgery. This would in turn obviate the need to subject the patient to the discomfort by such additional treatment during the immediate post-operative period of residual periodontal tissue tenderness.

There exists also the possible option of an elective vital root resection, with the objective of maintaining pulpal vitality (Haskell, 1966). A subsequent publication (Haskell, 1969), described the technique and presented the results of the resection of either the mesiobuccal or distobuccal roots of 10 maxillary molars, coupled with occlusal adjustment to relieve stresses. In nine instances the pulp remained vital for periods of up to 6 years (see Chapter 18). However, Allen and Gutman (1977) have reported internal root resorption as a potential complication of vital root resection. It was suggested that this might have been produced by a chronic retrograde pulpitis, the calcium hydroxide capping material (Seltzer and Bender, 1975), or the trauma of the resection itself.

Accessory furcation canals and endodontic–periodontal lesions

In the early 1970s the possibility of pulpal disease affecting the periodontal tissue and the reverse was realized. This may be either by infection via lateral canals existing along root surfaces or, of greater relevance here, within the pulp chamber floor of molar teeth via accessory canals. This led to Bender and Seltzer (1972) describing a new syndrome, the pulpodontic–periodontic syndrome. However, in presenting a classification of these so-called endodontic–periodontal lesions, Simon *et al.* (1972) cited several references to their existence dating back almost a decade (e.g. Schilder, 1963).

The frequency with which furcation accessory canals occur is not clear. The findings of investigations carried out on extracted teeth differ markedly, although some of the differences might be explained by the different experimental methods. Thus, for example, Gutman (1978) reported an incidence of 28.8% of furcation accessory canals, Vertucci and Anthony (1986) between 12 and 36%, Vertucci and Williams (1974) 46%, Lowman *et al.* (1973) 59% and Burch and Hulen (1974) 76%. Furthermore, as the reasons for extraction were not given it is conceivable that the samples were biased and that the very existence of furcation canals, leading to pulpal or periodontal symptoms, might have been responsible for the extraction. Indeed, even the lowest claimed incidence seems high, bearing in mind the infrequency with which pulpal symptoms seem to occur in molars with surgically exposed furcations. This is endorsed by the finding that endodontic therapy was required at only 14 out of 387 maxillary molars with involved furcations (Ross and Thompson, 1978). On the other hand, it must be acknowledged that such canals might well exist more frequently than is implied here but are occluded by secondary dentine or by cementum and only become exposed to the oral microflora following root planing as shown by Vertucci and Anthony (1986). However, as suggested by Lowman *et al.* (1973), the chances of doing so within the furcation are slim because of the technical difficulties of furcation instrumentation.

Finally, there have been a number of clinical reports of the healing of the periodontal component of combined lesions following endodontic therapy alone. The most impressive of these was presented by Prichard (1972). However, it is not known whether the clinical and radiographic signs of bony regeneration observed in these cases are associated with an initial loss of connective tissue attachment to the root or not. If there is initial connective tissue loss it is also not known whether attachment occurs or if the interposition of epithelium takes place instead.

References

Abrams, L. and Trachtenberg, D. I. (1974) Hemisection – technique and restoration. *Dent. Clin. North Am.* **18**, 415–444

Allen, A. L. (1977) Internal root resorption after vital root resection. *J. Endodontol.* **3**, 438–440

Allen, A. L. and Gutmann, J. L. (1977) Internal root resorption after vital root resection. *J. Endodontol.* **3**, 438–440

Appleton, I. E. (1980) Restoration of root-resected teeth. *J. Prosthet. Dent.* **44**, 150–153

Arvins, A. N. (1961) Changing concepts in periodontal prognosis. *J. Dent. Med.* **16**, 133–139

Basaraba, N. (1969) Root amputation and tooth hemisection. *Dent. Clin. North Am.* Jan. 121–131

Bender, I. B. and Seltzer, S. (1972) Conference on the biology of the humandental pulp. *Oral Surg.* **33**, 458–474

Bergenholtz, A. (1972) Radectomy of multirooted teeth. *J. Am. Dent. Assoc.* **85**, 870–875

Björn, A.-L. and Hjort, P. (1982) Bone loss of furcated mandibular molars. A longitudinal study. *J. Clin. Periodontol.* **9**, 402–408

Black, G. V. (1915) *Special Dental Pathology*, pp. 205–206. Medico-Dental Publishing Co. Chicago

Booker, B. W. III and Loughlin, D. M. (1985) A morphologic study of the mesial root surface of the adolescent maxillary first bicuspid. *J. Periodontol.* **56**, 666–670

Bower, R. C. (1979a) Furcation morphology relative to periodontal treatment: Furcation entrance architecture. *J. Periodontol.* **50**, 23–27

Bower, R. C. (1979b) Furcation morphology relative to periodontal treatment: Furcation root surface anatomy. *J. Periodontol.* **50**, 366–374

Burch, J. G. and Hulen, S. (1974) A study of the presence of accessory foramina and the topography of molar furcations. *Oral Surg.* **38**, 451–455

Erpenstein, H. (1983) A 3-year study of hemisectioned molars. *J. Clin. Periodontol.* **10**, 1–10

Everett, F. G., Jump, E. B., Holder, T. D. and Williams, G. C. (1958) The intermediate bifurcational ridge: a study of the morphology of the bifurcation of the lower first molar. *J. Dent. Res.* **37**, 162–169

Everett, F. G. and Stern, I. B. (1969) When is tooth mobility an indication for extraction. *Dent. Clin. North Am.* **13**, 791–799

Farrar, J. M. (1884) Radical and heroic treatment of alveolar abscess byamputation of roots of teeth. *Dental Cosmos* **26**, 79–81

Gantes, B., Martin, M., Garrett, S. and Egelberg, J. (1988) Treatment of periodontal furcation defects. (II) Bone regeneration in mandibular class II defects. *J. Clin. Periodontol.* **15**, 232–239

Gher, M. E. and Vernino, A. R. (1980) Root morphology – clinical significance in pathogenesis and treatment of periodontal disease. *J. Am. Dent. Assoc.* **101**, 627–633

Goldman, H. M. (1958) Therapy of the incipient bifurcation involvement. *J. Periodontol.* **29**, 112–116

Goldman, H. M. and Cohen, D. W. (1980) *Periodontal Therapy*, 6th Edition, pp. 415–422. C. V. Mosby Co. St Louis, MO

Goldman, H. M., Shuman, A. M. and Isenberg, G. A. (1968) Management of the partial furcation involvement. *Periodontics* **6**, 197–206

Grant, D. A., Stern, I. B. and Everett, F. G. (1979) *Periodontics*. 5th Edition, pp. 488–497. C. V. Mosby Co. St Louis, MO

Green, E. N. (1986) Hemisection and root amputation. *J. Am. Dent. Assoc.* **112**, 511–518

Gutmann, J. L. (1978) Prevalence, location, and patency

of accessory canals in the furcation region of permanent molars. *J. Periodontol.* **49**, 21–26

Hamp, S.-E., Nyman, S. and Lindhe, J. (1975) Periodontal treatment of multirooted teeth. Results after 5 years. *J. Clin. Periodontol.* **2**, 126–135

Haskell, E. W. (1966) Vital root resection on maxillary multirooted teeth. *J. S. Calif. Dent. Assoc.* **34**, 509–512

Haskell, E. W. (1969) Vital root resection. *Endodontics.* **27**, 266–274

Helfer, A. R., Melnick, S. and Schilder, H. (1972) Determination of the moisture content of vital and pulpless teeth. *Oral Surg.* **34**, 661–670

Highfield, J. E. (1978) Periodontal treatment of multirooted teeth. *Aust. Dent. J.* **23**, 91–98

Hirschfeld, L. and Wasserman, B. (1978) A long-term survey of tooth loss in 600 treated periodontal patients. *J. Periodontol.* **49**, 225–236

Hou, G.-L. and Tsai, C.-C. (1987) Relationship between periodontal furcation involvement and molar cervical enamel projections. *J. Periodontol.* **58**, 715–721

Klavan, B. (1975) Clinical observations following root amputation in maxillary molar teeth. *J. Periodontol.* **46**, 1–5

Langer, B., Stein, S. D. and Wagenberg, B. (1981) An evaluation of root resections. A ten-year study. *J. Periodontol.* **52**, 719–722

Larato, D. C. (1975) Some anatomical factors related to furcation involvements. *J. Periodontol.* **46**, 608–609

Leon, L. E. and Vogel, R. I. (1987) A comparison of the effectiveness of hand scaling and ultrasonic debridement in furcations as evaluated by differential dark-field microscopy. *J. Periodontol.* **58**, 86–94

Lindhe, J. and Nyman, S. (1975) The effect of plaque control and surgical pocket elimination on the establishment and maintenance of periodontal health. A longitudinal study of periodontal therapy in cases of advanced disease. *J. Clin. Periodontol.* **2**, 67–79

Lowman, J. V., Burke, R. S., and Pelleu, G. B. (1973) Patent accessory canals: Incidence in molar furcation region. *Oral Surg.* **36**, 580–584

Martin, M., Gantes, B., Garrett, S. and Egelberg, J. (1988) Treatment of periodontal furcation defects. (I) Review of the literature and description of a regenerative surgical technique. *J. Clin. Periodontol.* **15**, 227–231

Masters, D. H. and Hoskins, S. W. (1964) Projection of cervical enamel into molar furcations. *J. Periodontol.* **35**, 49–53

Matia, J., Bissada, N., Maybury, J. and Ricchetti, R. (1985) Scaling and root planing of the bifurcation area with and without surgical access. *J. Dent. Res.* **64**, 335 (abstract No. 1447)

Messinger, T. F. and Orban, B. (1954) Elimination of periodontal pockets by root amputation. *J. Periodontol.* **25**, 213–215

Newell, D. H. (1981) Current status of the management of teeth with furcation invasions. *J. Periodontol.* **52**, 559–568

Nordland, P., Garrett, S., Kiger, R., Vanooteghem, R., Hutchens, L. H. and Egelberg, J. (1987) The effect of plaque control and root debridement in molar teeth. *J. Clin. Periodontol.* **14**, 231–236

Nyman, S. and Lindhe, J. (1976) Considerations in the treatment of patients with multiple teeth with furcation involvements. *J. Clin. Periodontol.* **3**, 4–13

Nyman, S. and Lindhe, J. (1979) A longitudinal study of combined periodontal and prosthetic treatment of patients with advanced periodontal disease. *J. Periodontol.* **50**, 163–169

Nyman, S., Lindhe, J. and Lundgren, D. (1975) The role of occlusion for the stability of fixed bridges in patients with reduced periodontal tissue support. *J. Clin. Periodontol.* **2**, 53–66

Payot, P., Bickel, M. and Cimasoni, G. (1987) Longitudinal quantitative radiodensitometric study of treated and untreated lower molar furcation involvements. *J. Clin. Periodontol.* **14**, 8–18

Pihlstrom, B. L., Oliphant, T. H. and McHugh, R. B. (1984) Molar and nonmolar teeth compared over 6½ years following two methods of periodontal therapy. *J. Periodontol.* **55**, 499–504

Pontoriero, R., Lindhe, J., Nyman, S., Karring, T., Rosenberg, E. and Sanavi, F. (1988) Guided tissue regeneration in degree II furcation-involved mandibular molars. *J. Clin. Periodontol.* **15**, 247–254

Pontoriero, R., Lindhe, J., Nyman, S., Karring, T., Rosenberg, E. and Sanavi, F. (1989) Guided tissue regeneration in the treatment of furcation defects in mandibular molars. *J. Clin. Periodontol.* **16**, 170–174

Prichard, J. F. (1972) *Advanced Periodontal Disease and Surgical and Prosthetic Management,* 2nd Edition, pp. 535–565. W. B. Saunders Co. Philadelphia

Prichard, J. F. (1979) *The Diagnosis and Treatment of Periodontal Disease,* pp. 161–162. W. B. Saunders Co. Philadelphia

Ramfjord, S. P., Knowles, J. W., Morrison, E. C., Burgett, F. G. and Nissle, R. R. (1980) Results of periodontal therapy related to tooth type. *J. Periodontol.* **51**, 270–273

Rosen, H. and Gitnick, P. J. (1964) Integrating restorative procedures into the treatment of periodontal disease. *J. Prosthet. Dent.* **14**, 343–354

Rosen, H. and Gitnick, P. J. (1969) Separation and splinting of the roots of multirooted teeth. *J. Prosthet. Dent.* **21**, 34–38

Ross, I. F. (1980) Fracture susceptibility of endodontically treated teeth. *J. Endodontol.* **6**, 560–565

Ross, I. F. and Thompson, R. H. Jr. (1978) A long-term study of root retention in the treatment of maxillary molars with furcation involvement. *J. Periodontol.* **49**, 238–244

Ross, I. F. and Thompson, R. H. Jr. (1980) Furcation involvement in maxillary and mandibular molars. *J. Periodontol.* **51**, 450–454

Saadoun, A. P. (1985) Management of furcation involvement. *J. West Soc. Periodont. Periodont. Abstr.* **33**, 91–125

Saxe, S. R. and Carman, D. K. (1969) Removal or

retention of molar teeth: the problem of the furcation. *Dent. Clin. North Am.* **13**, 783–790

Schilder, H. (1963) The relationship of periodontics to endodontics. *Transactions of the Third International Conference on Endodontics* (Louis I. Grossman, Editor), University of Philadelphia, Philadelphia

Seltzer, S. and Bender, I. B. (1975) *The Dental Pulp,* pp. 234–252. J. B. Lippincott, Philadelphia

Simon, J. H. S., Glick, D. H. and Frank, A. L. (1972) The relationship of endodontic-periodontic lesions. *J. Periodontol.* **43**, 202–208

Smukler, H. and Tagger, M. (1976) Vital root amputation; a clinical and histological study. *J. Periodontol.* **47**, 324–330

Socransky, S. S., Haffajee, A. D., Goodson, J. M. and Lindhe, J. (1984) New concepts of destructive periodontal disease. *J. Clin. Periodontol.* **11**, 21–32

Staffileno, H. J. (1969) Surgical management of the furca invasion. *Dent. Clin. North Am.* 103–119

Tagger, M. and Smukler, H. (1977) Microscopic study of the pulps of human teeth following vital root resection. *Oral Surg.* **44**, 96–105

Tal, H. (1982 a) Furcal defects in dry mandibles. Part 1: A biometric study. *J. Periodontol.* **53**, 360–363

Tal, H. (1982 b) Relationship between the depths of furcal defects and alveolar bone loss. *J. Periodontol.* **53**, 631–634

Tal, H. and Lemmer, J. (1982) Furcal defects in dry mandibles. Part II: Severity of furcal defects. *J. Periodontol.* **53**, 364–367

Vertucci, F. J. and Anthony, R. L. (1986) A scanning electron microscopic investigation of accessory foramina in the furcation and pulp chamber floor of molar teeth. *Oral Surg.* **62**, 319–326

Vertucci, F. J. and Williams, R. G. (1974) Furcation canals in the human mandibular first molar. *Oral Surg.* **38**, 308–314

Volchansky, A. and Cleaton-Jones, P. E. (1978) Bony defects in dried Bantu mandibles. *Oral Surg.* **45**, 647–653

Waerhaug, J. (1980) The furcation problem. Etiology, pathogenesis, diagnosis, therapy and prognosis. *J. Clin. Periodontol.* **7**, 73–95

Yuodelis, R. A. and Mann, W. V. Jr. (1965) The prevalence and possible role of nonworking contacts in periodontal disease. *Periodontics.* **3**, 219–223

31

Osseous therapy

The pattern of periodontal breakdown in any individual appears to reflect variations in the retention of bacterial plaque and its pathogenicity, at different sites. The direct or indirect destructive changes within the supracrestal tissues result in the progressive loss of periodontal attachment, the apical migration of epithelium along the root surface and the inevitable involvement of the subjacent crestal bone which undergoes resorption. A relationship appears to exist between the pattern of bone resorption and the supracrestal gingival inflammatory infiltration and/or the apical migration of the junctional epithelium. Thus, a narrow band of intact supra-alveolar connective tissue always exists between the base of the pocket epithelium and the crestal bone, regardless of the extent of disease (Waerhaug, 1952, 1979 a; Goldman, 1957). The underlying mechanism of the bone resorption in periodontal disease does, however, still remain unclear – for reviews see Hausmann and Ortman (1979), Johnson et al. (1985) and Wirthlin (1986). The nature of bony defects, their management and the role of bone in healing will now be considered.

The nature of bony defects

Histological features

The classic histological description of intrabony defects by Carranza and Glickman (1957) listed changes essentially comparable to those occurring in suprabony pockets. Thus, the epithelial downgrowth, the associated variable degrees of connective tissue inflammation and degradation is separated from the intrabony crest (see Figure 19.1) by a narrow band of intact supracrestal periodontal fibres. The bone surface within the defect is characterized by zones of osteoclastic resorption together with osteoblastic regeneration of previously resorbed areas. The remaining supracrestal periodontal fibres are longer than in health, extending from their attachment to cementum along the bony surface to the edge of the bony defect. From here they extend, as in the normal state, to gain insertion into the adjacent tooth as the transeptal fibres (Goldman, 1957). In addition, they extend into the gingival papilla, the facial and oral gingivae and the periosteum.

Pattern of defects

The particular pattern of bony resorption occurring at any one site has been attributed to occlusal stresses (Glickman, 1963; Glickman and Smulow, 1962, 1965, 1967; Svanberg, 1974), alveolar bony morphology (Prichard, 1967; Saari et al., 1968; Larato, 1970; Manson, 1976; Waerhaug, 1979 a and b; Tal, 1984 a); to tooth anatomy and position (Goldman and Cohen, 1958; Lee et al., 1969; Nielsen et al., 1980; Tal, 1984 b) and to furcation morphology (see also Chapter 28 – Furcation involvements). The last of these appears to be of major importance as stressed in Part II.

There is a long-held but unsubstantiated clinical impression that sites devoid of bone, such as bony dehiscences, are more susceptible to loss of attachment than sites without developmental defects (Gartrell and Mathews, 1976) (see also Chapter 32). Experimentally produced sites having long suprabony connective tissue attachment have been shown to sustain no greater attachment losses than control sites to plaque-induced disease (Nyman *et al.*, 1984). Similarly Årtun *et al.* (1986) reported that closely approximated anterior teeth with thin interdental bone were not susceptible to more rapid periodontal breakdown than neighbouring or contralateral teeth with a normal width of bone between the roots. These findings suggest that attachment loss is unrelated to the presence or absence of a bony component to the periodontium.

Overhanging interproximal restoration margins have also been incriminated in the pathogenesis of intrabony defects and indeed significant correlations exist with alveolar bone losses (Björn *et al.*, 1969; Gilmore and Sheiham, 1971; Highfield and Powell, 1978; Hakkarainen and Ainamo, 1980; Jeffcoat and Howell, 1980). However, the influence of these margins upon intrabony defects *per se* on the natural history of periodontal disease is not clear. Gilmore (1970) failed to demonstrate a relationship between intrabony defects and overhanging margins or with open interproximal tooth contacts. Similarly, for open contacts Larato (1971) found, in a study on dry skulls, that only 18% of intrabony defects were associated with factors able to cause food impaction, whilst Koral *et al.* (1981), concluded that open contacts might not be associated with a greater degree of bone loss than elsewhere.

Classification

The principle of using truly graphic terms, like that of the 'col', introduced by Cohen (1959), to describe the soft tissue depression between the facial and oral gingival papillae, might also have been usefully applied to the description of the rather complex and varied pattern of bony resorption encountered in disease. Instead, the rather less graphic classification based upon the number (one, two or three) of bony walls bounding the intrabony defects about periodontally involved roots, suggested by Goldman and Cohen (1958), has generally been used (see also *Glossary of Periodontic Terms*, 1986). Although such classic defects do occur in most instances, they can also present as combinations of these three types (Ellegaard, 1976), which leads to difficulties with terminology. The use of descriptive terms, like crater, trench, moat, ramp and plane have been proposed recently by Karn *et al.* (1984) as an alternative terminology. As the function of terminology is primarily for clear communication and record purposes, use is made of readily understood everyday terms in Part II.

The treatment of intrabony defects

Physiological form

A concept was evolved in the 1950s that the gingival contour depended on the form of the underlying bone (Schluger, 1949; Friedman, 1955; Ochsenbein, 1958) and moreover, 'physiologic' gingival contour was necessary for the maintenance of periodontal health (Goldman, 1950). As a result of this concept, surgical remodelling of bony defects was undertaken to create the required anatomical foundation for the gingiva. Osteoplasty was introduced by Friedman (1955), to achieve surgical reshaping without loss of supporting bone; also osteoectomy, the removal of supporting bone to eliminate the bony component to the pocket, thereby establishing physiological contours.

The need for osseous correction has been questioned following a number of investigations. Firstly, the healed gingiva does not necessarily follow the contour of the underlying bone and it may even be true that gingiva actually governs the bone contour (Glickman *et al.*, 1963; Zander and Matherson, 1963). Secondly, Lobene and Glickman (1963) and Pennel *et al.* (1967), reported that further bone loss occurred following osseous therapy, so that the ultimate contour may differ from that created at operation. An alternative view was presented by Matherson and Zander (1963), who reported no bony change during a 6-month postoperative assessment. Thirdly, Patur and Glickman (1962); Donnenfeld *et al.* (1970) found that bone was able to remodel spontaneously following the removal of deposits on the related teeth and the additional removal of inflamed connective tissues from intrabony defects. Finally, Rosling *et al.* (1976) showed that, with a high standard of cleaning, disease could be halted independently of bone removal at the time of different pocket surgical techniques. Indeed, the most favourable healing of bone could be achieved if bone removal was avoided altogether.

The importance claimed for 'deflecting contours for proper form and function' of the gingiva (Schluger, 1949) and of gaining 'physiologic' gingival form (Goldman, 1950), and which was ratified by the development of an index of gingival architectural form (MacLeod *et al.*, 1965), has yet to be substantiated. Indeed, as stated in Part II, the fact that such a gingival morphology exists *de novo* in most individuals, coupled with the widespread nature of marginal gingival disease, indicates that optimal gingival form *per se* does not bestow any special benefits against the onset of plaque-induced disease. Furthermore, Nyman *et al.* (1975) showed that the creation of acceptable gingival form by surgery did not avoid recurrent disease in the absence of a high standard of oral hygiene. More importantly, Zamet (1975) demonstrated that 'good healing, followed by a high standard of oral hygiene may overcome the presence of gingival and marginal osseous deformities'. It was also observed by Smith *et al.* (1980), that health could be maintained post-surgically despite 'non-physiologic' gingival and osseous contours. Similarly, Newman (1984) has questioned the importance of good gingival contour for the maintenance of periodontal health.

Surgical mucosal coverage

The importance of post-surgical mucosal coverage of bone upon bony healing has been endorsed by the findings of Rosling *et al.* (1976). Such optimal flap adaptation may however sometimes be complicated at the back of the palate by the existence of palatal bony exostoses presenting as nodules, spikes or ridges (Larato, 1972). Consequently, the removal of these exostoses may be indicated. The benefits of periosteal retention (split thickness flap) are not clear; earlier claims of improved healing (see Staffileno, 1974) are countered by the finding of greater bone losses following partial rather than full-thickness flaps (Wood *et al.*, 1972). In addition, Johnson (1976) concluded that the risk of sloughing at split thickness flaps, resulting in bony denudation, outweighed any possible advantages of the technique. This dilemma is also discussed in Part II. The risks of damaging anatomical structures during any flap preparation have also been stressed; these and other anatomical hazards involved in periodontal surgery have been considered by Clarke and Bueltmann (1971).

Surgical elimination of intrabony defects

The retention of intrabony defects (as advocated in Chapter 19) cannot be reconciled with the intended surgical elimination of the pocket. However, the resection of bone necessary to achieve such pocket elimination also sacrifices supporting bone about both the involved teeth and the adjacent teeth. The methods of bone resection and the tissue response to this are now reviewed briefly. (See also Wirthlin, 1987.)

Bone resection techniques

Files, chisels and burs (high and low speed steel and diamond abrasive) have been advocated (Schluger, 1949; Fox, 1955; Ochsenbein, 1958). The importance of a coolant spray and the need to flush away debris when using ultraspeed burs has been emphasized by Costich *et al.* (1964). On the other hand Hall (1965) has shown that high-speed cutting with a light touch and without a water coolant, did not cause thermal necrosis of bone. More recently, Horton *et al.* (1981) demonstrated that Cavitron ultrasonic instruments removed bone with ease and precision and without any detrimental effects clinically or histologically. It is expedient to note here that no adverse effects have been reported following the use of ultrasonic devices for root planing during flap surgery by Walsh and Waite

(1978) or Glick and Freeman (1980). It should also be noted here that, although contact with bone is not intended during electrosurgical soft tissue pocket resection, accidental contact will result in osseous necrosis (Azzi *et al.*, 1983; Krejci *et al.*, 1987).

Effects of bone resection

It must at the outset be realized that mean losses of crestal bone height ranging between 0.5–1.0 mm have been reported following inverse bevel flap procedures alone (Review: Tavtigian, 1970). Sites with thin labial bone sustain the most severe bone losses whereas little or no loss occurs at sites with thick labial bone, or interproximally. The possible reasons for these differences are discussed in Part II.

Losses of bone sustained following the resection of supporting bone have been found to be in excess of the amount actually removed at surgery. This has been shown in humans (Rosling *et al.*, 1976; Smith *et al.*, 1980), and also in animal models (Wilderman *et al.*, 1970; Caton and Nyman, 1981) in which histologic losses of connective tissue attachment were also observed. However, Caffesse *et al.* (1968) detected no changes in bone height or attachment levels in monkeys. It must be concluded, in agreement with Barrington (1981), that while 'osseous contouring will eliminate discrepancies in bony architecture . . . there is no general agreement on the role of osseous contouring in periodontal therapy.' Furthermore, following a failure to achieve clinically significant bony regeneration in humans, Isidor *et al.* (1985) concluded that, if the establishment of shallow pockets is a desirable goal of treatment, osseous surgery must be carried out. In an effort to avoid further loss of support by bone resection, various surgical methods have evolved, which have aimed at correcting the intrabony defect have evolved by using bony regeneration instead.

Intrabony defect healing

It has been well established by numerous investigations both in animals and in humans, that intrabony defects are capable of becoming filled in by bone regeneration ('bone fill'), although the relationship of this regenerated bone to the previous pathologically involved root surface is not clear.

The term reattachment has often been used to describe the regeneration of all the tooth supporting structures. However, the term new attachment is preferable, as new connective tissue and cementum must also form, and reattachment is then reserved for the reunion of healthy periodontal tissues following surgical or traumatic separation (Kalkwarf, 1974). Unfortunately it is difficult to establish clinically whether healing within intrabony defects is via new attachment or simply bone fill. This is because each will appear similar, radiographically, to probing and indeed even when exposed surgically at re-entry operations. Only histological analysis will reveal the nature of the healed tissue.

The earliest attempts to gain attachment used a combination of root surface debridement and curettage (for Reviews see Ellegaard, 1976; Wirthlin, 1981 and 1987). With the renewed interest in the flap technique in the 1950s, the bony defects were carefully curetted to remove all granulation tissue and transeptal fibres (Carranza and Glickman, 1957; Goldman and Cohen, 1958; Prichard, 1967). This has since been carried out as a routine measure even though the rationale has never been altogether clear. Recent findings by Lindhe and Nyman (1985) have however questioned the need to remove granulation tissue, apart from in rapidly progressing lesions in which bacterial penetration might occur (*cf.* Curettage, Chapter 29). In addition, possible barriers to tissue proliferation from the marrow spaces by the removal of underlying transeptal fibres, (Carranza and Glickman, 1957; Goldman and Cohen, 1958), or the perforation of sclerotic bony walls to facilitate ingress of osteogenic marrow cells (see Wirthlin, 1981), has been carried out preceding optimal flap adaptation.

The most favourable healing reported in humans under these conditions, has occurred in three-walled defects (Ellegaard and Löe, 1971; Prichard, 1972), although recent findings by Renvert *et al.* (1985a) suggest the outcome of intra-osseous therapy based upon evaluation of defect characteristics is difficult to predict. Rosling *et al.* (1976) and Polson and Heijl (1978) have, in turn, reported mean bony regeneration of 80% and 77% respectively, in conjunction with some marginal bone resorption within both two- and three-walled defects, in the presence of a high standard of post-surgical plaque control and optimal mucosal coverage of the bone as advocated in Part II. In direct contrast, Prichard (1983) has stressed the importance of avoiding any post-surgical coverage of intrabony defects and furthermore, of not removing any root surface cementum during debridement and also achieved comparably favourable healing. This has been endorsed more recently by Becker *et al.* (1986). The above impressive findings have not been consistently achieved by others since (e.g. Froum *et al.*, 1982; Renvert *et al.*, 1985c; Isidor *et al.*, 1985) even in the presence of high standards of oral hygiene.

Histologic examination of the sites treated by Froum and co-workers revealed healing was primarily by soft tissue adhesion with insignificant crestal osteogenesis (Stahl *et al.*, 1982).

Animal model investigations have confirmed that the essential prerequisite for bony regeneration is resolution of the plaque-induced connective tissue inflammatory infiltrate associated with intrabony

pockets (Polson *et al.*, 1979; Kantor, 1980). The importance of good oral hygiene has been endorsed by the research of van Dijk and Wright (1983).

Surgical flap margin positioning in relation to the crestal bone appears to be critical in healing. Thus, Klinge *et al.* (1981) demonstrated new attachment and bony regeneration within canine furcation defects, following coronally positioned flaps, but not when the flap margins were replaced at the cemento-enamel junction. In the latter, the tissues receded early in healing, apparently counteracting optimal healing. This was endorsed by the subsequent animal model finding that suturing attached to the crown could prevent gingival recession and also favour the formation of new attachment (Klinge *et al.*, 1985a). (See also Chapter 30 – The efficacy of therapy.) As the crown shape of human teeth permits neither technique, an attempt was made to provide support for the flap by using various implants and was assessed by Klinge *et al.* (1985b). New attachment was achieved inconsistently with autogenous bone and not at all with non-bony implant materials. The development of a more predictable technique is clearly required.

The benefits of coronal flap positioning in gaining new attachment appear to relate primarily to the obstacle presented by the greater distance the epithelial cells must migrate and with the greater chance consequently provided for periodontal ligament cells to migrate (Gottlow *et al.*, 1986). On the other hand, this also increases the risk of root resorption as shown by Bogle *et al.* (1985) following coronally positioned flaps in dogs. The more coronally located cervical resorption adjacent to gingival connective tissue appeared progressive and resulted in loss of significant portions of dentine within the crown. Resorption taking place more apically, in areas of newly formed bone, was in turn associated with ankylosis and usually appeared to have become arrested (see also below).

The results of investigations on bony regeneration in animal models must be viewed with some caution. In the first place bony repair has been attributed by Lindhe and Ericsson (1978), Caton and Zander (1976), Caton and Nyman (1980) and Caton *et al.* (1980) to periodontal therapy, for no repair was observed following removal of ligatures used to induce experimental bony defects (Caton and Zander, 1975; Lindhe and Ericsson, 1978). Yet others have reported comparable spontaneous reduction of severity of periodontal inflammation and alveolar bone repair following ligature removal alone Jansen (1982, 1983) and Jansen *et al.* (1982). This would then complicate any interpretation of the effects of periodontal therapy. Secondly, Caton and Zander (1976), Caton and Nyman (1980) and Caton *et al.* (1980) have shown that osseous repair following therapy in monkeys develops in conjunction with a junctional epithelium on the root surface without new attachment of connective tissue. This was also observed by Jansen *et al.* (1982), in the absence of therapy and in a histological assessment of an autogenous bone graft in humans (Moskow *et al.*, 1979). Thirdly, the development of new attachment should not, according to Caton and Zander (1976), be based upon re-entry procedures, probing measurements or radiographs, for none are reliable indicators thereof. This implies that histological measurement verification alone will suffice which makes things difficult as this is feasible only experimentally and is not possible clinically. Even histological evaluation of new attachment is still open to question, because any pre-operative clinical recording of the apical extension of the pocket epithelium cannot be related to that observed histologically, following treatment. This difficulty was overcome by Cole *et al.* (1980) by notching the root through the most apical extent of the subgingival calculus located at pocket surgery.

The reparative potential of existing bone in the healing of an intrabony defect is considered only after that of the use of bone grafting and root surface demineralization to enhance healing.

Bone grafting

The use of bone grafts stems from the fact long recognized in orthopaedic surgery, that fresh autogenous bone grafts will provide a scaffold for ossification and supply the cellular elements capable of forming new bone. The first use of grafts in periodontics, has been attributed to Hegedus (1923), although Cross (1955, 1957) can be credited with making the first significant contribution to an era of research in which a great number of investigations have been carried out, both in humans and in animal models. The origins of the different techniques and their clinical benefits are considered here briefly. (For reviews see Ellegaard, 1976; Schallhorn, 1977; Gara and Adams, 1981.)

The cortical shaving technique introduced by Nabers and O'Leary (1965) was modified by Robinson (1969) to become the osseous coagulum technique. The bone removed, by burring at sites in the surgical field requiring osteoplasty, was harvested in a blood coagulum. The apparently limited osteogenic potential of this, primarily cortical bone, was enhanced by perforating into the trabecular and marrow bone of the defect. Diem *et al.* (1972) introduced the bone blending technique in which any bone fragments obtained at operation were pulverized and blended together in a dental amalgamator. Froum *et al.* (1976) reported greater levels of regeneration in intrabony defects by the use of osseous coagulum bone blends than by surgical debridement alone. Ewen (1965) introduced the technique of bone swaging or contiguous osseous grafting, whereby the bony wall of the defect is forcibly impacted into direct contact with the root surface, whilst maintaining some continuity at the base of the deflected bone (see also Sussman and Ewen, 1969).

Intra-oral cancellous bone as donor material has had the most extensive use of all because of its claimed osteo-inductive potential. This donor bone can be obtained from the maxillary tuberosity, retromolar sites, edentulous ridges, 8-10-week post-healing extraction sockets (Rosenberg, 1971; Hiatt and Schallhorn, 1973; Soehren and van Swol, 1979; Evian *et al.*, 1982) or from newly forming bone within surgically created alveolar defects (Halliday, 1969). In this context, Amler (1984) has demonstrated, in an animal model, that bony regeneration is markedly more favourable with regenerating than mature marrow. Average bone fills of 3.4 mm and 3.07 mm were observed by Hiatt and Schallhorn (1973) and Carraro *et al.* (1976) respectively, using this technique. Most recently, Renvert *et al.* (1985 c) showed that osseous grafting from the maxillary tuberosity did not enhance the limited benefits of citric acid conditioning (see below). This regenerative surgery was frequently associated with post-operative soft interdental craters, thus endorsing previous findings by Dragoo and Kaldahl (1983). Takei *et al.* (1985) described the 'papilla preservation technique' designed to overcome this complication with favourable results over a 6-month healing period.

The limited amount of bone available from intra-oral sites led to the use of donor material derived from extra-oral sites, usually the iliac crest (Schallhorn, 1967, 1968; Schallhorn *et al.*, 1970; Dragoo and Sullivan, 1973 a, b). Although this haemopoetic bone affords the most favourable results (Schallhorn, 1977; Hiatt *et al.*, 1978), the patient is involved in an additional surgical procedure with its potential risks and the greater expense. In addition, the possible complication of root resorption and ankylosis exists (Schallhorn, 1972; Burnett, 1972; Dragoo and Sullivan, 1973; Ellegaard, 1976) although, according to Schallhorn *et al.* (1970), this occurs only with fresh but not with frozen marrow material. This so-called 'replacement resorption' as described by Andreasen and Hjörting-Hansen (1966), represents a continuous replacement of cementum and dentine with bone tissue, which was found to follow re-implantation of extracted or accidentally luxated teeth. Indeed Karring *et al.* (1984), has since concluded that bone grafting is contraindicated in periodontal surgery because granulation tissue derived from bone consistently favoured subsequent root resorption and ankylosis (Karring *et al.*, 1980) rather than new attachment. Furthermore, the comparative infrequency of replacement resorption following bone grafting was attributed by Karring *et al.* (1980) to the migration of periodontal ligament cells coronally and, more especially, dentogingival epithelium apically along the root surface, before cells derived from bone establish contact with the root. The epithelium thus functions as a protective barrier against replacement resorption (see below). Karring *et al.* (1984) also stated that the thin layer of ankylosing bone observed along the root surface does, in some instances, resemble newly formed cementum which might be misinterpreted as new attachment.

Allogenic marrow grafts, frozen to preserve the bone but to inhibit the antigenic potential, has been used with some success (Hiatt and Schallhorn, 1971; Schallhorn and Hiatt, 1972; Hiatt *et al.*, 1978), but problems of tissue incompatability remain. Freeze-dried bone appears to be a rather less favourable material, (Mellonig *et al.*, 1976; Sepe *et al.*, 1978; Sanders *et al.*, 1983), although recent findings by Bowers *et al.* (1985) and Mabry *et al.* (1985) are encouraging.

Non-bone materials like sclera (Klingsberg, 1972, 1974), cartilage (Chodroff and Ammons, 1984), heterogenic bone, e.g. 'Kielbone' (Sigurdson, 1972) and calcium phosphate ceramics (Reviewed by Han *et al.*, 1984) have also been used. Of these, the last, in both its hydroxyapatite and tricalcium phosphate forms, appears to be the most promising. Yukna *et al.* (1984, 1985) have demonstrated at least compa-rable and often better results, Meffert *et al.* (1985) significantly better defect elimination and fill and Kenney *et al.* (1985) significant clinical parameter improvements than by the use of surgical debride-ment alone. More recent human histologic evidence does however suggest neither bone formation nor new attachment is induced. Instead the material merely functions as a filler which becomes well encapsulated by gingival connective tissue (Stahl and Froum, 1986; Ganeles *et al.*, 1986). The risk of root resorption has been reported by Ibbott (1985). It is also of interest to note here that the predictable use of hydroxyapatite for localized alveolar ridge augmentation has been claimed (Allen *et al.*, 1985).

Acid conditioning

The principle of enhanced cementogenesis on root surfaces following demineralization during pocket surgery was introduced by Register and Burdick (1975 a). The rationale for this is based on the findings of Urist (1971), that new bone or cementum can be induced to form on the surface of implants of demineralized enamel and dentine. Furthermore, studies on the healing of surgically detached periodontal tissues (Morris and Thomson, 1963; Frank *et al.*, 1974; Nalbandian and Frank, 1980), demonstrated that superficial dentinal demineraliza-tion is an important step in the natural healing

process. Register and Burdick (1975 b) showed dentine tubules were widened by citric acid de-mineralization, facilitating the entry of anchoring pins of cementum. The recent finding of tissue cell processes extending into dentinal tubules, might prove to be significant in this respect (Polson and Frederick, 1985).

It is claimed that citric acid demineralization exposes the dentinal matrix collagen fibrils, which subsequently become interdigitated or spliced with collagen fibrils of the adjacent tissues (Garrett *et al.*, 1978; Ririe *et al.*, 1980; Selvig *et al.*, 1981; Polson and Proye, 1982). A comparable sequence has been demonstrated with phosphoric acid by Heritier (1983, 1984). Willey and Steinberg (1984) reported a greater exposure of dentinal collagen and possibly enhanced healing by the additional treatment with various enzymes. Findings by Gottlow *et al.* (1984) do, however, suggest that this splicing concept may only be valid where the wound is repopulated by periodontal ligament cells, but not by cells from gingiva or alveolar bone, when root resorption and ankylosis will follow.

It has been postulated that acid 'conditioning' creates an environment comparable to that existing in cutaneous incisional wounds (Polson and Proye, 1983). In this situation the closely related dentinal and periodontal tissue fibrils facilitate an initial fibrin linkage involving the plasma protein fibronec-tin which has a strong affinity for collagen and fibrin (for reviews see Holden and Smith, 1983; Terranova and Wikesjö, 1987). An enhanced fibroblast attach-ment to demineralized root surfaces observed *in vitro* by Boyko *et al.* (1980) was attributed to fibronectin. This has been supported by the laboratory culture findings of Fernyhough and Page (1983) and the results of healing in animal models (Caffesse *et al.*, 1985, 1987; Caton *et al.*, 1986; Nasjleti *et al.*, 1986, 1987; Smith *et al.*, 1987). The possibility that citric acid treatment may have an indirect inhibitory effect upon epithelial down-growth is suggested by Crigger *et al.* (1978), Ririe *et al.* (1980), Klinge *et al.* (1981), Polson and Proye (1982), Magnusson *et al.* (1985 a), Hanes *et al.* (1985) and Polson *et al.* (1986). On the other hand, the greater distance the epithelial cells would have to migrate as a result of coronal flap displacement in some of these studies, might also be significant (Gottlow *et al.*, 1986). In the event of such epithelial inhibition, wound repopulation would be predomi-nantly of gingival connective tissue and bony origins which could induce root resorption (Karring *et al.*, 1980, 1984, 1985; Nyman *et al.*, 1980; Gottlow *et al.*, 1984 a; Bogle *et al.*, 1985; Magnusson *et al.*, 1985 a). This might also explain the more extensive resorp-tion observed at acid treated sites when compared to controls (Nyman *et al.*, 1985).

It has been postulated that root surface demineral-ization enhances fibroblast migration and attachment so facilitating new attachment (Pitaru and Melcher, 1983; Pitaru *et al.*, 1984 a, b). Furthermore, that collagen exposed by cemental demineralization may regulate the physiological organization of adjacent connective tissue cells during the early stages of wound healing (Pitaru and Melcher, 1987).

The findings of citric acid conditioning of periodontally diseased root surfaces vary greatly. Some investigators have shown new connective tissue attachment following pocket surgery. (For review see Holden and Smith, 1983; and more recently, Bogle *et al.*, 1983; Klinge *et al.*, 1985.) Cementogenesis with new connective tissue attachment has also been demonstrated on acid conditioned dentine, previously exposed to periodontal pockets, implanted into human buccal mucosa (Lopez, 1984). This was not the case with non-acid conditioned, previously healthy roots, that were surgically denuded of periodontal ligament tissue (Lopez and Belvederessi, 1983). Aukhil *et al.* (1986 a) concluded that partial demineralization of roots implanted into palatal connective tissues in dogs did not promote new attachment. Others have reported inconsistent reparative responses in which new attachment was either not enhanced by conditioning or where epithelial downgrowth occurred instead (for review see Holden and Smith, 1983). More recent endorsement of these findings is derived from investigations in humans (Froum *et al.*, 1983; Stahl *et al.*, 1983; Frank *et al.*, 1983; Kashani *et al.*, 1984; Parodi and Esper, 1984; Marks and Mehta, 1986; Smith *et al.*, 1986 and Moore *et al.*, 1987) and in animal models (Gottlow *et al.*, 1986 a; Issidor *et al.*, 1985 b; Nyman *et al.*, 1985; Gottlow *et al.*, 1986 b; Lai *et al.*, 1986; Dreyer and van Heerden, 1986; Pettersson and Aukhil, 1986). In addition, Cogen *et al.* (1983, 1984) observed no enhanced attachment of gingival fibroblasts in cell cultures to acid conditioned, planed root fragments.

The questionable benefits of citric acid conditioning on the healing of surgically treated non-furcation involved intrabony defects in humans, has been shown recently in a series of investigations. A limited but unpredictable bony regeneration was observed following acid treatment in periodontal flap surgery alone (Renvert *et al.*, 1985 a, b), when coupled with intra-oral bone grafting (Renvert *et al.*, 1985 c) and both non-resective and resective bony techniques (Chamberlain *et al.*, 1985). Root resorption has been observed in several investigations, following citric acid conditioning, as noted above, and in an uncontrolled study by Bogle *et al.* (1985), but also, albeit to a lesser extent, at non-conditioned control surfaces (Proye and Polson, 1982 a; Magnusson *et al.*, 1985 a; Nyman *et al.*, 1985; Petterson and Aukhil, 1986; Aukhil *et al.*, 1986 b). The reduced epithelial downgrowth also observed, implies an enhanced selective wound repopulation by cells

derived from gingival connective tissue and bone bringing with them a greater risk of resorption. In this context, (Isidor *et al.*, 1985) have pointed out the possibility that the collagen fibres closely related to these areas of resorption might have been misinterpreted by others as new attachment, following citric acid treatment. On the other hand, Stahl and Tarnow (1985) endorse the view that root resorption probably occurs as part of normal post-surgical gingival repair (Nalbandian and Frank, 1980), the resulting 'unmasked' dentinal collagen fibrils becoming 'spliced' with fibrils from gingival collagen.

A surface smear layer demonstrated by scanning electron microscope, commonly occurs following root surface instrumentation (Jones *et al.*, 1972). This layer of microcrystalline debris virtually occludes the dentinal tubules and, if not removed, might possibly inhibit new attachment. Its appearance could be misinterpreted as an initial connective tissue deposit during cementogenesis (Polson *et al.*, 1984). Citric acid has been shown *in vitro* to remove most of this smear layer but, at the same time, markedly increasing dentinal permeability (Pashley *et al.*, 1981; Lasho *et al.*, 1983), and as a result, the surface area available for bacterial penetration into the pulp (Michelich *et al.*, 1980). Ryan *et al.* (1984) have demonstrated post-surgical bacterial invasion of dentinal tubules in conditioned, but not control, teeth in cats and attributed this as the cause of the more severe pulpal reactions observed. These workers concluded that as gingival recession is a common finding following periodontal surgery and acid demineralization (Cole *et al.*, 1980), the technique might best be avoided where difficulties in post-surgical plaque control are anticipated and restricted to only those sites where recession and subsequent exposure to oral microflora can be controlled. The possible antibacterial (Daly, 1982) and detoxifying (Lasho *et al.*, 1983; Sarbinoff *et al.*, 1983; Olson *et al.*, 1985) properties of citric acid might be effective when any contaminated cementum remains following incomplete mechanical debridement.

The use of citric acid conditioning in the repair of localized gingival recession is also worth considering here. Yukna (1980) showed significantly greater amounts of both root coverage and of connective tissue attachment with laterally repositioned flaps, in baboons, following acid conditioning. Liu and Solt (1980) demonstrated successful root coverage by coronally positioned flaps following root surface conditioning. Common and McFall (1983) showed a tendency for greater root surface coverage following laterally positioned flaps at acid conditioned experimental teeth. Oles *et al.* (1985) and Ibbott *et al.* (1985) have on the other hand, concluded that there was no clinical justification for citric acid treatment in either laterally positioned pedicle flaps or free gingival autografts respectively, in the coverage of denuded roots.

In conclusion, although the benefits of root surface conditioning by acid have not been clearly established, and there may be a possible indirect adverse pulpal effect and predisposition to root resorption, its potential advantages and the fact that no detrimental effects have been demonstrated upon soft tissues (Seymour *et al.*, 1983; Crigger *et al.*, 1983) or pulp (Nilveus and Selvig, 1983) warrants further investigation.

The role of bone in new attachment

The long-held clinical impression that bone is critical to the establishment of new attachment has been questioned increasingly by recent investigations. These have in turn demonstrated the all-importance of periodontal ligament cells in healing (Review: Egelberg, 1987). The studies have involved tooth reimplantation and transplantation, implantation of diseased root specimens into the periodontal tissues and finally the selective exclusion of the different periodontal tissue cell types allowing preferential cell repopulation during healing.

Tooth reimplantation/transplantation

Teeth which have been extracted and reimplanted or autotransplanted within a short time, heal with a normal periodontal ligament (Löe and Waerhaug, 1961; Andreasen, 1980, 1981; Proye and Polson, 1982 a, b). Optimal healing depends on maintaining vitality of periodontal ligament cells on the extracted root surfaces. Consequently, following selective experimental root surface alterations, it has been possible to investigate the effects of these alterations upon healing.

Proye and Polson (1982 b) demonstrated that, despite close approximation of reimplanted root surgically divested of its periodontal fibres to bony socket, new connective tissue attachment failed to form and epithelium migrated over the root surfaces. Epithelial downgrowth was however prevented by citric acid conditioning (Polson and Proye, 1982 a) and a new supracrestal connective tissue attachment established without cementum formation. The extensive root resorption, observed along the intra-alveolar part of the reimplanted root, was attributed to the effects of extraction trauma on the periodontal ligament cells (Andreasen, 1980), a lack of an epithelial migration, and wound healing by cells derived from bone. Thus, the healed attachment relationship is dependent upon the progenitor cells that repopulate the wound (Melcher, 1976; Nyman *et al.*, 1980; Boyko *et al.*, 1981).

The lack of evidence supporting a regenerative potential for bone was demonstrated in another investigation in monkeys (Polson and Caton, 1982). An incisor affected by periodontitis was transplanted into the extraction socket of its contralateral tooth where a normal periodontium had existed previously. No new attachment occurred and epithelium migrated apically between the diseased parts of the root and the bone. These workers concluded however that root surface alterations, rather than lack of adjacent progenitor cell populations, inhibited the potential for new attachment. Lindskog *et al.* (1983) observed only limited new attachment within experimental cavities prepared on the middle third of monkey incisor roots immediately after they had been extracted and then promptly reimplantated.

Lindhe *et al.* (1984) observed no fibrous reattachment to reimplanted tooth root surfaces that had been surgically stripped of periodontal ligament before reimplantation, either in the presence, or following the removal, of part of the alveolar bony socket. The former situation of the complete bony socket indicates that bone is not essential for optimal healing and further questions the rationale for bone grafting. In the latter situations, a limited coronal regrowth of bone occurred within the gingival components of the sockets, but only in conjunction with reattachment to uninstrumented parts of the root surfaces with a residual periodontal ligament layer. This confirmed the findings of Nyman and Karring (1979) and further emphasized the minimal influence of bone upon the biological conditions determining the nature of healing. Indeed, in a similar subsequent investigation (Nyman *et al.*, 1985) connective tissue attachment again failed to form on most reimplanted (and transplanted) root surfaces deprived of their periodontal ligament tissue, despite acid conditioning. Healing was instead most frequently characterized by root resorption and ankylosis.

Root implantation

The failure of alveolar bone *per se* to create a new attachment has been clearly demonstrated in dogs by Karring *et al.* (1980). Root surfaces previously exposed to periodontal pockets were thoroughly root planed, implanted into bony cavities prepared in edentulous ridges, and covered completely by a mucoperiosteal flap. This coverage was designed to exclude reinfection by plaque and any possibility of epithelial downgrowth, as shown in previous investigations to interfere with attempted new attachment (Caton and Zander, 1976; Caton and Nyman, 1980; Caton *et al.*, 1980). Despite the intimate relationship achieved between implanted root and bone, no new attachment developed at previously diseased surfaces and healing was characterized by replacement resorption (Andreasen and Hjörting-Hansen, 1966). Similar responses have also been reported at implanted healthy roots in baboons that had been surgically denuded of their investing periodontal tissues (Dreyer and van Heerden, 1986) and roots in dogs exposed to advanced periodontal disease (Aukhil *et al.*, 1986 b).

In a further similar investigation (Nyman *et al.*, 1980), roots were implanted into prepared shallow bony troughs and then covered with the gingival connective tissue of the overlying mucoperiosteal flap. Once again, no new fibrous attachment formed adjacent to bone or indeed in relation to the gingival connective tissue. Replacement resorption occurred, as above, in the former sites and resorption lacunae containing multinucleated cells were commonly noted adjacent to gingiva. These findings indicated that gingival connective tissue cells, in common with bone, not only lack the ability to form new attachment but might also lead to root resorption; this phenomenon had also been described by Andreasen (1981) and Boyko *et al.* (1981). The failure of gingival flap connective tissue cells to form new attachment has also been demonstrated in another animal model investigation in which healing by bony and periodontal ligament derived granulation tissue had been excluded by the placement of a Nuclepore membrane physical barrier (Aukhil *et al.*, 1987).

The relative infrequency with which replacement resorption does actually occur following clinical attempts to gain new attachment, is presumably the result of the protective epithelial barrier (Karring *et al.*, 1980) forming before the granulation tissue derived from bone and gingiva makes contact with the root thus preventing resorption. This assumption was confirmed by a further implantation experiment (Karring *et al.*, 1984), in which the coronal parts of roots partially embedded in bony sockets, were in contact with gingival connective tissue. After an initial healing phase the overlying mucosa was cut away to allow epithelial migration into the wound. Extensive resorption was a consistent observation, adjacent to both bone and gingival connective tissue, during healing but was prevented where apical downgrowth of the epithelium had occurred along the root.

Preferential repopulation investigations

Animal model experiments designed to give preference to periodontal ligament cell repopulation of wounds have shown that periodontal ligament cells alone are capable of forming new attachment on root surfaces whether previously diseased or surgically divested of ligament. In the first of these experiments by Nyman *et al.* (1982 a), based on a model system developed by Melcher (1970), a semilunar shaped mucoperiosteal flap, not involving

the marginal periodontal attachment, was reflected. The underlying buccal bony plate was then removed to expose the root surfaces, from which periodontal ligament and cementum was curetted. A Millipore filter was placed over this bony fenestration to prevent the connective tissue of the replaced flap coming into contact with the root during healing. New cementum with inserting collagen fibres was observed on the curetted root surfaces, endorsing data from an earlier study in cats by Nalbandian and Frank (1980). The findings thus revealed that preferential repopulation of the healing wound by periodontal ligament cells results in a connective tissue attachment. In addition, the extensive bony regeneration, without evidence of replacement resorption, indicated that periodontal ligament cell proliferated over the root in advance of those derived from bone. However, new attachment observed by others using similar experimental models (Petterson and Aukhil, 1986; Caton *et al.*, 1987), has been accompanied by root resorption and ankylosis. In a further investigation Aukhill *et al.* (1986 c) concluded that contact with root dentine may be necessary for progenitor cell differentiation into formative cells like cementoblasts.

The potential for new attachment, stemming from the remaining periodontal ligament tissue, upon root surfaces associated with long-standing disease was then demonstrated clinically (Nyman *et al.*, 1982 b) and in animal model investigations (Aukhil *et al.*, 1983, 1986 d) using the Millipore filter technique. This excluded epithelium and gingival connective tissue cells from healing following periodontal flap surgery. In the former clinical investigation, at a lower incisor scheduled for extraction, a block biopsy was performed at 3 months revealing new attachment up to a level of 5 mm coronal to the presurgical alveolar crest. In addition, although bone regenerated within the pre-existing angular bony defect, no coronal bone growth occurred, endorsing earlier observations that the formation of a new attachment is not necessarily accompanied by any coronally directed regeneration of alveolar bone (Nyman and Karring, 1979). In a composite investigation using root reimplantation, decoronation and complete mucoperiosteal flap coverage of the buried roots together with some bone removal, Houston *et al.* (1985) confirmed that new attachment can form without a concomitant build-up of alveolar bone. This in turn implies that bone tissue regrowth and periodontal ligament regeneration may be unrelated phenomena.

It should be noted that the findings of Nyman *et al.* (1982 b) appear to invalidate the long held concept (Ratcliff, 1966) that the root surface affected by periodontitis is the major factor preventing new attachment. Similarly, Isidor *et al.* (1985 c) in an investigation on healing following reconstructive periodontal surgery, demonstrated comparable fibrous attachment healing potentials on planed root surfaces that had previously been exposed to periodontal disease (giving new attachment) and those surgically divested of their attachment apparatus (giving reattachment).

The predictability of new attachment using the Millipore membrane technique was then evaluated by Gottlow *et al.* (1984 b). The crowns of periodontally diseased teeth were removed and the root surfaces affected by disease carefully debrided. A membrane was then placed over the debrided roots which were then completely covered with coronally repositioned mucoperiosteal flaps. Extensive amounts of new attachment resulted from the ingrowth of the adjacent periodontal ligament tissue and, once more, no replacement resorption occurred. The inference is that the periodontal ligament cell migration rate is at least as high as that of the regenerating bone. No relationship however was found between the amount of new cementum and the degree of coronal regrowth of bone corroborating the findings of Bogle *et al.* (1983) and Lindhe *et al.* (1984), that the formation of new attachment is unrelated to the presence or absence of adjacent alveolar bone.

In a further 'Millipore filter' investigation, Magnusson *et al.* (1985 b) repeated the clinical technique performed by Nyman *et al.* (1982) on monkeys, demonstrating new attachment approximately half way up the formerly exposed 'diseased' root surfaces. The majority of control surfaces showed no such healing, having been inhibited by epithelial downgrowth. Root resorption was however noted in some control specimens, indicating that granulation tissue derived from the overlying gingival connective tissue flap had established contact with the root prior to any epithelial downgrowth or periodontal ligament proliferation in a coronal direction. These workers thus confirmed that the problem of obtaining new attachment is not related to the state of the root surface, but to guiding wound repopulation by periodontal ligament cells possessing the biological capacity to regenerate new attachment. This has been endorsed by the finding that placement of physical barriers (like semipermeable silicone membranes) between root surface and surgical flaps facilitate coronal migration of progenitor cells from the periodontal ligament (Aukhil *et al.*, 1986 d).

Finally, the formation of new attachment has been investigated in an ingenious animal model experiment (Karring *et al.*, 1985) which involved submerging decoronated roots and covering them with mucoperiosteal flaps to exclude wound epithelialization. The contaminated cementum of the diseased root surfaces related to intrabony defects was burred away prior to flap closure. New attachment formed at the apical parts of the roots within bony defects, the new cementum being in direct continuity with that already *in situ*. This implies that new attachment has been formed by the coronal migration of cells originating in the periodontal ligament. This has since been endorsed by the finding that prevention of coronal growth of the periodontal ligament by the use of tightly adapted elastic ligatures about the root at the bottom of the defect in this model, inhibited the formation of new attachment (Isidor *et al.*, 1986).

The resorption noted at the more coronal aspects of the roots in each of these investigations indicates that tissues derived from other sources (alveolar bone and gingival connective tissue) had invaded the wound and endorses the protective role of epithelial downgrowth in clinical therapy in preventing resorption (Karring *et al.*, 1984; Houston *et al.*, 1985), albeit at the expense of the possible development of a new attachment. Consequently, if new attachment is to be achieved, the use of a membrane to exclude both epithelium and granulation tissue from cell sources other than those from the periodontal ligament appears to be essential. The principles of guided tissue regeneration (Gottlow *et al.*, 1986 b; Nyman *et al.*, 1987; Pontoriero *et al.*, 1987) and so-called root isolation (Becker *et al.*, 1987) in the restitution of the attachment apparatus lost in periodontal disease has been convincingly demonstrated in humans and warrants further investigation (see also Chapter 30). On the other hand, Caton *et al.* (1987) have emphasized the risk of root resorption as a complication of this technique and that long-term clinical trials in humans are essential before widespread clinical application of guided tissue regeneration can be recommended.

Impacted third molar post-extraction healing

The possible effects of the surgical removal of impacted mandibular third molars on the distal periodontal support of the second molar are considered briefly here. There appears to be a consensus of opinion that some loss of attachment is sustained (Review: Chin Quee, 1985), but that some reduction of any pre-extraction pocketing is achieved in the process (Szmyd and Hester, 1963; Groves and Moore, 1970; Gröndahl and Lekholm, 1973; Stephens *et al.*, 1983). Such pocket reductions have, by way of comparison, also been reported at tooth surfaces adjacent to extraction sites elsewhere in the arches (Grassi *et al.*, 1987). Ash *et al.* (1962) have on the other hand, reported a high incidence of periodontal pocketing on the distal surface of the second molar and an increase of this incidence with age. It also appears that surgical flap design for third molar removal is not critical to post-surgical attachment levels, although Groves and Moore

(1970) concluded that it may influence post-surgical pocket reduction. Debridement of the second molar immediately following removal of the adjacent impacted third molar was found to be of little benefit to post-healing crevicular depths or attachment levels (Osborne *et al.*, 1982).

It is difficult to draw any definitive conclusions from the variable findings of these investigations. This is due, in part, to inadequate experimental design, lack of statistical analyses and a failure of some of the studies to separate data derived from fully or partially impacted third molars. Furthermore, the major stumbling block, as noted in Part II, is the difficulty of assessing the pre-extraction attachment levels of the second molar by clinical probing or even by radiographs because of interference from the impacting tooth. Nevertheless, it is evident from the previous section that periodontal ligament integrity is of paramount importance and where loss has already been sustained prior to surgery, new attachment depends solely upon its proliferative potential. This periodontal ligament tissue is located apically as well as at the buccal and lingual aspects of the denuded second molar root surface.

References

Allen, E. P., Gainza, C. S., Farthing, G. G. and Newbold, D. A. (1985) Improved technique for localized ridge augmentation. *J. Periodontol.* **56**, 195–199

Amler, M. H. (1984) The effectiveness of regenerating versus mature marrow in physiologic autogenous transplants. *J. Periodontol.* **55**, 268–272

Andreasen, J. O. (1980) A time-related study of periodontal healing and root resorption activity after replantation of mature permanent incisors in monkeys. *Swed. Dent. J.* **4**, 101–110

Andreasen, J. O. (1981) Periodontal healing after replantation and autotransplantation of permanent incisors. *Int. J. Oral Surg.* **60**, 54–61

Andreasen, J. O. and Hjörting-Hansen, E (1966) Replantation of teeth. II. Histological study of 22 replanted anterior teeth in humans. *Acta Odontol. Scand.* **24**, 287–306

Årtun, J., Osterberg, S. K. and Kokich, V. G. (1986) Long-term effect of thin interdental alveolar bone on periodontal health after orthodontic treatment. *J. Periodontol.* **57**, 341–346

Ash, M. M. Jr., Costitch, E. R. and Hayward, J. R. (1962) A study of periodontal hazards of third molars. *J. Periodontol.* **33**, 209–219

Aukhil, I., Greco, G., Suggs, C. and Torney, D. (1986a) Root resorption potentials of granulation tissue from bone and flap connective tissue. *J. Periodont. Res.* **21**, 531–542

Aukhil, I., Pettersson, E. and Suggs, C. (1986b) Guided tissue regeneration. An experimental procedure in beagle dogs. *J. Periodontol.* **57**, 727–734

Aukhil, I., Simpson, D. M., Suggs, C. and Pettersson, E. (1986c) *In vivo* differentiation of progenitor cells of the periodontal ligament. *J. Clin. Periodontol.* **13**, 862–868

Aukhil, I., Suggs, C. and Pettersson, E. (1986d) Healing following implantation of partially-demineralized roots in palatal connective tissue. *J. Periodont. Res.* **21**, 569–575

Aukhil, I., Pettersson, E. and Suggs, C. (1987) Periodontal wound healing in the absence of periodontal ligament cells. *J. Periodontol.* **58**, 71–77

Aukhil, I., Simpson, D. M. and Schaberg, T. V. (1983) An experimental study of new attachment procedure in beagle dogs. *J. Periodont. Res.* **18**, 643–654

Azzi, R. (1981) Electrosurgery in periodontics: a literature review. *J. West Soc. Periodont. Periodont. Abstr.* **29**, 4–10

Azzi, R., Kenney, E. B., Tsao, T. F. and Carranza, F. A. Jr. (1983) The effect of electrosurgery on alveolar bone. *J. Periodontol.* **54**, 96–100

Barrington, E. P. (1981) An overview of periodontal surgical procedures. *J. Periodontol.* **52**, 518–528

Becker, W., Becker, B. E., Berg, L. and Samsam, C. (1986) Clinical and volumetric analysis of three-wall intrabony defects following open flap debridement. *J. Periodontol.* **57**, 277–285

Becker, W., Becker, B. E., Prichard, J. F., Caffesse, R., Rosenberg, E. and Gian-Grasso, J. (1987) Root isolation for new attachment procedures. A surgical and suturing method: 3 case reports. *J. Periodontol.* **58**, 819–826

Björn, A.-L., Björn, H. and Grkovic, B. (1969) Marginal fit of restorations and its relation to periodontal bone level. Part I. Metal fillings. *Odont. Revy.* **20**, 311–321

Bogle, G., Garrett, S., Crigger, M. and Egelberg, J. (1983) New connective tissue attachment in beagles with advanced natural periodontitis. *J. Periodont. Res.* **18**, 220–228

Bogle, G., Claffey, N. and Egelberg, J. (1985) Healing of horizontal circumferential periodontal defects following regenerative surgery in beagle dogs. *J. Clin. Periodont.* **12**, 837–849

Bowers, G. M., Granet, M., Stevens, M., Emerson, J., Corio, R., Mellonig, J., Lewis, S. B., Peltzman, B., Romberg, E. and Risom, L. (1985) Histologic evaluation of new attachment in humans. *J. Periodontol.* **56**, 381–396

Boyko, G. A., Brunette, D. M. and Melcher, A. H. (1980) Cell attachment to demineralized root surfaces *in vitro*. *J. Periodont. Res.* **15**, 297–303

Boyko, G. A., Melcher, A. H. and Brunette, D. M. (1981) Formation of new periodontal ligament by periodontal ligament cells implanted in vivo after culture *in vitro*. A preliminary study of transplanted roots in the dog. *J. Periodont. Res.* **16**, 73–88

Burnette, E. W. (1972) Fate of an iliac crest graft. *J. Periodontol.* **43**, 88–90

Caffesse, R. G., Ramfjord, S. P. and Nasjleti, C. E. (1968) Reverse bevel periodontal flaps in monkeys. *J. Periodontol.* **39**, 219–235

Caffesse, R. G., Holden, M. J., Kon, S. and Nasjleti C. E. (1985) The effect of citric acid and fibronectin application on healing following surgical treatment of naturally occurring periodontal disease in beagle dogs. *J. Clin. Periodontol.* **12**, 578–590

Caffesse, R. G., Smith, B. A., Nasjleti, C. E. and Lopatin, D. E. (1987) Cell proliferation after flap surgery, root conditioning and fibronectin application. *J. Periodontol.* **58**, 661–666

Carraro, J. J., Sznajder, N. and Alonso, C. A. (1976) Intraoral cancellous bone autografts in the treatment of infrabony pockets. *J. Clin. Periodontol.* **3**, 104–109

Carranza, F. A. Jr., and Glickman, I. (1957) Some observations on the microscopic features of intrabony pockets. *J. Periodontol.* **28**, 33–36

Caton, J. and Nyman, S. (1980) Histometric evaluation of periodontal surgery. I. The modified Widman flap procedure. *J. Clin. Periodontol.* **7**, 212–223

Caton, J. and Nyman, S. (1981) Histometric evaluation of periodontal surgery. II. The effect of bone resection on the connective tissue attachment level. *J. Periodontol.* **52**, 405–409

Caton, J. and Zander, H. A. (1975) Primate model for testing periodontal treatment procedures. I. Histologic investigation of localized periodontal pockets produced by orthodontic elastics. *J. Periodontol.* **46**, 71–77

Caton, J. and Zander, H. A. (1976) Osseous repair of an infrabony pocket without new attachment of connective tissue. *J. Clin. Periodontcl.* **3**, 54–58

Caton, J., Nyman, S. and Zander, H. (1980) Histometric evaluaton of periodontalsurgery. II. Connective tissue attachment levels after four regenerative procedures. *J. Clin. Periodontol.* **7**, 224–231

Caton, J. G., Polson, A. M., Pini Prato, G., Bartolucci, E. G. and Clauser, C. (1986) Healing after application of tissue-adhesive material to denuded and citric acid-treated root surfaces. *J. Periodontol.* **57**, 385–390

Caton, J., Defuria, E. L., Polson, A. M. and Nyman, S. (1987) Periodontal regeneration via selective cell re-population. *J. Periodontol.* **58**, 546–552

Chamberlain, H., Garrett, S., Renvert, S. and Egelberg, J. (1985) Healing after treatment of periodontal intraosseous defects. *J. Clin. Periodontol.* **12**, 525–539

Chin Quee, T. A., Gosselin, D., Millar, E. P. and Stamm, J. W. (1985) Surgical removal of the fully impacted mandibular third molar. The influence of flap design and alveolar bone height on the periodontal status of the second molar. *J. Periodontol.* **56**, 625–630

Chodroff, R. E. and Ammons, W. F. (1984) Periodontal repair after surgical debridement with and without cartilage allografts. *J. Clin. Periodontol.* **11**, 295–312

Clarke, M. A. and Bueltmann, K. W. (1971) Anatomical considerations in periodontal surgery. *J. Periodontol.* **42**, 610–625

Cogen, R. B., Garrison, D. C. and Weatherford, T. W. (1983) *J. Periodontol.* **54**, 277–282

Cogen, R. B., Al-Joburi, W., Gantt, D. G. and Denys, F. R. (1984) Effect of various root surface treatments on the attachment and growth of human gingival fibro-blasts: histologic and scanning electron microscopic evaluation. *J. Clin. Periodontol.* **11**, 531–539

Cohen, B. (1959) Morphologic factors in the pathogenesis of periodontal disease. *Br. Dent. J.* **107**, 31–39

Cole, R. T., Crigger, M., Bogle, G., Egelberg, J. and Selvig, K. A. (1980) Connective tissue regeneration to periodontally diseased teeth. *J. Periodontol. Res.* **15**, 1–9

Common, J. and McFall, W. T. Jr. (1983) The effects of citric acid on attachment of laterally positioned flaps. *J. Periodontol.* **54**, 9–18

Costich, E. R., Youngblood, P. J. and Walden, J. M. (1964) A study of the effects of high-speed rotary instruments on bone repair in dogs. *Oral Surg.* **17**, 563–571

Crigger, M., Bogle, G., Nilveus, R., Egelberg, J. and Selvig, K. A. (1978) The effect of topical citric acid application on the healing of experimental furcation defects in dogs. *J. Periodont. Res.* **13**, 538–549

Crigger, M., Renvert, S. and Bogle, G. (1983) The effect of topical citric acid application on surgically exposed periodontal attachment. *J. Periodont. Res.* **18**, 303–305

Cross, W. G. (1955) Bone grafts in periodontal disease. *Dent. Pract.* **6**, 91–101

Cross, W. G. (1957) Bone implants in periodontal diseases – a further study. *J. Periodontol.* **28**, 184–191

Daly, C. G. (1982) Anti-bacterial effect of citric acid treatment of periodontally diseased root surfaces *in vitro. J. Clin. Periodontol.* **9**, 386–392

Diem, C. R., Bowers, G. M. and Moffitt, W. C. (1972) Bone blending: a technique for osseous implants. *J. Periodontol.* **43**, 295–297

Donnenfeld, O. W., Hoag, P. M. and Weissman, D. P. (1970) A clinical study on the effects of osteoplasty. *J. Periodontol.* **41**, 131–141

Dragoo, M. R. and Kaldahl, W. B. (1983) Clinical and histological evaluation of alloplasts and allografts in regenerative periodontal surgery in humans. *Int. J. Periodont. Rest. Dent.* **2**, 9–29

Dragoo, M. R. and Sullivan, H. C. (1973a) A clinical and histological evaluation of autogenous iliac bone grafts in humans: Part I. Wound healing 2 to 8 months. *J. Periodontol.* **44**, 599–613

Dragoo, M. R. and Sullivan H. C. (1973b) A clinical and histologic evaluation of autogenous iliac bone grafts in humans: Part II. External root resorption. *J. Periodontol.* **44**, 614–625

Dreyer, W. P. and van Heerden, J. D. (1986) The effect of citric acid on the healing of periodontal ligament-free, healthy roots, horizontally implanted against bone and gingival connective tissue. *J. Periodont. Res.* **21**, 210–220

Egelberg, J. (1987) Regeneration and repair of periodontal tissues. *J. Periodont. Res.* **22**, 233–242

Ellegaard, B. (1976) Bone grafts in periodontal attachment procedures. *J. Clin. Periodontol.* **3**, 5–54

Ellegaard, B. and Löe, H. (1971) New attachment of periodontal tissues after treatment of intrabony lesions. *J. Periodontol.* **42**, 648–652

Evian, C. I., Rosenberg, E. S., Coslet, J. G. and Corn, H. (1982) The osteogenic activity of bone removed from healing extraction sockets in humans. *J. Periodontol.* **53**, 81–85

Ewen, S. J. (1965) Bone swaging. *J. Periodontol.* **36**, 57–63

Fernyhough, W. and Page, R. C. (1983) Attachment, growth and synthesis by human gingival fibroblasts on demineralized or fibronectin-treated normal and diseased tooth roots. *J. Periodontol.* **54**, 133–140

Fox, L. (1955) Rotating abrasives in the management of periodontal soft and hard tissues. *Oral Surg.* **8**, 1134–1138

Frank, R. M., Fiore-Dunno, G., Cimasoni, G. and Matter, J. (1974) Ultrastructural study of epithelial and connective gingival reattachment in man. *J. Periodontol.* **45**, 626–635

Frank, R. M., Fiore-Donno, G. and Cimasoni, G. (1983) Cementogenesis and soft tissue attachment after citric acid treatment in a human. An electron microscopic study. *J. Periodontol.* **54**, 389–401

Friedman, N. (1955) Periodontal osseous surgery: osteoplasty and osteoectomy. *J. Periodontol.* **26**, 257–269

Froum, S. J., Coran, M., Thaller, B., Kushner, L., Scopp, I. W. and Stahl, S. S. (1982) Periodontal healing following open debridement flap procedures. I. Clinical assessment of soft tissue osseous repair. *J. Periodontol.* **53**, 8–14

Froum, S. J., Kushner, L. and Stahl, S. S. (1983) Healing responses of human intraosseous lesions following the use of debridement, grafting and citric acid root treatment. I. Clinical and histologic observations six months postsurgery. *J. Periodontol.* **54**, 67–76

Froum, S. J., Ortiz, M., Witkin, R. T., Thaler, R., Scopp, I. W. and Stahl, S. S. (1976) Osseous autografts. III. Comparison of osseous coagulum-bone blend implants with open curettage. *J. Periodontol.* **47**, 287–294

Ganeles, J., Listgarten, M. A. and Evian, C. I. (1986) Ultrastructure of durapatite-periodontal tissue interface in human intrabony defects. *J. Periodontol.* **57**, 133–140

Gara, G. G. and Adams, D. F. (1981) Implant therapy in human intrabony pockets: A review of the literature. *J. West Soc. Periodont. Periodont. Abstr.* **29**, 32–47

Garrett, J. S., Crigger, M. and Egelberg, J. (1978) Effects of citric acid on diseased root surfaces. *J. Periodont. Res.* **13**, 155–163

Gartrell, J. R. and Mathews, D. P. (1976) Gingival recession. The condition, process and treatment. *Dent. Clin. North Am.* **20**, 199–213

Gilmore, N. D. (1970) An epidemiological investigation of vertical osseous defects in periodontal disease. Thesis, Ann Arbor, Michigan

Gilmore, N. D. and Sheiham, A. (1971) Over-hanging dental restorations and periodontal disease. *J. Periodontol.* **42**, 311–321

Glick, D. H. and Freeman, E. (1980) Postsurgical bone loss following root planing by ultrasonic and hand instruments. *J. Periodontol.* **51**, 510–512

Glickman, I. (1963) Inflammation and trauma from occlusion, codestructive factors in chronic periodontal disease. *J. Periodontol.* **34**, 5–10

Glickman, I. and Smulow, J. B. (1962) Alterations in the pathway of gingival inflammation into the underlying tissues induced by excessive occlusal forces. *J. Periodontol.* **33**, 7–13

Glickman, I. and Smulow, J. B. (1965) Effect of excessive occlusal forces upon the pathway of gingival inflammation in humans. *J. Periodontol.* **36**, 141–147

Glickman, I. and Smulow, J. B. (1967) Further observations on the effects of trauma from occlusion in humans. *J. Periodontol.* **38**, 280–293

Glickman, I., Smulow, J. B., O'Brien, T. and Tannen, R. (1963) Healing of the periodontium following mucogingival surgery. *Oral Surg.* **16**, 530–538

Glossary of Periodontic Terms (1986) Supplement *Journal of Periodontology,* Nov. The American Academy of Periodontology

Goldman, H. M. (1950) The development of physiological gingival contours by gingivoplasty. *Oral Surg.* **3**, 879–888

Goldman, H. M. (1957) The behavior of transseptal fibers in periodontal disease. *J. Dent. Res.* **36**, 249–254

Goldman, H. and Cohen, D. W. (1958) The infrabony pocket: classification and treatment. *J. Periodontol.* **29**, 272–291

Gottlow, J., Nyman, S. and Karring, T. (1984a) Healing following citric acid conditioning of roots implanted into bone and gingival connective tissue. *J. Periodont. Res.* **19**, 214–220

Gottlow, J., Nyman, S., Karring, T. and Lindhe, J. (1984b) New attachment formation as the result of controlled tissue regeneration. *J. Clin. Periodontol.* **11**, 494–503

Gottlow, J., Nyman, S., Karring, T. and Lindhe, J. (1986a) Treatment of localized gingival recessions with coronally displaced flaps and citric acid. An experimental study in the dog. *J. Clin. Periodontol.* **13**, 57–63

Gottlow, J., Nyman, S., Lindhe, J., Karring, T. and Wennström, J. (1986b) New attachment formation in the human periodontium by guided tissue regeneration. *J. Clin. Periodontol.* **13**, 604–616

Grassi, M., Tellenbach, R. and Lang, N. P. (1987) Periodontal conditions of teeth adjacent to extraction sites. *J. Clin. Periodontol.* **14**, 334–339

Gröndahl, H. G. and Lekholm, U. (1973) Influence of mandibular third molars on related supporting tissues. *Int. J. Oral Surg.* **2**, 137–142

Groves, B. J. and Moore, J. R. (1970) The periodontal implications of flap design in lower third molar extractions. *Dent. Pract.* **20**, 297–304

Hakkarainen, K. and Ainamo, J. (1980) Influence of overhanging posterior tooth restorations on alveolar bone height in adults. *J. Clin. Periodontol.* **7**, 114–120

Hall, R. M. (1965) The effect of high-speed bone cutting without the use of water coolant. *Oral Surg.* **20**, 150–153

Halliday, D. G. (1969) The grafting of newly formed autogenous bone in the treatment of osseous defects. *J. Periodontol.* **40**, 511–514

Han, T., Carranza, F. A. and Kenney, E. B. (1984) Calcium phosphate ceramics in dentistry: a review of the literature. *J. West Soc. Periodont. Periodont. Abstr.* **32**, 88–108

Hanes, P. J., Polson, A. M. and Ladenheim, S. (1985) Cell and fiber attachment to demineralized dentin from normal root surfaces. *J. Periodontol.* **56**, 752–765

Hausmann, E. and Ortman, L. (1979) Present status of bone resorption in human periodontal disease. *J. Periodontol. Special Issue.* 7–10

Hegedus, Z. (1923) The rebuilding of the alveolar processes by bone transplantation. *Dent. Cosmos.* **65**, 736–742

Heritier, M. (1983) Ultrastructural study of new connective tissue attachment following phosphoric acid application on human root dentin. *J. Periodontol.* **54**, 515–521

Heritier, M. (1984) Effects of phosphoric acid on root dentin surface. A scanning and transmission electron microscopic study. *J. Periodont. Res.* **19**, 168–176

Hiatt, W. H. and Schallhorn, R. G. (1971) Human allografts of iliac cancellous bone marrow in periodontal osseous defects. I. Rationale and methodology. *J. Periodontol.* **42**, 642–647

Hiatt, W. H. and Schallhorn, R. G. (1973) Intraoral transplants of cancellous bone and marrow in periodontal lesions. *J. Periodontol.* **44**, 194–208

Hiatt, W. H., Schallhorn, R. G. and Aaronian, A. J. (1978) The induction of new bone and cementum formation. IV. Microscopic examination of the periodontium following human bone and marrow allograft, autograft, and nongraft periodontal regenerative procedures. *J. Periodontol.* **49**, 495–512

Highfield, J. E. and Powell, R. N. (1978) Effects of removal of posterior overhanging metallic margins of restorations upon the periodontal tissues. *J. Clin. Periodontol.* **5**, 169–181

Holden, M. J. and Smith, B. A. (1983) Citric acid and fibronectin in periodontal therapy. *J. West Soc. Periodont. Periodont. Abstr.* **31**, 45–56

Horton, J. E., Tarpley, T. M. Jr. and Jacoway, J. R. (1981) Clinical applications of ultrasonic instrumentation in the surgical removal of bone. *Oral Surg.* **51**, 236–242

Houston, F., Sarhed, G., Nyman, S., Lindhe, J. and Karring, T. (1985) Healing after root reimplantation in the monkey. *J. Clin. Periodontol.* **12**, 716–727

Ibbott, C. G. (1985) Root resorption associated with placement of a ceramic implant. Report of a case. *J. Periodontol.* **56**, 419–421

Ibbott, C. G., Oles, R. D. and Laverty, W. H. (1985) Effects of citric acid treatment on autogenous free graft coverage of localized recession. *J. Periodontol.* **56**, 662–665

Isidor, F., Attström, R. and Karring, T. (1985a) Regeneration of alveolar bone following surgical and non-surgical periodontal treatment. *J. Clin. Periodontol.* **12**, 687–696

Isidor, F., Karring, T., Nyman, S. and Lindhe, J. (1985b) New attachment formation on citric acid treated roots. *J. Periodont. Res.* **20**, 421–430

Isidor, F., Karring, T., Nyman, S. and Lindhe, J. (1985c) New attachment – reattachment following reconstructive periodontal surgery. *J. Clin. Periodontol.* **12**, 728–735

Isidor, F., Karring, T., Nyman, S. and Lindhe, H. (1986) The significance of coronal growth of periodontal ligament tissue for new attachment formation. *J. Clin. Periodontol.* **13**, 145–150

Jansen, J. (1982) Artificial periodontal defects around incisor teeth of beagle dogs. A clinical and histometrical analysis. *J. Periodont. Res.* **17**, 210–218

Jansen, J. (1983) Histopathology of artificial periodontal defects in beagle dogs before and after ligature removal. *J. Periodont. Res.* **18**, 262–275

Jansen, J., van Dijk, J. and Pilot, T. (1982) Histometric analysis of ligature-induced periodontal defects in beagle dogs. Longitudinal evaluation following ligature removal. *J. Periodont. Res.* **17**, 202–209

Jeffcoat, M. K. and Howell, T. H. (1980) Alveolar bone destruction due to overhanging amalgam in periodontal disease. *J. Periodontol.* **51**, 599–602

Johnson, N. W., Iino, Y. and Hopps, R. M. (1985) Bone resorption in periodontal diseases: role of bacterial factors. *Int. Endodont. J.* **18**, 152–157

Johnson, R. H. (1976) Basic flap management. *Dent. Clin. North Am.* **20**, 3–31

Jones, S. J., Lozdan, J. and Boyde, A. (1972) Tooth surfaces treated in situ with periodontal instruments. Scanning electron microscopic studies. *Br. Dent. J.* **132**, 57–64

Kalkwarf, K. L. (1974) Periodontal new attachment without the placement of osseous potentiating grafts. *J. West Soc. Periodont. Periodont. Abstr.* **12**, 53–62

Kantor, M. (1980) The behavior of angular bone defects following reduction of inflammation. *J. Periodontol.* **51**, 433–436

Karn, K. W., Shockett, H. P., Moffitt, W. C. and Gray, J. L. (1984) Topographic classification of deformities of the alveolar process. *J. Periodontol.* **55**, 336–340

Karring, T., Isidor, F., Nyman, S. and Lindhe, J. (1985) New attachment formation on teeth with a reduced but healthy periodontal ligament. *J. Clin. Periodontol.* **12**, 51–60

Karring, T., Nyman, S. and Lindhe, J. (1980) Healing following implantation of periodontitis affected roots into bone tissue. *J. Clin. Periodontol.* **7**, 96–105

Karring, T., Nyman, S., Lindhe, J. and Sirirat, M. (1984) Potentials for root resorption during periodontal wound healing. *J. Clin. Periodontol.* **11**, 41–52

Kashani, H. G., Magner, A. W. and Stahl, S. S. (1984) The effect of root planing and citric acid applications on flap healing in humans. *J. Periodontol.* **55**, 679–683

Kenney, E. B., Lekovic, V., Han, T., Carranza, F. A. Jr., and Dimitrijevic, B. (1985) The use of porous hydroxylapatite implant in periodontal defects. *J. Periodontol.* **56**, 82–88

Klinge, B., Nilveus, R., Kiger, R. D. and Egelberg, J. (1981) Effect of flap placement and defect size on healing of experimental furcation defects. *J. Periodont. Res.* **16**, 236–248

Klinge, B., Nilveus, R., Bogle, G., Badersten, A. and Egelberg, J. (1985a) Effect of implants on healing of experimental furcation defects in dogs. *J. Clin. Periodontol.* **12**, 321–326

Klinge, B., Nilveus, R. and Egelberg, J. (1985b) Effect of crown-attached sutures on healing of experimental furcation defects in dogs. *J. Clin. Periodontol.* **12**, 369–373

Klinge, B., Nilveus, R. and Egelberg, J. (1985c) Bone regeneration pattern and ankylosis in experimental furcation defects in dogs. *J. Clin. Periodontol.* **12**, 456–464

Klingsberg, J. (1972) Preserved sclera in periodontal surgery. *J. Periodontol.* **43**, 634–639

Klingsberg, J. (1974) Periodontal scleral grafts and combined grafts of sclera and bone: two year appraisal. *J. Periodontol.* **45**, 262–272

Koral, S. M., Howell, T. H. and Jeffcoat, M. K. (1981) Alveolar bone loss due to open interproximal contacts in periodontal disease. *J. Periodontol.* **52**, 447–450

Krejci, R. F., Kalkwarf, K. L. and Krause-Hohenstein, U. (1987) Electrosurgery – a biological approach. *J. Clin. Periodontol.* **14**, 557–563

Lai, H., O'Leary, T. J. and Kafrawy, A. H. (1986) The effect of different treatment modalities on connective tissue attachment. *J. Periodontol.* **57**, 604–612

Larato, D. C. (1970) Intrabony defects in the dry human skull. *J. Periodontol.* **41**, 496–498

Larato, D. C. (1971) Relationship of food impaction to interproximal intrabony lesions. *J. Periodontol.* **42**, 237–238

Larato, D. C. (1972) Palatal exostoses of the posterior maxillary alveolar process. *J. Periodontol.* **43**, 486–489

Lasho, D. J., O'Leary, T. J. and Kafrawy, A. H. (1983) A scanning electron microscope study of the effects of various agents on instrumented periodontally involved root surfaces. *J. Periodontol.* **54**, 210–220

Lee, K. W., Lee, F. C. and Poon, K. Y. (1969) Palato-gingival grooves in maxillary incisors. *Br. Dent. J.* **124**, 14–18

Lindhe, J. and Ericsson, I. (1978) Effect of ligature placement and dental plaque on periodontal tissue breakdown in the dog. *J. Periodontol.* **49**, 343–350

Lindhe, J. and Nyman, S. (1985) Scaling and granulation tissue removal in periodontal therapy. *J. Clin. Periodontol.* **12**, 374–388

Lindhe, J., Nyman, S. and Karring, T. (1984) Connective tissue reattachment as related to presence or absence of alveolar bone. *J. Clin. Periodontol.* **11**, 33–40

Lindskog, S., Blomlöf, L. and Hammarström, L. (1983) Repair of periodontal tissues *in vivo* and *in vitro*. *J. Clin. Periodontol.* **10**, 188–205

Liu, W. J-L. and Solt, C. W. (1980) A surgical procedure for the treatment of localized gingival recession in conjunction with root surface citric acid conditioning. *J. Periodontol.* **51**, 505–509

Lobene, R. R. and Glickman, I. (1963) The response of

alveolar bone to grinding with rotary diamond stones. *J. Periodontol.* **34**, 105–119

Löe, H. and Waerhaug, J. (1961) Experimental replantation of teeth in dogs and monkeys. *Arch. Oral Biol.* **3**, 176–184

Lopez, N. J. (1984) Connective tissue regeneration to periodontally diseased roots, planed and conditioned with citric acid and implanted into the oral mucosa. *J. Periodontol.* **55**, 381–390

Lopez, N. J. and Belvederessi, M. (1983) Healing following implantation of healthy roots, with and without periodontal ligament tissue, in the oral mucosa. *J. Periodontol.* **54**, 283–290

Mabry, T. W., Yukna, R. A. and Sepe, W. W. (1985) Freeze-dried bone allografts combined with tetracycline in the treatment of juvenile periodontitis. *J. Periodontol.* **56**, 74–81

MacLeod, K. M., Betz, P. K. and Ratcliff, P. A. (1965) An index of gingival architectural form. *J. Periodontol.* **36**, 413–416

Magnusson, I., Claffey, N., Bogle, G., Garrett, S. and Egelberg, J. (1985a) Root resorption following periodontal flap procedures in monkeys. *J. Periodont. Res.* **20**, 79–85

Magnusson, I., Nyman, S., Karring, T. and Egelberg, J. (1985b) Connective tissue attachment formation following exclusion of gingival connective tissue and epithelium during healing. *J. Periodont. Res.* **20**, 201–208

Manson, J. D. (1976) Bone morphology and bone loss in periodontal disease. *J. Clin. Periodontol.* **3**, 14–22

Marks, S. C. Jr. and Mehta, N. R. (1986) Lack of effect of citric acid treatment of root surfaces on the formation of new connective tissue attachment. *J. Clin. Periodontol.* **13**, 109–116

Matherson, D. G. and Zander, H. A. (1963) Evaluation of osseous surgery in monkeys. *J. Dent. Res.* **42**, 116 (IADR Abstr. No. 325)

Meffert, R. M., Thomas, J. R., Hamilton, K. M. and Brownstein, C. N. (1985) Hydroxyapatite as an alloplastic graft in the treatment of human periodontal osseous defects. *J. Periodontol.* **56**, 63–73

Melcher, A. H. (1970) Repair of wounds in the periodontium of the rat. Influence of the periodontal ligament on osteogenesis. *Arch. Oral Biol.* **15**, 1183–1204

Melcher, A. H. (1976) On the repair potential of periodontal tissues. *J. Periodontol.* **47**, 256–260

Mellonig, J. R., Bowers, G. M., Bright, R. W. and Lawrence, J. J. (1976) Clinical evaluation of freeze-dried bone allografts in periodontal osseous defects. *J. Periodontol.* **47**, 125–131

Michelich, V. J., Schuster, G. S. and Pashley, D. H. (1980) Bacterial penetration of human dentin *in vitro*. *J. Dent. Res.* **59**, 1398–1403

Moore, J. A., Ashley, F. P. and Waterman, C. A. (1987) The effect on healing of the application of citric acid during replaced flap surgery. *J. Clin. Periodontol.* **14**, 130–135

Morris, M. L. and Thomson, R. H. (1963) Healing of

human periodontal tissues surgical detachment. *Periodontics* **1**, 189–195

Moskow, B. S., Karsh, F. and Stein, S. D. (1979) Histological assessment of autogenous bone graft. A case report and critical evaluation. *J. Periodontol.* **50**, 291–300

Nabers, C. L. and O'Leary, T. J. (1965) Autogenous bone transplants in the treatment of osseous defects. *J. Periodontol.* **36**, 5–14

Nalbandian, J. and Frank, R. M. (1980) Electron microscopic study of the regeneration of cementum and periodontal connective tissue attachment in the cat. *J. Periodont. Res.* **15**, 71–89

Nasjleti, C. E., Caffesse, R. G., Castelli, W. A., Lopatin, D. E. and Kowalski, C. J. (1986) Effect of lyophilized autologous plasma on periodontal healing of replanted teeth. *J. Periodontol.* **57**, 568–578

Nasjleti, C. E., Caffesse, R. G., Castelli, W. A., Smith, B. A., Lopatin, D. E. and Kowalski, C. J. (1987) Effect of citric acid and lyophilized autologous plasma on healing following periodontal flap surgery in monkeys. *J. Periodontol.* **58**, 770–779

Newman, P. S. (1984) The effects of the inverse bevel flap procedure on gingival contour and plaque accumulation. *J. Clin. Periodontol.* **11**, 361–366

Nielsen, I. M., Glavind, L. and Karring, T. (1980) Interproximal periodontal intrabony defects. Prevalence, localization and etiological factors. *J. Clin. Periodontol.* **7**, 187–198

Nilveus, R. and Selvig, K. A. (1983) Pulpal reactions to the application of ciric acid to root-planed dentin in beagles. *J. Periodont. Res.* **18**, 420–428

Nyman, S. and Karring, T. (1979) Regeneration of surgically removed buccal alveolar bone in dogs. *J. Periodont. Res.* **14**, 86–92

Nyman, S., Rosling, B. and Lindhe, J. (1975) Effect of professional tooth cleaning on healing after periodontal surgery. *J. Clin. Periodontol.* **2**, 80–86

Nyman, S., Karring, T., Lindhe, J. and Plantén, S. (1980) Healing following implantation of periodontitis-affected roots into gingival connective tissue. *J. Clin. Periodontol.* **7**, 394–401

Nyman, S., Gottlow, J., Karring, T. and Lindhe, J. (1982a) The regenerative potential of the periodontal ligament. An experimental study in the monkey. *J. Clin. Periodontol.* **9**, 257–265

Nyman, S., Lindhe, J., Karring, T. and Rylander, H. (1982b) New attachment following surgical treatment of human periodontal disease. *J. Clin. Periodontol.* **9**, 290–296

Nyman, S., Ericsson, I., Runstead, L. and Karring,T. (1984) The significance of alveolar bone in periodontal disease. An experimental study in the dog. *J. Periodont. Res.* **19**, 520–525

Nyman, S., Houston, F., Sarhed, G., Lindhe, J. and Karring, T. (1985) Healing following reimplantation of teeth subjected to root planing and citric acid treatment. *J. Clin. Periodontol.* **12**, 294–305

Nyman, S. Gottlow, J., Lindhe, J., Karring, T. and

Wennström, J. (1987) New attachment formation by guided tissue regeneration. *J. Periodont. Res.* **22**, 252–254

Ochsenbein, C. (1958) Osseous resection in periodontal surgery. *J. Periodontol.* **29**, 15–26

Oles, R. D., Ibbott, C. G. and Laverty, W. H. (1985) Effects of citric acid treatment on pedicle flap coverage of localized recession. *J. Periodontol.* **56**, 259–261

Olson, R. H., Adams, D. F. and Layman, D. L. (1985) Inhibitory effect of periodontally diseased root extracts on the growth of human gingival fibroblasts. *J. Periodontol.* **56**, 592–596

Osborne, W. H., Snyder, A. J. and Tempel, T. R. (1982) Attachment levels and crevicular depths at the distal of mandibular second molars following removal of adjacent third molars. *J. Periodontol.* **53**, 93–95

Parodi, R. J. and Esper, M. E. (1984) Effect of topical application of citric acid in the treatment of furcation involvement in human lower molars. *J. Clin. Periodontol.* **11**, 644–651

Pashley, D. H., Michelich, V. and Kehl, T. (1981) Dentin permeability: effects of smear layer removal. *J. Prosthet. Dent.* **46**, 531–537

Patur, B. and Glickman, I. (1962) Clinical and roentgenographic evaluation of post-treatment healing of infrabony pockets. *J. Periodontol.* **33**, 164–171

Pennel, B. M., King, O. K., Wilderman, M. H. and Barron, J. M. (1967) Repair of the alveolar process following osseous surgery. *J. Periodontol.* **38**, 426–500

Pettersson, E. C. and Aukhil, I. (1986) Citric acid conditioning of roots affects guided tissue regeneration in experimental periodontal wounds. *J. Periodont. Res.* **21**, 543–552

Pitaru, S. and Melcher, A. H. (1987) Organization of an oriented fibre system *in vitro* by human gingival fibroblasts attached to dental tissue: Relationship between cells and mineralized and demineralized tissue. *J. Periodont. Res.* **22**, 6–13

Pitaru, S., Gray, A., Aubin, J. E. and Melcher, A. H. (1984a) The influence of the morphological and chemical nature of dental surfaces on the migration, attachment and orientation of human gingival fibroblasts *in vitro*. *J. Periodont. Res.* **19**, 408–418

Pitaru, S., Aubin, J. E., Gray, A., Metzger, Z. and Melcher, A. H. (1984b) Cell migration attachment and orientation *in vitro* are enhanced by partial demineralization of dentin and cementum and inhibited by bacterial endotoxin. *J. Periodont. Res.* **19**, 661–665

Polson, A. M. and Caton, J. (1982) Factors influencing periodontal repair and regeneration. *J. Periodontol.* **53**, 617–625

Polson, A. M. and Frederick, G. T. (1985) Cell processes in dentin tubules during early phases of attachment to demineralized periodontitis-affected surfaces. *J. Clin. Periodontol.* **12**, 162–169

Polson, A. M. and Heijl, L. C. (1978) Osseous repair in infrabony periodontal defects. *J. Clin. Periodontol.* **5**, 13–23

Polson, A. M. and Proye, M. P. (1982) Effect of root

surface alterations on periodontal healing. II. Citric acid treatment of the denuded root. *J. Clin. Periodontol.* **9**, 441–454

Polson, A. M. and Proye, M. P. (1983) Fibrin linkage: a precursor for new attachment. *J. Periodontol.* **54**, 141–147

Polson, A. M., Kantor, M. E. and Zander, H. A. (1979) Periodontal repair after reduction of inflammation. *J. Periodont. Res.* **14**, 520–525

Polson, A. M., Frederick, G. T., Landenheim, S. and Hanes, P. J. (1984) The production of a root surface smear layer by instrumentation and its removal by citric acid. *J. Periodontol.* **55**, 443–446

Polson, A. M., Ladenheim, S. and Hanes, P. J. (1986) Cell and fibre attachment to demineralized dentin from periodontitis-affected root surfaces. *J. Periodontol.* **57**, 235–246

Pontoriero, R., Nyman, S., Lindhe, J., Rosenberg, E. and Sanavi, F. (1987) Guided tissue regeneration in the treatment of furcation defects in man. *J. Clin. Periodontol.* **14**, 618–620

Prichard, J. F. (1967) The etiology, diagnosis and treatment of the intrabony defect. *J. Periodontol.* **38**, 455–465

Prichard, J. F. (1972) *Advanced Periodontal Disease, Surgical and Prosthetic Management,* 2nd Edition, pp. 512–601. W. B. Saunders Co. Philadelphia

Prichard, J. F. (1983) The diagnosis and management of vertical bony defects. *J. Periodontol.* **54**, 29–35

Proye, M. P. and Polson, A. M. (1982a) Repair in different zones of the periodontium after tooth reimplantation. *J. Periodontol.* **53**, 379–389

Proye, M. P. and Polson, A. M. (1982b) Effect of root surface alterations on periodontal healing. I. Surgical denudation. *J. Clin. Periodontol.* **9**, 428–440

Ratcliff, P. A. (1966) Periodontal therapy – review of the literature. In *World Workshop in Periodontics,* p. 277. Editors Ramfjord, S. P., Kerr, D. H. and Ash, M. M. American Academy of Periodontology and University of Michigan, Ann Arbor

Register, A. A. and Burdick, F. A. (1975) Accelerated reattachment with cementogenesis to dentin, demineralized in situ. I. Optimum range. *J. Periodontol.* **46**, 646–655

Register, A. A. and Burdick, F. A. (1976) Accelerated reattachment with cementogenesis to dentin, demineralized in situ. II. Defect repair. *J. Periodontol.* **47**, 497–505

Renvert, S., Nilveus, R. and Egelberg, J. (1985a) Healing after treatment of periodontal intraosseous defects. V. Effect of root planing versus flap surgery. *J. Clin. Periodontol.* **12**, 619–629

Renvert, S., Garrett, S., Nilveus, R., Chamberlain, A. D. H. and Egelberg, J. (1985b) Healing after treatment of periodontal intraosseous defects. VI. Factors influencing the healing response. *J. Clin. Periodontol.* **12**, 707–715

Renvert, S., Garrett, S., Shallhorn, R. G. and Egelberg, J. (1985c) Healing after treatment of periodontal intraos-

seous defects. III. Effect of osseous grafting and citric acid conditioning. *J. Clin. Periodontol.* **12**, 441–455

Ririe, C. M., Crigger, M. and Selvig, K. A. (1980) Healing of periodontal connective tissues following surgical wounding and application of citric acid in dogs. *J. Periodont. Res.* **15**, 314–327

Robinson, R. E. (1969) Osseous coagulum for bone induction. *J. Periodontol.* **40**, 503–510

Rosenberg, M. M. (1971) Free osseous tissue autografts as a predictable procedure. *J. Periodontol.* **42**, 195–209

Rosling, B., Nyman, S. and Lindhe, J. (1976a) The effect of systematic plaque control on bone regeneration in infrabony pockets. *J. Clin. Periodontol.* **3**, 38–53

Rosling, B., Nyman, S., Lindhe, J. and Jern, B. (1976b) The healing potential of the periodontal tissues following different techniques of periodontal surgery in plaque-free dentitions. A 2-year clinical study. *J. Clin. Periodontol.* **3**, 233–250

Ryan, P. C., Newcomb, G. M., Seymour, G. J. and Powell, R. N. (1984) The pulpal response to citric acid in cats. *J. Clin. Periodontol.* **11**, 633–643

Saari, J. T., Hurt, W. C. and Biggs, N. L. (1968) Periodontal bony defects on the dry skull. *J. Periodontol.* **39**, 278–283

Sanders, J. J., Sepe, W. W., Bowers, G. M., Koch, R. W., Williams, J. E., Lekas, J. S., Mellonig, J. T., Pelleu, G. B. Jr. and Gambill, V. (1983) Clinical evaluation of freeze-dried bone allografts in periodontal osseous defects. Part III. Composite freeze-dried bone allografts with and without autogenous bone grafts. *J. Periodontol.* **54**, 1–8

Sarbinoff, J. A., O'Leary, T. J. and Miller, C. H. (1983) The comparative effectiveness of various agents in detoxifying diseased root surfaces. *J. Periodontol.* **54**, 77–80

Schallhorn, R. G. (1967) Eradication of bifurcation defects utilising frozen autogenous hip marrow implants. *Periodont. Abstr.* **15**, 101–105

Schallhorn, R. G. (1968) The use of autogenous hip marrow biopsy implants for bony crater defects. *J. Periodontol.* **39**, 145–147

Schallhorn, R. G. (1972) Postoperative problems associated with iliac transplants. *J. Periodontol.* **43**, 3–9

Schallhorn, R. G. (1977) Present status of osseous grafting procedures. *J. Periodontol.* **48**, 570–576

Schallhorn, R. G. and Hiatt, W. H. (1972) Human allografts of iliac cancellous bone and marrow in periodontal osseous defects. II. Clinical observations. *J. Periodontol.* **43**, 67–81

Schallhorn, R. G., Hiatt, W. H. and Boyce, W. (1970) Iliac transplants in periodontal therapy. *J. Periodontol.* **41**, 566–580

Schluger, S. (1949) Osseous resection – a basic principle in periodontal surgery. *Oral Surg.* **2**, 316–325

Selvig, K. A., Ririe, C. M., Nilveus, R. and Egelberg, J. (1981) Fine structure of new connective tissue attachment following acid treatment of experimental furcation pockets in dogs. *J. Periodont. Res.* **16**, 123–129

Sepe, W. W., Bowers, G. M., Lawrence, J. J., Friedlander, G. E. and Koch, R. W. (1978) Clinical evaluation of freeze-dried bone allografts in periodontal osseous defects. II. *J. Periodontol.* **49**, 9–14

Seymour, G. J., Romaniuk, K. and Newcomb, G. M. (1983) Effect of citric acid on soft tissue healing in the rat palate. *J. Clin. Periodontol.* **10**, 182–187

Sigurdson, A. (1972) Orala benimplantat. *Swed. Dent. J.* **65**, 33–40

Smith, B. A., Mason, W. E., Morrison, E. C. and Caffesse, R. G. (1986) The effectiveness of citric acid as an adjunct to surgical re-attachment procedures in humans. *J. Clin. Periodontol.* **13**, 701–708

Smith, B. A., Smith, J. S., Caffesse, R. G., Nasjleti, C. E., Lopatin, D. E. and Kowalski, C. J. (1987) Effect of citric acid and various concentrations of fibronectin on healing following periodontal flap surgery in dogs. *J. Periodontol.* **58**, 667–673

Smith, D. H., Ammons, W. F. Jr., and van Belle, G. (1980) A longitudinal study of periodontal status comparing osseous recontouring with flap curettage. I. Results after 6 months. *J. Periodontol.* **51**, 367–375

Soehern, S. E. and van Swol, R. L. (1979) The healing extraction: a donor area for periodontal grafting material. *J. Periodontol.* **50**, 128–133

Staffileno, H. (1974) Significant differences and advantages between the full thickness and split thickness flaps. *J. Periodontol.* **45**, 421–425

Stahl, S. S. and Froum, S. (1986) Histological evaluation of human intraosseous healing responses to the placement of tricalcium phosphate ceramic implants. I. Three to eight months. *J. Periodontol.* **57**, 211–217

Stahl, S. S. and Tarnow, D. (1985) Root resorption leading to linkage of dentinal collagen and gingival fibers? A case report. *J. Clin. Periodontol.* **12**, 399–404

Stahl, S. S., Froum, S. J. and Kushner, L. (1982) Periodontal healing following open debridement flap procedures. II. Histologic observations. *J. Periodontol.* **53**, 15–21

Stahl, S. S., Froum, S. J. and Kushner, L. (1983) Healing responses of human intraosseous lesions following the use of debridement, grafting and citric acid root treatment. II. Clinical and histologic observations: one year postsurgery. *J. Periodontol.* **54**, 325–338

Stephens, R. J., App, G. R. and Foreman, D. W. (1983) Periodontal evaluation of two mucoperiosteal flaps used in removing impacted mandibular third molars. *J. Maxillofac. Surg.* **41**, 719–724

Sussmann, H. I. and Ewen, S. J. (1969) A case of bone swaging. *N.Y. State Dent. J.* **35**, 157–161

Svanberg, G. (1974) Experimental trauma from occlusion in the dog. Thesis. Göteborg

Szmyd, L. and Hester, W. (1963) Crevicular depth of the second molar in impacted third molar surgery. *J. Oral Surg.* **21**, 185–189

Takei, H. H., Han, T. J., Carranza, F. A. Jr., Kenney, E. B. and Lekovic, V. (1985) Flap technique for periodontal bone implants. Papilla preservation technique. *J. Periodontol.* **56**, 204–210

Tal, H. (1984a) The prevalence and distribution of intrabony defects in dry mandibles. *J. Periodontol.* **55**, 149–154

Tal, H. (1984b) Relationship between the interproximal distance of roots and the prevalence of intrabony pockets. *J. Periodontol.* **55**, 604–607

Tavtigian, R. (1970) The height of the facial radicular alveolar crest following apically positioned flap operations. *J. Periodontol.* **41**, 412–418

Terranova, V. P. and Wikesjö, U. M. E. (1987) Extracellular matrices and polypeptide growth factors as mediators of functions of cells of the periodontium. A review. *J. Periodontol.* **58**, 371–380

Urist, M. R. (1971) Bone histogenesis and morphogenesis in implants of demineralized enamel and dentin. *J. Oral Surg.* **29**, 88–102

van Dijk, L. J. and Wright, W. H. (1983) Effects of oral hygiene on the results of periodontal surgery in beagle dogs with artificially created defects. *J. Periodontol.* **54**, 291–298

Waerhaug, J. (1952) The gingival pocket. *Odontol. Tidskr.* **60**, Suppl. 1

Waerhaug, J. (1979a) The angular bone defect and its relationship to trauma from occlusion and downgrowth of subgingival plaque. *J. Clin. Periodontol.* **6**, 61–82

Waerhaug, J. (1979b) The infrabony pocket and its relationship to trauma from occlusion and subgingival plaque. *J. Periodontol.* **50**, 355–365

Walsh, T. F. and Waite, I. M. (1978) A comparison of postsurgical healing following debridement by ultrasonic or hand instruments. *J. Periodontol.* **49**, 201–205

Wilderman, M. N., Pennel, B. M., King, K. and Barron, J. M. (1970) Histogenesis of repair following osseous surgery. *J. Periodontol.* **41**, 551–565

Willey, R. and Steinberg, A. D. (1984) Scanning electron microscopic studies of root dentin surfaces treated with citric acid, elastase, hyaluronidase, pronase and collagenase. *J. Periodontol.* **55**, 592–596

Wirthlin, M. R. (1981) The current status of new attachment therapy. *J. Periodontol.* **52**, 529–544

Wirthlin, M. R. (1986) Review of bone biology in periodontal disease. *J. Western Soc. Periodont.* **34**, 125–143

Wirthlin, M. R. (1987) Resective and regenerative osseous surgery. *J. West. Soc. Periodont.* **35**, 5–21

Wood, D. L., Hoag, P. M., Donnenfeld, O. W., Rosenfeld, L. D. (1972) Alveolar crest reduction following full and partial thickness flaps. *J. Periodontol.* **43**, 141–144

Yukna, R. A., Mayer, E. T. and Brite, D. V. (1984) Longitudinal evaluation of durapatite ceramic as an alloplastic implant in periodontal osseous defects after 3 years. *J. Periodontol.* **55**, 633–637

Yukna, R. A., Harrison, B. G., Caudill, R. F., Evans, G. H., Mayer, E. T. and Miller, S. (1985) Evaluation of durapatite ceramic as an alloplastic implant in periodontal osseous defects. II. Twelve month reentry results. *J. Periodontol.* **56**, 540–547

Zamet, J. S. (1975) A comparative clinical study of three

periodontal surgical techniques. *J. Clin. Periodontol.* **2**, 87–97

Zander, H. A. and Matherson, D. G. (1963) The effect of osseous surgery on interdental tissue morphology in monkeys. *J. Dent. Res.* **41**, 117 (IADR Abstract no. 326)

32

Mucogingival considerations

Introduction

It has long been believed, on the strength of clinical impressions, that a certain width of keratinized attached gingiva is necessary for the maintenance of gingival health, the prevention of gingival recession and attachment loss and to withstand marginal tissue retraction during movement of the alveolar mucosa (Friedman, 1962), so preventing food particles and bacteria from entering the gingival sulcus. It has also been assumed that prominent frenal insertions, especially in association with a shallow vestibule, predisposed to gingival inflammation by impeding oral hygiene (for review see Wennström, 1982).

Research findings over the past decade have questioned the validity of these traditional beliefs. Consequently, many of the surgical techniques that have evolved to correct these mucogingival inadequacies (for review, see Nery and Davies, 1976; Schmid, 1976; Guinard and Caffesse, 1977; Hall, 1981) have fallen into disuse and remain of mainly historical interest. These techniques will therefore be referred to only in their basic forms when assessing the clinical significance of gingival dimensions *per se,* the so-called functional adequacy of the gingiva and, lastly, vestibular sulcus morphology. It would be instructive to first consider the aetiology of gingival recession about which much of mucogingival philosophy revolves.

Aetiology of recession

The incidence of recession has been studied extensively in both children and adults, increasing in

prevalence and severity with age (for reviews, see Woofter, 1969; Guinard and Caffesse, 1977). However the aetiology and pathogenesis of recession remains unclear. This is due primarily to difficulties in obtaining human material and designing a satisfactory animal model, and to the predominance of clinical impressions over scientific evidence. Many factors have been implicated, including plaque-induced marginal gingival inflammation and faulty toothbrushing (referred to in Chapters 13 and 21 respectively), tooth position, developmental crestal bony deformities (dehiscences) and thin gingival morphology, frenal attachments and narrow zones of gingiva, traumatic occlusion and impingement of restoration margins. Of these, thin gingival tissue with bony dehiscences alone and in conjunction with tooth malpositioning appear to be prerequisites for the development of recession. Two major factors, toothbrush trauma and plaque-induced inflammation may then cause marginal recession at such sites. Once developed, localized sites of recession may then lead to or perpetuate plaque-induced disease due to impaired accessibility to normal toothbrushing. The evidence relating to each of these possible factors is considered.

Plaque-induced inflammation

The role of inflammation was first described by Goldman and Cohen (1973) in relation to gingival cleft formation following the inflammatory proliferation and anastomosis of pocket lining epithelial rete ridges with the oral epithelium. A similar mechanism was cited by Novaes *et al.* (1975), in the development of periodontal clefts following mucosal fenestration (see also Lane, 1977). This was endorsed by Baker and Seymour (1976) who demonstrated the importance of the volume of the affected tissue. Thus, where the gingiva is thin the plaque-induced inflammatory infiltrate would occupy the major portion of the connective tissue of the free gingiva (Ericsson and Lindhe, 1984). Destruction of this very small connective tissue component and its replacement by epithelial rete ridges could in turn be accomplished quickly producing rapid recession. Where in contrast to this the tissue is thick, the inflammation would be confined to the region of the sulcus and would not destroy the outer gingival tissue, which would therefore persist as the wall of a pocket (see Figure 13.2). Thus, although recession does not always occur concomitantly with the development of periodontal disease, it is still a common feature (Lindhe and Nyman, 1980) which is related to the tissue morphology (Wennström, 1985).

Direct trauma

Gorman (1967), O'Leary *et al.* (1971), Sagnes and Gjermo (1976) reported that individuals with good oral hygiene had a higher frequency of gingival recession than subjects with poor oral hygiene. Surface abrasion and friction associated with over-zealous toothbrushing wearing away the gingival crest or even direct inadvertent trauma can be readily incriminated. The apparent inconsistency with the inflammatory hypothesis could be explained by the existence of subclinical inflammation as a result of toothbrush trauma increasing epithelial permeability (Baker and Seymour, 1976). On the other hand, the co-existence of a plaque-induced inflammation might simply not be recognized clinically, because as shown by Lindhe *et al.* (1978), the clinical and histological parameters used to assess the degrees of gingivitis do not always agree. The lack of a significant correlation between oral hygiene and gingival recession in preclinical dental students (Tenenbaum, 1982), could be interpreted to support both inflammatory and direct traumatic aetiological factors. Niemi *et al.* (1984, 1987) demonstrated a greater frequency of gingival abrasions with a combination of a hard brush held with a palm grip than a soft one with a pen grip to support the possible role of repeated trauma.

Breitenmoser *et al.* (1979) found that 'cut' toothbrush bristles caused greater gingival abrasions than 'rounded' ones. Smukler and Landsberg (1984) have presented histological data on toothbrush trauma. Finally, the possibility of self-inflicted gingival injuries causing recession should not be discounted (for review see Pattison, 1983).

Tooth malposition

The strong correlations shown between malaligned teeth and gingival recession (e.g. Parfitt and Mjor, 1964; Trott and Love, 1966; Gorman, 1967) should be viewed with some caution. This is because in many instances, the impression of gingival recession, created by disparities in gingival heights at neighbouring units and which is so commonly encountered in adolescents (Stoner and Mazdyasna, 1980), has not been differentiated from true recession in which loss of attachment and exposure of root surface occurs. Thus, for example, Stoner and Mazdyasna (1980) reported true recession in only 1% of a sample of 1003 15-year-olds, whereas 17% presented with pseudogingival recession, while a bias towards recession is shown in a longitudinal study on isolated gingival recession in children (Powell and McEniery, 1982). The latter investigators make no reference to root surface exposure in the criteria used for case selection, and the clinical case illustrations are predominantly of altered rates of gingival maturation (or of passive eruption) rather than true recession. It should, in this context, be realized that clinical crown heights may increase by a process of continued passive eruption to at least early adulthood (Volchansky *et al.*, 1979) and that variations of the rates at adjacent teeth may give the impression of gingival recession. Furthermore, it is also possible that the reduced gingival dimensions reported at malposed teeth (Rose and App, 1973; Mazeland, 1980) may be interpreted as true rather than pseudogingival recession.

It is, however, clear that more prominent tooth position in the arch would predispose to brushing trauma. In addition the frequently associated thin overlying mucosa coupled with bony dehiscences, means that the 'supracrestal' attachment could be readily damaged and lead to loss of attachment and marginal tissue recession. This is endorsed by the significant correlation shown between gingival recession and bony dehiscences (Bernimoulin and Curilovic, 1977) and between the depths of recession and of dehiscences (Löst, 1984).

Orthodontic movement

The relationship between orthodontic realignment of teeth and the development of gingival recession remains controversial. The association might be purely coincidental or due to appliances complicating cleaning and leading to plaque-induced or inadvertent traumatic gingival recession. This and the bony changes following orthodontic movement are considered in Chapter 33.

Frenal attachment

Frena are frequently incriminated in gingival recession especially at mandibular central incisors (e.g.

Gottsegen, 1954; Gormon, 1967; Rose, 1967). In contrast, Trott and Love (1966) observed that frena were not directly associated with any of a number of sites exhibiting gingival recession, while Placek *et al.* (1974) concluded that the pathogenic influence of the frenal attachment manifested itself only within certain subjects. The claimed relationship might simply reflect gingival margin recession, occurring quite independently, to the level of the frenal insertion (Gottsegen, 1954). The possible roles of the likely interference of the frenum with oral hygiene measures especially in the mandible, as suggested by the findings of Addy *et al.* (1987), and that of the associated thin gingival form at the affected site and its predisposition to inadvertent trauma leading to the gingival recession cannot be discounted.

Gingival dimensions

A narrow zone of gingiva in a site exhibiting recession may be considered a cause of recession (e.g. Hall, 1977), but the opposite may well be true. That is, the narrow gingival zone is the result of loss of marginal tissue during the development of recession. The investigations relating to reduced gingival width are considered separately below.

Occlusal trauma

The relationship between occlusal trauma and recession is also unclear. Stillman (1921) first implicated occlusal trauma in the development of gingival clefts which are V-shaped sites of gingival recession. Rose (1967) claimed that recession at mandibular incisors could be attributed to occlusal trauma. Novaes *et al.* (1975) suggested that bony resorption resulting from occlusal trauma could, in the presence of plaque-induced gingival inflammation, lead to recession. This hypothesis appears to be supported by the finding that gingival clefts apparently underwent spontaneous repair following occlusal analysis and subsequent adjustment (Solnit and Stambaugh, 1983). On the other hand, Emslie (1958) found no evidence to support the role of occlusal trauma, while Parfitt and Mjör (1964) observed no occlusal contacts in over half the mandibular incisors with recession and 'heavy occlusion' in only 15% of instances. Similarly 'trauma from occlusion' was observed in only 10% and 20% of cases with recession in the investigations of Trott and Love (1966) and Gormon (1967). Bernimoulin and Curilovic (1977) found no significant correlation between tooth mobility and gingival recession. The possible association of tooth to soft tissue trauma and gingival recession in deep overbites is considered in Chapters 21 and 33.

Restorative and prosthetic treatment

Subgingival margins of restorations will inevitably accumulate bacterial plaque (see also Chapter 24 – Periodontal restorative relationships) and thereby result in inflammation. As this inflammatory cell infiltrate will occupy the major portion of the free gingival connective tissue in situations with thin narrow zones of keratinized tissue, recession is likely to occur (Ericsson and Lindhe, 1984). On the other hand, although higher levels of gingival inflammation were observed in relation to submarginal restoration sites in the presence of narrow than wide zones of keratinized tissue (see also below 'Relevance of gingival deficiencies'), this was not accompanied by significant differences in attachment levels (Stetler and Bissada, 1987). This, in turn, suggests greater difficulties in plaque control at the former sites or that the tissue thickness, which was not stated, minimized the likelihood of gingival recession over the mean 4–5-year period of this investigation. The claim that 3 mm of attached gingiva (namely 4-5 mm of keratinized tissue) is necessary for restorative treatment (Maynard and Wilson, 1979) has yet to be substantiated and tissue thickness would seem to be more critical. If this can be shown, the principle of bilaminar subepithelial connective tissue grafting (see below 'Historical perspective') to increase marginal tissue bulk, would seem to be promising.

Donaldson (1974) evaluated the reasons for gingival recession associated with temporary crowns and concluded that direct operative trauma predominated. Removable partial prostheses may both facilitate plaque-induced disease and result in direct trauma leading to recession at vulnerable tissue sites (see also Chapter 34 – Restorative/prosthetic implications). For example, a poorly-supported mandibular free end saddle dentures is liable to traumatize the underlying mucosa, especially if thin (Farnoush and Schonfeld, 1983) and cause marginal tissue recession. This potential, together with its management by free gingival grafting, has been described by Schokking (1976), Langer and Calagha (1978) and Dello Russo (1982).

The assessment of gingival dimensions

The clinical importance of gingiva depends upon it having different tissue characteristics from that of the contiguous alveolar mucosa and the fact that gingival dimensions appear to decrease as a result of gingival recession.

Assessment of mucogingival junction

The junction has been defined by Lozdan and Squier (1969) as that point where a sudden marked increase of elastic fibres occurs in the corium. This, in turn, supplies a rational explanation for the mobility of alveolar mucosa. Change in distribution of acid phosphatase, non-specific esterase and glycogen (Ten Cate, 1963) also takes place at this junction. Other changes with respect to keratinization and the shape of the epithelial ridges (Orban, 1948) are less clearly defined. Bernimoulin *et al.* (1971) compared the anatomical, functional (wrinkle method – Coppes, 1972) and histochemical methods of defining the mucogingival junction. They concluded that staining with Schiller's IKI (iodine) solution which stains the glycogen within alveolar mucosa brown (Fasske and Morgenroth, 1958) was the most reliable. This method was used by Grevers (1977) and Wennström (1982) in their comprehensive investigations on gingival dimensions in relation to gingival health. The reproducibility of the 'wrinkle' method was demonstrated by Mazeland (1978).

Measurement of gingival dimensions

There have been several clinical studies on the width of attached gingiva at the facial aspects measured from the mucogingival junction to the horizontal projection at the base of the gingival crevice (Bowers 1963; Ainamo and Löe, 1966; Coppes, 1972; Lang and Löe, 1972). The dimensions of lingual attached gingiva have also been recorded by Coppes (1972), Lang and Löe (1972) and Voight *et al.* (1978). Coatoam *et al.* (1981) observed increased width of the keratinized tissue at some teeth during orthodontic therapy in adolescents. Furthermore, the increases in clinical crown heights observed were not accompanied by significant reductions in gingival dimensions. Tenenbaum and Tenenbaum (1986) examined the width of attached gingiva in the deciduous transitional and permanent dentitions, reporting a gradual increase in attached gingiva related to a concomitant decrease in gingival sulcus depth. The keratinized gingival width does however not change significantly (*cf.* Chapter 33 – The effects of therapy).

As changes in the position of the mucogingival junction cannot be determined clinically in longitudinal assessments, Talari and Ainamo (1976) developed an orthopantomographic method of assessing gingival dimensions. Alterations in the position of the gingival margins following recession have been recorded by most researchers by using the cemento-enamel junctions as a fixed point for measurement, although more recently soft acrylic occlusal overlays have been increasingly used (*cf.* Chapter 28). Tenenbaum *et al.* (1984) have described a standardized and reproducible photometric method of measuring gingival recession.

Influence of gingival recession

The reductions in gingival dimensions following marginal recession do not necessarily reflect the degree of recession sustained. Thus, Ainamo and Löe (1966) reported comparable gingival widths in adults regardless of whether the marginal gingiva was located at the cemento-enamel junctions or were markedly receded. Tenenbaum (1982), in turn, demonstrated that the mean width of attached gingiva in 100 preclinical dental students was only slightly lower, but not significantly different, in individuals with some gingival recession when compared to those with little or no recession. These findings suggest that the mucogingival junction moves apically at the receded sites. This possibility is also reflected in studies on periodontal disease in dogs in which the loss of attachment was always accompanied by gingival recession (to an extent that deep pockets do not form), but without the development of a commensurate decrease in gingival dimensions (Wennström *et al.*, 1981).

On the other hand, it has been claimed that gingival dimensions increase with age (Ainamo and Talari, 1976; Ainamo and Ainamo, 1978; Mazeland, 1980) and moreover that the location of the mucogingival junction remains constant (Ainamo and Talari, 1976; Ainamo, 1978). This increase in gingival dimensions has been attributed to continuous eruption of the teeth to compensate for occlusal wear (Ainamo and Ainamo, 1978) and to increases in lower anterior face height occurring with vertical growth within the alveolar processes (Mazeland, 1980). This passive tooth eruption (Manson, 1963) involves occlusal movement of both tooth and supporting tissues, i.e. the gingival attachment remains at the cemento-enamel junction as it does in supra-erupted teeth (Ainamo and Ainamo, 1978).

The ultimate effect of gingival recession on gingival dimensions *per se* has yet to be clearly demonstrated and must depend on longitudinal evaluation. Currently available data (see below) coupled with clinical observations do however indicate that a minimal residual band of keratinized tissue either persists or reforms as clinical crown height increases following recession of the marginal tissues.

Gingival dimensions and gingival health
Lack of physiological gingival width

The claimed importance of a certain physiological width of keratinized gingiva in the maintenance of health (see Nery and Davies, 1976; Hall, 1981) has yet to be substantiated. Thus, although Lang and Löe (1972) concluded from an investigation on dental students that 1 mm of attached gingiva (corresponding to 2 mm of keratinized tissue) is necessary to maintain health, many others have reported clinical health at sites with less than 1 mm of attached gingiva in humans (e.g. Bowers, 1963; Grevers, 1972; Miyasato *et al.*, 1977; Kennedy *et al.*, 1985) as well as in animal models (Wennström *et al.*, 1981; Wennström and Lindhe, 1983). Lindhe and Nyman (1980) have demonstrated convincingly in a 10-11-year post-surgical maintenance investigation that an absence of keratinized gingiva does not jeopardize periodontal health. This has also been endorsed by the results of longitudinal investigations on the management by plaque control measures alone of sites exhibiting true or pseudogingival recession and minimal levels or an absence of attached gingiva (Powell and McEniery, 1982; Schoo and van der Velden, 1985; Kisch *et al.*, 1986; Eaton and Kieser, 1986; Salkin *et al.*, 1987; Wennström, 1987) as well as at similarly treated control sites in subjects treated with free gingival grafts (Hangorsky and Bissada, 1980; De Trey and Bernimoulin, 1980; Dorfman *et al.*, 1980, 1982; Kennedy *et al.*, 1985). Thus, marginal tissue health with no further gingival recession or loss of attachment can be maintained, despite the lack of attached gingiva, by controlling gingival inflammation. Whilst increased gingival dimensions resulted from the grafts, the recipient sites responded in the same fashion as the controls. Furthermore, the few instances of further recession were equally distributed between grafted and control sites. When this is coupled with the fact that further recession has also been noted at sites with adequate gingival dimensions in the investigations by Wennström (1983), Schoo and Van der Velden (1985); Kisch *et al.* (1986), Eaton and Kieser (1986) and Wennström (1987), the rationale for increasing the width of gingiva at receded sites to prevent further progression must be questioned (Wennström, 1985).

Outcome of gingival grafting

Gingival grafting would seem to have a limited role in clinical practice although it certainly is an effective and predictable means of increasing the gingival dimensions in humans (Rateitschak *et al.*, 1979; Dorfman *et al.*, 1980; De Trey and Bernimoulin, 1980; Hangorsky and Bissada, 1980; Kennedy *et al.*, 1985) and in animal models (Wennström and Lindhe, 1983). Moreover, a slight coronal migration of the gingival margin, 'creeping attachment' (Goldman and Cohen, 1964), has been observed following free gingival grafting (Ward, 1976; Matter and Cimasoni, 1976; Dorfman *et al.*, 1982; Kennedy *et al.*, 1985). The resulting reduction in clinical crown height has been as much as 3.5 mm, whilst Pollack (1984) reported unusual changes of 7–9 mm in one individual over a 4-year period. This phenomenon of 'creeping' should, however, be differentiated from that of 'bridging' in which the root surface is intentionally covered with graft tissue at operation and following which some coronal creeping has also been reported (Bell *et al.*, 1978; Matter, 1980, 1982; Holbrook and Ochsenbein, 1983). The bridging effect appears to be enhanced by the use of a bilaminar graft comprised of a free gingival connective tissue graft with an overlying gingival pedicle flap (Langer and Langer, 1985; Miller, 1987; Nelson, 1987) and has the advantage of a closer colour blend of the healed graft with the adjacent tissues. On the other hand, a coronal regrowth of the gingival margin (of about 1 mm) has also been observed following periodontal flap surgery (Lindhe and Nyman, 1980), occlusal therapy (Solnit and Stambaugh, 1983) and following plaque control measures alone (Eaton and Kieser, 1986; Wennström, 1987), so questioning the influence of tissue grafting *per se*.

Regeneration of keratinized tissue

The tissue growth reported by Lindhe and Nyman (1980) following periodontal surgery occurred during a 10–11-year maintenance period at sites of gingival recession. Some of the sites developed keratinized tissue even though none had existed at the start of the study. This was attributed to the potential of connective tissue derived from periodontal ligament to induce keratinization on its surface epithelium during healing following surgical excision of the overlying mucosa (Karring *et al.*, 1975 a and b). Thus, regeneration of keratinized marginal tissues was encountered consistently, following the complete surgical excision of keratinized tissue in monkeys (Karring *et al.*, 1975 b), dogs (Wennström and Lindhe, 1983) and in humans (Wennström, 1983). It is of interest that the existence of keratinized tissue was not detected at first, because the initial thinness of the keratin layer of the newly formed mucosa (Wennström *et al.*, 1981; Wennström and Lindhe, 1983) made it difficult to distinguish clinically between alveolar mucosa and gingiva. Only with maturation of the regenerated gingival tissue and concomitant progressive thickening of the keratin layer did it become possible to do so. It is also significant that irrespective of the surgical technique used (internal or external bevel resection) that the length of the supracrestal connective tissue attachment was similar to that of non-operated control units (Wennström, 1983; Wennström and Lindhe, 1983). This corroborated earlier findings (Ramfjord *et al.*, 1966; Karring *et al.*, 1975 a) that a free gingival margin will reform and will be in most respects clinically and histologically similar to that of the normal healthy dentogingival unit.

Tissue inductive potential

The properties of the regenerating tissue, following mucogingival surgery, are dictated by the origins of the reparative granulation tissue (Karring *et al.*, 1975 a). This observation stems from earlier investigations by Smith (1970 a and b) and Karring *et al.* (1971, 1972), which confirmed that the characteristic features of epithelium are determined genetically rather than arising from functional adaptation. The mechanism of tissue specificity rests within the connective tissues (e.g. Billingham and Silvers, 1968), so that tissue derived from alveolar mucosa forms non-keratinized epithelium whereas that from gingival connective tissue and, as noted above, periodontal ligament produces keratinized gingival epithelium.

The extent to which periodontal ligament contributes to the healing will be dictated by the degree of post-surgical crestal bony resorption (Karring *et al.*, 1975 a), which is, in turn, influenced by the thickness of the bone (see Chapters 19 and 20 and also 31 – Osseous therapy). Thus, where thin alveolar bony plates exist, as at buccal aspects of the jaws, a considerable loss of crestal bone height is sustained and larger portions of periodontal ligament become engaged in forming granulation tissue. This then results in the development of a wider band of keratinized tissue (Wennström, 1983). Furthermore, it is at such sites especially when in association with initially shallow pockets that post-surgical loss of attachment is most likely to occur (Knowles *et al.*, 1979; Lindhe *et al.*, 1982). However, the fact that this loss was sustained almost exclusively in the first postoperative month (Wennström, 1983), suggests that surgical intervention rather than any associated lack of keratinized tissue has been responsible. In this context, health was maintained independently of the presence or absence of attached gingiva or the width of keratinized tissue. It can therefore be concluded that there is no minimal width of keratinized tissue necessary for the maintenance of marginal tissue health and that the level of plaque control practised by the patient remains the critical factor. It does also seem that, at sites displaying gingival recession, a very narrow zone of keratinized tissue at least will always remain (or reform if removed by toothbrushing or surgical resection), in the presence of an intact dentomucosal junction. The significance of such tissue junctions in the development of recurrent plaque-induced disease is considered next.

Gingival dimensions and plaque-induced disease

Relevance of gingival deficiencies

Lang and Loë (1972) suggested that sites with minimal amounts or a lack of attached gingiva would facilitate subgingival plaque formation because the movable gingival margins would favour the introduction of microorganisms into the gingival crevices. Miyasato *et al.* (1977), on the other hand, found no difference in the development of clinical gingival inflammation following the withdrawal of oral hygiene measures over a 25-day period, at sites with minimal (< 1 mm) or appreciable (> 2 mm) width of keratinized tissue. Similar findings were reported by Grevers (1977) from an experimental gingivitis study and by Dorfmann and Kennedy (1981) in a comparable investigation in which some of the sites with a lack of attached gingiva were rectified with free gingival grafts. These workers therefore concluded that deficiencies in keratinized gingiva did not predispose to inflammation. This has also been demonstrated histologically in dogs (Wennström *et al.*, 1982; Wennström and Lindhe, 1983) and in monkeys (Kure *et al.*, 1984); dentogingival units with both a narrow zone and a total lack of gingiva were no more susceptible to plaque-induced inflammation than units with a wide zone of attached gingiva. The finding that the clinical signs of gingivitis were more pronounced in the former sites appeared to be somewhat inconsistent. However, this was explained by a combination of the relative thinness of the keratin layer of the marginal oral epithelium and of the marginal tissues overall in a bucco-lingual plane, making the signs of connective tissue inflammation clinically more obvious. Consequently, caution must be exercised when using the clinical signs of persistent inflammation as indications for increasing the gingival dimensions surgically as proposed by for, example, De Trey and Bernimoulin (1980) and Hall (1981).

Historical perspective of corrective surgery

The surgical resection of pockets related to and extending beyond the mucogingival junction would result in margins of alveolar mucosa. These would then, according to Goldman (1953), predispose to further breakdown, because first and foremost the tissue was claimed to be fragile, non-keratinized and less endowed structurally to withstand physiological forces and oral hygiene procedures. Secondly, the close proximity of muscle attachments and frena, with or without a shallow vestibule, were thought to create tensional retraction of the mucosal margin, initiation of the inflammatory process with proliferation of junctional epithelium and pocket formation.

The foregoing impressions heralded an era of reconstructive mucogingival surgical procedures. (For Review see Nery and Davies, 1976; Schmid, 1976). Initially, these techniques involved the resection of the suprabony pocket wall tissue and denudation of the bone which led to irreversible bony resorption and attachment loss (e.g. Wilderman *et al.*, 1960). It was found, however, that this damage could be reduced by retaining periosteum on the bone (e.g. Staffileno *et al.*, 1966), whilst preservation of postoperative mucosal coverage of the vulnerable marginal and radicular bone overlying the roots of the teeth ensured optimal healing (e.g. Friedman and Levine, 1964). (See also Chapter 31, Osseous therapy.)

The claimed need to retain the keratinized tissue component of the pocket was first suggested by Nabers (1954) and applied in the technique of repositioning the attached gingiva. Friedman (1962) subsequently proposed the term apically repositioned flap. Thus, suprabony pocket elimination could be achieved whilst at the same time conserving the entire mucogingival tissue complex and displacing the base of the vestibule apically. Where, however, little or no keratinized tissue existed this was corrected by separate surgical exercises using pedicle or free gingival grafts (for review see Guinard and Caffesse, 1977). The principles of the latter technique are well described by Sullivan and Atkins (1968 a). The relative insignificance of both periosteal retention or bony denudation and of the exposure of bony fenestrations and dehiscences at recipient sites in the healing of free gingival grafts has been demonstrated in a clinical evaluation by Dordick *et al.* (1976 a and b). This is supported by the finding that revascularization of gingival wounds is mainly via new capillaries from the surrounding epithelium whilst that derived from periosteum and the Volkman canals progressed very slowly (Nobuto *et al.*, 1987). Root coverage by free gingival grafts was introduced by Nabers (1966) and subsequently described as 'bridging' by Sullivan and Atkins (1968 b). (See also Sullivan and Atkins, 1969; Miller, 1987.) It is self evident that the grafted donor tissue incorporates a connective tissue base. As the epithelial tissue specificity depends on this, gingival connective tissue devoid of surface epithelium has also been used by several investigators (e.g. Edel, 1974; Donn, 1978) with comparable success. Similarly 'bridging' has been demonstrated with free gingival connective tissue grafts in conjunction with a recipient bed mucosal envelope (Raetzke, 1985) and with pedicle grafting (Langer and Langer, 1985; Nelson, 1987).

Numerous pedicle type graft techniques and variations thereof have been described to cover root surfaces resulting from gingival recession. The basic techniques are the lateral sliding flap (Grupe and Warren, 1956), the split-thickness pedicle flap (Staffileno, 1964), the oblique rotated flap (Pennel *et al.*, 1965), the double papillary flap (Cohen and Ross, 1968) and the coronally repositioned flap (Harvey, 1965). The latter can also be carried out in conjunction with free gingival grafting (Harvey, 1970; Bernimoulin *et al.*, 1975). A simplified modification of the coronally repositioned flap has been described by Tarnow (1986).

The results of the above surgical methods have been reviewed by Guinard and Caffesse (1977). More recently reported 3-year follow-up findings on laterally and coronally repositioned flaps (Caffesse and Guinard, 1980) have confirmed that about 2–3 mm (65–70%) of root surface coverage might be achieved and be maintained. Thus, where coverage of root surfaces is desired, gingival pedicle flap surgery is well justified. Healing is by a combination of new connective tissue attachment (which develops from the periodontal ligament located apically and laterally to the receded site) and a long junctional epithelium (Caffesse *et al.*, 1984). The donor sites following lateral sliding flaps sustained about 1 mm irreversible loss of marginal tissue (recession).

Functional adequacy of gingiva

This concept revolved about that amount of attached gingiva deemed sufficient to prevent the free gingiva from being retracted from the tooth by the frenum or the alveolar mucosa (Friedman, 1962). Thus, the intervening firmly bound down gingival tissue dissipated the pull from the contiguous vestibular tissues and the gingival dimensions in turn, then expressed in terms of functional adequacy rather than in millimetres. The functional adequacy of gingiva was judged subsequently (Glickman, 1972) by assessing the effects of artificial tension on the attached gingiva by retracting the lips and cheeks laterally. If the marginal gingiva is pulled away from the teeth in this tension test, the attached gingiva is considered to be inadequate. Blanching of the marginal tissues may also be noted at such sites. However, as blanching may occur even in the absence of visible marginal retraction, it was regarded as the earliest sign of a developing mucogingival problem (Carman and Kopczyk, 1973).

The tension test was shown in an investigation in children (Kopczyk and Saxe, 1974) to be somewhat subjective and affected by the amount of tension applied. The blanching test was also deemed unreliable as an indicator of gingival adequacy, because it might be influenced by variations of gingival collagen tissue density occurring with the development of inflammation. This is supported by the strong correlation between both tension and blanching tests and minimal gingival dimensions, in the presence of plaque-induced inflammation but not at uninflamed sites as demonstrated by Chapple (1980). Vincent *et al.* (1976) in turn observed no relationship between the results of the tension test and the clinical measurements of the attached gingiva, whilst Ramfjord and Ash (1979) deemed these clinical tests meaningless and possibly even misleading for blanching may occur even in the presence of gingival health.

Grevers (1977) devised a marginal gingiva mobility index to evaluate the functional quality of the gingiva. No relationship was observed between this index and the development or resolution of experimental plaque-induced gingivitis in humans. The retraction effect on the marginal tissue via frenal insertions has been termed the 'pull syndrome' by Placek *et al.* (1974). The localized gingival ischaemia, manifested clinically as blanching, produced by such frenal insertions was assessed by Gaberthüel and Mormann (1978) using fluorescein angiography. They concluded that, as ischaemia was unrelated to attached gingival widths, blanching could not be used to determine functional gingival adequacy.

Conclusions

The conclusions drawn by Wennström (1982) from the series of experiments carried out in dogs and in humans are also applicable to the findings of other investigations and so are presented here:

(1) Following periodontal surgery, using gingivectomy, flap or grafting procedures, a free gingiva will reform which is in most respects clinically as well as histologically similar to that of a 'normal' dentogingival unit.
(2) Subsequent to the experimental surgical excision of the entire zone of gingiva a keratinized free gingiva regenerates consistently, whereas reformation of attached gingiva is unpredictable.
(3) Soft tissue grafting is an effective and predictable means of increasing the width of attached gingiva, and so too of the keratinized gingiva, but it does not enhance the quality of the dentogingival junction with respect to periodontal tissue health.
(4) With effective mechanical plaque control, gingival health can be maintained without the development of recession or attachment loss at sites lacking in attached or keratinized gingivae.
(5) A dentogingival unit with a narrow and poorly keratinized gingiva has an equal capacity for inflammatory response against bacterial plaque as a unit with a wide zone of properly keratinized gingiva.
(6) A free gingiva supported by loosely attached alveolar mucosa is no more susceptible to bacterial plaque infection than a free gingiva supported by a wide zone of attached gingiva.

The above conclusions mean that mucogingival surgical procedures have little role in contemporary clinical practice. However, it must be stressed as advocated by Wennström (1985) that the techniques may still be indicated in situations where gingival recession creates aesthetic problems or where gingival coverage of exposed root surfaces is desirable. Finally, it can be confirmed on the basis of these research findings that there is no longer any clinical reason to differentiate between free and attached gingiva, so that the use of the term gingiva, recommended by the WHO Scientific Group (1978), is appropriate for the description of the soft tissue located between the gingival margin and the mucogingival junction.

Vestibular morphology

Vestibular dimensions

The close proximity of the vestibular tissue muscle attachments to the dentogingival junctions has been indicted in the development of plaque-induced disease (Goldman, 1953) but has yet to be substantiated. Similarly the claimed need to deepen the shallow vestibule to facilitate plaque control and minimize mechanical and microbial irritation of the marginal periodontium (e.g. Wade, 1969; Schmid *et al.,* 1979; Lange, 1980) is supported by clinical impressions alone. In contrast, others have concluded that there is no justification for performing vestibular extension surgery simply to correct a vestibule considered too shallow for efficient oral hygiene (Bergenholtz and Hugoson, 1967). Indeed, Ward (1976 b) showed that gingival health may be maintained even where the vestibule is shallow, so that surgical deepening of the vestibule is not justified on the basis of vestibular and gingival dimensions alone (Grevers, 1977). Finally, as it has never been shown that a certain vestibular depth is needed for effective toothbrushing, there is no valid reason for vestibular extension on these grounds alone (Ramfjord and Ash, 1979). This has been endorsed by the findings of Addy *et al.* (1987).

Finally, as gingival tissue *per se* appears not to be necessary for either the maintenance of marginal tissue health or to disperse any functional pulling movements of vestibular tissues, the reasons for conserving this tissue, during pocket elimination surgery by apically repositioning the gingival flap (as advocated in Part II), rather than simply resecting it might reasonably be questioned. It must be conceded that the gingiva is conserved primarily because it is intrinsic to the periodontium and so presumably serves some specific, if not clearly determined, purpose.

Thus the inherent toughness of gingiva would seem to be advantageous by withstanding more effectively any possible trauma sustained during mastication of hard, fibrous foods or during mechanical tooth cleaning. Furthermore, gingiva appears to function as a fixed barrier between the dentogingival junction and the mobile vestibular mucosal tissue, thereby displacing any possible interference from the latter during routine cleaning.

Put another way, the presence of a broad zone of gingiva effectively deepens the vestibular sulcus and may facilitate plaque control.

Evaluation of vestibular interference

Any clinical assessment of the role of the vestibular tissues in disease is inevitably complicated by several difficulties. Firstly, that of distinguishing between the potential influences of gingival dimensions on the one hand, and of vestibular depth and form on the other. Secondly, the frequent lack of any definite dividing line between surgical procedures designed for vestibular fornix extension and those for increasing the zone of attached gingiva. Thus, apart from the investigations on surgical vestibular deepening procedure (Wade, 1969; Bergenholtz and Hugoson, 1973; Schmid *et al.*, 1979; Marggraf, 1985) based upon the technique of Edlan and Mejchar (1963) in which no increased gingival dimension is intended, the majority of corrective techniques have also involved the gingiva. Consequently any post-surgical benefits observed could be due to any one or a combination of altered gingival dimensions, improved vestibular form or greater vestibular depth. This in turn reflects the final difficulty of assessment, which concerns the lack of documented data about the proportions of the overall vestibular mucosal morphology occupied by each component before and after corrective surgery. In this context it must be appreciated that, unlike that of gingival dimensions described earlier, a reproducible method of measuring vestibular dimensions has yet to be developed. Ward (1976 a) has reviewed the various methods of vestibular depth measurement used by others and presented a radiographic contrast medium technique that is applicable to the mandibular anterior region. The gingival component of the vestibule was thus shown to vary from a mean of 34% in the canine region to approximately 55 and 60% at the central and lateral incisors respectively (Ward, 1976 b).

Surgical technique

The vestibular extension technique (Corn, 1962) and its numerous modifications (for review see Schmid, 1976) are now mainly of historical interest, for it has been replaced by free gingival grafting (Nabers, 1966). The technique essentially denudes labial bone by displacing the overlying mucosa apically (from an alveolar crestal incision or from one related to the mucogingival junction) and then leaving this bone to granulate over. The pattern of healing depended upon the origins of the granulation tissue (Karring *et al.*, 1975 a and b). Because of the extensive bony resorption (see Chapter 31, Osseous therapy) plus the possible presence of bony

fenestrations and dehiscences at thin labial plates, a considerable proportion of the reparative tissue is derived from the exposed periodontal ligament (see Figure 22.1). This results in increased amounts of keratinized tissue. Whereas, with retention of periosteum to minimize bony resorption and its accompanying marked postoperative pain, and in situations with thick bone and over inter-radicular bone the necrosis is largely contained within bone. Little or no granulation tissue then originates from periodontal ligament, so that the healed mucosa is comprised mainly of alveolar mucosa. The variations in healing reported in different studies are thus readily explained.

The major disadvantage of the vestibular extension technique is the strong tendency for relapse during healing with a return of the displaced tissue towards its presurgical position (Schmid, 1976). For example, Jenkins and Stephen (1979) reported a 50% relapse of vestibular depth gained at operation within 6 months compared with that of only 17% following free grafting. The greater predictability of the surgical outcome when combined with free grafting (as described in Part II), coupled with reduced postoperative symptoms has been largely responsible for the clinical abandonment of vestibular extension surgery as a surgical entity. It should, however, be pointed out that greater degrees of shrinkage following free grafting have been reported by others, as cited by Jenkins and Stephen (1979). This loss has extended up to almost half the initial graft dimensions and can be attributed in part to the thicker tissues used (Sullivan and Atkins, 1968 a).

In conclusion, there can, in common with gingival dimensions, be no linear measurement that will form a positive indication for vestibular surgery. Rather, if the patient is unable to keep a gingival area free of inflammation and feels that access for oral hygiene is being impeded by a shallow vestibule (including any frenum) then vestibular extension by gingival grafting should be considered.

References

Addy, M., Dummer, P. M. H., Hunter, M. L., Kingdon, A. and Shaw, W.C. (1987) A study of the association of fraenal attachment, lip coverage, and vestibular depth with plaque and gingivitis. *J. Periodontol.* **58**, 752–757

Ainamo, A. (1978) Influence of age on the location of the maxillary mucogingival junction. *J. Periodont. Res.* **13**, 189–193

Ainamo, A. and Ainamo, J. (1978) The width of attached gingiva on supraerupted teeth. *J. Periodont. Res.* **13**, 194–198

Ainamo, J. and Löe, H. (1966) Anatomical characteristics of gingiva. A clinical and microscopic study of the free and attached gingiva. *J. Periodontol.* **37**, 5–12

Ainamo, J. and Talari, A. (1976) The increase with age of

the width of attached gingiva. *J. Periodont. Res.* **11**, 182–188

Baker, D. L. and Seymour, G. J. (1976) The possible pathogenesis of gingival recession. *J. Clin. Periodontol.* **3**, 208–219

Bell, L. A., Valluzzo, T. A., Garnick, J. J. and Pennel, B. M. (1978) The presence of 'creeping attachment' in human gingiva. *J. Periodontol.* **49**, 513–517

Bergenholtz, A. and Hugoson, A. (1967) Vestibular sulcus extension surgery in cases with periodontal disease. *J. Periodont. Res.* **2**, 221–226

Bergenholtz, A. and Hugoson, A. (1973) Vestibular sulcus extension surgery in the mandibular front region. The Edlan–Mejchar Method – a five-year follow-up study. *J. Periodontol.* **44**, 309–311

Bernimoulin, J.-P. and Curilovic, Z. (1977) Gingival recession and tooth mobility. *J. Clin. Periodontol.* **4**, 107–114

Bernimoulin, J. P., Son, S. and Regolati, B. (1971) Biometric comparison of three methods for determining the mucogingival junction. *Helv. Odont. Acta* **15**, 118–120

Bernimoulin, J.-P., Lüscher, B. and Mühlemann, H. R. (1975) Coronally repositioned periodontal flap. Clinical evaluation after one year. *J. Clin. Periodontol.* **2**, 1–13

Billingham, R. E. and Silvers, W. K. (1968) Dermo-epidermal interactions and epithelial specificity. In *Epithelial-Mesenchymal Interactions,* pp. 252–266. (Editors Fleischmajer, R. and Billingham, R. E.) Williams & Wilkins Co., Baltimore

Bowers, G. M. (1963) A study of the width of attached gingiva. *J. Periodontol.* **34**, 201–209

Breitenmoser, J., Mörmann, W. and Mühlemann, H. R. (1979) Damaging effects of toothbrush bristle end form on gingiva. *J. Periodontol.* **50**, 212–216

Caffesse, R. G. and Guinard, E. A. (1980) Treatment of localized gingival recessions. Part IV. Results after three years. *J. Periodontol.* **51**, 167–170

Caffesse, R. G., Kon, S., Castelli, W. A. and Nasjleti, C. E. (1984) Revascularization following the lateral sliding flap procedure. *J. Periodontol.* **55**, 352–358

Carman, D. K. and Kopczyk, R. A. (1973) Periodontal treatment in the child. *Dent. Clin. North Am.* **17**, 67–76

Chapple, C. C. (1980) Clinical tests for gingival functional adequacy. MSc. Thesis, University of London

Coatoam, G. W., Behrents, R. G. and Bissada, N. F. (1981) The width of keratinized gingiva during orthodontic treatment: its significance and impact on periodontol status. *J. Periodontol.* **52**, 307–313

Cohen, D. W. and Ross, S. E. (1968) The double papillae repositioned flap in periodontal therapy. *J. Periodontol.* **39**, 65–70

Coppes, L. (1972) Routine-sulcusdieptemetingen in de parodontologie. *Academisch Proefschrift.* 117–135

Corn, H. (1962) Periosteal separation – its clinical significance. *J. Periodontol.* **33**, 140–153

De Trey, E. and Bernimoulin, J.-P. (1980) Influence of free gingival grafts on the health of the marginal gingiva. *J. Clin. Periodontol.* **7**, 381–393

Dello Russo, N. M. (1982) Gingival autografts as an adjunct to removable partial dentures. *J. Am. Dent. Assoc.* **104**, 179–181

Donaldson, D. (1974) The etiology of gingival recession associated with temporary crowns. *J. Periodontol.* **45**, 468–471

Donn, B. J. (1978) The free connective tissue autograft: A clinical and histologic wound healing study in humans. *J. Periodontol.* **49**, 253–260

Dordick, B., Coslet, J. G. and Seibert, J. S. (1976a) Clinical evaluation of free autogenous gingival grafts placed on alveolar bone. Part 1. Clinical predicatability. *J. Periodontol.* **47**, 559–567

Dordick, B., Coslet, J. G. and Seibert, J. S. (1976b) Clinical evaluation of free autogenous gingival grafts placed on alveolar bone. Part II. Coverage of nonpathologic dehiscences and fenestrations. *J. Periodontol.* **47**, 568–573

Dorfman, H. and Kennedy, J. (1981) Gingival parameters associated with varying widths of attached gingiva. *J. Dent. Res.* **60**, (Special Issue A) 386 (IADR Abstract no. 301)

Dorfman, H. S., Kennedy, J. E. and Bird, W. C. (1980) Longitudinal evaluation of free autogenous gingival grafts. *J. Clin. Periodontol.* **7**, 316–324

Dorfman, H. S., Kennedy, J. E. and Bird, W. C. (1982) Longitudinal evaluation of free autogenous gingival grafts. A four year report. *J. Periodontol.* **53**, 349–352

Eaton, K. A. and Kieser, J. B. (1986) A conservative approach to the management of gingival recession and other gingival 'inadequacy'. *Restorative Dentistry.* March, 29–35

Edel, A. (1974) Clinical evaluation of free connective tissue grafts used to increase the width of keratinised gingiva. *J. Clin. Periodontol.* **1**, 185–196

Edlan, A. and Mejchar, B. (1963) Plastic surgery of the vestibulum in periodontal therapy. *Int. Dent. J.* **13**, 593–596

Emslie, R. D. (1958) Localized gingival recession. *Int. Dent. J.* **8**, 18 (abstract)

Ericcson, I. and Lindhe, J. (1984) Recession in sites with inadequate width of the keratinized gingiva. An experimental study in the dog. *J. Clin. Periodontol.* **11**, 95–103

Farnoush, A. and Schonfeld, S. E. (1983) Rationale for mucogingival surgery: A critique and update. *J. West Soc. Periodont. Periodont Abstr.* **31**, 125–130

Fasske, T. and Morgenroth, K. (1958) Comparative stomatoscopic and histochemical studies of the marginal gingiva in man. *Parodontologie* **12**, 151–160

Friedman, N. (1957) Mucogingival surgery. *Tex. Dent. J.* **75**, 358–362

Friedman, N. (1962) Mucogingival surgery: The apically repositioned flap. *J. Periodontol.* **33**, 328–240

Friedman, N. and Levine, H. L. (1964) Mucogingival surgery: Current status. *J. Periodontol.* **35**, 5–21

Gaberthüel, T. W. and Mörmann, W. (1978) The angiographic tension test in mucogingival surgery. *J. Periodontol.* **49**, 395–399

Gartrell, J. R. and Mathews, D. P. (1976) Gingival recession. The condition, process and treatment. *Dent. Clin. North Am.* **20**, 199–213

Glickman, I. (1972) *Clinical Periodontology*, 4th Edition, pp. 712–714. W. B. Saunders Co., Philadelphia

Goldman, H. M. (1953) *Periodontia*, 3rd Edition, pp. 552–561. C. V. Mosby Co., St Louis, MO

Goldman, H. M. and Cohen, D. W. (1964) *Periodontal Therapy*, 3rd Edition, pp. 546–562. C. V. Mosby Co., St Louis, MO

Goldman, H. M. and Cohen, D. W. (1973) *Periodontal Therapy*, 5th Edition, pp. 66–71. C. V. Mosby Co., St Louis, MO

Gorman, W. J. (1967) Prevalence and etiology of gingival recession. *J. Periodontol.* **38**, 316–322

Gottsegen, R. (1954) Frenum position and vestibule depth in relation to gingival health. *Periodontia* 1069–1078

Grevers, A. (1977) Width of attached gingiva and vestibular depth in relation to gingival health. Thesis, University of Amsterdam

Grupe, H. E. and Warren, R. F. (1956) Repair of gingival defects by a sliding flap operation. *J. Periodontol.* **27**, 92–95

Guinard, E. A. and Caffesse, R. G. (1977a) Localized gingival recessions: I. Etiology and prevalence. *J. West Soc. Periodont. Periodont. Abstr.* **25**, 3–9

Guinard, E. A. and Caffesse, R. G. (1977b) Localized gingival recessions: II. Treatment. *J. West Soc. Periodont. Periodont. Abstr.* **25**, 10–21

Hall, W. B. (1977) Present status of soft tissue grafting. *J. Periodontol.* **48**, 587–597

Hall, W. B. (1981) The current status of mucogingival problems and their therapy. *J. Periodontol.* **52**, 569–575

Hangorsky, U. and Bissada, N. F. (1980) Clinical assessment of free gingival graft effectiveness on the maintenance of periodontal health. *J. Periodontol.* **51**, 274–278

Harvey, P. M. (1965) Management of advanced periodontitis. Part I. Preliminary report of a method of surgical reconstruction. *N.Z. Dent. J.* **61**, 180–187

Harvey, P. M. (1970) Surgical reconstruction of the gingiva. Part II. Procedures. *N.Z. Dent. J.* **66**, 42–52

Holbrook, T. and Ochsenbein, C. (1983) Complete coverage of the denuded root surface with a one-stage gingival graft. *Int. J. Periodont. Rest. Dent.* **3**, 9–27

Jenkins, W. M. M. and Stephen, K. W. (1979) A clinical comparison of two gingival extension procedures. *J. Dent.* **7**, 91–97

Karring, T., Östergaard, E. and Löe, H. (1971) Conservation of tissue specificity after heterotopic transplantation of gingiva and alveolar mucosa. *J. Periodont. Res.* **6**, 282–293

Karring, T., Lang, N. P. and Löe, H. (1972) Role of connective tissue in determining epithelial specificity. *J. Dent. Res.* **51**, 1303 (IADR Abstract 1)

Karring, T., Cumming, B. R., Oliver, R. C. and Löe, H. (1975a) The origin of granulation tissue and its impact on postoperative results of mucogingival surgery. *J. Periodontol.* **46**, 577–585

Karring, T., Lang, N. P. and Löe, H. (1975b) The role of gingival connective tissue in determining epithelial differentiation. *J. Periodont. Res.* **10**, 1–11

Kennedy, J. E., Bird, W. C., Palcanis, K. G. and Dorfman, H. S. (1985) A longitudinal evaluation of varying widths of attached gingiva. *J. Clin. Periodontol.* **12**, 667–675

Kisch, J., Badersten, A. and Egelberg, J. (1986) Longitudinal observation of 'unattached' mobile gingival areas. *J. Clin. Periodontol.* **13**, 131–134

Knowles, J., Burgett, F., Nissle, R., Shick, R., Morrison, E. and Ramfjord, S. (1979) Results of periodontal treatment related to pocket depth and attachment level. Eight years. *J. Periodontol.* **50**, 225–233

Kopczyk, R. A. and Saxe, S. R. (1974) Clinical signs of gingival inadequacy: The tension test. *J. Dent. Child.* 352–355

Kure, K., Mera, T., Nishihara, T., Lin, C., Kimura, Y., Noguchi, T. and Kinoshita, S. (1984) Influences of attached gingiva on plaque accumulation and gingival inflammation in monkeys. *J. Dent. Res.* **63**, 555. (Abstract no. 17)

Lane, J. J. (1977) Gingival fenestration. *J. Periodontol.* **48**, 225–227

Lang, N. P. and Löe, H. (1972) The relationship between the width of keratinized gingiva and gingival health. *J. Periodontol.* **43**, 623–627

Lange, D. E. (1980) Efficacy of mucogingival surgery. In *Efficacy of Treatment Procedures in Periodontics*, pp. 99–110. (Editor Shanley, D. B.). Quintessence Publishing Co. Chicago

Langer, B. and Calagna, L. (1978) The alteration of lingual mucosa with free gingival grafts. *J. Periodontol.* **42**, 646–648

Langer, B. and Langer, L. (1985) Subepithelial connective tissue graft technique for root coverage. *J. Periodontol.* **56**, 715–720

Lindhe, J. and Nyman, S. (1980) Alterations of the position of the marginal soft tissue following periodontal surgery. *J. Clin. Periodontol.* **7**, 525–530

Lindhe, J., Parodi, R., Liljenberg, B. and Fornell, J. (1978) Clinical and structural alterations characterizing healing gingiva. *J. Periodont. Res.* **13**, 410–424

Lindhe, J., Westfelt, E., Nyman, S., Socransky, S., Heijl, L. and Bratthall, G. (1982) Healing following surgical/non-surgical treatment of periodontal disease. A clinical study. *J. Clin. Periodontol.* **9**, 115–128

Löst, C. (1984) Depth of alveolar bone dehiscences in relation to gingival recessions. *J. Clin. Periodontol.* **11**, 583–589

Lozdan, J. and Squier, C. A. (1969) The histology of the muco-gingival junction. *J. Periodont. Res.* **4**, 83–93

Manson, J. D. (1963) Passive eruption. *Dent. Pract.* **14**, 2–9

Marggraf, E. (1985) A direct technique with a double lateral bridging flap for coverage of denuded root surface and gingiva extension. Clinical evaluation after 2 years. *J. Clin. Periodontol.* **12**, 69–76

Matter, J. (1980) Creeping attachment of free gingival

grafts. A five-year follow-up study. *J. Periodontol.* **51**, 681–685

Matter, J. (1982) Free gingival grafts for the treatment of gingival recession. A review of some techniques. *J. Clin. Periodontol.* **9**, 103–114

Matter, J. and Cimasoni, G. (1976) Creeping attachment after free gingival grafts. *J. Periodontol.* **47**, 574–579

Maynard, J. G. and Wilson, R. D. K. (1979) Physiologic dimensions of the periodontium significant to the restorative dentist. *J. Periodontol.* **50**, 170–174

Mazeland, G. R. J. (1978) Jaws and gums. The mucogingival complex in relation to alveolar process height and lower anterior face height in man. *Academisch proefschrift*, Universiteit van Amsterdam

Mazeland, G. R. J. (1980a) The mucogingival complex in relation to alveolar process height and lower anterior face height. *J. Periodont. Res.* **15**, 345–352

Mazeland, G. R. J. (1980b) Longitudinal aspects of gingival width. *J. Periodont. Res.* **15**, 429–433

Miller, P. D. (1987) Root coverage with the free gingival graft. Factors associated with incomplete coverage. *J. Periodontol.* **58**, 674–681

Miyasato, M., Crigger, M. and Egelberg, J. (1977) Gingival condition in areas of minimal and appreciable width of keratinized gingiva. *J. Clin. Periodontol.* **4**, 200–209

Nabers, C. L. (1954) Repositioning the attached gingiva. *J. Periodontol.* **25**, 38–39

Nabers, J. M. (1966) Free gingival grafts. *Periodontics* **4**, 243–245

Nelson, S. W. (1987) The subpedical connective tissue graft. A bilaminar reconstructive procedure for the coverage of denuded root surfaces. *J. Periodontol.* **58**, 95–102

Nery, E. B. and Davies, E. E. (1976) The historical development of mucogingival surgery. *J. West Soc. Periodont. Periodont. Abstr.* **24**, 149–161

Niemi, M.-L., Ainamo, J. and Etemadzadeh, H. (1987) The effect of toothbrush grip on gingival abrasion and plaque removal during toothbrushing. *J. Clin. Periodontol.* **14**, 19–21

Niemi, M.-L., Sandholm, L. and Ainamo, J. (1984) Frequency of gingival lesions after standardized brushing as related to stiffness of toothbrush and abrasiveness of dentifrice. *J. Clin. Periodontol.* **11**, 254–261

Nobuto, T., Tokioka, T., Imai, H., Suwa, F., Ohta, Y. and Yamaoka, A. (1987) Microvascularization of gingival wound healing using corrosion casts. *J. Periodontol.* **58**, 240–246

Novaes, A. B., Ruben, M. P., Kon, S., Goldman, H. M. and Novaes, A. B. Jr. (1975) The development of the periodontal cleft. A clinical and histopathologic study. *J. Periodontol.* **46**, 701–709

O'Leary, T. J., Drake, R. B., Crump, P. P. and Allen, M. F. (1971) The incidence of recession in young males: A further study. *J. Periodontol.* **42**, 264–267

Orban, B. (1948) Clinical and histologic study of the surface characteristics of the gingiva. *Oral Surg.* **1**, 827–841

Parfitt, G. J. and Mjör, I. A. (1964) A clinical evaluation of local gingival recession in children. *J. Dent. Child.* **31**, 257–262

Pattison, G. L. (1983) Self-inflicted gingival injuries: Literature review and case report. *J.Periodontol.* **54**, 299–304

Pennel, B. M., Higgason, J. D., Towner, J. D., King, K. O., Fritz, B. D. and Salder, J. F. (1965) Oblique rotated flap. *J. Periodontol.* **36**, 305–309

Placek, M., Skach, M. and Mrklas, L. (1974) Significance of the labial frenum attachment in periodontal disease in man. Part I. Classification and epidemiology of the labial frenum attachment. *J. Periodontol.* **45**, 891–894

Placek, M., Skach, M. and Mrklas, L. (1974) Significance of the labial frenum attachment in periodontal disease in man. Part II. An attempt to determine the resistance of periodontium. *J. Periodontol.* **45**, 895–897

Pollack, R. P. (1984) Bilateral creeping attachment using free mucosal grafts. A case report with 4-year follow-up. *J. Periodontol.* **55**, 670–672

Powell, R. N. and McEniery, T. M. (1982) A longitudinal study of isolated gingival recession in the mandibular central incisor region of children aged 6-8 years. *J. Clin. Periodontol.* **9**, 357–364

Raetzke, P. B. (1985) Covering localized areas of root exposure employing the 'envelope' technique. *J. Periodontol.* **56**, 397–402

Ramfjord, S. P., Engler, W. O. and Hiniker, J. J. (1966) A radio-autographic study of healing following simple gingivectomy. II. The connective tissue. *J. Periodontol.* **37**, 179–189

Ramfjord, S. P. and Ash, M. M. (1979) *Periodontology and Periodontics*, pp. 613–614. W. B. Saunders Co. Philadelphia

Rateitschak, K. H., Egli, U. and Fringeli, G. (1979) Recession: A 4-year longitudinal study after free gingival grafts. *J. Clin. Periodontol.* **6**, 158–164

Rose, G. J. (1967) Receding mandibular labial gingiva on children. *Angle Orthod.* **37**, 147–150

Rose, S. T. and App, G. R. (1973) A clinical study of the development of the attached gingiva along the facial aspect of the maxillary and mandibular anterior teeth in the deciduous, transitional and permanent dentitions. *J. Periodontol.* **44**, 131–139

Salkin, L. M., Freedman, A. L., Stein, M. D. and Bassiouny, M. A. (1987) A longitudinal study of untreated mucogingival defects. *J. Periodontol.* **58**, 164–166

Sangnes, G. and Gjermo, P. (1976) Prevalence of oral soft and hard tissue lesions related to mechanical toothcleaning procedures. *Commun. Dent. Oral Epidemiol.* **4**, 77–83

Schmid, M. O. (1976) The subperiosteal vestibule extension literature review, rationale and technique. *J. West Soc. Periodont. Periodont. Abstr.* **24**, 89–99

Schmid, M. O., Mörmann, W. and Bachmann, A. (1979) Mucogingival surgery. The subperiostal vestibule extension. Clinical results 2 years after surgery. *J. Clin. Periodontol.* **6**, 22–32

Schokking, C. C. (1976) Free grafts of palatal mucosa on the lingual aspect of the mandible. *J. Clin. Periodontol.* **3**, 251–255

Schoo, W. H. and Van der Velden, U. (1985) Marginal soft tissue recessions with and without attached gingiva. A five year longitudinal study. *J. Periodont. Res.* **20**, 209–211

Silness, J. and Røynstrand, T. (1985) Effects of the degree of overbite and overjet on dental health. *J. Clin. Periodontol.* **12**, 389–398

Smith, R. M. (1970a) A study of the intertransplantation of gingiva. *Oral Surg.* **29**, 169–177

Smith, R. M. (1970b) A study of the intertransplantation of alveolar mucosa. *Oral Surg.* **29**, 328–340

Smukler, H. and Landsberg, J. (1984) The toothbrush and gingival traumatic injury. *J. Periodontol.* **55**, 713–719

Solnit, A. and Stambaugh, R. V. (1983) Treatment of gingival clefts by occlusal therapy. *Int. J. Periodont. Restorat. Dent.* **3**, 39–55

Staffileno, H. Jr. (1964) Management of gingival recession and root exposure problems associated with periodontal disease. *Dent. Clin. North Am.* 111–120

Staffileno, H., Levy, S. and Gargiulo, A. (1966) Histologic study of cellular mobilization and repair following a periosteal retention operation via split thickness mucogingival flap surgery. *J. Periodontol.* **37**, 117–131

Stetler, K. J. and Bissada, N. B. (1987) Significance of the width of keratinized gingiva on the periodontal status of teeth with submarginal restorations. *J. Periodontol.* **58**, 696–700

Stillman, P. R. (1921) Early clinical evidences of disease in the gingiva and pericementum. *J. Dent. Res.* **3**, xxv–xxxi

Stoner, J. E. and Mazdyasna, S. (1980) Gingival recession in the lower incisor region of 15-year old subjects. *J. Periodontol.* **51**, 74–76

Sullivan, H. C. and Atkins, J. H. (1968a) Free autogenous gingival grafts. I. Principles of successful grafting. *Periodontics* **6**, 121–129

Sullivan, H. C. and Atkins, J. H. (1968b) Free autogenous gingival grafts. III. Utilization of grafts in the treatment of gingival recession. *Periodontics* **6**, 152–160

Sullivan, H. C. and Atkins, J. H. (1969) The role of free gingival grafts in periodontal therapy. *Dent. Clin. North Am.* 133–148

Talari, A. and Ainamo, J. (1976) Orthopantomographic assessment of the width of attached gingiva. *J. Periodont. Res.* **11**, 177–181

Tarnow, D. P. (1986) Semilunar coronally repositioned flap. *J. Clin. Periodontol.* **13**, 182–185

Ten Cate, A. R. (1963) The distribution of acid phosphatase, non-specific esterase and lipid in oral epithelium in man and the macaque monkey. *Arch. Oral Biol.* **8**, 747–753

Tenenbaum, H. (1982) A clinical study comparing the width of attached gingiva and the prevalence of gingival recessions. *J. Clin. Periodontol.* **9**, 86–92

Tenenbaum, H. and Tenenbaum, M. (1986) A clinical

study of the width of the attached gingiva in the deciduous, transitional and permanent dentitions. *J. Clin. Periodontol.* **13**, 270–275

Tenenbaum, H., Herr, P., Bercy, P. and Klewansky, P. (1984) A photometric test method for the control of gingival recessions. *J. Periodont. Res.* **19**, 199–201

Trott, J. R. and Love, B. (1966) An analysis of localized gingival recession in 766 Winnipeg High School students. *Dent. Practit.* **16**, 209–213

Vincent, J. W., Machen, J. B. and Levin, M. P. (1976) Assessment of attached gingiva using the tension test and clinical measurements. *J. Periodontol.* **47**, 412–414

Voigt, J. P., Goran, M. L. and Fleisher, R. M. (1978) The width of lingual mandibular attached gingiva. *J. Periodontol.* **49**, 77–80

Volchansky, A., Cleaton-Jones, P. and Fatti, L. P. (1979) A 3-year longitudinal study of the position of the gingival margin in man. *J. Clin. Periodontol.* **6**, 231–237

Wade, A. B. (1969) Vestibular deepening by the technique of Edlan and Mejchar. *J. Periodont. Res.* **4**, 300–313

Ward, V. J. (1974) A clinical assessment of the use of the free gingival graft for correcting localized recession associated with frenal pull. *J. Periodontol.* **45**, 78–83

Ward, V. J. (1976a) A technique of measurement of the depth of the vestibular fornix in the mandibular anterior region. *J. Periodontol.* **47**, 525–530

Ward, V. J. (1976b) The depth of the vestibular fornix in the mandibular anterior region in health. *J. Periodontol.* **47**, 651–655

Wennström, J. L. (1982) Keratinized and attached gingiva. Regenerative potential and significance for periodontal health. Thesis, University of Gothenburg

Wennström, J. L. (1983) Regeneration of gingiva following surgical excision. A clinical study. *J. Clin. Periodontol.* **10**, 287–297

Wennström, J. L. (1985) Status of the art in mucogingival surgery. *Acta Parodontologica* **95**, 343–347

Wennström, J. L. (1987) Lack of association between width of attached gingiva and development of soft tissue recession. A 5-year longitudinal study. *J. Clin. Periodontol.* **14**, 181–184

Wennström, J. and Lindhe, J. (1983a) Role of attached gingiva for maintenance of periodontal health. Healing following excisional and grafting procedures in dogs. *J. Clin. Periodontol.* **10**, 206–221

Wennström, J. and Lindhe, J. (1983b) Plaque-induced gingival inflammation in the absence of attached gingiva in dogs. *J. Clin. Periodontol.* **10**, 266–276

Wennström, J., Lindhe, J. and Nyman, S. (1981) Role of keratinized gingiva for gingival health. *J. Clin. Periodontol.* **8**, 311–328

Wennström, J., Lindhe, J. and Nyman, S. (1982) The role of keratinized gingiva in plaque-associated gingivitis in dogs. *J. Clin. Periodontol.* **9**, 75–85

WHO (1978) *Epidemiology, etiology and prevention of periodontal disease,* pp. 47–54. Technical Report Series No. 621. Geneva

Wilderman, M., Wentz, F. and Orban, B. (1960)

Histogenesis of repair after mucogingival surgery. *J. Periodontol.* **31**, 283–299

Woofter, C. (1969) The prevalence and etiology of gingival recession. *J. West Soc. Periodont. Periodont. Abstr.* **17**, 45–50

33

Occlusion and the periodontal tissues

Introduction

There is a long-held clinical belief stemming from the early findings of Box (1935) and Stones (1938) that a direct relationship exists between occlusal forces and the pattern and progression rate of plaque-induced periodontal destruction. This belief was endorsed by the findings of Macapanpan and Weinman (1954) and Glickman and Smulow (1962) and then, most importantly, by the observations of Glickman and Smulow (1965) on two autopsy cases, upon which it was postulated that 'gingival inflammation and trauma from occlusion . . . exert a combined co-destructive effect which produces angular bone defects and intrabony defects.' This 'co-destructive' concept has since been used by many periodontists, and more especially by prosthodontists, to justify the role of occlusal equilibration and splinting in periodontal therapy. On the other hand, many clinicians have, as advocated in Chapter 23, refrained from any form of occlusal therapy without apparently prejudicing the outcome of periodontal treatment.

   The evidence relating to the above controversial issue clearly demands examination. Similarly the influence of increased mobility upon units with reduced periodontal support, under conditions of marginal tissue health and during post-surgical healing must also be considered. In doing so it must however be appreciated that the establishment of any correlation between clinical and radiographic findings and the all-important histological changes, will be handicapped by the inevitable difficulties of

obtaining suitable human material. Furthermore, the alternative use of animal experimental models presents problems of differences of species and the reproduction of representative occlusal forces. The extrapolation of any results from animals to humans must therefore be effected with caution.

Occlusal trauma and the pattern of periodontal breakdown

Autopsy material findings

Attempts to correlate occlusal traumatism and chronic periodontitis, using human autopsy material, have been inconclusive. Glickman and Smulow (1965) claimed such a relationship existed whilst Waerhaug (1979 a) found no evidence, in 64 sets of human jaws, that functional (traumatic) forces can act as co-factors. Thus, bony defects were not only associated invariably with the downgrowth of subgingival plaque but also occurred just as commonly in sites adjacent to non-traumatized teeth as to those that were traumatized. The specific pattern of breakdown was attributed instead (Prichard, 1967; Manson, 1976) to the interplay between the form and volume of the alveolar bone and the variable extent of the apical downgrowth of the microbial plaque on the affected root surfaces. In a further investigation, on extracted teeth in advanced disease, Waerhaug (1979 b) endorsed the consistent aetiological relationship that exists between the subgingival plaque front and the alveolar crest and marginal attachment. In addition, the radiographic evidence of intrabony pocketing did not justify the diagnosis of trauma from occlusion. Nearly half of the extracted teeth had demonstrated physiological mobility and, where hypermobility had been present, it proved to be mostly orientated buccolingually whereas the intrabony pockets were located mesially and distally. Waerhaug thus concluded that there are no reliable clinical or radiological criteria upon which the diagnosis of trauma from occlusion can be based. Further, there is no reliable basis for the philosophy of splinting of teeth and eliminating cuspal interferences as an essential element of periodontal therapy.

Animal model findings

Early efforts to produce occlusal stresses in animal models by placing a wedge between the two teeth (Macapanpan and Weinman, 1954), demonstrated that the lesion of CIPD could not be produced by occlusal trauma alone. This was confirmed by Bhaskar and Orban (1955), who produced traumatism with premature contact from high crowns on monkey premolars and by Wentz *et al.* (1958) who introduced jiggling trauma, in which the experimental traumatic forces were created to act alternately in one direction and then in another, to reproduce the traumatic forces occurring in humans. Subsequent investigations by Svanberg (1974) and Polson *et al.* (1976 a) reinforced the belief that trauma from occlusion is incapable of causing pocket formation in animal models with normal gingiva or even with an overt gingivitis.

Other similar model investigations showed that attachment loss failed to occur in the presence of 'co-destructive' factors (Comar *et al.*, 1969), and that bruxism did not appear to cause progression of gingivitis to destructive chronic marginal periodontitis (Budtz-Jørgensen, 1980). Furthermore, Hanamura *et al.* (1987) failed to show any significant effect of bruxism on the periodontal status of individuals with moderate to severe periodontal disease and concluded that the two phenomena are in general not closely associated.

The tissue changes that occur in response to occlusal overloading, represent a physiological adaptation to altered functional demands (Svanberg, 1974; Polson *et al.*, 1976 a). This response consists of an initial traumatic phase of increasing tooth mobility followed by a post-traumatic phase of permanently increased mobility. The former is characterized by an initially increased vascularity and vascular permeability, enhanced osteoclastic activity, together with a gradually increasing periodontal ligament space and tooth mobility. In the later adapted phase, the periodontal ligament space is increased but with normal constituents and activity. All these changes are confined to the subcrestal tissues and therefore do not compromise the integrity of the marginal attachment. It has also been shown that these adaptive changes are almost completely reversible following the cessation of jiggling forces (Polson *et al.*, 1976 b). Thus, a marked regeneration of bone (i.e. an increase in bone volume) occurred and no detectable mobility persisted. As will be shown later, no such reversibility exists in the presence of marginal inflammation.

The relationship between occlusal overloading and the pattern of destruction in a co-existing plaque-induced periodontitis was then examined in a further series of experiments in beagle dogs and squirrel monkeys. In the former, a ligature-induced plaque-associated chronic marginal periodontitis (ad modum Swenson, 1947), was first established and jiggling forces then applied (Lindhe and Svanberg, 1974). An enhanced rate of attachment loss and downgrowth of pocket epithelium was observed compared to the control side with periodontitis alone. In contrast, Meitner (1975) assessed the effects of repetitive mechanical trauma on a marginal periodontitis (induced ad modum Kennedy and Polson, 1973) in the squirrel monkey, but observed an aggravating effect in only one out of four instances. The associated pocketing was always suprabony in nature. In addition, it was shown that with the jiggling type of trauma, there was a single extended traumatic phase of progressively increasing mobility. This was characterized by a gradual widening of the periodontal ligament space which contained an increased number of vessels having increased permeability. This suggested that adaptation to the altered functional demand had not been achieved. When, in the interests of comparability with the dog model, Polson and Zander (1983) repeated the monkey experiment in the presence of intrabony pockets increased bone loss was sustained, but this was not associated with greater attachment loss at the experimental sites.

The influence of a progressive tooth mobility on the rate of ongoing destructive periodontitis has also been investigated in the animal model (Review: Ericsson, 1986). Nyman *et al.* (1978) produced increasing mobility by periodic jiggling forces applied with an elevator. An increased rate of attachment loss occurred. The mechanism is not clear, but it was suggested that progressively increasing mobility might have favoured an apical proliferation of the microbial plaque which in turn caused further destruction. On the other hand, the influence of the high level of traumtic forces produced in this investigation bordered on an extraction force and may have been more significant. Furthermore such forces cannot be accepted readily as a clinical analogy. This possibility was acknowledged by Ericsson and Lindhe (1982), as a result of the enhanced rate of destruction observed with longstanding jiggling in the presence of an ongoing periodontitis. The experimental teeth become intruded into their alveolar bony housing which, together with the markedly increased mobility, indicates that the magnitude of the forces used experimentally was much greater than that encountered with occlusal trauma in humans. Consequently, it was stated that 'no immediate conclusions regarding the effects of trauma from occlusion in the human dentition should be allowed.'

It is of interest that Yumet and Polson (1985) observed in squirrel monkeys, a marked epithelial downgrowth into incisional wounds in gingivae inflamed by plaque. The possibility therefore exists that a similarly marked apical migration of pocket epithelium might also follow from the highly artificial and excessive trauma induced in the dog experiments, which would help to explain the enhanced rate of destruction. The possibility that the periodontal pocket flora might, under conditions of occlusal trauma, change to become more aggressive thereby increasing the rate of loss of attachment, was investigated in beagle dogs (Kaufman *et al.*, 1984). However these workers concluded that the mechanism for this increased attachment loss appeared not to be bacterial.

The differences between the findings of the animal investigations reviewed above might be explained by differences in individual animal models, experimental techniques to produce disease, methods of inducing and maintaining the mechanical trauma and, finally, the duration of the experiments. Whatever the significance of these differences and the interpretation of the findings any extrapolation to the human clinical situation must be made with caution. This is especially so, as the trauma invoked in these investigations did not correspond to clinical levels.

Conclusion

It is not possible at present on the basis of the available evidence, to draw any firm conclusions about the role of occlusal trauma in progressive disease in humans. Further carefully controlled research in humans is necessary to confirm the claimed effects and without this support, the rationale for occlusal therapy in the management of progressive plaque-induced disease must be deemed to be questionable (see also Polson, 1980; Ramfjord and Ash, 1981).

Occlusal trauma and reduced periodontal support

Periodontal health

Ericsson and Lindhe (1977) investigated the effect of 'jiggling' on markedly reduced (as a result of previous disease) but non-inflamed periodontal tissues in dogs. An expected increased tooth mobility and angular bony resorption resulted but with no apical shift of the dentogingival epithelium or intrabony pocketing. The periapical radiolucencies produced were regarded, in line with earlier findings (Lindhe and Svanberg, 1974), as an adaptation to increased functional demands. Perrier and Polson (1982) confirmed the ability of a reduced but healthy periodontium to withstand the effects of occlusal trauma without incurring any loss of attachment. In addition, the histological appearance was similar to that occurring when a normal periodontal support is stressed and confined to the subcrestal tissues. There is therefore no scientific basis for considering that hypermobility should be reduced in order to preserve periodontal health.

Marginal periodontitis

In the presence of a plaque-induced periodontitis, jiggling forces have resulted in much greater degrees of tooth mobility and bone resorption in both squirrel monkeys (Polson *et al.*, 1976 a) and beagle dogs (Lindhe and Svanberg, 1974). The latter experimental model it should be recalled, also sustained greater attachment losses. Following the discontinuation of the jiggling there was neither a regeneration of bone nor an improvement in the levels of tooth hypermobility over a 10-week assessment period (Polson *et al.*, 1976 b). On the other hand, when the cessation of jiggling was accompanied by rigorous oral hygiene measures (Kantor *et al.*, 1976), there followed a progressive decrease in hypermobility and a significant regeneration of alveolar bone. Consequently, it was postulated that the presence of marginal periodontal inflammation in some way inhibits the potential for the regeneration of bone (*cf.* Chapter 31 – Intrabony defect healing).

Lindhe and Ericsson (1982) observed that, when the jiggling was maintained following resolution of the supracrestal plaque-induced inflammatory lesion, the hypermobility persisted but no further loss of attachment was sustained. In addition, when the jiggling force was removed this resulted in a marked decrease in the mobility of the teeth. Histologic and histometric analysis revealed a constant zone (width 315–875 µm) of non-infiltrated connective tissue, lying between the inflamed supracrestal connective tissue adjacent to the microbial plaque, and the alveolar bone and periodontal ligament. It has been suggested that this zone of connective tissue serves as a protective barrier for the marginal periodontal ligament. The above findings show clearly that jiggling alone will not cause further destruction of the connective tissue attachment, even when periodontal support is reduced. It also implies (as has been advocated in Part II) that occlusal adjustment *per se* and any associated reduction in tooth hypermobility that might be achieved by this will not improve the periodontal condition.

Recurrent periodontitis

The influence of a permanently increased mobility, with its associated widened periodontal ligament and bony resorption, on the pattern of recurrent plaque-induced disease was investigated in beagle dogs by Ericsson and Lindhe (1984). Jiggling trauma was produced on the test teeth followed by experimental ligature-induced periodontitis at both test and control sites. The degree of periodontal breakdown was found to be similar at both sites. It was concluded that the progression of plaque-associated lesions appears unrelated to the degree of horizontal tooth mobility. This does not appear consistent with the earlier findings of Lindhe and Svanberg (1974).

Hypermobility and periodontal healing

Effect of plaque control

Significant reductions in tooth mobility have been observed following resolution of marginal inflammation in periodontitis in squirrel monkeys (Polson *et al.*, 1979) and in the management of moderate to advanced periodontal disease in humans (Lindhe and Nyman, 1975; Rosling *et al.*, 1976; Polson and Heijl, 1978; Fleszar *et al.*, 1980; Persson, 1980; Kerry *et al.*, 1982). The morphological reason for reduced mobility associated with the suprabony pockets in the former animal model was attributed to the associated alveolar repair following marked reductions in the supracrestal connective tissue inflammatory infiltrate. As an increased bone density (i.e. bone volume) plus a decreased width of the periodontal ligament occurred, with no associated alterations in crestal bone height, it would suggest that bone density and ligament width may be of greater significance, regarding tooth mobility, than crestal height itself. On the other hand, the supracrestal tissues appear to provide a proportionately greater support as loss of alveolar bone occurs with progressive periodontal destruction (Gillespie *et al.*, 1979). The supportive role of even inflamed supracrestal tissue is also demonstrated by the immediate increase in mobility (of about 20%) recorded following gingivectomy (Burch *et al.*, 1968). Persson (1981 a) reported rather smaller post-gingivectomy increases of about 13%. Although this increased mobility and that of up to 80% observed after flap procedures, coupled with the gradual decreases to the pre-treatment levels in the presence of optimal oral hygiene, were attributed to the effects of surgical trauma itself

(Persson, 1981 b), the influence of supracrestal tissue damage and then of repair cannot be overlooked. In another investigation, Polson *et al.* (1983) demonstrated bone regeneration, even in the presence of active and continued tooth hypermobility, following resolution of inflammation. Furthermore, this active hypermobility appeared to have no detrimental effect on the resolution of inflammation taking place following removal of the local aetiological factors.

Together with reduction in the height of the attachment apparatus in long-standing untreated disease there is a gradual apical displacement of the fulcrum for the movement of the crown of the tooth (Ericsson and Lindhe, 1984), associated with a progressive increase of the horizontal tooth mobility (Lindhe and Ericsson, 1976). Investigations concerning the significance of this hypermobility on healing, following periodontal surgical treatment, have produced conflicting results. Although Lindhe and Ericsson (1976) claimed that jiggling type occlusal trauma and tooth hypermobility are not factors which detrimentally affect healing following surgery, more favourable gains in connective tissue attachment were reported in teeth with normal mobility. In another animal model investigation Klinge *et al.* (1985) found that periodontal healing of furcation defects created experimentally in dogs did not seem to be affected by tooth displacement following reconstructive surgery. Fleszar *et al.* (1980) analysed the influence of tooth mobility on periodontal treatment carried out in an 8-year longitudinal study at Michigan (Ramfjord *et al.*, 1973, 1975). They concluded that pockets at clinically mobile teeth did not respond as well to periodontal treatment as those at firm teeth exhibiting the same severity of disease at baseline. Rosling *et al.* (1976) and Polson and Heijl (1978) have, on the other hand, demonstrated in clinical trials that increased tooth mobility had no adverse effect on healing of intrabony pockets following periodontal surgery in the presence of optimal plaque control. The differences between the results of these clinical investigations might be in part due to the less than ideal oral hygiene levels in the Michigan study.

Lindhe and Nyman (1975) showed following therapy significant reductions in the number of teeth with initial mobility scores of '2' or '3', although 26% of all teeth still exhibited some mobility (the majority with a score of '1') after 5 years. A substantial reduction in tooth mobility was also observed in subjects with moderate periodontal disease, shortly after the institution of oral hygiene procedures (Persson, 1980). Kerry *et al.* (1982) in another study, reported slight reductions in tooth mobility over the 2-year maintenance period, regardless of treatment methods. There were, however, significant reductions in mobility following initial nonsurgical therapy but, as occlusal adjustments were also carried out, the extent to which this was due to the resolution of inflammation (as suggested by the animal experimental studies) cannot be judged.

Shefter and McFall (1984) have reported on the occlusal relations and the periodontal status of an adult population. As no significant deleterious influence on the status of the periodontium due to occlusal disharmonies could be detected, they concluded (as advocated in Part II) that it would seem prudent to minimize the role of the correction of occlusal disharmonies in routine periodontal therapy. In this context, Volmer and Rateitschak (1975) showed that while selective grinding of occlusally traumatized teeth reduced tooth mobility it had no effect on the degree of gingival inflammation. Similarly, Hakkarainen (1986) demonstrated that occlusal adjustment had no effect on the marginal periodontium, as reflected by the rate of sulcular fluid flow. Finally Pihlstrom *et al.* (1986) were unable to show any association between various occlusal contact patterns and the severity of disease.

Conclusions

Much of current knowledge relating to the role of occlusal forces in periodontal breakdown and in its treatment has been obtained from animal experimental models. Caution must therefore be exercised when extrapolating results from these studies to the clinical management of patients, but the following conclusions may be drawn:

(1) Resolution of marginal inflammation will lead invariably to a significant decrease in tooth mobility. Any residual tooth hypermobility may be due to the loss of periodontal support, resulting from periodontal disease.

(2) Intrabony pockets associated with hypermobile teeth will undergo significant bony regeneration when the marginal periodontal lesion has been resolved. This will occur even in the presence of hypermobility, although healing might possibly be more favourable in its absence.

(3) Where inflammatory resolution is not achieved, due to inaccessible subgingival plaque retention sites, there is no reliable evidence that any associated tooth hypermobility will further compromise the periodontal attachment. Thus the evidence in support of a co-destructive effect of occlusal trauma in periodontitis is unconvincing and emphasizes the importance of the effective control of the associated plaque-induced disease.

(4) Trauma from occlusion does result in radiographic signs of alveolar bone resorption (but with no loss of attachment) and increased tooth mobility. Each should be regarded as a physiological adaptive response to an altered functional demand and must not be confused clinically with the often similar radiographic appearances of plaque-induced intrabony defects and the increased mobility related to the associated inflammatory disease.

(5) Treatment directed at occlusal trauma alone (i.e. occlusal adjustment or splinting) may reduce increased mobility of traumatized teeth but will not arrest the plaque-induced breakdown of the supporting tissues. Progressively increasing mobility usually indicates progessive disease for which plaque control measures rather than occlusal therapy are required.

(6) The role of occlusion on the progression of disease in humans is unproven and current research findings, as stated by Polson (1986), place decreased emphasis upon the management of tooth mobility and increased emphasis upon resolution of marginal inflammation.

Clinical implications

Firstly, the management of periodontal disease in conjunction with hypermobility should, as advocated in Part II, be based first and foremost upon resolution of the plaque-induced marginal inflammation. Secondly, there is no reason to splint teeth with reduced support after periodontal treatment in order to preserve periodontal health. Thirdly, reduced attachment levels can be maintained by plaque control measures alone. Fourthly, any increased mobility at such teeth can be accepted for a physiological adaptation to environmental forces as residual mobility will not affect the attachment levels. There may however be limiting factors relating to patient comfort, function and aesthetics. In these cases the forces are such that the adaptation results in a degree of mobility incompatible with mastication, or that the adapative capacity of the periodontium is exceeded. The result may be drifting of the teeth with their consequent poor appearance or even the spontaneous avulsion of teeth. The prevention of these sequelae provides a biological justification for splinting (see also Chapter 34 – Fixed or removable prosthesis.)

Orthodontic therapy and the periodontium

The significance of crowding

While the orthodontic realignment of imbricated teeth is most frequently carried out on functional and cosmetic grounds (Review: Shaw *et al.*, 1980), the reasons for doing so in the interests of periodontal health are less clear. Thus, a correlation between crowding, plaque accumulation and the degree of periodontal disease has been claimed by some (Poulton and Aaronson, 1961; Suomi, 1969; Alexander and Tipnis, 1970; Buckley, 1972; Ainamo, 1972; Behlfelt *et al.*, 1981; Griffith and Addy, 1981; Silness and Røynstrand, 1985 a), others report no such relationship (Beagrie and James, 1962; Geiger, 1962; Gould and Picton, 1966; Geiger *et al.*, 1973; Ingervall *et al.*, 1977), while there seem to be only minor differences in periodontal status between crowded and well-aligned incisors of individuals with good oral hygiene when assessed 10 years following orthodontic treatment (Årtun and Osterberg, 1987).

Overbite and overjet relationships

The relationship between vertical overbite and horizontal overjet and disease has yet to be clearly established. Poulton and Aaronson (1961) and Gould and Picton (1966) reported higher disease indices with increased overbite and overjet, while Alexander and Tipnis (1970), Tipnis *et al.* (1971) and Geiger *et al.* (1973) observed no such changes. However, a trend towards more disease existed with a severe overbite and overjet (Geiger *et al.*, 1973) and individuals with high overbite/overjet ratios displayed more favourable periodontal conditions than those with lower ratios (Silness and Røystrand, 1985 b).

No correlation has been found between the amount of overbite and the degree of gingival recession in children (Parfitt and Mjör, 1964; Rose, 1967). Similarly, Silness and Røystrand (1985 b) observed no traumatic impingement on the gingivae from deep overbites in adolescents and concluded that interceptive orthodontic treatment, occlusal adjustment and/or restorative procedures was not indicated from a periodontal point of view. However, as there is a risk of damage following the loss of posterior teeth, periodic evaluation of the occlusal relationships was considered necessary.

Mouthbreathing

It is expedient to include a brief review here of the possible effects of mouthbreathing. Individuals with a lip-apart posture may present with a so-called mouthbreathing gingivitis (Lite *et al.*, 1958). The mechanism of the erythematous enlargement of the mucosa observed is not clear. The possible drying effect of the air so often cited, (e.g. Lite *et al.*, 1955; Jacobson, 1973; Addy *et al.*, 1987), would seem to be countered by the failure of experimental drying of rat gingiva to lead to inflammation (Klingsberg *et al.*, 1961). Difficulties of removing the dried-out bacterial plaque may however be significant (Goldman and Cohen, 1973). Alexander (1970) reported a

significant correlation between habitual mouthbreathing and gingival inflammation in individuals attending for routine treatment, but the findings of a comparable study in a rather younger group of dental students did not support the assumption that mouthbreathing causes gingival inflammation. Jacobson (1973) in turn, observed more severe gingivitis in mouthbreathers than non-mouthbreathers, while Jacobson and Linder-Aronson (1972) demonstrated a correlation between gingivitis and crowding in mouthbreathing. Sutcliffe (1968), on the other hand, considered mouthbreathing to be unimportant in the aetiology of gingivitis. Further investigations are required.

The effects of therapy

General considerations

There are differences of opinion about the effects of orthodontic therapy upon periodontal tissue integrity. Baxter (1967), Rateitschak (1968), Kloehn and Pfeifer (1974), Eliasson *et al.* (1982), Polson and Reed (1984) and Polson (1984) reported no discernible effect on periodontal health; Sjolien and Zachrisson (1973), Zachrisson and Alnaes (1973, 1974), Zachrisson (1975), Hollender *et al.* (1980) and Hamp *et al.* (1982) some detrimental effects; whilst Alstad and Zachrisson (1979) observed no statistically significant differences in periodontal conditions of treated and untreated individuals. Brown (1982) has reviewed the nature of root resorption following orthodontic therapy.

The influence of plaque

Fixed appliance therapy undoubtedly complicates oral hygiene measures (Zachrisson, 1974). Methods of plaque control for orthodontic patients have been evaluated by Zachrisson (1974) and Lundström *et al.* (1980). Banding may increase subgingival plaque retention (Zachrisson and Zachrisson, 1972; Zachrisson and Alnaes, 1973, 1974; Tersin, 1973, 1975) and as a result possibly convert a gingivitis into a periodontitis. Thus as shown by Diamanti-Kipioti *et al.* (1987) bands will, in the absence of optimal oral hygiene promote the growth of subgingival plaque and cause specific shifts in its bacteriological composition, resulting in the establishment of accentuated pathological conditions. Tooth intrusion may have a similar effect by carrying the supragingival plaque subgingivally (Ericsson *et al.*, 1977, 1986).

Development of gingival recession

Pearson (1968) reported greater degrees of recession (but without any mention of attachment loss) at mandibular central incisors following orthodontic treatment compared with untreated controls. Maynard and Ochsenbein (1975) demonstrated gingival recession in a number of instances following orthodontic therapy, but without implicating tooth movement *per se*. Furthermore, as no recession occurred when free gingival grafts were placed prior to orthodontic treatment, prophylactic mucogingival surgery was advocated at sites with insufficient keratinized tissue (see also Maynard and Wilson, 1980). On the other hand, Årtun *et al.* (1986) demonstrated that labially erupted canines with minimal or no attached gingiva resisted the stresses associated with a full period of fully-banded orthodontic appliance therapy as well as those during a 16-year post-orthodontic period without significant attachment losses. Boyd (1978), Dorfman (1978) and Coatoam *et al.* (1981) have discussed mucogingival changes including gingival recession, incident to mandibular incisor tooth movement. The potential for both decreased and increased gingival dimensions appears to exist post-orthodontically. Coatoam *et al.* (1981) stressed however that an increase in crown lengths (passive eruption) should not be misinterpreted as gingival recession.

Foushee *et al.* (1985) reported clinically significant gingival recession in six out of 24 patients following orthognathic therapy in the mandibular anterior area. This recession did however tend to occur at sites at which the gingiva and underlying bone appeared thin and was coupled with gingival inflammation in some instances. Post-orthodontic loss of attachment and gingival recession have been observed in animal model investigations by Batenhorst *et al.* (1974) and Steiner *et al.* (1981) but not by Wingard and Bowers (1976). Finally, the observation of Wennström *et al.* (1987) in the animal model, suggest that plaque-induced inflammation and the thickness (volume) of the marginal soft tissue, rather than the apicocoronal width of the gingiva, are the determining factors in the development of gingival recession and attachment loss during orthodontic therapy (see also Chapter 32 – Mucogingival considerations).

Creation of dehiscences

It has been reported that bony dehiscences (Reitan, 1957; Batenhorst *et al.,* 1974) and also an associated loss of attachment (Batenhorst *et al.,* 1974), result from the orthodontic tipping of teeth. However others consider that a compensatory bone formation occurs (Elliott and Bowers, 1963; Gaudet, 1970; Wingard and Bowers, 1976). More recently, Karring *et al.* (1982) showed that alveolar bone dehiscences, produced by orthodontic tipping forces in dogs, persisted whilst the tilted teeth were proclined but the bone regenerated once the teeth had been moved back into their original positions. No

attachment losses were sustained, supporting the findings of Svanberg (1974) and Polson *et al.* (1976) that traumatic forces including 'repetitive trauma to the periodontium incident to orthodontic tooth movement' will not induce downgrowth of junctional epithelium. Complete bony regeneration implies that cells derived from bone must have invaded the area for according to Melcher (1976) only these are capable of forming bone. The failure of compensatory bone formation following tooth proclination suggests that degradation of both the inorganic and organic bony components occurs as a result of trauma. Alternatively, any osteogenic progenitor cells within dehiscences are incapable of forming bone outside the normal architecture of the jaw bone. The former possibility is supported by the effects of surgically removing the soft tissue within alveolar bony dehiscences produced by jiggling forces (Nyman *et al.*, 1982). Markedly reduced coronal regrowth of bone was observed when the forces were discontinued, whereas considerable regeneration occurred following surgical flap reflection and replacement alone at the control sites.

Influence of extraction sites

It has been claimed that orthodontic movement of teeth into bicuspid extraction sites may be detrimental to long term periodontal health of the related teeth (e.g. Prichard, 1975; Robertson *et al.*, 1977; Hamp *et al.*, 1982). The 10-year post-orthodontic therapy findings by Reed *et al.* (1985) demonstrated no significant differences for clinical attachment levels, pocket depths or recession at these sites. Furthermore the gingival bunching and clefting reported by others appears to be only transient, undergoing resolution with time.

Other orthodontic objectives

Correction of intrabony defects

Substantial improvements in intrabony pocket morphology suggestive of bone regeneration have been produced and improved connective tissue attachment levels claimed, by orthodontically moving the involved tooth into the defect (Geraci, 1973; Brown, 1973; Gazit and Lieberman, 1980). Polson *et al.* (1984) have confirmed that intrabony defects on the pressure side were transformed, giving the appearance of a more coronal level of alveolar bone, but demonstrated the presence of epithelium interposed between this bone and the root surface. Angular defects on the tension side were in turn transformed into suprabony pockets, as a result of the bodily movement of the tooth away from the defect.

Molar uprighting

The uprighting of tilted molars has been advocated to facilitate plaque control, reduce periodontal osseous defects and to improve axial and occlusal relationships in prosthodontic therapy (Brown, 1973; Tulloch, 1982). Evaluation of this type of treatment is, however, complicated by the lack of fixed reference points and of suitable controls. Brown (1973) and Kraal *et al.* (1980) demonstrated some pocket reductions, but no improvement in gingival health was observed when compared with untreated controls (Kraal *et al.*, 1980).

Forced eruption

The principle of forced eruption has been described for the correction of isolated intrabony defects (Ingber, 1974), and has been used with some success in the management of roots fractured below the alveolar crest (Heithersay, 1973; Ingber, 1976; Heithersay and Moule, 1982).

References

Addy, M., Dummer, P. M. H., Hunter, M. L., Kingdon, A. and Shaw, W. C. (1987) A study of the association of fraenal attachment, lip coverage, and vestibular depth with plaque and gingivitis. *J. Periodontol.* **58**, 752–757

Ainamo, J. (1972) Relationship between malalignment of the teeth and periodontal disease. *Scand. J. Dent. Res.* **80**, 104–110

Alexander, A. G. (1970) Habitual mouthbreathing and its effect on gingival health. *Periodontologie* **24**, 49–55

Alexander, A. G. and Tipnis, A. K. (1970) The effect of irregularity of teeth and the degree of overbite and overjet on the gingival health. *Br. Dent. J.* **128**, 539–544

Alstad, S. and Zachrisson, B. U. (1979) Longitudinal study of periodontal condition associated with orthodontic treatment in adolescents. *Am. J. Orthod.* **76**, 277–286

Årtun, J. and Osterberg, S. K. (1987) Periodontal status of secondary crowded mandibular incisors. Long-term results after orthodontic treatment. *J. Clin. Periodontol.* **14**, 261–266

Årtun, J., Osterberg, S. K. and Joondeph, D. R. (1986) Long-term periodontal status of labially erupted canines following orthodontic treatment. *J. Clin. Periodontol.* **13**, 856–861

Batenhorst, K. F., Bowers, G. M. and Williams, J. E. (1974) Tissue changes resulting from facial tipping and extrusion of incisors in monkeys. *J. Periodontol.* **45**, 660–668

Baxter, D. H. (1967) The effect of orthodontic treatment on alveolar bone adjacent to the cemento-enamel junction. *Angle Orthod.* **37**, 35–47

Beagrie, G. S. and James, G. A. (1962) The association of posterior tooth irregularity and periodontal disease. *Br. Dent. J.* **113**, 239–243

Behlfelt, K., Ericsson, L., Jacobson, L. and Linder-Aronson, S. (1981) The occurrence of plaque and gingivitis and its relationship to tooth alignment within the dental arches. *J. Clin. Periodontol.* **8**, 329–337

Bhaskar, S. and Orban, B. (1955) Experimental occlusal trauma. *J. Periodontol.* **26**, 270–284

Box, H. K. (1935) Experimental traumatogenic occlusion in sheep. *Oral Health* **25**, 9–15

Boyd, R. L. (1978) Mucogingival considerations and their relationship to orthodontics. *J. Periodontol.* **49**, 67–76

Brown, I. S. (1973) The effect of orthodontic therapy on certain types of periodontal defects. *J. Periodontol.* **44**, 742–754

Brown, W. A. B. (1982) Resorption of permanent teeth. *Br. J. Orthodont.* **9**, 212–220

Buckley, I. A. (1972) The relationship between malocclusion and periodontal disease. *J. Periodontol.* **43**, 415–417

Budtz-Jørgensen, E. (1980) Bruxism and trauma from occlusion. *J. Clin. Periodontol.* **7**, 149–162

Burch, J. G., Conroy, C. W. and Ferris, R. T. (1968) Tooth mobility following gingivectomy. A study of gingival support of the teeth. *Periodontics.* **6**, 90–94

Coatoam, G. W., Behrents, R. G. and Bissada, N. F. (1981) The width of keratinized gingiva during orthodontic treatment: its significance and impact on periodontal status. *J. Periodontol.* **52**, 307–313

Comar, M. D., Kollar, J. A. and Gargiulo, A. W. (1969) Local irritation and occlusal trauma as co-factors in the periodontal disease process. *J. Periodontol.* **40**, 193–200

Diamanti-Kipioti, A., Gusberti, F. A. and Lang, N. P. (1987) Clinical and microbiological effects of fixed orthodontic appliances. *J. Clin. Periodontol.* **14**, 326–333

Dorfman, H. S. (1978) Mucogingival changes resulting from mandibular incisor tooth movement. *Am. J. Orthod.* **74**, 286–297

Eliasson, L., Hugoson, A., Kurol, J. and Siwe, H. (1982) The effects of orthodontic treatment on periodontal tissues in patients with reduced periodontal support. *Eur. J. Orthod.* **4**, 1–9

Elliott, J. R. and Bowers, G. M. (1963) Alveolar dehiscence and fenestration. *Periodontics*, **1**, 245–248

Ericsson, I. (1986) The combined effects of plaque and physical stress on periodontal tissues. *J. Clin. Periodontol.* **13**, 918–922

Ericsson, I. and Lindhe, J. (1977) Lack of effect of trauma from occlusion on the recurrence of experimental periodontisis. *J. Clin. Periodontol.* **4**, 115–127

Ericsson, I. and Lindhe, J. (1982) Effect of longstanding jiggling on experimental marginal periodontitis in the beagle dog. *J. Clin. Periodontol.* **9**, 497–503

Ericsson, I. and Lindhe J. (1984) Lack of significance of increased tooth mobility in experimental periodontitis. *J. Periodontol.* **55**, 447–452

Ericsson, I., Thilander, B., Lindhe, J. and Okamoto, H. (1977) The effect of orthodontic tilting movements on the periodontal tissues of infected and non-infected dentitions in dogs. *J. Clin. Periodontol.* **4**, 278–293

Fleszar, T. J., Knowles, J. W., Morrison, E. D., Burgett, F. G., Nissle, R. R. and Ramfjord, S. P. (1980) Tooth mobility and periodontal therapy. *J. Clin. Periodontol.* **7**, 495–505

Foushee, D. G., Moriarty, J. D. and Simpson, D. M. (1985) Effects of mandibular orthognathic treatment on mucogingival tissues. *J. Periodontol.* **56**, 727–733

Gaudet, E. L. Jr. (1970) Tissue changes in the monkey following root torque with the Begg technique. *Am. J. Orthod.* **58**, 164–178

Gazit, E. and Lieberman, M., (1980) Occlusal and orthodontic considerations in the periodontally involved dentition. *Angle Orthod.* **50**, 346–349

Geiger, A. M. (1962) Occlusal studies in 188 consecutive cases of periodontal disease. *Am. J. Orthod.* **48**, 330–360

Geiger, A. M., Wasserman, B. H. and Turgeon, L. R. (1973) Relationship of occlusion and periodontal disease. Part VI. Relation of anterior overjet and overbite to periodontal destruction and gingival inflammation. *J. Periodontol.* **44**, 150–157

Geraci, T. F. (1973) Orthodontic movements of teeth into artificially produced infrabony defects in the rhesus monkey: a histological report. In *Report Annual Meeting of the American Academy of Periodontology – 1972.* (Editor Winslow, M. B.) *J. Periodontol.* **44**, 110–123

Gillespie, B. R., Chasens, A. I., Brownstein, C. N. and Alfano, M. C. (1979) The relationship between the mobility of human teeth and their supracrestal fibre support. *J. Periodontol.* **50**, 120–124

Glickman, I. and Smulow, J. B. (1962) Alterations in the pathway of gingival inflammation into the underlying tissues induced by excessive occlusal forces. *J. Periodontol.* **33**, 7–13

Glickman, I. and Smulow, J. B. (1965) Effect of excessive occlusal forces upon the pathway of gingival inflammation in humans. *J. Periodontol.* **36**, 141–147

Goldman, H. M. and Cohen D. W. (1973) *Periodontal Therapy*, 5th Edition, pp. 213–214. C. V. Mosby Co., St Louis, MO

Gould, M. S. E. and Picton, D. C. A. (1966) The relation between irregularities of the teeth and periodontal disease. *Br. Dent. J.* **121**, 20–23

Griffiths, G. S. and Addy, M. (1981) Effects of malalignment of teeth in the anterior segments on plaque accumulation. *J. Clin. Periodontol.* **8**, 481–490

Hakkarainen, K. (1986) Relative influence of scaling and root planing and occlusal adjustment on sulcular fluid flow. *J. Periodontol.* **57**, 681–684

Hamp, S., Lundstrom, F. and Nyman, S. (1982) Periodontal conditions in adolescents subjected to multiband orthodontic treatment with controlled oral hygiene. *Eur. J. Orthod.* **4**, 77–86

Hanamura, H., Houston, F., Rylander, H., Carlsson, G. E., Haraldson, T. and Nyman, S. (1987) Periodontal status and bruxism. A comparative study of patients with periodontal disease and occlusal parafunctions. *J. Periodontol.* **58**, 173–176

Heithersay, G. S. (1973) Combined endodontic-orthodontic treatment of transverse root fractures in the region of the alveolar crest. *Oral Surg.* **36**, 404–415

Heithersay, G. S. and Moule, A. J. (1982) Anterior subgingival fractures: A review of treatment alternatives. *Aust. Dent. J.* **27**, 368–376

Hollender, L., Ronnerman, A. and Thilander, B. (1980) Root resorption, marginal bone support and clinical crown length in orthodontically treated patients. *Eur. J. Orthod.* **2**, 197–205

Ingber, J. S. (1974) Forced eruption: Part I. A method of treating isolated one and two wall infrabony osseous defects – rationale and case report. *J. Periodontol.* **45**, 199–206

Ingber, J. S. (1976) Forced eruption: Part II. A method of treating non-restorable teeth – periodontal and restorative considerations. *J. Periodontol.* **47**, 203–216

Ingervall, B., Jacobson, U. and Nyman, S. (1977) A clinical study of the relationship between crowding of teeth, plaque and gingival condition. *J. Clin. Periodontol.* **4**, 214–222

Jacobson, L. (1973) Mouthbreathing and gingivitis. 1. Gingival conditions in children with epipharyngeal adenoids. *J. Periodontol.* **8**, 269–277

Jacobson, L. and Linder-Aronson, S. (1972) Crowding and gingivitis: a comparison between mouthbreathers and nosebreathers. *Scand. J. Dent. Res.* **80**, 500–504

Kantor, M., Polson, A. M. and Zander, H. A. (1976) Alveolar bone regeneration after removal of inflammatory and traumatic factors. *J. Periodontol.* **47**, 687–695

Karring, T., Nyman, S., Thilander, B. and Magnusson, I. (1982) Bone regeneration in orthodontically produced alveolar bone dehiscences. *J. Periodont. Res.* **17**, 309–315

Kaufman, H., Carranza, F. A. Jr., Endres, B., Newman, M. G. and Murphy, N. (1984) The influence of trauma from occlusion on the bacterial repopulation of periodontal pockets in dogs. *J. Periodontol.* **55**, 86–92

Kennedy, J. E. and Polson, A. M. (1973) Experimental marginal periodontitis in squirrel monkeys. *J. Periodontol.* **44**, 140–144

Kerry, G. J., Morrison, E. C., Ramfjord, S. P., Hill, R. W., Caffesse, R. G., Nissle, R. R. and Appleberry, E. A. (1982) Effect of periodontal treatment on tooth mobility. *J. Periodontol.* **53**, 635–638

Klinge, B., Nilveus, R. and Egelberg, J. (1985) Effect of periodic tooth displacement on healing of experimental furcation defects in dogs. *J. Clin. Periodontol.* **12**, 239–246

Klingsberg, J., Cancellaro, L. A. and Butcher, E. O. (1961) Effects of air drying on rodent oral mucous membrane: A histologic study of simulated mouth breathing. *J. Periodontol.* **32**, 38–42

Kloehn, J. S. and Pfeifer, J. S. (1974) The effect of orthodontic treatment on the periodontium. *Angle Orthod.* **44**, 127–134

Kraal, J. H., Digiancinto, J. J., Dail, R. A., Lemmerman, K. and Peden, J. W. (1980) Periodontal conditions in patients after molar uprighting. *J. Prosthet. Dent.* **43**, 156–162

Lindhe, J. and Ericsson, I. (1976) The influence of trauma from occlusion on reduced but healthy periodontal tissues in dogs. *J. Clin. Periodontol.* **3**, 110–122

Lindhe, J. and Ericsson, I. (1982) The effect of elimination of jiggling forces on periodontally exposed teeth in the dog. *J. Periodontol.* **53**, 562–567

Lindhe, J. and Nyman, S. (1975) The effect of plaque control and surgical pocket elimination in the establishment and maintenance of periodontal health. A longitudinal study of periodontal therapy in cases of advanced disease. *J. Clin. Periodontol.* **2**, 67–79

Lindhe, J. and Svanberg, G. (1974) Influence of trauma from occlusion on progression of experimental periodontitis in the beagle dog. *J. Clin. Periodontol.* **1**, 3–14

Lite, T., Di Maio, D. J. and Burman, L. R. (1958) Gingival pathosis in mouth breathers. *Periodontia* **8**, 382–391

Lundström, F., Hamp, S. E. and Nyman, S. (1980) Systematic plaque control in children undergoing long-term orthodontic treatment. *Eur. J. Orthod.* **2**, 27–39

Macapanpan, L. C. and Weinmann, J. P. (1954) The influence of injury to the periodontal membrane on the spread of gingival inflammation. *J. Dent. Res.* **33**, 263–272

Manson, J. D. (1976) Bone morphology and bone loss in periodontal disease. *J. Clin. Periodontol.* **3**, 14–22

Manson, J. D. and Nicholson, K. (1974) The distribution of bone defects in chronic periodontitis. *J. Periodontol.* **45**, 88–92

Maynard, J. G. and Ochsenbein, C. (1975) Mucogingival problems, prevalence and therapy in children. *J. Periodontol.* **46**, 543–551

Maynard, J. G. and Wilson, R. D. K. (1980) Diagnosis and management of mucogingival problems in children. *Dent. Clin. North Am.* **24**, 683–703

Meitner, S. (1975) Co-destructive factors of marginal periodontitis and repetitive mechanical injury. *J. Dent. Res.* **54**, (Special Issue C), C78–C85

Melcher, A. H. (1976) On the repair potential of periodontal tissues. *J. Periodontol.* **47**, 256–260

Nyman, S., Karring, T and Bergenholtz, G. (1982) Bone regeneration in alveolar bone dehiscences produced by jiggling forces. *J. Periodont. Res.* **17**, 316–322

Nyman, S., Lindhe, J. and Ericsson, I. (1978) The effect of progressive tooth mobility on destructive periodontitis in the dog. *J. Clin. Periodontol.* **5**, 213–225

Parfitt, G. J. and Mjör, I. A. (1964) A clinical evaluation of local gingival recession in children. *J. Dent. Child.* 257–262

Pearson, L. E. (1968) Gingival height of lower central incisors, orthodontically treated and untreated. *Angle Orthod.* **38**, 337–339

Perrier, M. and Polson, A. (1982) The effect of progressive and increasing tooth hypermobility on reduced but healthy periodontal supporting tissues. *J. Periodontol.* **53**, 152–157

Persson, R. (1980) Assessment of tooth mobility using small loads. II. Effect of oral hygiene procedures. *J. Clin. Periodontol.* **7**, 506–515

Persson, R. (1981a) Assessment of tooth mobility using small loads. III. Effect of periodontal treatment including a gingivectomy procedure. *J. Clin. Periodontol.* **8**, 4–11

Persson, R. (1981b) Assessment of tooth mobility using small loads. IV. The effect of periodontal treatment including gingivectomy and flap procedures. *J. Clin. Periodontol.* **8**, 88–97

Pihlström, B. L., Anderson, K. A., Aeppli, D. and Scaffer, E. M. (1986) Association between signs of trauma from occlusion and periodontitis. *J. Periodontol.* **57**, 1–6

Polson, A. M. (1980) Interrelationship of inflammation and tooth mobility (trauma) in pathogenesis of periodontal disease. *J. Clin. Periodontol.* **7**, 351–360

Polson, A. M. (1984) Long-term effect of orthodontic treatment on the periodontium. In *Orthodontic Treatment and the Periodontium*, pp. 89–100. (Editors J. A. McNamara, Jr. and K. A. Ribbens). Monograph 14 Craniofacial Growth Series, Center for Human Growth and Development, The University of Michigan, Ann Arbor

Polson, A. M. (1986) The relative importance of plaque and occlusion in periodontal disease. *J. Clin. Periodontol.* **13**, 923–927

Polson, A. M. and Heijl, L. C. (1978) Osseous repair in infrabony periodontal defects. *J. Clin. Periodontol.* **5**, 13–23

Polson, A. M. and Zander, H. A. (1983) Effect of periodontal trauma upon intrabony pockets. *J. Periodontol.* **54**, 586–591

Polson, A. M. and Reed, B. E. (1984) Long-term effect of orthodontic treatment on crestal alveolar bone levels. *J. Periodontol.* **55**, 28–34

Polson, A. M., Meitner, S. W. and Zander, H. A. (1976a) Trauma and progression of marginal periodontitis in squirrel monkeys. III. Adaption of interproximal alveolar bone to repetitive injury. *J. Periodont. Res.* **11**, 279–289

Polson, A. M., Meitner, S. W. and Zander, H. A. (1976b) Trauma and progression of marginal periodontitis in squirrel monkeys. IV. Reversibility of bone loss due to trauma alone and trauma superimposed upon periodontitis. *J. Periodont. Res.* **11**, 290–298

Polson, A. M., Kantor, M. E. and Zander, H. A. (1979) Periodontal repair after reduction of inflammation. *J. Periodont. Res.* **14**, 520–525

Polson, A. M., Adams, R. A. and Zander, H. A. (1983) Osseous repair in the presence of active tooth hypermobility. *J. Clin. Periodontol.* **10**, 370–379

Polson, A. M., Caton, J., Polson, A. P. Nyman, S., Novak, J. and Reed, B. (1984) Periodontal response after tooth movement into intrabony defects. *J. Periodontol.* **55**, 197–202

Poulton, D. R. and Aaronson, S. A. (1961) The relationship between occlusion and periodontal status. *Am. J. Orthod.* **47**, 690–699

Prichard, J. F. (1967) The etiology, diagnosis and treatment of the intrabony defect. *J. Periodontol.* **38**, 455–465

Prichard, J. F. (1975) The effect of bicuspid extraction orthodontics on the periodontium. *J. Periodontol.* **46**, 534–542

Ramfjord, S. P. and Ash, M. M. M. Jr. (1981) Significance of occlusion in the etiology and treatment of early, moderate and advanced periodontitis. *J. Periodontol.* **52**, 511–517

Ramfjord, S. P., Knowles, J. W., Nissle, R. R., Shick, R. A. and Burgett, F. G. (1973) Longitudinal study of periodontal therapy. *J. Periodontol.* **44**, 66–77

Ramfjord, S. P., Knowles, J. W., Nissle, R. R., Burgett, F. G. and Shick, R. A. (1975) Results following three modalities of periodontal therapy. *J. Periodontol.* **46**, 522–526

Rateitschak, K. H. (1968) Orthodontics and periodontology. *Int. Dent. J.* **18**, 108–120

Reed, B. E., Polson, A. M. and Subtelny, J. D. (1985) Long-term periodontal status of teeth moved into extraction sites. *Am. J. Orthod.* **88**, 203–208

Reitan, K. (1957) Some factors determining the evaluation of forces in orthodontics. *Am. J. Orthod.* **43**, 32–45

Robertson, P. B., Schultz, L. D. and Levy, B. M. (1977) Occurrence and distribution of interdental gingival clefts following orthodontic movement into bicuspid extraction sites. *J. Periodontol.* **48**, 232–235

Rose, G. J. (1967) Receding mandibular labial gingiva on children. *Angle Orthod.* **37**, 147–150

Rosling, B., Nyman, S. and Lindhe, J. (1976) The effect of systematic plaque control on bone regeneration in infrabony pockets. *J. Clin. Periodontol.* **3**, 38–53

Shaw, W. C., Addy, M. and Ray, C. (1980) Dental and social effects of malocclusion and effectiveness of orthodontic treatment: a review. *Commun. Dent. Oral Epidemiol.* **8**, 36–45

Shefter, G. J. and Mcfall Jr., W. T. (1984) Occlusal relations and periodontal status in human adults. *J. Periodontol.* **55**, 368–374

Silness, J. and Røynstrand, T. (1985a) Relationship between alignment conditions of teeth in anterior segments and dental health. *J. Clin. Periodontol.* **12**, 312–320

Silness J. and Røynstrand, T. (1985b) Effects of the degree of overbite and overjet on dental health. *J. Clin. Periodontol.* **12**, 389–398

Sjølien, T. and Zachrisson, B. U. (1973) Periodontal bone support and tooth length in orthodontically treated and untreated persons. *Am. J. Orthod.* **64**, 28–37

Steiner, G. G., Pearson, J. K. and Ainamo, J. (1981) Changes of the marginal periodontium as a result of labial tooth movement in monkeys. *J. Periodontol.* **52**, 314–320

Stones, H. H. (1938) An experimental investigation into the association of traumatic occlusion with periodontal disease. *Proc. R. Soc. Med.* **31**, 479–495

Suomi, J. D. (1969) Periodontal disease and oral hygiene in an institutionalized population: report of an epidemiological study. *J. Periodontol.* **40**, 5–10

Sutcliffe, P. (1968) Chronic anterior gingivitis. An epidemiological study in school children. *Br. Dent. J.* **125**, 47–55

Svanberg, G. (1974) Influence of trauma from occlusion on the periodontium of dogs with normal or inflamed gingivae. *Odont. Revy* **25**, 165–178

Swenson, H. M. (1947) Experimental periodontal pockets in dogs. *J. Dent. Res.* **26**, 273–275

Tersin, J. (1973) Studies on gingival conditions in relation to orthodontic treatment. I. The relationship between amounts of gingival exudate and gingival scores, plaque scores and gingival pocket depths in children undergoing orthodontic treatment. *Swed. Dent. J.* **66**, 165–177

Tersin, J. (1975) Studies of gingival conditions in relation to orthodontic treatment. II. Changes in amounts of gingival exudate in relation to orthodontic treatment. *Swed. Dent. J.* **68**, 102–210

Tipnis, A. K., Slatter, J. M. and Alexander, A. G. (1971) The relationship between anterior overbite and overjet and gingival crevice depth. A pilot study of 48 individuals. *Paradontologie* **25**, 19–23

Tulloch, J. F. C. (1982) Uprighting molars as an adjunct to restorative and periodontal treatment of adults. *Br. J. Orthod.* **9**, 122–128

Vollmer, W. H. and Rateitschak, K. H. (1975) Influence of occlusal adjustment by grinding on gingivitis and mobility of traumatized teeth. *J. Clin. Periodontol.* **2**, 113–125

Waerhaug, J. (1979a) The angular bone defect and its relationship to trauma from occlusion and downgrowth of subgingival plaque. *J. Clin. Periodontol.* **6**, 61–82

Waerhaug, J. (1979b) The infrabony pocket and its relationship to trauma from occlusion and subgingival plaque. *J. Periodontol.* **50**, 355–365

Wennström, J. L., Lindhe, J., Sinclair, F. and Thilander, B. (1987) Some periodontal tissue reactions to orthodontic tooth movement in monkeys. *J. Clin. Periodontol.* **14**, 121–129

Wentz, F. M., Jarabak, J. and Orban, B. (1958) Experimental occlusal trauma imitative cuspal interferences. *J. Periodontol.* **29**, 117–127

Wingard, C. E. and Bowers, G. M. (1976) The effect on facial bone from facial tipping of incisors in monkeys. *J. Periodontol.* **47**, 450–454

Yumet, J. A. and Polson, A. M. (1985) Gingival wound healing in the presence of plaque-induced inflammation. *J. Periodontol.* **56**, 107–119

Zachrisson, B. U. (1974) Oral hygiene for orthodontic patients: Current concepts and practical advice. *Am. J. Orthod.* **66**, 487–497

Zachrisson, B. U. (1975) Iatrogenic tissue damage following orthodontic treatment: clinical and radiographic findings. In: *Transactions of the Third International Orthodontic Congress*, pp. 488–501. Crosby Lockwood Staples

Zachrisson, B. U. and Alnaes, L. (1973) Periodontal condition in orthodontically treated and untreated individuals. I. Loss of attachment, gingival pocket depth and clinical crown height. *Angle Orthod.* **43**, 402–411

Zachrisson, B. U. and Alnaes. L. (1974) Periodontal condition in orthodontically treated and untreated individuals. *Angle Orthod.* **44**, 48–55

Zachrisson, S. and Zachrisson, B. U. (1972) Gingival condition associated with orthodontic treatment. *Angle Orthod.* **42**, 26–34

34

Restorative and prosthetic implications

Restorations and the marginal periodontal tissues
Removable prostheses and the periodontium
The dilemma of tooth replacement

Root caries
References

Restorations and the marginal periodontal tissues

Introduction

The long-established practice of placing the margins of restoration subgingivally as a means of protection against caries has been challenged by the finding that the incidence of recurrent caries at subgingival crown margins (3.5% of surfaces) was no less than at supragingivally placed margins (Valderhaug and Heløe, 1977). Moreover, Valderhaug (1980) has shown, in common with many others (for review of earlier investigations see Leon, 1977, and more recently, Gorzo et al., 1979; Gullo and Powell, 1979; Rodriguez-Ferrer et al., 1980; Arneberg et al., 1980; Keszthely and Szabo, 1984; Grasso et al., 1985), that subgingival restoration margins are associated with an increased incidence of gingival inflammation and pocketing. Overhanging restoration margins have, in turn, been shown to have a similar effect. It has also been claimed that gingival inflammation related to crown margins located at the gingival margin, is more pronounced than with supragingival margins, but less than with subgingival margins (Valderhaug and Birkeland, 1976; Valderhaug and Heløe, 1977; Valderhaug, 1980; Muller, 1986). The presence of anterior interproximal restorations has been shown to result in less favourable periodontal status compared with non-restored surfaces (Silness and Røynstrand, 1984). Finally, the greater attachment losses found at restored than at non-restored surfaces (Than et al., 1982) were considered too small to be of any biological or clinical significance.

The effects of restorations

The reasons for the gingival inflammation associated with subgingival margins have been attributed to:

(1) irritation from the restorative material,
(2) increased plaque-retaining potential of the restoration itself,
(3) imperfections at the junction between the restoration and the tooth,
(4) adverse cervical contours of the restoration,
(5) open contact points.

None of the traditionally used materials (amalgam, gold, porcelain and heat-cured acrylic) have been shown to be irritating in themselves (for reviews see Leon, 1977 a; Pennel and Keagle, 1977), and the more recently introduced composite resins have also been shown to be well tolerated by the gingivae (Blank et al., 1979). Thus van Dijken et al. (1987 a) observed no clinically measurable differences in the development of plaque and gingivitis in relation to enamel and composite resin-filled surfaces in a 7-day experimental gingivitis study in humans. This was endorsed in another study (van Dijken et al., 1987 b) comparing different types of composite materials over 12 months in individuals with relatively good oral hygiene. However, as the material surfaces deteriorated and became rougher over a 3-4-year period, higher plaque and gingival index scores developed. Furthermore, although small differences have been shown in the plaque-retaining capacity of different materials (Wise and Dykeman, 1975) and in the bacterial composition on such surfaces in contact with oral mucosa (Ørstavik et al., 1981), it is

518

the presence of bacterial plaque that is essential to the production of mucosal inflammation (Silness *et al.*, 1982). Consequently, the ease with which the plaque can be removed by the patient, will determine the outcome of any relationship between restorative material and gingival tissue relationship. This depends in part upon the operator's efforts in the placement and finishing of restorations. Thus mechanical imperfections at restoration margins and over-contoured cervical restoration form, particularly at proximal surfaces, may impede plaque removal (for review see Becker and Kaldahl, 1981). The extent of the former must however be kept in perspective, for the marginal deficiencies at even clinically well-fitting amalgam of at least 25 μm as shown by Wing and Lyell (1966) and Øilo (1976) and of no less than 40 μm at castings as demonstrated by Christensen (1966), are great compared with the sizes of the microorganisms involved. The significance of this is reinforced by the microbiological findings of Lang *et al.* (1983) which suggest that marginal periodontal lesions associated with overhanging restoration margins, may be due to alterations in subgingival flora rather than plaque mass *per se*. This in turn re-emphasizes the importance of the facility with which the developing microbial flora can be disrupted by mechanical plaque-control measures.

Open contacts and food impaction have also been implicated in the development of interproximal periodontal lesions, but the relationship with periodontal disease has yet to be clearly demonstrated. Thus, for example, Gould and Picton (1966) found teeth associated with open contacts had significantly more disease than elsewhere, whereas no differences were observed by Geiger *et al.* (1974). Similarly O'Leary *et al.* (1975) reported a high percentage of open or defective contacts in periodontally healthy young adults, whilst Silness and Roynstrand (1984) found a more favourable periodontal condition at anterior proximal surfaces without interdental contact. Hancock *et al.* (1980) have in turn reported significant relationships between pocket depths and food impaction, but not open contacts *per se*, whilst Jernberg *et al.* (1983) found both food impaction and attachment losses were related to open contacts (see also Chapter 31 – Pattern of defects). These differing observations must, however, be viewed primarily in the context of the influence of these factors upon the efficacy of mechanical methods of plaque control.

The correction of defective restorations

Significant improvements in gingival inflammation and probing depths have been reported following the recontouring of defective subgingival restoration margins, in conjunction with root surface instrumentation and improved patient oral hygiene (Highfield and Powell, 1978; Gorzo *et al.*, 1979; Rodriguez-Ferrer *et al.*, 1980). The fact that less improvement in gingival inflammation occurred with improved cleaning alone, than when coupled with recontouring (Highfield and Powell, 1978), appears to substantiate the significance of overhanging margins in gingival inflammation. On the other hand, Arneberg *et al.* (1980) found that the removal of overhangs had little influence on gingivitis and pocketing. This is consistent with the findings of insignificant differences in gingivitis scores at teeth with and without overhangs (Gilmore and Sheiham, 1971), with defective and good restoration margins (Leon, 1976), and the recent observation by Grasso *et al.* (1985), that improving the quality of restorations is unlikely to lead to significant gains in periodontal health.

The extent to which overhanging subgingival margins must be smoothed, to achieve gingival health, is also not clear. Laurell *et al.* (1982) have shown that the recontouring of such amalgam edges with motor-driven diamond tips (EVA-system Dentatus Sweden), conventional diamond burs (as advocated in Part II) and finishing burs, to permit adequate oral hygiene was no less effective than the additional use of polishing methods at these sites. Clinical ease and speed of removal of amalgam and composite overhangs and the smoothness produced, was found to be greatest with diamond tips, when compared to the sonic scaler and hand curettes (Spinks *et al.*, 1986).

The above findings support the pragmatic approach advocated in Part II of attending to any less than ideal subgingival margins, so commonly encountered in clinical practice, only when they can be shown to be preventing cleaning. This, it should be recalled, is manifested by the finding of persistent gingival inflammation within the immediately adjacent tissues alone.

The relevance of approximal carious lesions in the initiation and progression of attachment loss has not been clearly established. On the one hand, Ainamo (1970) concluded that carious lesions were more destructive to the periodontium than any plaque-retentive restoration or indeed dental calculus; while, on the other, Turgeon *et al.* (1972), Leon (1977 b) and Keszthelyi *et al.* (1985) found no significant differences in attachment loss between carious and sound approximal tooth surfaces.

The effects of gingival recession

The conversion of a subgingival margin to a supragingival position by gingival recession may lead to total resolution of any associated marginal gingival inflammation in a significant number of instances (Arneberg *et al.*, 1980). This beneficial effect upon the periodontium as part of the gingival response to plaque control has been stressed in Part

II. In a 5-year retrospective study on jacket crowns fitted with subgingivally placed margins, Turner (1982) showed that the margins became supragingival at 10.6% of interproximal aspects as opposed to 32.8% and 45.9% for labial and palatal surfaces respectively. This can be explained readily by the presence of plaque-induced marginal inflammation, the local tissue morphology predisposing to gingival recession and the poor marginal fit displayed by 67.2% of crowns. This was endorsed experimentally in an animal model (Ericsson and Lindhe, 1984). Valderhaug (1980), in turn, showed that of 150 buccal crown margins located subgingivally at cementation, 60% remained so after 1 year but only 29% were subgingival at the 10-year observation stage. In contrast, Jones (1972) encountered recession after a period of 5 years at only 15.7% of crowns which had subgingival margins initially. Thus, it is apparent that gingival recession is the predominant ultimate outcome of the subgingival placement of crown margins and the patient should be advised accordingly at the outset.

The effects of operative procedures

It is clear that operative procedures can lead to irreversible damage to the marginal gingival attachment (for review see Leon, 1977). More recent histological investigations by Ruel *et al.* (1980) and Dragoo and Williams (1981) have emphasized the need for great care during both tooth preparation and gingival retraction, whether using cords (with or without caustics and astringents), copper bands or electrosurgical techniques. The destructive potential of electrosurgery in periodontics, even in experienced hands, was endorsed by the clinical findings of Simon *et al.* (1976). For review see Azzi (1983).

Restorations, pontic form and the periodontium

The questions of axial contour and of pontic design have been the subject of numerous publications, but most have been based primarily on clinical experience (for reviews see Tjan *et al.*, 1980; Becker and Kaldahl, 1981). The importance of so-called protective contours to restorations has yet to be substantiated, although the traditional concept of self-cleansing and of cleansing by fibrous foods (e.g. Lindhe and Wicén, 1969) upon which it depends, have been invalidated. Readily cleansible contours are however required, as advocated in Part II. This has been endorsed by the finding that bacterial plaque will form on all materials used for bridge pontics (Silness *et al.*, 1982) and that problems of cleansibility alone remain the essential factor in the production of subpontic mucosal inflammation. This is true also (see below) for removable partial dentures (Bates and Addy, 1978).

Silness (1974) suggested that the frequent closure of the space between pontic and mucosa is due to plaque-induced inflammation. It was also found that the pontics increased plaque retention and gingival inflammation at the adjacent abutment tooth surface which was coupled with increased pocketing when the margins of the bridge retainers were placed subgingivally. Furthermore, where the bridge design used double abutments, the related interproximal periodontal status deteriorated when compared to non-splinted contralateral control sites, in individuals cleaning ineffectively and where subgingival retainer margins existed (Silness and Ohm, 1974).

Maintenance care

The longitudinal investigation of subjects with fixed prostheses, by Nyman and Lindhe (1979) and Valderhaug (1980) revealed that acceptable levels of oral health (i.e. minimal recurrent caries and periodontal breakdown) can be maintained for long periods with a well supervised oral hygiene regimen. The techniques of plaque control in such cases have been well illustrated by Balshi and Mingledorff (1977). The interdental brush was claimed by Waerhaug (1976) to be the most efficient tool for cleaning interdental spaces related to crown and bridge work.

Prerestorative periodontal surgery

The stability of the gingival crestal tissue following prerestorative periodontal surgery is critical, particularly in relation to the cosmetic presentation of crown margins. Schluger *et al.* (1977) have advocated delaying definitive crown replacement for a 6-month period lest an unexpected degree of shrinkage occurs. In a pilot investigation, Wise (1985) recommended waiting for at least 20 weeks after surgery before preparing teeth. Further investigation appears to be necessary for a definitive answer to this question. It is of interest that Lindhe and Nyman (1980) observed a tendency for a coronal regrowth of the gingival margin (1 mm) at supragingival crown margin sites, after an initial post-surgical healing period of 2 months. The effects of the elective lengthening of clinical crowns in periodontal health to expedite restorative procedures (see Kaldahl *et al.*, 1984), appears not to have been investigated. However, clinical observations suggest a tendency for post-surgical coronal proliferation of the marginal tissues exists (*cf.* Chapter 24).

Ridge augmentation

The augmentation of edentulous mucosal ridges to improve aesthetics and to enhance pontic adaptation has been achieved by both free gingival mucosal and subepithelial grafting and with hydroxylapatite implant material (e.g. Allen *et al.*, 1985).

Removable prostheses and the periodontium

The potential for damage

The long-held clinical view that removable partial dentures (RPD) are potentially damaging to periodontal health has been demonstrated in numerous investigations (for review see Carlsson *et al.*, 1970). However, while not dismissing the physically destructive effects of poorly designed RPDs (particularly those with little or no tooth support) upon the marginal tissues and the edentulous alveolar ridges, it is quite apparent that the outcome of prosthetic treatment depends more on biologic factors (Carlsson *et al.*, 1965). The adverse effects of wearing a partial denture have been described collectively as the biological price exacted from the oral tissues (Zarb and MacKay, 1980). Furthermore, as partially edentulous individuals frequently have progressive caries and periodontal disease because of poor attitudes or motivation, any RPD fitted will be inevitably and unjustifiably indicted as having caused further tooth loss (Zarb and MacKay, 1980). Thus, Bergman *et al.* (1977) demonstrated no significant deterioration in periodontal status, over a carefully supervised 6-year period, in individuals with a high standard of oral hygiene and well-designed RPDs. In addition, the number of new carious lesions was low. It was concluded that the widely accepted yet unproven opinion that RPDs *per se* will cause periodontal and carious lesions, could not be supported. This has been reinforced by the findings of Wilding and Reddy (1987).

Plaque retentive potential

Bates and Addy (1978) showed that RPDs worn by day only, or both day and night, did increase plaque accumulation significantly, compared with wearing no denture. This endorsed the view that RPDs are best restricted to those with satisfactory levels of oral hygiene and that such dentures should be as simple in design as possible, covering only essential hard and soft tissues. Where gingival margins are covered, relief is advocated by some (Bissada *et al.*, 1974; Bates and Addy, 1978), while others (Hobkirk and Strahan, 1979) advise the closest possible adaptation. Bissada *et al.* (1974) have demonstrated that acrylic resin denture bases led to greater gingival inflammation than metal, but little work has been undertaken in this field. It would seem possible that such tissue reaction is related primarily to an incidental plaque accumulation, for no evidence was found by Silness *et al.* (1982) to support the

superiority of any one material over another in avoiding inflammation. The recent renewed interest in overdentures (Davis *et al.*, 1981), coupled with the difficulties anticipated in plaque control at root stumps located level with the gingival margins, means that new and so far uninvestigated problems in maintenance therapy will arise.

The dilemma of tooth replacement

The traditional view that extracted teeth should be replaced demands re-evaluation (Zarb and MacKay, 1980). In this context, the statement by DeVan (1952) that: 'Our objective should be the perpetual preservation of what remains, rather than the meticulous restoration of what is missing' is salutory.

The risks of non-replacement

There has been surprisingly little attention to the effects of not replacing missing teeth. Both drifting and supra-eruption of posterior teeth into edentulous spaces are often encountered but the reasons for these changes have been inadequately investigated. Thus, Love and Adams (1971) showed that tooth movements are not only smaller than is commonly anticipated but are neither inevitable nor predictable. Waerhaug (1968) claimed that drifting is unlikely if the tissues are maintained free of inflammation, although this has neither been substantiated nor disproved. In another investigation, Silness *et al.* (1973) found reduced plaque accumulation, gingival inflammation and pocket depths, but less supporting bone, distal to pre-molar teeth following the loss of their distal neighbouring units, than at contralateral premolars in a continuous arch. Finally, the findings of Käyser (1975) and Battistuzzi *et al.* (1987) showed non-replacement of missing teeth to be of minimal clinical significance and that the decision to replace such teeth is best dictated by individual aesthetic and functional needs.

Fixed versus removable prostheses

This issue has been poorly investigated although numerous papers based on clinical impressions and opinions have been published. It does appear that while patient comfort, function and psychological considerations play a major role in these clinical decisions, economic implications will frequently dictate the final outcome.

The replacement of missing units, where retained teeth have markedly reduced support and demonstrate increasing mobility, is best accomplished by fixed prostheses (Lungren *et al.*, 1975; Nyman and Ericsson, 1982). This is because the bridge is considered more rigid and may provide more favourable distribution of the mastication forces over the remaining periodontium (Nyman and Lindhe, 1979). The designs of these fixed prostheses have furthermore questioned the traditionally accepted principles (Tylman and Tylman, 1960; Johnson *et al.*, 1971; Tylman and Malone, 1978), the most important of which, according to Johnson *et al.* (1971), being that abutment teeth in fixed bridgework must not only be favourably distributed, but their crown–root ratio or periodontal support should satisfy the criteria of the so-called 'Ante's Law' (Ante, 1938). Thus, Nyman and Ericsson (1982) reported on a random sample of 60 complex bridges in which 'Ante's Law' was satisfied in only 8% of instances and 57% of the bridge abutments had less than 50% of the support so demanded. Yet despite this, all the bridges which had been constructed 8-11 years previously based on alternative principles described by Nyman *et al.* (1975), Lindhe and Nyman (1975, 1977) and Nyman and Lindhe (1977), functioned properly without further loss of periodontal support.

The limitations for fixed bridgework in such cases appear to be related to technical and biomechanical problems in bridge construction (see Glantz and Nyman, 1983), rather than the biological capacity of the remaining periodontium to support bridges successfully (e.g. Karlsson, 1986; Randow *et al.*, 1986). Investigations analysing the relationships between occlusal force patterns during chewing and biting, and reduced periodontal support (Laurell and Lundgren, 1984, 1986; Lundgren and Laurell, 1984, 1986 a and b) have however indicated the possible risks of traumatic periodontal destruction, as a result of the intense and undue forces produced by bruxism and other parafunctions, and of fracture of abutments and cementation failure. In this context, the finding that non-vital teeth withstand higher cantilever load levels than vital teeth before causing periodontal pain, may lead to systematic relative occlusal overloading and, in turn, contribute to the higher frequency of fractures of the reconstructions, teeth and luting cements observed when distal abutment teeth were non-vital (Randow *et al.*, 1986). Bergenholtz and Nyman (1984) have revealed that pulpal necrosis, including periapical lesions, developed with a significantly higher frequency (15% versus 3%) in abutment teeth than in non-abutment teeth. This might stem from the extensive coronal tooth preparation to ensure optimal mechanical retention (Randow *et al.*, 1986).

Endosseous implants

Although dental implantology has been practised for some years, with the osseo-integration technique (Review: Adell *et al.*, 1981) most favoured, the periodontal implications have received little attention. Thus, for example only in 1986 have the requirements for Advanced Speciality Education Programs in Periodontics, as approved by the Commission on Dental Accreditation of the American Dental Association, incorporated the provision of instruction in the use of dental implants (see Meffert, 1986). The materials and methods used have been briefly reviewed by Meffert (1986) whilst stressing the importance of continuing research in this promising treatment modality. Smithloff and Fritz (1987) showed that bladevent endosteal implants can be maintained for up to 15 years with clinically insignificant levels of peri-implant disease, probably analogous to periodontal disease around natural teeth, occurring in about half the implants. It does appear that significant differences exist in the biomechanical conditions, but not in functional and tissue reactions, about osseo-integrated titanium fixtures and natural teeth when used as combined abutments for fixed-bridge restoorations (Ericsson *et al.*, 1986). Furthermore, Lekholm *et al.* (1986) demonstrated that in patients enrolled in a strict maintenance care programme, healthy conditions as determined microbiologically and histologically prevailed at both tooth and fixture abutments.

Root caries

An increasing proportion of elderly individuals in the population coupled with improved dental care, means that a new and progressively enlarging cohort of dental patients is developing. Many of these will have exposed root surfaces which present a greater risk for root caries. These patients thus represent a potentially major therapeutic problem.

Research into the aetiology, epidemiology and pathogenesis of root caries is rather limited. (Review: Nyvad and Fejerskov, 1982.) The lesions are most frequently encountered on approximal and buccal surfaces. They are yellowish and softened in active stages but become darkly stained and regain a hard texture during passive stages. Root caries appears typically as a superficial spreading lesion with a depth of only 0.5–1.0 mm. Microradiographically, the early lesion is similar to that occurring in enamel, presenting as a radiolucency deep to a hypermineralized surface zone of cementum. Bacterial penetration of dentinal tubules takes place early in the carious process but tends not to extend deeply and only progresses at a slow rate with minor accompanying pulpal change. No specific microorganism species, such as the *Streptococcus* and *Lactobacillus* species implicated in enamel caries, have been incriminated convincingly in root caries although the *Actinomyces* species have attracted considerable interest.

The prevalence of root caries is difficult to

establish because of the extreme diversity of the population samples studied and differences in the methods of assessment. It does, however, appear that the proportion of subjects affected by root surface caries increases with age. The optimal preventive methods for root caries have also not been established, although in common with enamel caries prevention, the importance of plaque removal has been cited. Thus, Lindhe and Nyman (1975) have shown that frequent professional cleaning, coupled with a high standard of plaque control is capable of almost totally preventing the development of root surface caries. Similarly, Ravald and Hamp (1981) reported new caries lesions in only 5% of exposed root surfaces following an extensive preventive programme over a 4-year observation period. The latter workers nevertheless concluded, in accord with the findings of Hix and O'Leary (1976), that oral hygiene status was not a reliable indicator of the likelihood of root surface caries and would in turn question the viability of an improved plaque control regime as a population strategy in the control of root caries. A strong correlation has been shown with previous root surface caries and low salivary secretion rates (Ravald and Hamp, 1981), whilst Banting *et al.* (1980) demonstrated a relationship between previous coronal caries and subsequent root surface caries incidence in the individual. Furthermore, Nyvad and Fejerskov (1982) concluded that 'root caries susceptibility is not related to unknown variations in tooth resistance or the presence of specific bacteria, but should rather be sought in a combination of dietary habits, quality of plaque removal and salivary flow rate.' Finally, Ravald *et al.* (1986) evaluated root surface caries 8 years following periodontal therapy. They observed not only considerable differences between the subjects in the possible variables cited in root caries, but also that no single variable could be incriminated in all the subjects. Further investigation of these variables is obviously necessary.

The role of fluorides in prevention and treatment of root caries also remains unclear although Fejerskov *et al.* (1981) concluded that its cariostatic action can be ascribed almost entirely to its topical effect of the ongoing caries processes. The use of topical fluoride plus dietary sugar control would seem to be the most efficient way of treating subclinical or established root caries, thereby preventing further development of the lesions (see Nyvad and Fejerskov, 1982). It is possible to reharden even extensive active root caries lesions and so avoid the need to restore such surfaces. Professionally applied fluoride varnishes (but not acidulated gel which may decalcify the root surface) or aqueous solutions of sodium fluoride for mouth rinses (0.05% for daily use or 0.2% solution for weekly use) would seem most appropriate.

The restoration of root caries is fraught with difficulties. These relate to problems of access, particularly at lesions within furcations which may be impossible to restore. Other difficulties are the establishment of well-defined cavity margins due to the extensive and uneven distribution of the lesions, the proximity of the pulp within the involved roots, and difficulties of removing the excess restorative material from the marginal areas due to the root surface anatomy. The last might in turn preclude subsequent plaque control and perpetuate periodontal lesions. The problem of marginal leakage with amalgam and composite fillings also exists. Glass ionomer cements appear to be promising (Munksgaard *et al.*, 1984; McLean *et al.*, 1985), but are complicated by the difficulties of moisture control during setting. The slow release of fluoride from the intrinsically high levels present within these cements, may also prove to be advantageous in preventing secondary caries.

References

Adell, R., Lekholm, U., Rockler, B. and Branemark, P-I. (1981) A 15-year study of osseointegrated implants in the treatment of the edentulous jaw. *Int. J. Oral Surg.* **10**, 387–416

Ainamo, J. (1970) Concomitant periodontal disease and dental caries in young adult males. *Suomen Hammaslääkäriseuran Toimituksia* **66**, 301–364

Allen, E. P., Gainza, C. S., Farthing, G. G. and Newbold, D. A. (1985) Improved technique for localized ridge augmentation. A report of 21 cases. *J. Periodontol.* **56**, 195–199

Ante, I. H. (1938) The fundamental principles, design and construction of bridge prosthesis. *Can. Dent. Assoc.* **10**, 1–9

Arneberg, P., Silness, J. and Nordbø, H. (1980) Marginal fit and cervical extent of class II amalgam restorations related to periodontal condition. *J. Periodont. Res.* **15**, 669–677

Azzi, R., Kenney, E. B., Tsao, T. F. and Carranza, F. A. Jr. (1983) The effect of electrosurgery on alveolar bone. *J. Periodontol.* **54**, 96–100

Balshi, T. J. and Mingledorff, E. B. (1977) Maintenance procedures for patients after complete fixed prosthodontics. *J. Prosthet. Dent.* **37**, 420–431

Banting, D. W., Ellen, R. P. and Fillery, E. D. (1980) Prevalence of root surface caries among institutionalized older persons. *Community Dent. Oral Epidemiol.* **8**, 84–88

Bates, J. F. and Addy, M. (1978) Partial dentures and plaque accumulation. *J. Dent.* **6**, 285–293

Battistuzzi, P., Käyser, A. and Kanters, N. (1987) Partial edentulism, prosthetic treatment and oral function in a Dutch population. *J. Oral Rehabil.* **14**, 549–555

Becker, C. M. and Kaldahl, W. B. (1981) Current theories of crown contour, margin placement, and pontic design. *J. Prosthet. Dent.* **45**, 268–277

Bergenholtz, G. and Nyman, S. (1984) Endodontic complications following periodontal and prosthetic treatment of patients with advanced periodontal diseaase. *J. Periodontol.* **55**, 63–68

Bergman, B. B., Hugoson, A. and Olsson, C-O. (1977) Caries and periodontal status in patients fitted with removable partial dentures. *J. Clin. Periodontol.* **4**, 134–146

Bissada, N. F., Ibrahim, S. I. and Barsoum, W. M. (1974) Gingival response to various types of removable partial dentures. *J. Periodontol.* **45**, 651–659

Blank, L. W., Caffesse, R. G. and Charbeneau, G. T. (1979) The gingival response to well-finished composite resin restorations. *J. Prosthet. Dent.* **42**, 626–632

Carlsson, G. E., Hedegard, B. and Koivumaa, K. K. (1965) Studies in partial dental prosthesis. *Acta Odontol. Scand.* **23**, 443–472

Carlsson, G. E., Hedegard, B. and Koivumaa, K. K. (1970) The current place of removable partial dentures in restorative dentistry. *Dent. Clin. North Am.* **14**, 553–568

Christensen, G. J. (1966) Marginal fit of gold inlay castings. *J. Prosthet. Dent.* **16**, 297–305

Davis, R. K., Renner, R. P., Antos, E. W. Jr., Schlissel, E. R. and Baer, P. N. A two-year longitudinal study of the periodontal health status of overdenture patients. *J. Prosthet. Dent.* **45**, 358–363

DeVan, M. M. (1952) The nature of the partial denture foundation: Suggestions for its preservation. *J. Prosthet. Dent.* **2**, 210–218

Dragoo, M. R. and Williams, G. B. (1981) Periodontal tissue reactions to restorative procedures. *Int. J. Periodont. Rest. Dent.* **1**, 9–23

Ericsson, I. and Lindhe, J. (1984) Recession in sites with inadequate width of keratinized gingiva. *J. Clin. Periodontol.* **11**, 95–103

Ericsson, I., Lekholm, U., Branemark, P-I., Lindhe, J., Glantz, P-O. and Nyman, S. (1986) A clinical evaluation of fixed bridge restorations supported by the combination of teeth and osseointegrated titanium implants. *J. Clin. Periodontol.* **13**, 307–312

Fejerskov, O., Thylstrup, A. and Larsen, M. (1981) Rational use of fluorides in caries prevention. *Acta Odontol. Scand.* **39**, 241–255

Geiger, A. M., Wasserman, B. H. and Turgeon, L. R. (1974) Relationship of occlusion and periodontal disease. Part VIII. Relationship of crowding and spacing to periodontal destruction and gingival inflammation. *J. Periodontol.* **45**, 43–49

Gilmore, N. and Sheiham, A. (1971) Overhanging dental restorations and periodontal disease. *J. Periodontol.* **42**, 8–12

Glantz, P. and Nyman, S. (1983) Technical and biophysical aspects of crown and bridge therapy in patients with reduced amounts of periodontal tissue support. In *Textbook of Clinical Periodontology*, pp. 466–479. (Editor Lindhe, J.). Munksgaard, Copenhagen

Gorzo, I., Newman, H. N. and Strahan, J. D. (1979) Amalgam restorations, plaque removal and periodontal health. *J. Clin. Periodontol.* **6**, 98–105

Gould, M. S. E. and Picton, D. C. A. (1966) The relation between irregularities of the teeth and periodontal disease. A pilot study. *Br. Dent. J.* **121**, 20–23

Grasso, J. E., Nalbandian, J., Sanford, C. and Bailit, H. (1985) Effect of restoration quality on periodontal health. *J. Prosthet. Dent.* **53**, 14–19

Gullo, C. A. O. and Powell, R. N. (1979) The effect of placement of cervical margins of class II amalgam restorations on plaque accumulation and gingival health. *J. Oral Rehabil.* **6**, 317–322

Hancock, E. B., Mayo, C. V., Schwab, R. R. and Wirthlin, M. R. (1980) Influence of interdental contacts on periodontal status. *J. Periodontol.* **51**, 445–449

Highfield, J. E. and Powell, R. N. (1978) Effects of removal of posterior overhanging metallic margins of restorations upon the periodontal tissues. *J. Clin. Periodontol.* **5**, 169–181

Hix, J. O. III and O'Leary, T. J. (1976) The relationship between cemental caries, oral hygiene status and fermentable carbohydrate intake. *J. Periodontol.* **47**, 398–404

Hobkirk, J. A. and Strahan, J. D. (1979) The influence on the gingival tissues of prostheses incorporating gingival relief areas. *J. Dent.* **7**, 15–21

Jernberg, G. R., Bakdash, M. B. and Keenan, K. M. (1983) Relationship between proximal tooth open contacts and periodontal disease. *J. Periodontol.* **54**, 529–533

Johnston, J. F., Philips, R. W. and Dykema, R. W. (1971) *Modern Practice in Crown and Bridge Prosthodontics*, 3rd Edition. W. B. Saunders Co., Philadelphia, London, Toronto

Jones, J. C. G. (1972) The success rate of anterior crowns. *Br. Dent. J.* **132**, 399–403

Kaldahl, W. B., Becker, C. M. and Wentz, F. M. (1984) Periodontal surgical preparation for specific problems in restorative dentistry. *J. Prosthet. Dent.* **51**, 36–41

Karlsson, S. (1986) A clinical evaluation of fixed bridges, 10 years following insertion. *J. Oral Rehabil.* **13**, 423–432

Käyser, A. F. (1975) Shortened tooth arches and oral functions. A clinical investigation of 118 adults. Thesis, University of Nijmegen

Keszthelyi, G. and Szabo, I. (1984) Influence of class II amalgam fillings on attachment loss. *J. Clin. Periodont.* **11**, 81–86

Keszthelyi, G., Szabo, I. and Strahan, J. D. (1985) Loss of attachment adjacent to class II carious lesions. *J. Clin. Periodont.* **12**, 405–410

Lang, N. P., Kiel, R. A. and Anderhalden, K. (1983) Clinical and microbiological effects of subgingival restorations with overhanging or clinically perfect margins. *J. Clin. Periodont.* **10**, 563–578

Laurell, L. and Lundgren, D. (1985) Periodontal ligament areas and occlusal forces in dentitions restored with cross-arch bilateral end abutment bridges. *J. Clin. Periodont.* **12**, 850–860

Laurell, L. and Lundgren, D. (1986) Periodontal ligament areas and occlusal forces in dentitions restored with cross-arch unilateral posterior two-unit cantilever bridges. *J. Clin. Periodont.* **13**, 33–38

Laurell, L., Rylander, H. and Pettersson, B. (1982) The effect of different levels of polishing of amalgam restorations on the plaque retention and gingival inflammation. *Swed. Dent. J.* (Suppl.). **12**, 45–53

Lekholm, U., Ericsson, I., Adell, R. and Slots, J. (1986) The condition of the soft tissues at tooth and fixture abutments supporting fixed bridges. A microbiological and histological study. *J. Clin. Periodontol.* **13**, 558–562

Leon, A. R. (1976) Amalgam restorations and periodontal disease. *Br. Dent. J.* **140**, 377–382

Leon, A. R. (1977a) The effect of approximal carious lesions on the periodontium. *Br. Dent. J.* **143**, 18–21

Leon, A. R. (1977b) The periodontium and restorative procedures. A critical review. *J. Oral Rehabil.* **4**, 105–117

Lindhe, J. and Nyman, S. (1975) The effect of plaque control and surgical pocket elimination on the establishment and maintenance of periodontal health. A longitudinal study of periodontal therapy in cases of advanced disease. *J. Clin. Periodontol.* **2**, 67–79

Lindhe, J. and Nyman, S. (1977) The role of occlusion in periodontal disease and the biological rationale for splinting in treatment of periodontitis. *Oral Sci. Rev.* **10**, 11–43

Lindhe, J. and Nyman, S. (1980) Alterations of the position of the marginal soft tissue following periodontal surgery. *J. Clin. Periodontol.* **7**, 525–530

Lindhe, J. and Wicén, P. O. (1969) The effects on the gingiva of chewing fibrous foods. *J. Periodont. Res.* **4**, 193–201

Love, W. D. and Adams, R. L. (1971) Tooth movement into edentulous areas. *J. Prosthet. Dent.* **25**, 271–277

Lundgren, D. and Laurell, L. (1984) Occlusal forces in prosthetically restored dentitions: a methodological study. *J. Oral Rehabil.* **11**, 29–37

Lundgren, D. and Laurell, L. (1986a) Occlusal force pattern during chewing and biting in dentisions restored with fixed bridges of cross-arch extention. I. Bilateral end abutment bridges. *J. Oral Rehabil.* **13**, 57–71

Lundgren, D. and Laurell, L. (1986b) Occlusal force pattern during chewing and biting in dentisions restored with fixed bridges of cross-arch extension. II. Unilateral posterior two-unit cantilever bridges. *J. Oral Rehabil.* **13**, 191–203

Lundgren, D., Nyman, S., Heijl, L. and Carlsson, G. E. (1975) Functional analysis of fixed bridges on abutment teeth with reduced periodontal support. *J. Oral Rehabil.* **2**, 105–116

McLean, J. W., Powis, D. R., Prosser, H. J. and Wilson, A. D. (1985) The use of glass-ionomer cements in bonding composite resins to dentine. *Br. Dent. J.* **158**, 410–414

Meffert, R. M. (1986) Endosseous dental implantology from the periodontist's viewpoint. *J. Periodontol.* **57**, 531–536

Müller, H.-P. (1986) The effects of artificial crown margins at the gingival margin on the periodontal conditions in a group of periodontally supervised patients treated with fixed bridges. *J. Clin. Periodontol.* **13**, 97–102

Munksgaard, E. C., Hansen, E. K. and Asmussen, E. (1984) Effect of five adhesives on adaptation of resin in dentin cavities. *Scand. J. Dent. Res.* **92**, 544–548

Nyman, S. and Ericsson, I. (1982) The capacity of reduced periodontal tissues to support fixed bridgework. *J. Clin. Periodontol.* **9**, 409–414

Nyman, S. and Lindhe, J. (1977) Considerations on the design of occlusion in prosthetic rehabilitation of patients with advanced periodontal disease. *J. Clin. Periodontol.* **4**, 1–15

Nyman, S. and Lindhe, J. (1979) A longitudinal study of combined periodontal and prosthetic treatment of patients with advanced periodontal disease. *J. Periodontol.* **50**, 163–169

Nyman, S., Lindhe, J. and Lundgren, D. (1975) The role of occlusion for the stability of fixed bridges in patients with reduced periodontal tissue support. *J. Clin. Periodontol.* **2**, 53–66

Nyvad, B. and Fejerskov, O. (1982) Roof surface caries, clinical, histopathological and microbiological features and clinical implications. *Int. Dent. J.* **32**, 311–326

Øilo, G. (1976) Adaptation of amalgams to cavity walls. *J. Oral Rehabil.* **3**, 227–236

O'Leary, T. J. Baudell, M. C. and Bloomer, R. S. (1975) Interproximal contact and marginal ridge relationships in periodontally healthy young males classified as to orthodontic status. *J. Periodontol.* **46**, 6–9

Ørstavik, D., Arneberg, P. and Valderhaug, J. (1981) Bacterial growth on dental restorative materials in mucosal contact. *Acta Odontol. Scand.* 267–274

Pennel, B. M. and Keagle, J. G. (1977) Predisposing factors in the etiology of chronic inflammatory periodontal disease. *J. Periodontol.* **48**, 517–532

Randow, K., Glantz, P-O. and Zöger, B. (1986) Technical failures and some related clinical complications in extensive fixed prosthodontics. *Acta Odontol. Scand.* **44**, 241–245

Ravald, N. and Hamp, S-E. (1981) Prediction of root surface caries in patients treated for advanced periodontal disease. *J. Clin. Periodontol.* **8**, 400–414

Ravald, N., Hamp, S-E. and Birkhed, D. (1986) Long-term evaluation of root surface caries in periodontally treated patients. *J. Clin. Periodontol.* **13**, 758–767

Rodriguez-Ferrer, H. J., Strahan, J. D. and Newman, H. N. (1980) Effect on gingival health of removing overhanging margins of interproximal subgingival amalgam restorations. *J. Clin. Periodontol.* **7**, 457–462

Ruel, J., Schuessler, P. J., Malament, K. and Mori, D. (1980) Effect of retraction procedures on the periodontium in humans. *J. Prosthet. Dent.* **44**, 508–515

Schluger, S., Yuodelis, R. A. and Page, R. C. (1977)

Periodontal Disease, pp. 661–665. Lea & Febiger, Philadelphia

Silness, J. (1974) Periodontal conditions in patients treated with dental bridges. *J. Periodont. Res.* **9**, 50–55

Silness, J. and Ohm, E. (1974) Periodontal conditions in patients treated with dental bridges. *J. Periodont. Res.* **9**, 121–126

Silness, J. and Røynstrand, T. (1984) Effects on dental health of spacing of teeth in anterior segments. *J. Clin. Periodontol.* **11**, 387–398

Silness, J., Gustavsen, F. and Mangersnes, K. (1982) The relationship between pontic hygiene and mucosal inflammation in fixed bridge recipients. *J. Periodont. Res.* **17**, 434–439

Silness, J., Hunsbeth, J. and Figenschou, B. (1973) Effects of tooth loss on the periodontal condition of neighbouring teeth. *J. Periodont. Res.* **8**, 237–242

Simon, B. I., Schuback, P., Deasy, M. J. and Kelner, R. M. (1976) The destructive potential of electrosurgery on the periodontium. *J. Periodontol.* **47**, 342–347

Smithloff, M. and Fritz, M. E. (1987) The use of blade implants in a selected population of partially edentulous adults. *J. Periodontol.* **58**, 589–593

Spinks, G. C., Carson, R. E., Hancock, E. B. and Pelleu, G. B. Jr. (1986) An SEM study of overhang removal methods. *J. Periodontol.* **57**, 632–636

Than, A., Duguid, R. and McKendrick, A. J. W. (1982) Relationship between restorations and the level of the periodontal attachment. *J. Clin. Periodontol.* **9**, 193–202

Tjan, A. H. L., Freed, H. and Miller, G. D. (1980) Current controversies in axial contour design. *J. Prosthet. Dent.* **44**, 536–540

Turgeon, J., Le May, L. P. and Cleroux, R. (1972) Periodontal effects of restoring proximal tooth surfaces with amalgam: a clinical evaluation in children. *Can. Dent. Assoc. J.* **38**, 255–256

Turner, C. H. (1982) A retrospective study of the fit of jacket crowns placed around gold posts and cores, and the associated gingival health. *J. Oral Rehabil.* **9**, 427–434

Tylman, S. D. and Malone, W. F. P. (1978) *Theory and Practice of Fixed Prosthodontics,* 7th Edition. C. V. Mosby Co., St Louis, MO

Tylman, S. D. and Tylman, S. G. (1960) *Theory and Practice of Crown and Bridge Prosthodontics,* 4th Edition. C. V. Mosby Co., St Louis, MO

Valderhaug, J. (1980) Periodontal conditions and carious lesions following the insertion of fixed prostheses: a 10-year follow-up study. *Int. Dent. J.* **30**, 296–304

Valderhaug, J. and Birkeland, J. M. (1976) Periodontal conditions in patients 5 years following insertion of fixed prostheses. *J. Oral Rehabil.* **3**, 237–243

Valderhaug, J. and Heløe, L. A. (1977) Oral hygiene in a group of supervised patients with fixed prostheses. *J. Periodontol.* **48**, 221–224

van Dijken, J. W. V., Sjöström, S. and Wing, K. (1987a) The effect of different types of composite resin fillings on marginal gingiva. *J. Clin. Periodontol.* **14**, 185–189

van Dijken, J. W. V., Sjöström, S. and Wing, K. (1987b) Development of initial gingivitis around different types of composite resin. *J. Clin. Periodontol.* **14**, 257–260

Waerhaug, J. (1968) Periodontology and partial prosthesis. *Int. Dent. J.* **18**, 101–107

Waerhaug, J. (1976) The interdental brush and its place in operative and crown and bridge dentistry. *J. Oral Rehabil.* **3**, 107–113

Wilding, R. J. C. and Reddy, J. (1987) Periodontal disease in partial denture wearers – a biological index. *J. Oral Rehabil.* **14**, 111–124

Wing, G. and Lyell, J. S. (1966) The marginal seal of amalgam restorations. *Aust. Dent. J.* **11**, 81–86

Wise, M. D. (1985) Stability of gingival crest after surgery and before anterior crown placement. *J. Prosthet. Dent.* **53**, 20–23

Wise, M. D. and Dykema, R. W. (1975) The plaque-retaining capacity of four dental materials. *J. Prosthet. Dent.* **33**, 178–190

Zarb, G. A. and MacKay, H. F. (1980) The partially edentulous patient. I. The biologic price of prosthodontic intervention. *Aust. Dent. J.* **25**, 63–68

35

Chemical plaque control

M. Addy

Introduction

The association of bacteria with periodontal diseases (Review: Helderman and van Palenstein, 1981) is by no means a modern concept and the non-specific plaque hypothesis dates back to the end of the nineteenth century. Perhaps not surprisingly, therefore, references to the use of a variety of chemicals for the control of periodontal disease may be found around this time (Review: Gold, 1985). Some compounds, notably acids and alkalis, clearly had the potential to produce more harm than good to the teeth and supporting structures. Nevertheless, antiseptic formulations were proposed specifically to remove or destroy pathogenic organisms from the supra- and subgingival areas. Unfortunately, as with virtually all supposedly therapeutic agents, no attempt was made to determine efficacy scientifically. Recommendations for use were based only on subjective clinical impressions.

The late 1960s saw a considerable renewal of interest in chemical plaque control of periodontal disease, which has persisted to date. Several factors appear responsible for the extensive research efforts in this field. Firstly, the convincing evidence for the major aetiological role of bacterial plaque in the development of chronic gingivitis (Löe et al., 1965). Secondly, the association of microorganisms with the advancing lesions of chronic periodontitis (Reviews: Socransky, 1977; Slots, 1979; Tanner et al., 1984). Thirdly, the observation that many individuals appear unable to maintain, by mechanical methods, a level of oral hygiene consistent with gingival health. In this latter respect, many attempts have been made to improve techniques of oral hygiene instruction and the aids used for tooth cleaning. There is little evidence to indicate that any one technique or tooth cleaning aid has advantages over another (Sheiham, 1977). If improvements in oral hygiene are to be obtained they will be dependent upon improved performance by people using any of the accepted methods of oral hygiene aids (Frandsen, 1986).

Chemical plaque control measures appear to hold promise as adjuncts to toothbrushing by overcoming some of the deficiencies of mechanical methods. In theory chemical plaque control could be used as an alternative to mechanical methods but to date no one, totally satisfactory, compound has been discovered. For the purpose of discussion, as with mechanical cleaning, chemical plaque control will be considered under two headings, namely (1) supragingival plaque control for the prevention of disease or treatment of early gingivitis where there is little or no deepening of the gingival crevice, and (2) subgingival plaque control for the treatment of established disease. Further subdivision of chemical plaque control can be made, depending whether the agent is delivered locally or systemically.

However, with few exceptions, the systemic use of antiplaque agents at the present time for the treatment of chronic periodontal disease, and more particularly the prevention of chronic gingivitis, is open to question and criticism (Genco, 1981). Most advantages of such an approach appear to be outweighed by the potential disadvantages, particularly in respect of the systemic antimicrobial drugs. Attention has, therefore, been directed at the local delivery of compounds to the supra- and subgingival areas.

Supragingival plaque control

The mode of action of compounds used for the chemical inhibition of plaque formation on a tooth surface may be considered under three headings, accepting that for individual compounds, overlap in the mode of action may occur: (1) antimicrobial effect, (2) alteration of plaque biochemistry, (3) alteration of tooth surfaces to prevent bacterial adhesion.

In evaluating the literature on antiplaque agents or the claims made for various compounds it is important to appreciate that chemical agents may have quantitative or qualitative effects. Thus quantitative reductions in plaque by chemicals may not necessarily be sufficient to reduce disease. Conversely, alterations in plaque pathogenicity by chemicals may not be reflected in a reduction in the measurable amounts of plaque present.

Antiplaque agents

Of the very large range of compounds studied, most attention and most success has been with those achieving an effect mediated primarily by an antimicrobial action (Reviews: Hull, 1980; Kornman, 1985). Many were of interest for a possible role in preventing caries but also showed plaque inhibitory effects and reductions in gingivitis.

Antibiotics

A number of antibiotics used topically or systemically have been studied for effects on dental disease. These have included penicillin, vancomycin, kanamycin, erythromycin, niddomycin and spiromycin. Reductions in plaque and gingivitis have been reported, as well as beneficial effects on caries increments (Review: Shankwalker, 1975). However, the risk of resistant organisms, candidal suprainfection or patient hypersensitivity reactions must preclude the routine or long-term use of systemic and more particularly topical antibiotics for supragingival plaque control in the prevention and treatment of chronic gingivitis.

Enzymes

To date, two interesting and quite different approaches for plaque inhibition by enzymes have been considered. The first is the interference with bacterial attachment mechanisms to prevent adherence of the initial plaque-forming bacteria to the tooth surface or to disaggregate established plaque. Based on this attractive concept, proteolytic enzymes and enzymes directed at the bacterial insoluble extracellular polysaccharides (Robinson *et al.*, 1975) for example, dextranase and mutanase (Lobene, 1971) were used. However, the results were disappointing and convincingly effective formulations are still awaited. Side effects, particularly erosion of the oral mucosa, also were noted with some topically applied formulations.

The second concept is the use of enzymes to potentiate the naturally present antimicrobial activity of saliva. Under normal circumstances, lactoperoxidase in saliva catalyses, with the aid of hydrogen peroxide produced by bacteria, the formation of hypothiocyanite from salivary thiocyanate (Hoogendoorn *et al.*, 1977). Hypothiocyanite is claimed to have a significant effect upon bacterial growth. Potentiation of the salivary lactoperoxidase system has been attempted using the enzymes amyloglucosidase and glucose oxidase, to produce sufficient hydrogen peroxide in saliva to activate the lactoperoxidase system. Such chemical reactions have been demonstrated in the laboratory (Hoogendoorn and Moorer, 1973) but not in the mouth. Clinical evidence for beneficial effects on plaque, gingivitis and caries of a toothpaste containing the enzyme system, is inconclusive and contradictory. The effects in reducing caries are also confused by the presence of fluoride in the toothpaste formulation.

Antiseptics

Bisbiguanides

The most encouraging findings for the chemical inhibition of supragingival plaque have been derived from studies of various antiseptics. In 1970 it was reported that, in the absence of mechanical plaque control, a twice daily rinse with 10 ml of 0.2% chlorhexidine gluconate prevented plaque formation and the development of chronic gingivitis (Löe and Schiott, 1970). Numerous investigations into the use of antiseptics have been carried out since, which indicate that chlorhexidine is the most effective of the available antiseptics (Reviews: Gjermo, 1974; Hull, 1980), despite the fact that many possess equivalent or superior antibacterial activity (Gjermo *et al.*, 1970). A number of bisbiguanide antiseptics, other than chlorhexidine, also possess considerable antiplaque activity (Gjermo *et al.*, 1973). The most recently studied have been alexidine and octenidine but data on clinical effects and safety for prolonged use is very limited by comparison with chlorhexidine. The mode of action of chlorhexidine is attributable to the dicationic nature of the molecule. This enables the antiseptic, as with other bisbiguanides, to adsorb to oral surfaces from which they exert a prolonged bacteriostatic effect (Rolla and Melsen, 1975).

Unfortunately, despite freedom from systemic side effects, chlorhexidine produces local effects which, although not serious, reduce acceptability to individual users (Flotra *et al.*, 1971). Firstly, it has an unpleasant taste which cannot totally be masked by flavouring agents and in some individuals alters taste sensation. Secondly, and perhaps more importantly, chlorhexidine results for many individuals, in a brown discoloration of the teeth and dorsum of the tongue. Some controversy exists concerning the aetiology of the staining (Review: Eriksen *et al.,* 1985). However, the importance of chromogenic factors derived from the diet and precipitated onto the tooth surface, has been demonstrated by a large number of clinical and laboratory studies (Review: Addy and Moran, 1984). In particular, tea, coffee and red wine will all rapidly produce discoloration in the presence of chlorhexidine. Thirdly, chlorhexidine occasionally produces mucosal erosion which is concentration dependent. The effect can often be avoided by diluting the preparation but increasing the volume of the rinse in order to maintain plaque inhibition. Finally, parotid swelling has also been reported but is so rare as to make a study of a direct cause and effect relationship almost impossible.

In view of the local side effects, long-term usage for most individuals is unacceptable, particularly since staining is difficult to remove. Short- to medium-term oral use is nevertheless of considerable benefit in a number of ways (Review: Gjermo, 1974; Addy, 1986), including (1) an adjunct to mechanical oral hygiene in initial periodontal therapy, (2) post-surgical care, including that following periodontal surgery, (3) patients with intermaxillary fixation, (4) physically and mentally handicapped individuals, (5) medically compromised patients predisposed to oral disease, (6) high caries risk patients, (7) recurrent oral ulceration, (8) removable and fixed orthodontic appliance wearers, (9) denture stomatitis, and (10) post-irradiation.

Quaternary ammonium compounds

Cetyl pyridinium chloride and benzylconium chloride are the most studied quaternary antiseptics and exhibit moderate plaque-reducing effects. Interestingly, although they show greater oral retention and equivalent antibacterial activity to chlorhexidine, they are not as effective in reducing plaque formation (Gjermo *et al.,* 1970). Possible explanations have been that, once adsorbed, the antibacterial activity of these compounds is reduced considerably (Moran and Addy, 1984), presumably due to their monocationic nature and additionally they appear to rapidly desorb from oral sites (Bonesvoll and Gjermo, 1978).

Phenolic compounds

Phenols, either alone or in combination, have been available in mouth rinses and lozenges for many years. Commercial rinses containing phenols appear from studies to have little effect on established plaque but do reduce plaque formation (Lusk *et al.,* 1974; Fornell *et al.,* 1975). There is, at present, insufficient data to indicate whether the inhibitory effect on plaque accumulation is sufficient to reduce gingivitis. However, the safety of these preparations is well established and they have been used over prolonged periods as adjuncts to toothbrushing with encouraging results on plaque accumulation (Fine *et al.,* 1985). Further investigation into possible benefits on gingivitis would seem warranted, indeed worthwhile.

Natural antiseptics

A few studies have been carried out on the plant extract sanguinarine chloride, with moderate reductions in plaque reported (Klewansky and Vernier, 1984). However, the specific effects of sanguinarine are unclear because of the presence of zinc in the formulations. More recent investigations have questioned the plaque inhibitory effects of sanguinarine alone (Etemadadeh and Ainamo, 1986). Moreover sanguinarine/zinc mouthwashes when compared with chlorhexidine were very much less effective at inhibiting plaque and did not prevent the onset of gingivitis (Etemadzadeh and Ainamo, 1986; Moran and Addy, 1987).

Fluorides and metal ions

Despite the considerable evidence supporting the benefits of fluoride in reducing dental caries (Review: Murray, 1976), there is little to indicate that this is attributable to an antimicrobial or antiplaque effect. Not surprisingly therefore, there is no clinical or epidemiological evidence to indicate that the fluoride ion has any benefit in preventing gingivitis. Stannous fluoride is an exception to this and possesses antiplaque effects (Tinanoff *et al.,* 1980). However, these are almost certainly derived from the stannous rather than fluoride ion. Other metals, including zinc and copper also have moderate quantitative effects upon plaque accummulation (Fischman *et al.,* 1973), although additional qualitative effects on plaque may occur. Convincing evidence for effects of metal ions in reducing gingivitis is awaited. Furthermore, of interest, has been the observation that combinations of metals and antiseptics, for example, zinc and hexetidine, appear to produce additive or synergistic effects in reducing plaque accummulation (Waller and Rolla, 1980). Although there has been little information produced for the value of toothpastes containing zinc and hexetidine, the results for the combination of zinc and triclosan in a toothpaste on plaque and gingivitis are encouraging (Saxton *et al.,* 1987).

Oxygenating agents

Most interest in oxygenating agents for the control of supragingival plaque have been concerned with the management of acute necrotizing gingivitis with beneficial results reported for hydrogen peroxide and a proprietary peroxyborate rinse (Wade *et al.*, 1966). The effects of oxygenating agents in the treatment of acute necrotizing gingivitis presumably results from the susceptibility to oxygen of the obligate anaerobes, *Fusiform fusiformis* and spirochaete *vincenti*, associated with this condition. Moreover the release of nascent oxygen from these agents is potentiated by the necrotic gingival tissue and some physical debridement may aid in the removal or destruction of the microorganisms. Limited data also indicate that oxygenating agents may retard supragingival plaque growth (Wennstrom and Lindhe, 1979) but benefits to inhibiting chronic gingivitis require further study.

Other antiseptics

A considerable number of other antiseptics have been investigated in the short term for their effects on plaque accumulation. Of these, because of their commercial availability, two deserve comment. Firstly, hexetidine, as a 0.1% mouth rinse, has some plaque inhibitory activity but this is small by comparison to chlorhexidine (Bergenholtz and Hannstrom, 1974). Secondly, povidone iodine, is available as a 1% mouthwash and is suggested for use in various oral conditions, including gingivitis. Clinical studies, however, demonstrated no antiplaque activity (Addy *et al.*, 1977) and no benefit in the treatment of acute necrotizing gingivitis (Addy and Llewelyn, 1978). Furthermore, the absorption of significant levels of iodine with potential detrimental effects on thyroid function may make this compound unsatisfactory for prolonged usage in the oral cavity (Ferguson *et al.*, 1978).

Surface active agents

Attempts have been made to block the forces on the tooth surface which appear responsible for bacterial adherence. Particular attention has centred on substituted amino alcohols such as octopinol, including short-term studies in humans (Attström *et al.*, 1983). At this time the data are insufficient to indicate whether this interesting approach to plaque inhibition is feasible in humans.

Subgingival plaque control

In established chronic periodontitis the presence of pocketing provides an ideal environment for the proliferation of the bacterial species associated with the disease and a barrier to most personal oral hygiene methods. Pocketing also makes debridement of the root surface difficult so that surgical exposure is considered necessary by many to allow adequate access for cleaning. In view of potential patient and operator problems associated with such approaches to treatment, coupled with the recognition of the importance of microorganisms to the advancing lesions of chronic periodontitis, there has been considerable research in the use of antimicrobial drugs for treatment. Such compounds have been used systemically or locally, usually as adjuncts to mechanical treatments.

Systemic antimicrobial therapy

Particular attention has been paid to tetracycline and metronidazole which, when used alone, have resulted in short-term improvements in the bacteriological and clinical parameters of chronic periodontitis. However, when used as adjuncts to root planing with or without surgery, questionable benefits were shown. Thus, some investigators demonstrated significant improvements while others reported little, if any, added benefit from their concomitant use with surgery (Review: Genco, 1981).

For this reason, and the possibility for the emergence of resistant organisms, the routine use of systemic antimicrobials in the routine treatment of chronic periodontal disease cannot be recommended. However, in specific periodontal conditions, notably localized juvenile periodontitis, rapidly advancing or refractory periodontal disease, consideration may be given to the use of systemic antimicrobials. In localized juvenile periodontitis, tetracycline, 250 mg three or four times a day for 2–3 weeks, coinciding with periodontal surgery, has been recommended (Lindhe, 1982) and endorsed by subsequent findings (Lindhe and Liljenberg, 1984). The rationale for this regimen is the frequent association of *Actinobacillus actinomycetemcomitans* with lesions of this condition (Review: Zambon, 1985), coupled with the fact that this organism is very sensitive to tetracycline (Walker *et al.*, 1981) and the antibiotic concentrates in the periodontal pocket (Gordon *et al.*, 1981). Similarly, Slots and Rosling (1983) demonstrated that a substantial suppression of subgingival *Actinobacillus actinomycetemcomitans* was not accomplished by root surface debridement alone but was achieved when combined with systemic tetracycline therapy. The latter suppression also proved to be more predictable than that occurring after the surgical removal of granulation tissue by curettage or the modified Widman flap (Christersson *et al.*, 1985). On the other hand, localized juvenile periodontitis has also been successfully treated by both subgingival debridement alone and that associated with surgical techniques without recourse to systemic antimicrobial therapy (Wennström *et al.*, 1986; Saxen *et al.*, 1986). An overview of the treatment of localized juvenile periodontitis has been presented by Krill and Fry (1987).

In adult chronic periodontitis the presence of certain microorganisms in subgingival plaque may act as indicators of disease progression. These include *Actinobacillus actinomycetemcomitans*, *Bacteroides gingivalis* and *Bacteroides intermedius* (Slots *et al.*, 1986; Bragd *et al.*, 1987). Such data lend support to the specific plaque hypothesis of chronic periodontal disease. However, a cause and effect relationship between these microorganisms and chronic periodontitis is not established and at this time would not be an indication for the routine use of systemic antimicrobial drugs. Consequently, if and when specific pathogens can be shown as causally related to advancing lesions of chronic periodontitis, the use of systemic antimicrobials with specific spectra of activity, may have to be reconsidered. This would however require the routine availability of considerably simpler diagnostic bacteriological techniques. However, it is unlikely that systemic antimicrobial drugs will be used alone in the treatment, present information indicates that benefits are short lived unless supported by mechanical debridement techniques (Walsh *et al.*, 1986) (*cf.* Chapter 5).

Local antimicrobial therapy

Antimicrobial drugs used in mouth washes or pastes show little or no penetration into periodontal pockets (Flotra *et al.*, 1972). For this reason their application by conventional means has no place in the treatment of established chronic periodontiis. The relatively recent 'salt out' or Keyes technique using bicarbonate, salt and hydrogen peroxide mixtures, has only been proven to be of benefit when the paste is introduced into the pocket area (Rosling *et al.*, 1983). Apparent benefits when used at the gingival margin were almost certainly derived from the concomitant mechanical debridement of the root surface.

The local delivery of antimicrobial agents into periodontal pockets is not a new idea, although recently the number of delivery methods for the antimicrobial agents has increased. This has been extensively reviewed by Newman (1986). Vehicles for the antimicrobial drugs include (1) hollow fibres (Goodson *et al.*, 1979), (2) monolithic fibres (Goodson *et al.*, 1983), (3) direct irrigation using blunt needles attached to syringes or irrigating devices (Rathbun, 1974 and Review: Greenstein, 1987), (4) slow release materials, for example acrylic (Addy *et al.*, 1982) or ethyl cellulose polymers

(Golomb *et al.*, 1984). The latter slow release materials are placed into pockets for several days during which time the contained drug diffuses out into the pocket area. This gives a more prolonged delivery of the antimicrobial by comparison with hollow or monolithic fibres where the release is measured in hours rather than days.

The antimicrobial agents delivered by such methods have included chlorhexidine, metronidazole and tetracycline. All combinations of delivery methods and contained drugs so far evaluated, have produced advantageous antibacterial and clinical effects of varying duration. In some cases the local antimicrobial therapy alone has been shown as effective as root planing. However, until further evidence is available this form of therapy appears most suited as an adjunct to subgingival debridement, particularly where such procedures are made difficult by accessibility.

The choice of vehicle or drug to use at present depends on several factors, not the least of which is availability of materials. Syringes or irrigating devices can easily be obtained either by the profession for use in the surgery or supplied to the patient for home irrigation of pockets. Furthermore, chlorhexidine is available commercially for use in such irrigation devices. Intravenous metronidazole solution when used for pocket irrigation is a useful preparation but would have to be obtained by the dental surgeon. Tetracycline, cannot readily be used for irrigation because of its very low water solubility. Of the other delivery systems, few if any are available at present and would have to be made up by the dental surgeon. However, for some systems particularly the acrylic strips, preparation is not a difficult task. The powdered antimicrobial is simply polymerized into a cold cured acrylic sheet which is then cut into strips for insertion.

A further consideration must be the efficacy of the individual antimicrobial drugs. In the absence of routine bacteriological screening of periodontal pockets the choice of which antimicrobial drug to employ is somewhat arbitrary, and again largely dictated by availability. Although chlorhexidine has been shown to produce encouraging results when used locally, either alone or combined with root planing, clinical and bacteriological findings suggest it is less effective than metronidazole (Review: Addy, 1986). Similarly, Wennström *et al.* (1987 a and b) failed to demonstrate any significant therapeutic effect or bacterial changes from professionally performed periodic subgingival irrigation with chlorhexidine, used alone or in combination with mechanical debridement.

Thus chlorhexidine, arguably the most effective agent for the control of supragingival plaque, appears less effective on subgingival plaque. Possible explanations are that chlorhexidine has limited action where bacterial plaque is established, since its cationic nature prevents absorption to the deeper organisms within the plaque. Additionally, although most gingival bacteria are susceptible to chlorhexidine (Wade and Addy, 1987), the protein which is invariably present in crevicular fluid may greatly reduce the activity of this antiseptic.

The potential advantages of local antimicrobial therapy are several but have to be weighed against the possible disadvantages. The advantages are:

(1) delivery directly to the lesion,
(2) considerably reduced dosage by comparison with the systemic route,
(3) the possibility of using effective antimicrobials which cannot be delivered by the systemic route,
(4) the possibility of using systemic antimicrobials which do not reach therapeutic levels via the gingival crevicular fluid,
(5) avoidance or minimization of side effects known to occur when drugs are used systemically,
(6) simple to use requiring minimal operator skill and time by comparison with techniques such as root planing,
(7) in some cases the treatment can be patient delivered, as with irrigation techniques.

The potential disadvantages are, in turn:

(1) emergence of resistant strains of organisms to the antimicrobial used,
(2) patient hypersensitivity reactions,
(3) tissue damage from the delivery system. The damage in this case may arise from the antimicrobial drugs, such as chlorhexidine, being forced into the tissues due to high pressures arising from certain irrigation systems, or following accidental needle penetration,
(4) slow release vehicles may be difficult to recover from the pocket area and if unrecovered could act as a nidus to infection at a later date.

Until further information is available, certain guidelines may be proposed. Local antimicrobial therapy should be used as an adjunct to mechanical debridement techniques particularly for sites which are difficult to treat mechanically or appear refractory to normal techniques. Protracted or repeated use of any one antimicrobial drug should be avoided to reduce the risk of bacterial resistance arising. At present, antiseptics such as chlorhexidine should be used, primarily because of available evidence for efficacy, lack of emergence of resistant organisms, safety and availability. Moreover, antiseptics do not have a place in the treatment of human systemic disease, which is not true of the many other antimicrobials considered for local treatment of periodontal disease. In this respect, consideration should be given to the evaluation of other antimicrobial compounds which have little or no indication for use in other diseases. An example

is niridazole, an antimicrobial previously only employed in the treatment of schistosomiasis, but which is highly effective against periodontopathic bacteria (Wade *et al.*, 1986).

As with mechanical debridement techniques, the duration of the effects produced by local antimicrobial drugs cannot be assumed to be permanent. Moreover, the long-term success of such treatments are dependent upon continued good supragingival plaque control by the patient. At present there are no accurate means of detecting periodontal disease activity. However, techniques such as dark field microscopy and clinical signs, including bleeding on probing, may be useful in monitoring the duration of any treatment effects produced by local antimicrobials so that the need for further treatment can be assessed.

In conclusion, studies to date indicate that chemical plaque control methods for the prevention of chronic gingivitis have a role either alone or as adjuncts to mechanical cleaning. The local side effects of the most effective agents largely preclude protracted use but many short- to medium-term applications can be considered. Further breakthrough in this area over and above that seen for the cationic antiseptics, particularly chlorhexidine, do not appear imminent. Local antimicrobial drugs similarly appear to have a limited role to play in the treatment of periodontal disease. Delivery systems are likely to increase in both number and sophistication and should become more readily available to the profession. Unfortunately, until our knowledge of the connection between bacterial specificity and the progress of chronic periodontal disease is increased, all subgingival chemical and mechanical debridement techniques will remain largely nonspecific with the aim of rendering all the pockets as near sterile as possible. Such a goal is probably impossible to reach and even unnecessary for periodontal health.

References

Addy, M. (1986) Chlorhexidine compared with other locally delivered antimicrobials: A short review. *J. Clin. Periodontol.* **13**, 957–964

Addy, M. and Llewelyn, J. (1978) Use of chlorhexidine gluconate and povidone iodine mouthwashes in the treatment of acute ulcerative gingivitis. *J. Clin. Periodontol.* **5**, 272–277

Addy, M. and Moran, J. (1984) The formation of stains on acrylic surfaces by the interaction of antiseptic mouthwashes and tea. *J. Biomed. Mat. Res.* **18**, 631–641

Addy, M., Griffiths, C. and Isaac, R. (1977) The effect of povidone iodine on plaque and salivary bacteria – a double blind cross-over trial. *J. Periodontol.* **48**, 730–732

Addy, M., Rawle, L., Handley, R., Newman, H. N. and Coventry, R. (1982) The development and *in vitro* evaluation of acrylic strips and dialysis tubing for local drug delivery. *J. Periodontol.* **53**, 693–699

Attström, P., Matsson, L., Edwardson, S., Willard, L. G. and Klinge, B. (1983) The effect of octopinol on dentogingival plaque and developoment of gingivitis. III. Short term studies in humans. *J. Periodont. Res.* **18**, 445–451

Bergenholtz, A. and Hanstrom, L. (1974) The plaque inhibiting effect of Hexetidine (Oraldene^R) mouthwash compared to that of chlorhexidine. *Comm. Dent. Oral Epidemiol.* **2**, 70–74

Bonesvoll, P. and Gjermo, P. (1978) A comparison between chlorhexidine and some quaternary ammonium compound mouthrinses. *Arch. Oral Biol.* **23**, 289–294

Bragd, L., Dahlén, G., Wilkstrom, M. and Slots, J. (1987) The capability of Actinobacillus actinomycetemcomitans, Bacteroides gingivalis and Bacteroides intermedius to indicate progressive periodontitis; a retrospective study. *J. Clin. Periodontol.* **14**, 95–99

Christersson, L. A., Slots, J., Rosling, B. G. and Genco, R. J. (1985) Microbiological and clinical effects of surgical treatment of localised juvenile periodontitis. *J. Clin. Periodontol.* **12**, 465–476

Eriksen, H. M., Nordbo, H., Kantanen, H. and Ellingsen, J. E. (1985) Chemical plaque control and extrinsic tooth discolouration: A review of possible mechanisms. *J. Clin. Periodontol.* **12**, 345–350

Etemadzadeh, H. and Ainamo, J. (1986) Lacking antiplaque efficacy of 2 sanguinarine mouthrinses. *J. Clin. Periodontol.* **14**, 176–180

Ferguson, M. M., Geddes, D. A. M. and Wray, D. (1978) The effect of a povidone iodine mouthwash upon thyroid function and plaque accumulation. *Br. Dent. J.* **144**, 14–16

Fine, D. H., Leticia, J. and Mandel, I. D. (1985) The effect of rinsing with Listerine antiseptic on the properties of developing dental plaque. *J. Clin. Periodontol.* **12**, 660–666

Fischman, S. L., Picozzi, A., Cancro, L. P. and Pader, M. (1973) The inhibition of plaque by two experimental oral rinses. *J. Periodontol.* **44**, 100–102

Flotra, L., Gjermo, P., Rolla, G. and Waerhaug, J. (1971) Side effects of chlorhexidine mouthwashes. *Scand. J. Dent Res.* **79**, 119–125

Flotra, L., Gjermo, P., Rolla, G. and Waerhaug, J. (1972) A 4 month study on the effects of chlorhexidine mouthwashes on 50 soldiers. *Scand. J. Dent. Res.* **80**, 10–17

Fornell, J., Sundin, Y. and Lindhe, J. (1975) Effect of Listerine on dental plaque and gingivitis. *Scand. J. Dent. Res.* **83**, 18–25

Frandsen, A. (1986) Mechanical oral hygiene practices. In *Dental Plaque Control Measures and Oral Hygiene Practices Workshop*, pp. 93–116. (Editor H. Löe and D. V. Kleinman). IRL Press, Oxford, Washington, DC

Genco, R. J. (1981) Antibiotics in the treatment of human periodontal disease. *J. Periodontol.* **52**, 545–558

Gjermo, P. (1974) Chlorhexidine in dental practice. *J. Clin. Periodontol.* **1**, 143–152

Gjermo, P., Baastad, K. L. and Rolla, G. (1970) The plaque-inhibitory capacity of 11 antibacterial com pounds. *J. Periodont. Res.* **5**, 102–109

Gjermo, P., Rolla, G. and Arkaug, L. (1973) Effect on dental plaque formation and some *in vitro* properties of 12 bisbiguanides. *J. Periodont. Res.* **8**, (Suppl. 12), 81–88

Gold, S. I. (1985) Periodontics. The past – Part III Microbiology. *J. Clin. Periodontol.* **12**, 257–269

Golomb, G., Friedman, M., Soskolne, A., Stabholz, A. and Sela, M. N. (1984) Sustained release device containing metronidazole for periodontal use. *J. Dent. Res.* **63**, 1149–1153

Goodson, J. M., Haffajee, A. and Socransky, S. S. (1979) Periodontal therapy by local delivery of tetracycline. *J. Clin. Periodontol.* **6**, 83–92

Goodson, J. M., Holborow, D., Dunn, R., Hogan, P. and Dunham, S. (1983) Monolithic tetracycline containing fibres for control delivery to periodontal pockets. *J. Periodontol.* **54**, 575–579

Gordon, J. M., Walker, C. B., Murphy, J. C., Goodson, J. M. and Socransky, S. S. (1981) Tetracycline: levels achievable in gingival crevice fluid and in vitro effect on subgingival organisms. I. Concentrations in crevicular fluid after repeated doses. *J. Periodontol.* **52**, 609–612

Greenstein, G. (1987) Effects of subgingival irrigation on periodontal status. *J. Periodontol.* **58**, 827–836

Helderman, W. H. and Van Palenstein (1981) Microbial aetiology of periodontal disease. *J. Clin. Periodontol.* **8**, 261–280

Hoogendoorn, H. and Moorer, W. (1973) Lactoperoxidase in the prevention of plaque accummulation gingivitis and dental caries. (1) Effect on oral streptococci and lactobacilli. *Odontol. Rev.* **24**, 355–366

Hoogendoorn, H., Piessens, J. P., Scholtes, W. and Stoddars, L. S. (1977) Hypothiocyanate, the inhibitor formed by the system lactoperoxidase – thiocyanate – hydrogen peroxide. *Caries Res.* **11**, 77–84

Hull, P. (1980) Chemical inhibition of plaque. *J. Clin. Periodontol.* **7**, 431–442

Klewansky, P. and Vernier, D. (1984) Sanguinarine and the control of plaque in dental practice. *Compend. Contin. Educ. Dent.* (Suppl.) **5**, 394–397

Kornman, K. (1985) Antimicrobial agents. In *Dental Plaque Control Measures and Oral Hygiene Practices Workshop*. Bethesda, Maryland, USA

Krill, D. B. and Fry, H. R. (1987) Treatment of localised juvenile periodontitis (periodontosis). *J. Periodontol.* **58**, 1–8

Lindhe, J. (1982) Treatment of localised juvenile periodontitis in host-parasite interactions in periodontal diseases. In *Proceedings of a Symposium of the American Society for Microbiology*, pp. 382–394. (Editors Genco, R. J. and Mergenhagen, S. E.)

Lindhe, J. and Liljenberg, B. (1984) Treatment of localised juvenile periodontitis. *J. Clin. Periodontol.* **11**, 399–410

Lobene, P. R. (1971) A clinical study of the effect of

dextranase on human dental plaque. *J. Am. Dent. Assoc.* **82**, 132–135

Löe, H. and Schiott, R. C. (1970) The effect of mouthrinse and topical application of chlorhexidine on the development of dental plaque and gingivitis in man. *J. Periodont. Res.* **5**, 79–83

Löe, H., Theilade, E. and Jensen, S. B. (1965) Experimental gingivitis in man. *J. Periodontol.* **36**, 177–187

Lusk, S. S., Bowers, G. M., Tow, H. D., Watson, W. J. and Moffitt, W. C. (1974) Effects of an oral rinse on experimental gingivitis, plaque formation and formed plaque. *J. Am. Prev. Soc.* **4**, 31–37

Moran, J. and Addy, M. (1984) The effect of surface adsorption and staining reactions on the antimicrobial properties of some cationic antiseptic mouthwashes. *J. Periodontol.* **55**, 282–285

Moran, J. and Addy, M. (1987) Comparison between chlorhexidine and sanguinarine mouthrinses on plaque and gingivitis. *J. Dent. Res.* **66**, 278. (Abstract 1381)

Murray, J. J. (1976) Fluorides in caries prevention. *Dental Practitioner Handbook* No. 20, pp. 60–90. John Wright and Sons, Bristol

Newman, H. N. (1986) Modes of application of anti- plaque chemicals. *J. Clin. Periodontol.* **13**, 965–974

Rathbun, W. E., Crigger, M. and Oliver, R. (1974) The effect of chlorhexidine and oxytetracycline irrigation on the subgingival microbiota. *J. Dent. Res.* **53** (Special Issue) 271 (Abstract 867)

Robinson, R. J., Stoller, N. H. and Vilardi, G. (1975) Clinical evaluation of the effect of a protealytic enzyme mouthwash on plaque and gingivitis in young adults. *Comm. Dent. Oral Epidemiol.* **3**, 271–275

Rolla, G. and Melsen, B. (1975) On the mechanism of plaque inhibition by chlorhexidine. *J. Dent. Res.* **54**, (Special Issue) 57–62

Rosling, B. G., Slots, J., Webber, R. L., Christersson, L. A. and Genco, R. J. (1983) Microbiological and clinical effects of topical subgingival antimicrobial treatment on human periodontal disease. *J. Clin. Periodontol.* **10**, 487–514

Saxen, L., Asikainen, S., Sandholm, L. and Kari, K. (1986) Treatment of juvenile periodontitis without antibiotics. A follow up study. *J. Clin. Periodontol.* **13**, 714–719

Saxton, C. A. Lane, R. M. and Van der Ouderaa, F. (1987) The effects of a dentifrice containing zinc salt and a non-cationic antimicrobial agent on plaque and gingivitis. *J. Clin. Periodontol.* **14**, 144–148

Shankwalker, R. (1975) Anticalculus and antiplaque agents and their trials. *J. Indian Dent. Assoc.* **47**, 303–310

Sheiham, A. (1977) Prevention and control of periodontal disease. In *International Conference on Research in the Biology of Periodontal Disease*, pp. 309–368. Klavan, B. *et al.* University of Illinois, pp. 369–376 and Committee Report

Slots, J. (1979) Subgingival microflora and periodontal disease. *J. Clin. Periodontol.* **6**, 351–382

Slots, J. and Rosling, B. G. (1983) Suppression of periodontopathic microflora in localised juvenile periodontitis by systemic tetracycline. *J. Clin. Periodontol.* **10**, 465–486

Slots, J., Bragd, L., Wilkinson, M. and Dahlen, G. (1986) The occurrence of *Actinobacillus actinomycetemcomitans*, *Bacteroides gingivalis* and *Bacteroides intermedius* in destructive periodontal disease in adults. *J. Clin. Periodontol.* **13**, 570–577

Socransky, S. S. (1977) Microbiology of periodontal disease. Present status and future considerations. *J. Periodontol.* **48**, 497–504

Tanner, A. C. R., Socransky, S. S. and Goodson, J. M. (1984) Microbiota of periodontal pockets losing crestal alveolar bone. *J. Periodont. Res.* **19**, 279–291

Tinanoff, N., Hock, Camosci, D. and Hellden, L. (1980) Effect of stannous fluoride mouthrinse on dental plaque formation. *J. Clin. Periodontol.* **7**, 1–10

Wade, W. and Addy, M. (1987) Susceptibility of subgingival bacteria to Corsodyl. *J. Dent. Res.* **66**, 837 (Abstract) 23

Wade, A. B., Blake, G. C. and Mirza, K. B. (1966) Effectiveness of metronidazole in treating the acute phase of ulcerative gingivitis. *Dent. Pract.* 440–443

Wade, W., Bishop, P. and Addy, M. (1986) Niridazole, an alternative antimicrobial agent for topical subgingival use in chronic periodontitis. *J. Dent. Res.* **65**, 408 (Abstract) 204

Walker, C. B., Gordon, J. M., McQuilkin, S. J., Niebloom, T. A. and Socransky, S. S. (1981). Tetracycline: levels achievable in gingival crevice fluid and *in vitro* effect on subgingival organisms. II. Susceptibilities of periodontal bacteria. *J. Periodontol.* **52**, 613–616

Waller, S. M. and Rolla, G. (1980) Plaque inhibition effect of combinations of chlorhexidine and metal ions zinc and tin. *Acta Odontol. Scand.* **38**, 213–217

Walsh, M. M., Buchanen, S. A., Hoover, C. I., Newbrun, E., Taggert, E. J., Armatage, G. C. and Robertson, P. B. (1986) Clinical and microbiological effects of a single-dose metronidazole or scaling and root planing in treatment of adult periodontitis. *J. Clin. Periodontol.* **13**, 151–157

Wennström, J. L. and Lindhe, J. (1979) Effect of hydrogen peroxide on developing plaque and gingivitis in man. *J. Clin. Periodontol.* **6**, 115–130

Wennström, J. L., Heijl, L., Dahlén, G. and Gröndahl, K. (1987a) Periodic subgingival antimicrobial irrigation of periodontal pockets. (I) Clinical observations. *J. Clin. Periodontol.* **14**, 541–550

Wennström, J. L., Heijl, L., Dahlen, G. and Gröndahl, K. (1987b) Periodic subgingival antimicrobial irrigation of periodontal pockets. (II) Microbiological and radiographical observations. *J. Clin. Periodontol.* **14**, 573–580

Wennström, A., Wennström, J. and Lindhe, J. (1986) Healing following surgical and non-surgical treatment of juvenile periodontitis. *J. Clin. Periodontol.* **13**, 869–882

Zambon, J. J. (1985) *Actinobacillus actinomycetemcomitans* in human periodontal disease. *J. Clin. Periodontol.* **12**, 1–20

Index